Locomotion and Posture in Older Adults

Fabio Augusto Barbieri • Rodrigo Vitório
Paulo Cezar Rocha dos Santos
Editors

Locomotion and Posture in Older Adults

The Role of Aging and Movement Disorders

Second Edition

Springer

Editors
Fabio Augusto Barbieri
Human Movement Research Laboratory (MOVI-LAB), Department of Physical Education, School of Sciences
São Paulo State University (UNESP)
Bauru, São Paulo, Brazil

Rodrigo Vitório
Department of Sport, Exercise & Rehabilitation
Northumbria University
Newcastle upon Tyne, UK

Paulo Cezar Rocha dos Santos
IDOR/Pioneer Science Initiative
Rio de Janeiro, Rio de Janeiro, Brazil

ISBN 978-3-031-74125-8 ISBN 978-3-031-74123-4 (eBook)
https://doi.org/10.1007/978-3-031-74123-4

This Springer imprint is published by the registered company Springer Nature Switzerland AG
The registered company address is: Gewerbestrasse 11, 6330 Cham, Switzerland

Contents

Part I

Background Concepts to Motor Control in Aging and Movement Disorders

Clinical Aspects of Movement Disorders: Effects on Walking and Posture

1

Henrique Ballalai Ferraz and Roberta Arb Saba

Abstract

Movement disorders are a group of syndromes that include parkinsonism, chorea, dystonia, myoclonus, tremor, and tics. Many of the diseases of this group manifest disturbances of gait and posture along with other abnormalities. Parkinsonism is characterized by rest tremors, muscular rigidity, bradykinesia, flexed trunk posture, and loss of postural reflexes. Parkinson's disease (PD) is the most prevalent of the diseases of this group and patients usually manifest problems of gait and posture in late phases. On the other hand, atypical parkinsonism diseases (multiple-system atrophy, progressive supranuclear palsy, dementia with Lewy bodies, and corticobasal ganglionic degeneration) manifest gait problems and falls very early and are much more incapacitating than PD. Vascular parkinsonism manifests itself with lower limb rigidity and bradykinesia and affects gait very early. Huntington's disease is a genetic disorder characterized by behavioral and cognitive disturbances associated with chorea, dystonia, and loss of equilibrium. Sometimes, especially in subjects with the juvenile form of the disease, Huntington's disease may manifest with very severe parkinsonism. Movement disorders may cause severe disturbances of posture and gait and health professionals should be attentive to them.

H. B. Ferraz (✉)
Movement Disorders Unit, Department of Neurology, Escola Paulista de Medicina, Universidade Federal de São Paulo, São Paulo, Brazil
e-mail: hbferraz@unifesp.br

R. A. Saba
Movement Disorders Unit, Department of Neurology, Escola Paulista de Medicina, Universidade Federal de São Paulo, São Paulo, Brazil

Hospital do Servidor Público Estadual de São Paulo, São Paulo, Brazil

F. A. Barbieri et al. (eds.), *Locomotion and Posture in Older Adults*,
https://doi.org/10.1007/978-3-031-74123-4_1

Some of the diseases of the spectrum of movement disorders are associated with abnormalities of posture and locomotion. We can mention the multiple forms of Parkinsonism, Huntington's disease, and generalized dystonia among others. Posture and walking may be affected by involuntary movements per se or by degeneration or lesions of neural pathways involved in tonus and balance. In this chapter, we will present some of the diseases associated with abnormal involuntary movements and impairment of posture and gait.

Parkinsonism

Parkinsonism is a syndrome characterized by the combination of bradykinesia, also called akinesia, with any of the three: muscular rigidity, rest tremor, or impairment of postural reflexes.

Bradykinesia is the reduction of the global repertoire of automatic movements, and the decrease of the amplitude and the speed of the voluntary movements. We can detect bradykinesia in a parkinsonian patient either by observing the lack of facial expression while talking or listening with the examiner or by the reduced arms and hand gestures during a conversation. In other words, bradykinetic patients tend to have a poor repertoire of body language [1].

Muscular rigidity is observed by resistance while manipulating a joint of a limb. Resistance is present both during passive flexion or extension of a limb. We can also feel the sensation of manipulating a lead pipe, and sometimes this is associated with the clinical sign called "cogwheel rigidity." This is perceived as an intermittent and short-lived resistance release during a full extension or flexion movement [2].

Rest tremors can be observed in any part of the body. Hand tremors manifest as a rhythmic flexion and extension of the fingers and it is called "pill-rolling tremor." Tremors can also affect the lower limbs, trunk, chin, head, and larynx. It may cycle in a fashion varying from 4 to 6 Hz. Sometimes, parkinsonian patients may present with a postural and kinetic hand tremor associated or not with the resting tremor [1].

Impairment of postural reflexes is characterized by an inability to correct sudden shifts of the normal upright position. People with this kind of impairment usually have frequent falls and assume a stooped posture. To reduce the risk of falling, it's important to avoid bending the trunk too far forward. The further forward the trunk is bent, the greater the risk of falling [2].

The combination of these four cardinal symptoms results in the typical parkinsonian gait and posture. Patients tend to flex the trunk forward and the arms are flexed close to the level of the hip. The arms do not harmonically sway while the body is moving. The turning of the body is made by slow and fragmented successive short movements. The length of the steps is very short, and the heels drag to the floor. Sometimes, due to the flexed posture, parkinsonian people tend to fall forward, and to avoid it they shift the slow steps to a running pace. This is called festination or festinating gait, and when present is a classical manifestation of parkinsonism [1].

Too many clinical conditions may precipitate parkinsonism. The most frequent is idiopathic Parkinson's disease (PD). Other situations are pharmacologically induced parkinsonism (mainly antipsychotics), metal or poison exposure (manganese, pesticides, carbon monoxide), vascular lesions of the central nervous system (CNS), hereditary diseases, some dementia syndromes (Alzheimer's disease and frontotemporal dementia) and other degenerative diseases called atypical parkinsonism or Parkinson-Plus syndromes (progressive supranuclear palsy, multiple systems atrophy, dementia with Lewy body and corticobasal ganglionic degeneration). We will discuss some of the specific diseases associated with parkinsonism.

Parkinson's Disease

PD is characterized by motor and nonmotor symptoms and is associated with progressive degeneration of neurons of the CNS. The degenerative process seems to start in the medulla and pons and progress to a wider distribution in the encephalon. Motor symptoms (parkinsonism) begin when dopaminergic neurons of the substantia nigra are affected. Nigral neurons become progressively scarce and there is the presence of Lewy bodies, an eosinophilic intraneuronal inclusion, the classic pathological hallmark of PD [3].

PD may affect adult individuals of both genders and at any age, although most frequently those with 50 or more years of age. Unilateral symptoms are the most common way of starting the disease and the other side tends to be affected in the following months or years [1]. Patients may manifest rest tremors in one arm or feel difficulty in moving one limb. In a few months, the symptoms tend to become more and more intense and eventually will interfere with daily activities. Difficulty in arising from a chair or bed is also a common complaint in the early phase of the disease. Gait and postural impairment are usually present after a few years of onset [4].

Fully manifested PD includes bradykinesia, rigidity, and postural abnormalities with gait and balance impairment. PD patients tend to have a shuffling gait and a tendency to have falls. Festinating gait is a classic parkinsonian sign and results from the combination of the flexed forward posture, the short steps, and the loss of postural reflexes. In this case, patients tend to accelerate the steps to catch up with the center of gravity abnormally placed forward.

Freezing of gait may be present in many patients and is characterized by difficulty in taking out the feet off the floor while attempting to start the gait. Freezing of gait is more frequent when patients try to turn around or during the passage of narrow spaces. The "pull test" is the clinical way to detect impairment of postural reflexes. Patients are put standing with feet comfortably apart. The doctor stands backward and pulls him or her briskly and forcefully. The balance is considered impaired if the patient must move backward for at least three steps of recovery. In severely affected patients the examiner must hold the patients to prevent the fall.

Considering only the clinical presentation of PD, there are two main subtypes: a tremor dominant form and a postural impairment with gait disturbance (PIGD). The first one is characterized by a more benign progression, with excellent response to levodopa and late development of cognitive decline. The PIGD form has a faster progression, with less response to levodopa and early development of falls and cognitive decline [5].

Nonmotor symptoms include mood disorders (depression), cognitive decline (in the late stages of the disease), olfaction impairment, and disturbances of autonomic function (also in the late stages). Sleep disorders, especially rapid-eye movement-behavioral disorders, are quite common and may be present years before the development of motor symptoms.

Treatment is based on dopaminergic repositioning. Levodopa is the mainstay of pharmacological treatment. The drug is taken by mouth and is converted into dopamine in the brain, particularly in neuron and glial cells. If the conversion to dopamine is made by a nigral dopaminergic neuron, it can be stored in vesicles inside the synaptic terminal and can be released afterward. If the conversion is made in glial cells or nondopaminergic neurons dopamine cannot be stored and is immediately released to the post-synaptic receptor. Long-term use of levodopa may be associated with motor fluctuations and dyskinesias. These complications are more common if higher doses of levodopa are used (more than 500 mg a day) and if patients are more severely affected. Dopamine agonists may be also prescribed and act directly at the post-synaptic receptors of the striatum. The most commonly prescribed dopamine agonists are pramipexole, ropinirole, and rotigotine. Other drugs are entacapone (catechol-o-methyl-transferase inhibitor), rasagiline or selegiline (monoamine oxidase inhibitor), amantadine (glutamate receptor inhibitor), and anticholinergics [6].

Surgery treatment is indicated when patients are optimized for receiving levodopa combined with other adjuvant medications but present uncontrolled motor fluctuations and dyskinesias. There are two main surgery procedures: ablative lesions and deep brain stimulation (DBS). The targets indicated are thalamic nuclei, subthalamic nucleus, and globus pallidus interna [7].

Physical and speech therapy are useful for any phase of the disease but are particularly indicated in patients experiencing balance disturbances and falls (physical therapy) and those with swallowing difficulties and significant dysartrophonia (speech therapy).

Atypical Parkinsonism

Atypical parkinsonism is a group of diseases sharing motor signs such as rest tremors, bradykinesia, rigidity, and postural abnormalities. The difference between PD and these diseases is that atypical parkinsonian patients manifest other neurological abnormalities, such as cerebellar ataxia, autonomic dysfunction, paralysis of the vertical gaze, early-phase cognitive decline, and behavioral disturbances. We can admit that postural and gait abnormalities are more prominent in atypical parkinsonism as compared to PD.

All the diseases of this group are neurodegenerative in origin and display neuronal loss in different structures of the central nervous system. None of the diseases of this group has a curative or evolution-modifying pharmacotherapy. Levodopa rarely produces benefits for this group of patients. Alpha-synuclein inclusions are seen in multiple-system atrophy and dementia with Lewy bodies, while tau-protein fibrils are seen in progressive supranuclear palsy and corticobasal ganglionic degeneration.

Multiple-System Atrophy

Characterized by the combination of parkinsonian signs with autonomic, pyramidal, and cerebellar signs. There are two forms: multiple-system atrophy (MSA) MSA-P (parkinsonism), with a predominance of parkinsonian signs, and MSA-C (cerebellar), in which cerebellar signs are predominant. The most common form is the MSA-P. The most common signs are dysautonomic: postural hypotension, constipation, urinary incontinence, erectile dysfunction, and cold and cyanotic extremities ("cold blue hands"). Parkinsonian signs are bilateral from the start with the absence of rest tremor. Gait ataxia and balance disturbances can arise from the very beginning, as well as frequent falls. Pyramidal signs such as the Babinski sign are present, and dysphagia and dysarthria also manifest in the early stage. Other symptoms such as laryngeal stridor, trunk dystonia, and cerebellar signs may be observed. Neuroimaging studies show atrophy of the pons and the cerebellum and usually the presence of the "hot-cross bun signal," which is a characteristic hyperintensity on Fluid attenuated inversion recovery on Magnetic resonance imaging (FLAIR) of the transverse fibers of the pons and cerebellar peduncle with normal sign of the corticospinal tract and pontine tegmentum [8].

Progressive Supranuclear Palsy

It was described in the 1960s by Steele, Richardson, and Olszewski. Patients manifest the first symptoms around 50–60 years and are characterized by gait disturbance block and trunk hyperextension, postural instability with falls, lower vertical gaze palsy, cognitive impairment, and no response to levodopa treatment. The classic form of Richardson syndrome occurs in about 55% of subjects and presents peculiar symptoms of *progressive supranuclear palsy (PSP)*, such as parkinsonism, paralysis of vertical gaze, bilateral bradykinesia, frequent falls, and cognitive decline. PSP-parkinsonism (PSP-P) is the way of presentation in 30% of the subjects and the clinical picture is very similar to PD and only in late stages do patients develop gaze palsy and prominent cognitive decline. Fifteen percent of PSP patients present atypical forms. On imaging techniques, particularly in magnetic resonance imaging (MRI), enlargement of the third ventricle and atrophy of the midbrain are prominent in the late phases of the disease [9].

Dementia with Lewy Bodies

Dementia with Lewy bodies (DLB) starts between 60 and 70 years and is characterized by the presence of parkinsonian signs closely resembling DP associated with cognitive decline. Cognitive symptoms precede or follow up to 12 months after parkinsonism starts. The patient may present, in addition to parkinsonism and dementia, behavioral symptomatology such as hallucinations, and delusions, with fluctuation of these symptoms (worse at night). It is quite common for patients to manifest great sensitivity to exposure to neuroleptics (rapid development of severe stiffness and tremor) and rapid eye-movement (REM) sleep behavioral disorder [10]. DLB is frequently confounded with PD at the very beginning of symptoms, but the main features helping to differentiate both conditions in the early phases are cognitive decline, frequent falls, and severe impairment of balance observed in DLB patients [11].

Corticobasal Ganglionic Degeneration

Corticobasal ganglionic degeneration (CBGD) is characterized by progressive and asymmetric stiffness associated with upper limb apraxia. The phenomenon of "alien limb" is commonly present and characterized by involuntary movements of the upper limb, with levitation. Most patients present aphasia, unilateral dystonia, myoclonus, and rapidly progressive dementia of the frontotemporal type. Asymmetric atrophy of the cerebral hemisphere, mainly in the parietal region is usually seen in MRI studies [1].

Vascular Parkinsonism

Vascular parkinsonism (VP) accounts for 2.5–5% of the total cases of parkinsonism. VP patients exhibit lower disease duration, older age at onset, and higher frequency of cardiovascular risk factors. This disease can be clinically distinguished from PD based on the sudden onset of parkinsonism at an older age, characterized by lower body predominance, urinary incontinence, pyramidal signs, postural instability with freezing of gait and falls, and dementia. The upper limbs in VP are less symptomatic in terms of parkinsonism throughout the course of the disease. This is in clinical contrast to PD, in which patients generally present with tremors, rigidity, or slowness of the upper limbs. Thus, VP is also called "lower body or lower half" parkin sonism. VP patients developed cognitive impairment in comparison with matched-age individuals. These patients had a global pattern of cognitive impairment, including executive function, verbal memory, and language [12].

In addition to PD, VP may resemble frontal lobe tumors, obstructive hydrocephalus, normal pressure hydrocephalus, and progressive supranuclear palsy.

Imaging studies serve two purposes in a VP patient. First, it rules out other causes of parkinsonism, both degenerative (progressive supranuclear palsy) and secondary (tumors, hydrocephalous). Second, may show ischemic lesions to support the clinical diagnosis. MRI or computerized tomography (CT) is supportive, but not conclusive, of the diagnosis of VP because there are no characteristic features of VP in CT/MRI. However, white matter lesions and lacunes are also common observations among older people who do not have parkinsonism. This causes difficulty in determining the etiological mechanisms of VP. A study showed that most patients with VP had brain MRI changes with multiple lacunar infarcts (66.7%) or extensive white-matter (WM) disease (26.7%) [13]. Others investigated the WM microstructure using diffusion tensor imaging in patients with VP and specific fiber tract involvement concerning clinical severity, showed disruption of the microstructural organization of frontal lobe WM is associated with the severity of VP [14]. These findings are by the frontal lobe disconnection hypothesis for gait problems and reinforce the paradigm that the involvement of fibers related to the prefrontal cortex is crucial for the core features of VP [14].

Clinical features of the VP phenotype are early postural instability and gait disturbances. Gait impairments as the initial symptom are significantly more common in VP than in PD [13]. Gait disturbances were reported as the initial symptom in 90% of patients with VP as compared to 7% of patients with PD [15]. The gait in VP is like a "parkinsonian-ataxic" gait. The stance is wide-based. The posture is upright at least in the earlier stages and a much lesser degree of flexion is seen at the knees and hips than in PD. Steps are slow, and short, with a tendency to shuffle, particularly at the start and while turning the corners [13]. Freezing of gait can be seen, but festination is absent. In severe cases, the patient is unable to initiate a step and the feet remain fixed on the floor (magnetic gait). Postural instability and falls dominate the gait at this advanced stage and render the patient unable to walk or even stand without support. Another factor contributing to impaired mobility in advanced stages is truncal ataxia. These patients also have truncal and axial immobility. Sideways turning of the head is limited and patients turn their heads, neck, and shoulder in a block to be able to look sideways. The change of posture while lying in bed is also difficult and limited. An interesting feature in obvious gait impairments, at least in the earlier stages, is that many patients can perform simple tasks with their legs, like imitating bicycling or walking movements, when seated or lying. However, these movements are also slow.

The treatment should be directed at secondary stroke prevention to halt further disease progression although, understandably, it would not reverse or provide symptomatic relief to the existing clinical manifestations. The management of conventional vascular risk factors such as diabetes, hypertension, dyslipidemia, and smoking cessation would probably have the maximal impact in this approach to treatment. The levodopa response rates in the VP vary from 20% to 40%. A dose of up to 1000 mg/day should be given for at least 3 months before labeling the patient as a nonresponder or poor responder. In good responders, the duration of sustained response is typically less than in PD, with the drug becoming nonbeneficial after 1 to 2 years [16].

Huntington's Disease

Huntington's disease (HD) is a progressive neurodegenerative disease, rare and fatal, characterized by a movement disorder mostly manifesting as choric and dystonic movements, psychiatric abnormalities, and cognitive decline [17]. HD is a genetic disease of autosomal dominant inheritance. An expansion occurs in the number of repeats of the CAG pair of nitrogenous bases (adenine, cytosine, guanine) in unstable regions of the DNA HTT gene, which is located on the short arm of chromosome 4 (4p16.3). Twenty-seven or fewer repetitions of CAG have a normal phenotype. Intermediate alleles with 27 to 35 CAG repeats are unstable and may be transmitted as an expanded allele to offspring. However, the carriers of the normal intermediate allele also have a normal phenotype. These intermediate expanded alleles occur, particularly, during male gametogenesis, as the same is subjected to a larger number of division cycles and duplication of genetic material. Thus, there is a greater likelihood of an error in DNA replication during spermatogenesis, which increases the risk of mutated alleles to be paternal inheritance [18]. Alleles with 36–39 CAG repeats indicate incomplete penetrance and can generate both normal phenotypes with the disease. Alleles with more than 39 CAG repeats have complete penetrance and inevitably cause, in any phase of life, the phenotype of HD.

Symptoms usually start between ages 35 and 55 and the duration of the disease can vary from 15 to 20 years. In some cases, it may manifest after 80 years of age or earlier, in adolescents or children, due to the anticipation phenomenon, which occurs in 20% of cases. Due to the variability of the clinical signs and symptoms, a molecular test is required for the diagnosis [17].

The most frequent isolated initial complaint is the lack of "coordination" and occasional involuntary tremors in several body segments, which usually can be attributed to the presence of chorea. Other early motor abnormalities include saccadic eye movements interrupted or slow, inability to sustain tongue protrusion, and difficulty in performing rapid alternating movements. Behavioral changes are often reported to precede movement disorder over a decade. Symptoms of emotional nature or personality changes may antedate these movements in at least half of patients with DH. Patients are excessively irritable, impulsive, unstable, and aggressive. The most common early symptoms are mental depression. In some of the cases, the opening frame can be a frank psychosis.

The most striking feature of HD is the presence of choric movements seen in approximately 90% of the affected individuals. At first, chorea may be mild, affecting only a face or distal portions of limbs, but, with time, it becomes widespread, interfering with any voluntary movement [17]. Gradually, with the progress of the disease, the patients are becoming slower in nature, taking an athetoid character and, subsequently, dystonic [19]. Other involuntary movements, such as tremors and intention myoclonus, can rarely be present. Dysarthria is another prominent symptom that appears early in the course of the disease, as slowing or hesitancy in speech, which gradually becomes explosive, irregular, interspersed with long silences, and an increase of chances for complete disorganization and mutism. Dysphagia, common in the advanced stages of HD, is often responsible for choking and aspiration, bronchopneumonia aspiration, being reported in up to 85% of mortality. The causes of death are related to complications of immobility, such as food or trauma, and asphyxia aspirations. The patient's gait is characteristic, constantly parasitized by choric movements, taking the uncoordinated character in appearance and it can become impossible.

Postural instability and primary changes in the balance, with frequent falls and fractures, are very frequent and impair quality of life. Falls may be early manifestations of the disease and some patients are only diagnosed after several injuries and fractures [20]. Bradykinesia, with or without stiffness, occurs in the later stages of disease with extreme slowness of all movements. This symptom is directly related to the patients's disability and it occurs regardless of chorea [17]. Sphincter incontinence, both urinary and anal, is common, especially in the terminal stages of HD. There is evidence of autonomic dysfunction as hyperhidrosis and changes in blood pressure regulation. Generalized tonic-clonic seizures may occur in up to 3% of adults with DH and approximately 40% of patients with early disease onset (under 20), as other types of seizures can happen [19].

Psychiatric and cognitive changes may precede the motor manifestations, accompany them, or occur after [21]. Dementia is considered one of the cardinal signs of the disease. Patients with HD are more impaired in learning, mental flexibility, and attention. Executive function is compromised and is noted early, even in the absence of complaints from patients or family members. It includes difficulty in planning, organizing, and scheduling activities. The executive functions are related to the frontal lobe and its connections. Cognitive functions are more strongly correlated with the functional capacity of the motor symptoms.

The psychiatric symptoms occur in about 35–70% of cases. Patients may present frameworks of personality change, mood disorders, and psychosis. The most found personality changes are psychiatric and include irritability, apathy, emotional lability, impulsivity, and aggressiveness. Depression may precede motor symptoms. The frequency of suicides in HD is four to six times higher than that in the general population. Suicidal ideation is present in approximately 10% of individuals diagnosed with HD. Episodes of mania can also be found, less commonly, and schizophreniform psychosis occurs in 6–25% of cases; this is characterized by paranoid tables with persecutory delusions, jealousy, and auditory hallucinations. Other psychiatric conditions include irritability, agitation and aggression, disorder and obsessive-compulsive behavior, psychosomatic complaints, anxiety, sexual paraphilias, and behavioral changes [22].

Symptomatic treatment reduces motor and behavioral symptoms and thus maximizes the functional capacity affected individual. The treatment is done with chorea antagonists dopaminergic with high affinity for D2 receptors. Among the drugs that may be used to control abnormal movements, there are risperidone, olanzapine (typical neuroleptic), and haloperidol (atypical neuroleptic). Tetrabenazine is also indicated for the control of choric movements. However, due to the high incidence of depression in patients treated with this drug, its use is limited. The dose should be individualized, starting always with low doses, and increasing until the control of involuntary movements is satisfactory from a functional point of view [23].

Recently, deutetrabenazine has been approved to treat chorea in HD patients. It is a far more effective and safer drug as compared to tetrabenazine, but, unfortunately, demonstrated no efficacy in cognitive, mood, and balance abnormalities [24].

Patients generally tolerate high doses of conventional neuroleptics, showing no symptoms of impregnation. The inhibitors of N-methyl-D-aspartate (NMDA) glutamate receptors, such as amantadine, can be used for the motor's movement control. Depression usually responds to classical antidepressants such as selective inhibitors or serotonin reuptake dual inhibitors. Excessive irritability can be treated with benzodiazepines. Aggressive patients can benefit from both antidepressants and neuroleptics. There is no specific treatment for HD dementia [23].

Final Remarks

Gait and balance are usually impaired in many neurodegenerative diseases, but parkinsonism and Huntington's diseases are the most frequent and those with a higher impact on the daily activities of patients. Although these conditions usually do not have a definite treatment to control axial symptoms, pharmacological and rehabilitation approaches are essential to improve patients' quality of life. We still need more effective ways to treat problems related to gait and balance in degenerative movement disorders.

References

1. Fahn S, Jankovic J. Principle and practice of movement disorders. Philadelphia: Churchill Livingstone; 2007. p. 652.
2. Campbell WW. De Jong's.The neurologic examination. 7th ed. Philadelphia: Lippincott Willians & Wilkins; 2013. p. 818.
3. Jellinger KA. Neuropathological spectrum of synucleinopathies. Mov Disord. 2003;18(suppl 6):S2–S12.
4. Kalia LV, Lang AE. Parkinson's disease. Lancet. 2015;386:896–912.
5. Jankovic J, McDermott M, Carter J, et al. Variable expression of Parkinson's disease: a baseline analysis of the DATATOP cohort. Neurology. 1990;41:1529–34.
6. Connolly BS, Lang AE. Pharmacological treatment of Parkinson's disease. A review. JAMA. 2014;311:1670–83.
7. Wagle Shukla A, Okun MS. Surgical treatment of Parkinson's disease: patients, targets, devices, and approaches. Neurotherapeutics. 2014;11:47–59.
8. Fanciulli A, Wenning GK. Multiple-system atrophy. N Engl J Med. 2015;372:249–63.
9. Golbi LI. Progressive supranuclear palsy. Semin Neurol. 2014;34:151–9.
10. Walker Z, Possin KL, Boeve BF, Aarsland D. Lewy body dementias. Lancet. 2015;386:1683–94.
11. Sarasso E, Filippi M, Agosta F. Clinical and MRI features of gait and balance disorders in neurodegenerative diseases. J Neurol. 2023;270:1798–807.
12. Benítez-Rivero S, Lama MJ, Huertas-Fernández I, et al. Clinical features and neuropsychological profile in vascular parkinsonism. J Neurol Sci. 2014;345:193–7.
13. Vale TC, Caramelli P, Cardoso F. Clinicoradiological comparison between vascular parkinsonism and Parkinson's disease. J Neurol Neurosurg Psychiatry. 2015;86(5):547–53.
14. Wang HC, Hsu JL, Leemans A. Diffusion tensor imaging of vascular parkinsonism: structural changes in cerebral white matter and the association with clinical severity. Arch Neurol. 2012;69:1340–8.
15. FitzGerald PM, Jankovic J. Lower body parkinsonism: evidence for vascular etiology. Mov Disord. 1989;4:249–60.
16. Constantinescu R, Richard I, Kurlan R. Levodopa responsiveness in disorders with parkinsonism: a review of the literature. Mov Disord. 2007;22:2141–8.
17. Tabrizi SJ, Langbehn DR, Leavitt BR, et al. TRACK-HD investigators, biological and clinical manifestations of Huntington's disease in the longitudinal TRACK-HD study: cross-sectional analysis of baseline data. Lancet Neurol. 2009;8:791–801.
18. Wheeler VC, Persichetti F, McNeil SM, et al. Factors associated with HD CAG repeat instability in Huntington disease. J Med Genet. 2007;44:695–701.
19. Cardoso F. Huntington disease and other choreas. Neurol Clin. 2009;27:719–36.
20. Talman LS, Hiller AL. Approach to posture and gait in Huntington's disease. Front Bioeng Biotechnol. 2021;9:668699.

21. Andrew SE, Goldberg YP, Kremer B, Telenius H, et al. The relationship between trinucleotide (CAG) repeat length and clinical features of Huntington's disease. Nat Genet. 1993;4:398–403.
22. Morreale MK. Huntington's disease: looking beyond the movement disorder. Adv Psychosom Med. 2015;34:135–42.
23. Bonelli RM, Hoffman P. A systematic review of the treatment studies in Huntington's disease since 1990. Expert Opin Pharmacother. 2007;8:141–53.
24. Gupta H, Perkins W, Stark C, Kikkeri S, Kakazu J, Kaye A, Kaye A. Deutetrabenazine for the treatment of chorea associated with Huntington's disease. Health Psychol Res. 2022;10:36040.

MoBI: Mobile Brain/Body Imaging to Understand Walking and Balance

2

Patrick J. Tait, Emily C. Timm, Joan O'Keefe, Tamlyn Watermeyer, Rodrigo Vitorio, Rosie Morris, and Samuel Stuart

Abstract

Research investigating aging and neurological disorders that affect gait and balance aims to increase the understanding of the underlying neural mechanisms involved in task performance. Traditional brain-imaging techniques are restricted in their use in studies assessing brain activity during real-time balance and walking tasks, often restrained to the use of mental imagery, virtual reality, or single-segment motor tasks (e.g., finger tapping, button pressing, or foot movement), which lack ecological validity. Recent developments in mobile brain imaging technologies like functional near-infrared spectroscopy (fNIRS) and electroencephalography (EEG) allow the assessment of cortical brain activity during actual walking and standing tasks. The use of these techniques, in conjunction with human movement tracking devices, is known as Mobile Brain/Body Imaging (MoBI). MoBI provides a noninvasive, cost-effective, and ecologically valid approach to the simultaneous study of brain and body function. This book chapter provides an overview of the technology involved in MoBI, in addition to the challenges relating to data collection, integration, and standardization. We

P. J. Tait · R. Vitorio · R. Morris
Department of Sport, Exercise and Rehabilitation, Northumbria University, Newcastle upon Tyne, UK

E. C. Timm · J. O'Keefe
Department of Anatomy & Cell Biology, Rush University Medical Center, Chicago, IL, USA

T. Watermeyer
Department of Psychology, Northumbria University, Newcastle upon Tyne, UK

S. Stuart (✉)
Department of Sport, Exercise and Rehabilitation, Northumbria University, Newcastle upon Tyne, UK

Department of Neurology, Oregon Health and Science University, Portland, Oregon, USA
e-mail: samuel2.stuart@northumbria.ac.uk

F. A. Barbieri et al. (eds.), *Locomotion and Posture in Older Adults*,
https://doi.org/10.1007/978-3-031-74123-4_2

also discuss the current knowledge of the neural mechanisms involved in balance and walking with aging and neurological disorders. MoBI research provides valuable insights into the neural networks involved in gait and balance impairments, potentially allowing for the development of more effective and personalized treatments or targeted interventions.

Introduction

Neurological impairment due to age, injury and disease impacts gait and balance in millions of people worldwide [1], which negatively impacts quality of life and independence of these individuals [2]. New insights into the brain activity occurring during walking and balance tasks, in healthy young or older adults, and neurological groups, would facilitate a more comprehensive understanding of the underlying mechanisms involved in deficits and support the development of tailored interventions. Furthermore, the ability to image the brain during human movement and during real-world tasks is essential to understand how the brain underpins typical behavioral and cognitive processes [3–5]. As a result, understanding the relationships between gait, balance, and cognitive cortical processes has been the focus of many research fields over the past century, such as human movement science, cognitive neuroscience, psychology, and neurology.

In the past, traditional imaging techniques including functional magnetic imaging (fMRI) [6], positron emission tomography (PET) [7], and single-photon emission computerized tomography (SPECT) [8] have been used to study brain structure and function in a range of clinical populations. However, the use of traditional imaging during actual walking or balance performance is currently impossible as the head is required to remain in a static position to use these techniques [3]. Due to these motion limitations, traditional imaging studies require proxies of actual human movement, such as mental imagery, virtual reality, or use of simple single-segment motor tasks (e.g., finger tapping, button pressing, or foot movement) within imaging scanners [5]. While such studies may be able to infer some elements of cortical or subcortical motor control, they do not truly represent real-time walking or balance. Additionally, many of the previous imaging studies have focused primarily on brain regions directly related to motor function (primary motor (M1), supplementary motor area (SMA), premotor (PMC), and sensorimotor cortices (SMC)), with relatively few studies focusing on cognitive brain regions (i.e., prefrontal cortex (PFC) [9]) known to mediate the corticovolitional loops in the neural control of gait and balance [10].

Progression in digital technology has allowed for the development of increasingly smaller and more sophisticated mobile imaging devices that can measure brain, particularly cortical, function during real-time walking or balance tasks within a range of healthy and clinical neurological populations. Specifically, mobile techniques of near infra-red spectroscopy (fNIRS) or electroencephalography (EEG) provide approaches that can be used separately or combined to investigate human behavior during dynamic tasks [11]. There is independence between electrical and optical measurement of brain activity, and fNIRS and EEG both have specific limitations, which has led to multimodal integration of EEG-fNIRS that can overcome limitations within single systems [12, 13]. The combination of mobile neuroimaging techniques with fNIRS or EEG and human movement tracking with 3D motion capture or wearable sensors within a synchronized research approach is termed Mobile Brain/Body Imaging (MoBI). MoBI allows for a relatively cost-effective, noninvasive, and ecologically valid monitoring of real-time brain and body function simultaneously, within laboratory or naturalistic environments where movement impairments may occur. MoBI may allow for more accurate characterization and monitoring of functional activity of neural networks involved in gait or balance impairment with aging and neurological conditions.

This chapter will provide an overview of MoBI techniques used to examine cortical brain activity during gait and balance to understand how age and neurological impairment can negatively impact locomotor control. We will discuss hardware and software and provide an overview of neural activation patterns underlying gait and balance, with specific reference to the impact of neurological impairment.

Hardware

Functional Near Infrared Spectroscopy (fNIRS)

The use of noninvasive mobile/wearable fNIRS devices for monitoring cortical activity has been ongoing for over 30 years, as it has been validated against traditional imaging techniques, which provides credibility in the use of this technique in a variety of populations [14, 15]. fNIRS measures hemodynamic changes in blood flow in the local capillary network caused by metabolic changes with neuronal firings, which is commonly referred to as neurovascular coupling [16, 17]. Specifically, near-infrared light (650-1000 nm) emitter-detector pairs to transmit light into the skull that diffuses through brain tissues (including blood capillaries), resulting in the scattering of multiple photons. Photons that are sent into the skull via emitter optodes exit the skull after passing through the cortex and then detector optodes measure the light intensity. Typically, photons penetrate to 1–2 cm depth, with an emitter-detector distance of 3–5 cm. Longer-channel separation leads to increased depth, but also impacts signal strength and quality. Oxygenated and deoxygenated hemoglobin are chromophores and have different absorption coefficients at different wavelengths of near-infrared light that can be specifically calculated with Beer-Lamberts law [18].

The original fNIRS systems were quite heavy and large, with the need for carts to transport the signal receiver and computer, which meant that movement tasks were very limited (e.g., finger tapping, cycling, or walking on a treadmill) [19]. However, advancements in technology have led to the miniaturization of the sensors and batteries, with modern mobile fNIRS systems allowing for fully mobile tasks within any environment. The majority of mobile fNIRS studies have been limited to covering prefrontal cortical regions due to the limited number of channels available in commercial systems (e.g., 1–8 optode channels), and the fixed location of the sensors (e.g., on a headband). However, more recent research-grade mobile fNIRS systems have been developed that have a greater density of channels (>20–30 optode channels) that can be diversely applied across headcaps (Fig. 2.1). These modern mobile fNIRS systems are typically lightweight and have small batteries on the actual device, with transmitters attached to the person and a receiver connected to a nearby laptop which receives signals via Bluetooth or Wi-Fi. There are limited

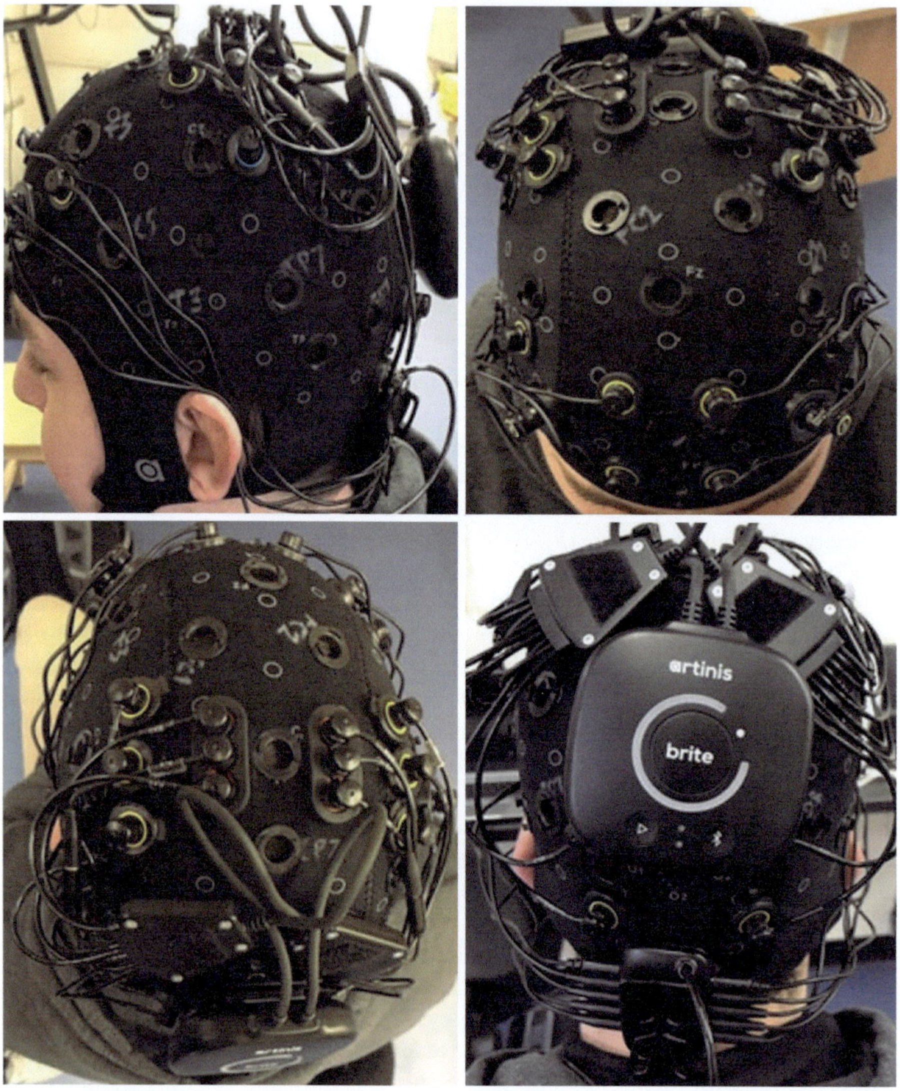

Fig. 2.1 Example of fNIRS headcap with optodes over prefrontal, motor, parietal, and occipital cortices (combined fNIRS Octamon and Brite 24, Artinis)

options for data logging systems. This has led to most studies of brain activation via fNIRS being conducted in laboratory settings.

Participant hair can negatively impact near-infrared light signals from fNIRS optode emitters, which is why the forehead was the location of choice for channels for many of the first fully mobile fNIRS systems. Advances in optical components have allowed for the development of optodes that emit near-infrared light that can travel through or be targeted around the hair on the head. This has allowed the extension of mobile fNIRS optode placement locations across the entire scalp. However, the increase in channel number and the ability to move channels to virtually any location across the scalp leads to several challenges, such as i) detector saturation (i.e., too much light due to either peripheral light or too many emitter optodes located near the detector), and ii) determining the location of the underlying brain regions that the fNIRS signal is measuring. To obtain the approximate cortical region that an fNIRS channel is measuring activity from, modern devices are able to synchronize with a 3D digitizer (e.g., Polhemus, Viper, or Patriot) that provides specific 3D locations on the scalp, of the channels that are referenced to specific anatomical landmarks including the nasion, inion, and preauricular regions (Fig. 2.2) [20, 21]. Accurate Brodman's areas of the cortex are obtained using specialized fNIRS software and the digitized 3D coordinates, which maps to Montreal Neurological Institute (MNI) coordinates of the standard brain model, a valid standard in the field [22–24].

Electroencephalography (EEG)

Noninvasive wearable EEG recording head-caps have been used more recently to study cortical activity during mobile activities, such as walking and balance tasks [5, 25–28]. The use of EEG for recording brain function during dynamic or real-world tasks allows for high temporal resolution data capture without limitation in movement capabilities. Mobile EEG systems are becoming increasingly smaller with lightweight amplifiers and wireless data transmission and more accessible,

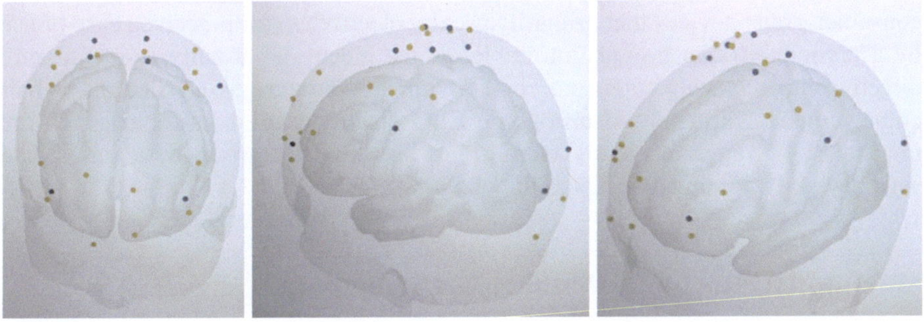

Fig. 2.2 Example of 3D digitized fNIRS optode locations (Polhemus Patriot digitizer with Artinis Oxysoft display)

allowing for nonexpert implementation and data collection. Technological advancements in EEG allow recording at higher resolution (>500 hz) for increasingly longer time periods (>8 h) via signal transmission from the head-mounted device to a laptop or a data logger built into the EEG system for extended recording without data loss.

There are both research-grade mobile EEG systems tailored to scientific or clinical research and consumer-grade systems targeting everyday self-use by novices, which differ in many respects, such as size (research-grade devices may require a backpack to carry amplifiers, but consumer-grade devices may be fully head-mounted) or electrode type (research-grade devices tend to use wet electrodes that require gel but consumer-grade devices may use dry electrodes for ease of application and self-use).

The number of EEG channels vary between systems [29], but typically research-grade mobile EEG systems use 32 or 64 electrodes, which is relatively fewer than tethered or static systems that can have up to 256 channels (such as the ActiveTwo system, Biosemi, ANT-Neuro) in their headcaps. Alternatively, consumer-grade EEG systems have substantially fewer channels than research-grade systems, typically ranging from 1 to 8 channels. The number of electrodes/channels may impact brain activity source localization [30, 31]. Ensuring scalp coverage is important for accurate reference channel set-up and artifact identification. However, at present, the selection of mobile EEG systems often relates to the cost of equipment (which may change with reduced costs over time), as systems with fewer electrodes are more affordable. Additionally, greater numbers of electrodes lead to increased set-up preparation time for participants, increasing data collection burden, as well as reduced comfort (caused by increased head-cap weight, etc.), which sometimes limits application for clinical populations. Set-up times can be particularly impacted by 3D digitization of channel locations (done in a similar manner to fNIRS), which typically takes a longer time with increased channel numbers and anatomical reference locations. However, accurately determining channel locations remains vital, as they directly influence the source-localization of the brain signals being detected.

Usability/user experience of the EEG system is important, particularly for clinical population deployment, to ensure suitability and that its implementation in clinical trials does not impact recruitment, retainment, or data collection. However, even consumer-grade devices that primarily use dry electrodes (for perceived ease of use by a participant) can be uncomfortable, as the electrodes usually exert pressure directly onto the scalp to ensure contact, which can cause skin irritation or hair entanglement. Ultimately, decisions on EEG electrode numbers for research are impacted by a range of factors and all must be weighed against the required data accuracy and participant acceptability of set-up.

Multimodal Functional (Mobile) Neuroimaging

Given that there is a lack of consensus guidelines on what mobile neuroimaging technique (fNIRS or EEG) should be used for specific walking, balance and/or cognitive tasks (see Table 2.1), a combination of devices may provide a pragmatic approach to obtain brain function data. Concurrent assessment of brain activity using fNIRS and EEG allows for examination of complementary features of brain activity, as they represent different physiological processes, i.e., neuronal electrical activity with EEG and hemodynamic responses with fNIRS, which provide a more comprehensive assessment of brain activity and function [32]. EEG-fNIRS systems have been applied to various neuroscientific projects, including clinical neurological populations such as Parkinson's disease, Alzheimer's disease and epilepsy, studies of infant development, and brain-computer interfaces to gather more robust data to more accurately classify brain signals [33].

Typically, multimodal mobile EEG-fNIRS systems are created through synchronizing separate EEG and fNIRS systems, which can often be challenging [33]. Challenges include: (i) difficulties with coupling and finding space for the electrodes and optodes on the subject's head (particularly for children or those with small head sizes); (ii) timing synchronization precision can be difficult due to the differences in the sampling frequencies of the devices; (iii) electrical cross-talk; and (iv) EEG gel impacting light detection of fNIRS optodes [34]. The wearability of the EEG-fNIRS system is a key challenge, particularly to studies that wish to examine mobile or habitual tasks within laboratory or real-world environments. Bulky or indiscrete EEG-fNIRS systems are challenging for the study of motor behavior, as the lack of wearability or usability can influence the behavior of the participant [35]. The advantages and disadvantages of using a combined mobile EEG-fNIRS system are summarized in Table 2.2.

Table 2.1 Comparison of mobile fNIRS and EEG systems

	Mobile fNIRS	Mobile EEG
Signal	Near infrared light	Electrical neural activity
Direct or indirect brain activity signal	Indirect	Direct
Temporal resolution (Hz)	1–50	1–2000
Spatial resolution (depth) (cm)	2–3	5–9
Impact of external tissue (e.g., skull etc.)	Some impact	Some impact
Invasiveness	No	No
Motion artifact tolerance	High	Signal impacted, needs data filtering
Size	Lightweight, depending on number of optodes	Lightweight, depending on number of electrodes
Preparation time	Can be long (especially in those with a lot of hair or with many optodes)	Very long (longer with more electrodes)
Portability	Portable (wireless within space or recording device)	Portable (wireless or can be logged)
Cost	Reasonable, depending on number of optodes	Reasonable, depending on number of electrodes

Table 2.2 Advantages and disadvantages of using a combined mobile EEG-fNIRS system

Advantages	Disadvantages
Complimentary spatial and temporal features (comprehensive) Near-infrared light does not directly impact electrical EEG measurement Can study neurovascular coupling Flexible, portable, noninvasive	Cortical level only Limited scalp surface for sensors Gel impact on light detection Patient discomfort may increase Long preparation times

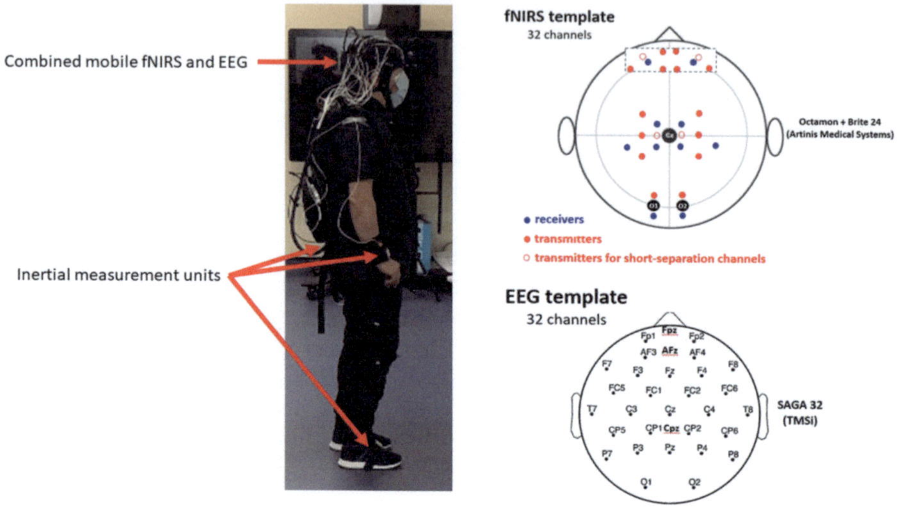

Fig. 2.3 Example of combined mobile fNIRS and EEG system with synchronized inertial measurement units for MoBI

To perform comprehensive MoBI assessment multimodal (or modular) EEG-fNIRS systems are frequently synchronized to movement analysis systems, such as 3D motion capture or wearable sensors (Fig. 2.3) [36]. This further allows for assessment of the underlying control of movement through mobile brain activity monitoring that is coupled with measurement of movement during walking or balance tasks. Wearable inertial measurement units enable the recording of fully mobile tasks in any environment. Motion capture systems, on the other hand, monitor or control tasks in controlled laboratory environments, offering greater insight into the neural control of specific human movement tasks.

Software and Analysis

Software and Analysis for fNIRS

There is currently no standardized and widely accepted signal processing method for fNIRS, and while there have been attempts at creating guidelines for particular methodologies, there are no comprehensive guidelines (unlike fMRI) [6]. This creates a challenge for researchers, particularly novice users, who wish to use fNIRS to monitor brain activity signals during various tasks. In order to provide relatively novice researchers with appropriate signal processing methods, commercial companies that develop fNIRS systems have developed their own ("black box") software platforms (e.g., Oxysoft, Artinis, Netherlands), but the lack of access to specific analysis methods could lead to false positives or negatives in results [37]. Due to the limitations in commercially developed analysis methods, academic researchers have developed open-source toolboxes (e.g., HOMER2, NIRS-SPM, Brain AnalyzIR, Brainstorm, LIONirs, NIRS-KIT, NIRSLab, etc.) that can be used through GUIs or within specific custom-made computer language scripts [24, 38–42].

One of the biggest progressions in fNIRS signal processing has been the ability to account for blood flow changes in the extra cortical layers (e.g., scalp, skull, etc.) of the head by removing heart rate, blood pressure/flow or sympathetic activation that can be influenced by human movement or psychological influences such as stress or anxiety [43–45]. Older fNIRS models had fixed optode holder positions and a standard set-up of locations for the sensors, whereas new fNIRS models allow for flexible application of optodes on the head, which allows for short-separation channels (0.5–2 cm distance between receiver and transmitter optodes to be deployed anywhere on the scalp [45]. Short-separation channels provide signals that can be used to remove signals that are not cerebral. This is done by taking the signal away from the long source-detector channels (3–4 cm separation) and using the short-separation channels as a reference and regressing them out [46]. Other approaches have been deployed in fNIRS signal processing to remove peripheral movement noise from cerebral signals when short-separation channels were not used, such as regression of single channels from long channels, principle component analysis, or independent component analysis [47], but these methods come with the caveat that peripheral physiological influences are not directly measured and therefore potentially not completely removed.

Software and Analysis for EEG

There have been significant advances in data analysis methodologies for EEG data over the past several decades, which have made EEG more accessible to a range of scientists and increased the uptake of this technology for clinical research. Increasingly more powerful computational tools have been created to deal with the signal noise that occurs with movement during walking or balance tasks, with open-source toolboxes such as EEGLAB available that can be exploited by a wide audience for EEG signal data analysis and interpretation [48–50]. EEG data is typically analyzed via either: (1) frequency domain (extracting power spectral densities of the signal typically across 1–70 Hz); (2) time domain (phase locking signal activity to specific stimuli or events, such as step-related potentials); or (3) combined time-frequency domain analysis that combines approaches to EEG signal processing [51].

One of the biggest progressions in EEG signal processing was spatial filtering using independent component analysis (ICA) that can separate temporally and functionally independent components of the signal into brain or nonbrain (i.e., eye, muscle, noise etc.) sources [52–54]. ICA has been used to filter motion artifacts from mobile EEG in a range of healthy and clinical population studies [55–58]. Additionally, the signal source separation progression has allowed for improved source localization processing methods to provide more accurate brain source anatomical locations, which are better with high-density systems [59–61]. Continual improvements in EEG signal processing methods are leading to more complex techniques that provide a wealth of information regarding functional brain activity, such as connectivity [62] and nonlinear signal processing [63], which may provide useful biomarkers within a variety of clinical conditions.

Underlying Mechanisms of Walking

Walking was assumed for many years to be a predominantly automatic motor function that involved only subcortical neural regions, but it is now known that diverse neural activity across cortical and subcortical regions is required for safe and effective walking [64]. Indeed, EEG studies have demonstrated that alterations in delta, theta, alpha, beta, and gamma power spectral densities are required within various cortical regions for effective gait cycle performance, stopping gait, response to different terrains, treadmill walking, and increasing or decreasing gait speeds in healthy individuals [11, 32, 65–76]. Many previous studies examining the underlying neural activity of walking have used either dual-task (performance of two tasks simultaneously, such as walking and talking/performing a cognitive task) or mental imagery (thinking about walking) during traditional fMRI [77], which have provided insights into the brain regions that may be required for walking under a variety of real world conditions. However, previous studies using mental imagery are limited as they do not record brain activity during actual walking and, therefore, only provide a proxy for actual brain activity deployed during locomotion. Recent studies employing MoBI techniques have significantly contributed to understanding underlying cortical mechanisms involved in walking with aging and neurological populations, including Parkinson's disease (PD), multiple sclerosis, traumatic brain injury (TBI), cognitive impairment/dementia, and stroke [78–80]. Typically, fNIRS has been used more predominantly within clinical populations to examine neural activity underlying mobile tasks, such as walking, likely due to the ease of application and analysis compared to EEG. Mobile EEG has primarily been used in healthy young and older adults, with limited application within clinical populations to date using only a few selective channels (1–4 channels) to examine brain activity. However, the evidence that has been generated within aging and neurological populations has demonstrated a shift from automatic processes used for single-task (ST) walking control toward more conscious control with executive-attentional deployment from the prefrontal cortex (PFC) required to overcome deficits in motor control regions [3], which reduces the neural resource ceiling available to deploy on more complex tasks such as DT walking, fast-paced walking, and obstacle navigation [81].

Within healthy young and older adults both fNIRS and EEG have been used to examine neural activity underpinning walking. The majority of previous fNIRS studies have been limited to only PFC recordings, due to the form factor of the devices with optodes over the forehead to avoid hair contact. Generally, MoBI findings during walking suggest an age-associated loss in flexible PFC cognitive resource allocation during ST and complex walking (DT, obstacle crossing, fast walking, etc.) [82, 83]. For example, older adults have been found to have increased PFC activity via fNIRS compared to young adults during walking when dual-tasking [83], although this is not consistent within the literature [84]. Similarly, event-related potentials (ERPs) from mobile EEG have been examined during walking under a dual-task (Go/No-Go response inhibition task) [64], showing that older adults modulate ERPs with increased P3 amplitudes in later stages of walking compared to young adults who had reduced N2 amplitudes and earlier P3 latencies. Findings generally suggest that there may be compensatory cortical mechanisms underpinning usual walking in older adults, with increased reliance on executive-attentional processing to walk [85]. Moreover, several studies have found that PFC activity (lower HbO2 levels) during walking was related with better gait measures, in older adults [83, 86] and people with PD [87]. While changes in neural circuits, consequential to natural aging, may lead to a decline in cognitive performance [88], recruiting additional brain regions or increasing neural activity within existing circuits may allow for the preservation of walking performance as people age. However, older adults that develop mild cognitive impairment have been shown to have an even greater reliance on PFC activity under ST and DT conditions but have worse gait than healthy older adults [89, 90], which highlights a potential neural resource ceiling effect (i.e., cortical activity may increase but resources may not be able to maintain effective gait performance).

As mobile EEG and fNIRS systems have been developing, there are new studies that have used full-cap fNIRS or combined EEG-fNIRS headcaps to study the underlying neural mechanisms involved in walking in various clinical conditions [91]. Generally, evidence suggests that reliance on increased cortical activity, particularly PFC activity, during usual walking and complex walking is further exacerbated compared to healthy older adults in those with neurological disorders such as PD [92], HD [93], multiple sclerosis [94], stroke [95], and cognitive impairment/dementia [89, 90]. To examine more specific underlying cortical activity involved in walking, research in neurological conditions have used various complex tasks. For example, these studies have examined more specific elements of gait, such as gait initiation, dual-tasking, acceleration of walking speed (slow, usual, fast), steady-state walking, turning, obstacle crossing, or walking with gait deficit interventions (cueing, robotic devices, or medications).

MoBI studies in PD have examined a range of walking activities to understand cortical control of gait in this condition. Specifically, MoBI data has been used to examine usual or treadmill walking [96, 97], dual-task walking [98–101], obstacle crossing [87, 92, 102–105], detection of freezing of gait [106–114], differentiation of disease subgroups [115], response to anti-parkinsonian medication [116–118], and response to cueing interventions [55, 119]. Additionally, MoBI (i.e., EEG) has been combined with electromyography to examine corticomuscular coherence in PD, highlighting the link between cortical activity and lower limb muscle activation [120]. MoBI has been less studied in other movement disorders, such as HD [121], but findings suggest commonalities across conditions. For example, people with HD also present with greater reliance on cortical activity via increases in P3 amplitude for DT walking [93]. Similarly, people with multiple sclerosis have also shown reliance on cortical activity, particularly within the PFC, under dual-task walking conditions [94, 122, 123]. Brain injuries, such as TBI or stroke, have also shown alterations in cortical activity during walking compared to controls. Dysfunctions in brain networks related to executive-attentional processing have been linked to poorer DT gait performance in patients with mild TBI [124], and robot-assisted gait has been shown to increase cortical activation in the PFC, bilateral premotor cortex (PMC) and motor cortex (M1) while walking in those with severe TBI [125]. MoBI studies in stroke have also shown that brain regions involved in executive-attentional (PFC), motor planning (supplementary motor area) and sensorimotor integration (sensorimotor cortex and the posterior parietal cortex) have greater activation during ST walking compared to young and older adults [126, 127], which changes (typically increases) with different walking complexities, including DT, various speeds or asymmetrical tasks [95, 128–130]. In addition, cortical activity during gait is modified by various interventions such as robot-assisted walking and whole body vibration used post-stroke [1, 128, 131]. In contrast to some neurological conditions, cortical activity during gait in dementia has received little attention, with more studies examining healthy older adults, or those at risk of dementia, especially those with mild cognitive impairment (MCI) [132]. However, a recent MoBI study reported altered activation patterns in PFC and sensorimotor regions for those with dementia compared to people with MCI or healthy older adults [133]. Ultimately, studies to date have shown that MoBI-derived cortical brain activity is a useful outcome for disease monitoring, subgrouping, and response to interventions, with findings indicating increased PFC, sensorimotor integration, and motor planning region activation required for walking in neurological conditions.

Neural Activity Involved in Balance

Balance or postural control requires diverse neural activity and interaction between cortical and subcortical brain regions, with differences seen in the activity of cortical structures under different conditions, including balance perturbations and modifying sensory inputs (and with declining age or progressive neurological disease or injuries [134]. Similar methodologies to gait research have been employed in the pursuit of understanding underlying neural mechanisms of balance control and their impairments in older adults and in those with neurological disease. For example, the same mobile neuroimaging techniques (fNIRS, EEG, or combined EEG-fNIRS) have been deployed with similar paradigms, such as cognitive dual-tasks or motor imagery [134–138]. However, unlike walking research, EEG rather than fNIRS has been used more frequently within studies that research the neural control of balance in real-time, which is likely due to its superior temporal resolution and limited motion artifacts occurring during static balance tasks. Investigation of the neural activity involved in balance has often used certain postural tasks to challenge specific balance domains and systems, such as sensory organization for the visual, vestibular, and proprioceptive system inputs into balance control or perturbation evoked potentials.

Sensory manipulation has been used to understand the input of various sensory systems into balance control (i.e., the weighting or organization of sensory input), which can decline with age or neurological disorders. This typically involves recording brain activity, often using MoBI, and assessing postural control in various standing conditions. These conditions may include feet together, in tandem, or on one leg, with eyes open or closed and on either a firm (stable) or foam (unstable) surface [139]. The goal of these different conditions is to test the impact of manipulating visual and/or proprioceptive inputs or challenging the vestibular system, both simultaneously and individually [140]. Studies in healthy young, middle-aged and older adults have found that there is greater attentional cortical region activation required with age during sensory manipulation balance tasks (e.g., re-weighting, optic flow tasks, etc.) [141–144].

Perturbation-evoked potentials, also known as mechanically evoked cerebral potentials [145, 146], are ERPs that are evoked by an expected or unexpected perturbation to balance. Perturbations can be induced by physical instruments such as force plates, tilt platforms or instrumented treadmills, or by sensory instruments such as virtual reality to provide visual cues or interruption of optical flow [147]. EEG is typically the preferred technique in these types of studies where it is important to assess more immediate effects on the brain with a high temporal resolution. Studies have found that there is cortical involvement in balance control in healthy adults and that this can be altered through aging or neurological impairment [148–153]. For example, within TBI, there is lower N1 amplitude compared to controls in response to balance perturbation [148]. This research provides further evidence of cortical involvement in postural control in healthy populations and people with neurological disorders.

Similar to gait research, studies in this field have assessed the effects of aging [154], but predominantly focus on the evaluation of individuals within a clinical population such as PD [137, 155, 156], HD [138], multiple sclerosis [136], TBI [157], and stroke [158]. These studies provide supporting evidence that there is an increased cortical reliance and involvement during postural control tasks, relative to healthy controls. Specifically, a recent systematic review highlighted that the dorsolateral prefrontal cortex, sensory motor area and superior temporal gyrus are activated during balance tasks in healthy individuals and further activated in aging or disease-related populations [159]. However, there are only a limited number of studies examining cortical control of balance with aging or neurological impairment, particularly relative to gait research [5]. Further work is necessary to increase the current understanding of the neural mechanisms underlying balance and postural control in clinical populations.

Challenges for MoBI in Clinical Research

Technological advancements have facilitated the proliferation of MoBI research. This has made a significant contribution to enhancing the knowledge of cortical brain activity and its relationship with gait and postural control with aging and neurological populations. However, MoBI studies do face several challenges and limitations. For example, MoBI research requires the integration of multiple data modalities (EEG/fNIRS data, clinical assessments, cognitive measures, and wearable sensors or motion tracking devices). The synchronization, management, and analysis of this range of data can be very time-consuming and complex, which limits the clinical application of these technologies within healthcare or clinical trial settings. In addition, as aforementioned, there is a lack of standardization in MoBI research and typically small sample sizes used (<30 participants per group) [1, 3, 5, 20, 32, 85, 88, 121, 128, 132, 134, 146, 160–168], which makes the comparison of findings between different studies difficult and limits generalizability to heterogeneous clinical populations. Moreover, even within groups of patients with the same neurological disorders, differences in disease stages, severity, and clinical presentations, make generalizability of MoBI outcomes difficult. To ensure that results are repeatable and comparable across conditions, there is a need to develop standard and consistent methodologies for examining cortical activity during gait and balance tasks across studies.

Future Directions

MoBI research provides valuable insights into the neural networks involved in gait and balance impairments, potentially allowing for development of more effective and personalized treatments to improve functional mobility within free-living environments. Past and future MoBI research will inform the design of future interventions to improve automaticity, reduce reliance on cognitive resources, improve gait, balance, cognitive function, and quality of life, and reduce fall risk for individuals with neurological disorders and older adults. For example, DT treadmill training in PD can reduce PFC activation during both ST and DT walking and has been linked to reduced falls, suggesting the intervention led to more efficient neural recruitment [169]. Other potential interventions include neuromodulation paradigms (e.g., transcranial magnetic stimulation or transcranial direct current stimulation), which have been shown to improve PFC activity, cognition, and gait in persons with PD [170–176].

Conclusions

In conclusion, technological developments in mobile brain imaging using portable, lightweight, and noninvasive fNIRS and EEG devices in conjunction with human movement tracking apparatus, have furthered the understanding of underlying cortical mechanisms involved in walking and balance. This methodology holds significant utility and importance in evaluating the impact of various factors, including cognitive dysfunction, genotype-phenotype relationships, and disease severity and its progression that may affect the motor control for gait and balance in neurological conditions and with the natural aging process. Findings suggest that walking and maintaining appropriate balance with age or neurological impairment engages cortical resources, potentially as a compensatory mechanism for impaired movement automaticity. However, MoBI studies do face certain challenges and limitations, including the lack of standardized data analysis and acquisition techniques, which require further research to develop.

Acknowledgments This work was funded in part by grants from the Parkinson's Foundation (PF-FBS-1898, PF-CRA-2073) (PI: Stuart), the Private Physiotherapy Educational Foundation (PPEF—#368) (PI: Stuart), a Northumbria University PhD studentship (PI: Morris), a Huntington's Disease Society of America Human Biology Project (PI: O'Keefe; 2021–2023), and a Rush University Rush Imaging Research Core pilot grant (PI: O'Keefe; 2023–2024).

References

1. Turner D, Murguialday AR, Birbaumer N, Hoffmann U, Luft A. Neurophysiology of robot-mediated training and therapy: a perspective for future use in clinical populations. Front Neurol. 2013;4:184.
2. Pirker W, Katzenschlager R. Gait disorders in adults and the elderly: a clinical guide. Wien Klin Wochenschr. 2017;129(3–4):81–95.
3. Vitorio R, Stuart S, Rochester L, Alcock L, Pantall A. fNIRS response during walking—artefact or cortical activity? A systematic review. Neurosci Biobehav Rev. 2017;83:160–72.
4. Menant JC, Maidan I, Alcock L, Al-Yahya E, Cerasa A, Clark DJ, et al. A consensus guide to using functional near-infrared spectroscopy in posture and gait research. Gait Posture. 2020;82:254–65.
5. Stuart S, Vitorio R, Morris R, Martini DN, Fino PC, Mancini M. Cortical activity during walking and balance tasks in older adults and in people with Parkinson's disease: a structured review. Maturitas. 2018;113:53–72.
6. Glover GH. Overview of functional magnetic resonance imaging. Neurosurg Clin N Am. 2011;22(2):133–9. vii
7. Jones T, Townsend D. History and future technical innovation in positron emission tomography. J Med Imaging (Bellingham). 2017;4(1):011013.
8. Crişan G, Moldovean-Cioroianu NS, Timaru DG, Andrieş G, Căinap C, Chiş V. Radiopharmaceuticals for PET and SPECT imaging: a literature review over the last decade. Int J Mol Sci. 2022;23(9)

9. Hamacher D, Herold F, Wiegel P, Hamacher D, Schega L. Brain activity during walking: a systematic review. Neurosci Biobehav Rev. 2015;57:310–27.
10. Takakusaki K. Functional neuroanatomy for posture and gait control. J Mov Disord. 2017;10(1):1–17.
11. Makeig S, Gramann K, Jung T-P, Sejnowski TJ, Poizner H. Linking brain, mind and behavior. Int J Psychophysiol. 2009;73(2):95–100.
12. Schmorrow DD, Estabrooke IV, Grootjen M. Foundations of augmented cognition. Neuroergonomics and operational neuroscience: 5th International Conference, FAC 2009, held as part of HCI International 2009 San Diego, CA, USA, July 19–24, 2009, Proceedings. Springer; 2009.
13. Muthalib M, Anwar AR, Perrey S, Dat M, Galka A, Wolff S, et al. Multimodal integration of fNIRS, fMRI and EEG neuroimaging. Clin Neurophysiol. 2013;124(10):2060–2.
14. Klein F, Debener S, Witt K, Kranczioch C. fMRI-based validation of continuous-wave fNIRS of supplementary motor area activation during motor execution and motor imagery. Sci Rep. 2022;12(1):3570.
15. Pinti P, Tachtsidis I, Hamilton A, Hirsch J, Aichelburg C, Gilbert S, et al. The present and future use of functional near-infrared spectroscopy (fNIRS) for cognitive neuroscience. Ann N Y Acad Sci. 2020;1464(1):5–29.
16. Phillips AA, Chan FH, Zheng MM, Krassioukov AV, Ainslie PN. Neurovascular coupling in humans: physiology, methodological advances and clinical implications. J Cereb Blood Flow Metab. 2016;36(4):647–64.
17. Quaresima V, Ferrari M. Functional Near-Infrared Spectroscopy (fNIRS) for assessing cerebral cortex function during human behavior in natural/social situations: a concise review. Organ Res Methods. 2016;22(1):46–68.
18. Kocsis L, Herman P, Eke A. The modified Beer–Lambert law revisited. Phys Med Biol. 2006;51(5):N91.
19. Ferrari M, Quaresima V. A brief review on the history of human functional near-infrared spectroscopy (fNIRS) development and fields of application. NeuroImage. 2012;63(2):921–35.
20. Pinti P, Aichelburg C, Gilbert S, Hamilton A, Hirsch J, Burgess P, et al. A review on the use of wearable functional near-infrared spectroscopy in naturalistic environments. Jpn Psychol Res. 2018;60(4):347–73.
21. Henschel A, Kent M, Leisten LM, Seelemeyer H, Timmerman R, Hortensius R, et al. A manual to digitising fNIRS probes with photogrammetry as described in Clausner et al. (2017). Zenodo. 2020; https://doi.org/10.5281/zenodo.
22. Singh AK, Okamoto M, Dan H, Jurcak V, Dan I. Spatial registration of multichannel multi-subject fNIRS data to MNI space without MRI. NeuroImage. 2005;27(4):842–51.
23. Tsuzuki D, Dan I. Spatial registration for functional near-infrared spectroscopy: from channel position on the scalp to cortical location in individual and group analyses. NeuroImage. 2014;85(Pt 1):92–103.
24. Ye JC, Tak S, Jang KE, Jung J, Jang J. NIRS-SPM: statistical parametric mapping for near-infrared spectroscopy. NeuroImage. 2009;44(2):428–47.
25. Oh K, Park J, Jo SH, Hong S-J, Kim W-S, Paik N-J, et al. Improved cortical activity and reduced gait asymmetry during poststroke self-paced walking rehabilitation. J Neuroeng Rehabil. 2021;18(1):60.
26. Gebel A, Lehmann T, Granacher U. Balance task difficulty affects postural sway and cortical activity in healthy adolescents. Exp Brain Res. 2020;238(5):1323–33.
27. Peterson SM, Ferris DP. Group-level cortical and muscular connectivity during perturbations to walking and standing balance. NeuroImage. 2019;198:93–103.
28. Roeder L, Boonstra TW, Kerr GK. Corticomuscular control of walking in older people and people with Parkinson's disease. Sci Rep. 2020;10(1):2980.
29. Niso G, Romero E, Moreau JT, Araujo A, Krol LR. Wireless EEG: a survey of systems and studies. NeuroImage. 2023;269:119774.

30. Sohrabpour A, Lu Y, Kankirawatana P, Blount J, Kim H, He B. Effect of EEG electrode number on epileptic source localization in pediatric patients. Clin Neurophysiol. 2015;126(3):472–80.
31. Koles ZJ. Trends in EEG source localization. Electroencephalogr Clin Neurophysiol. 1998;106(2):127–37.
32. Khan H, Naseer N, Yazidi A, Eide PK, Hassan HW, Mirtaheri P. Analysis of human gait using hybrid EEG-fNIRS-based BCI system: a review. Front Hum Neurosci. 2021;14:613254.
33. Uchitel J, Vidal-Rosas EE, Cooper RJ, Zhao H. Wearable, integrated EEG–fNIRS technologies: a review. Sensors. 2021;21(18):6106.
34. Yuan Z, Zhang X, Ding M. Techniques advances and clinical applications in fused EEG-fNIRS. Front Media SA. 2019:408.
35. Uchitel J, Vidal-Rosas EE, Cooper RJ, Zhao H. Wearable, integrated EEG-fNIRS technologies: a review. Sensors (Basel). 2021;21(18)
36. Jungnickel E, Gehrke L, Klug M, Gramann K. MoBI—mobile brain/body imaging. Neuroergonomics. 2019:59–63.
37. Tachtsidis I, Scholkmann F. False positives and false negatives in functional near-infrared spectroscopy: issues, challenges, and the way forward. Neurophotonics. 2016;3(3):031405.
38. Xu Y, Graber HL, Barbour RL, editors. nirsLAB: a computing environment for fNIRS neuroimaging data analysis. Biomedical Optics; 2014. Optica Publishing Group.
39. Hou X, Zhang Z, Zhao C, Duan L, Gong Y, Li Z, et al. NIRS-KIT: a MATLAB toolbox for both resting-state and task fNIRS data analysis. Neurophotonics. 2021;8(1):010802.
40. Santosa H, Zhai X, Fishburn F, Huppert T. The NIRS brain AnalyzIR toolbox. Algorithms. 2018;11(5):73.
41. Tadel F, Bock E, Niso G, Mosher JC, Cousineau M, Pantazis D, et al. MEG/EEG group analysis with brainstorm. Front Neurosci. 2019;13:76.
42. Tremblay J, Martínez-Montes E, Hüsser A, Caron-Desrochers L, Lepage C, Pouliot P, et al. LIONirs: flexible Matlab toolbox for fNIRS data analysis. J Neurosci Methods. 2022;370:109487.
43. Gagnon L, Cooper RJ, Yücel MA, Perdue KL, Greve DN, Boas DA. Short separation channel location impacts the performance of short channel regression in NIRS. NeuroImage. 2012;59(3):2518–28.
44. Gagnon L, Yücel MA, Boas DA, Cooper RJ. Further improvement in reducing superficial contamination in NIRS using double short separation measurements. NeuroImage. 2014;85:127–35.
45. Brigadoi S, Cooper RJ. How short is short? Optimum source–detector distance for short-separation channels in functional near-infrared spectroscopy. Neurophotonics. 2015;2(2):025005.
46. Goodwin JR, Gaudet CR, Berger AJ. Short-channel functional near-infrared spectroscopy regressions improve when source-detector separation is reduced. Neurophotonics. 2014;1(1):015002.
47. Virtanen J, Noponen T, Meriläinen P. Comparison of principal and independent component analysis in removing extracerebral interference from near-infrared spectroscopy signals. J Biomed Opt. 2009;14(5):054032–10.
48. Brunner C, Delorme A, Makeig S. Eeglab–an open source matlab toolbox for electrophysiological research. Biomed Eng/Biomedizinische Technik. 2013;58(SI-1-Track-G):000010151520134182.
49. Delorme A, Makeig S. EEGLAB: an open source toolbox for analysis of single-trial EEG dynamics including independent component analysis. J Neurosci Methods. 2004;134(1):9–21.
50. Delorme A, Mullen T, Kothe C, Acar ZA, Bigdely-Shamlo N, Vankov A, et al. EEGLAB, SIFT, NFT, BCILAB, and ERICA: new tools for advanced EEG processing. Comput Intell Neurosci. 2011;2011:10.
51. Roach BJ, Mathalon DH. Event-related EEG time-frequency analysis: an overview of measures and an analysis of early gamma band phase locking in schizophrenia. Schizophr Bull. 2008;34(5):907–26.

52. Grandchamp R, Braboszcz C, Makeig S, Delorme A, editors. Stability of ICA decomposition across within-subject EEG datasets. In 2012 Annual International Conference of the IEEE Engineering in Medicine and Biology Society; 2012. IEEE.
53. Mennes M, Wouters H, Vanrumste B, Lagae L, Stiers P. Validation of ICA as a tool to remove eye movement artifacts from EEG/ERP. Psychophysiology. 2010;47(6):1142–50.
54. Olbrich S, Jödicke J, Sander C, Himmerich H, Hegerl U. ICA-based muscle artefact correction of EEG data: what is muscle and what is brain?: Comment on McMenamin et al. NeuroImage. 2011;54(1):1–3.
55. Stuart S, Wagner J, Makeig S, Mancini M. Brain activity response to visual cues for gait impairment in Parkinson's disease: an EEG study. Neurorehabil Neural Repair. 2021;35(11):996–1009.
56. Bulea TC, Jonghyun K, Damiano DL, Stanley CJ, Hyung-Soon P. User-driven control increases cortical activity during treadmill walking: an EEG study. Annu Int Conf IEEE Eng Med Biol Soc. 2014;2014:2111–4.
57. Chaddad A, Wu Y, Kateb R, Bouridane A. Electroencephalography signal processing: a comprehensive review and analysis of methods and techniques. Sensors (Basel). 2023;23(14)
58. Heng HM, Lu MK, Chou LW, Meng NH, Huang HC, Hamada M, et al. Changes in balance, gait and electroencephalography oscillations after robot-assisted gait training: an exploratory study in people with chronic stroke. Brain Sci. 2020;10(11)
59. Pion-Tonachini L, Hsu S-H, Makeig S, Jung T-P, Cauwenberghs G, editors. Real-time eeg source-mapping toolbox (rest): Online ica and source localization. 2015 37th Annual International Conference of the IEEE Engineering in Medicine and Biology Society (EMBC); 2015. IEEE.
60. Ventouras EM, Ktonas PY, Tsekou H, Paparrigopoulos T, Kalatzis I, Soldatos CR. Independent component analysis for source localization of EEG sleep spindle components. Comput Intell Neurosci. 2010;2010:1.
61. Chikara RK, Ko L-W. Modulation of the visual to auditory human inhibitory brain network: an EEG dipole source localization study. Brain Sci. 2019;9(9):216.
62. Schoffelen JM, Gross J. Source connectivity analysis with MEG and EEG. Hum Brain Mapp. 2009;30(6):1857–65.
63. Hornero R, Abásolo D, Escudero J, Gómez C. Nonlinear analysis of electroencephalogram and magnetoencephalogram recordings in patients with Alzheimer's disease. Philos Trans R Soc A Math Phys Eng Sci. 1887;2009(367):317–36.
64. Malcolm BR, Foxe JJ, Butler JS, De Sanctis P. The aging brain shows less flexible reallocation of cognitive resources during dual-task walking: a mobile brain/body imaging (MoBI) study. NeuroImage. 2015;117:230–42.
65. Hortal E, Úbeda A, Iáñez E, Azorín JM, Fernández E. EEG-based detection of starting and stopping during gait cycle. Int J Neural Syst. 2016;26(07):1650029.
66. Jacobsen NSJ, Blum S, Witt K, Debener S. A walk in the park? Characterizing gait-related artifacts in mobile EEG recordings. Eur J Neurosci. 2021;54(12):8421–40.
67. Kline JE, Huang HJ, Snyder KL, Ferris DP. Isolating gait-related movement artifacts in electroencephalography during human walking. J Neural Eng. 2015;12(4):046022.
68. Lisi G, Morimoto J. EEG single-trial detection of gait speed changes during treadmill walk. PLoS One. 2015;10(5):e0125479.
69. Nathan K, Contreras-Vidal JL. Negligible motion artifacts in scalp electroencephalography (EEG) during treadmill walking. Front Hum Neurosci. 2016;9:708.
70. Nordin AD, Hairston WD, Ferris DP. Faster gait speeds reduce alpha and beta EEG spectral power from human sensorimotor cortex. IEEE Trans Biomed Eng. 2019;67(3):842–53.
71. Seeber M, Scherer R, Wagner J, Solis-Escalante T, Müller-Putz GR. EEG beta suppression and low gamma modulation are different elements of human upright walking. Front Hum Neurosci. 2014;8:485.
72. Seeber M, Scherer R, Wagner J, Solis-Escalante T, Müller-Putz GR. High and low gamma EEG oscillations in central sensorimotor areas are conversely modulated during the human gait cycle. NeuroImage. 2015;112:318–26.

73. Snyder KL, Kline JE, Huang HJ, Ferris DP. Independent component analysis of gait-related movement artifact recorded using EEG electrodes during treadmill walking. Front Hum Neurosci. 2015;9:639.
74. Weersink JB, Maurits NM, de Jong BM. EEG time-frequency analysis provides arguments for arm swing support in human gait control. Gait Posture. 2019;70:71–8.
75. Weersink JB, Maurits NM, van Laar T, de Jong BM. Enhanced arm swing improves Parkinsonian gait with EEG power modulations resembling healthy gait. Parkinsonism Relat Disord. 2021;91:96–101.
76. Jacobsen NSJ, Blum S, Scanlon JEM, Witt K, Debener S. Mobile electroencephalography captures differences of walking over even and uneven terrain but not of single and dual-task gait. Front Sports Act Living. 2022;4:945341.
77. Blumen HM, Holtzer R, Brown LL, Gazes Y, Verghese J. Behavioral and neural correlates of imagined walking and walking-while-talking in the elderly. Hum Brain Mapp. 2014;35(8):4090–104.
78. Clark DJ, Manini TM, Ferris DP, Hass CJ, Brumback BA, Cruz-Almeida Y, et al. Multimodal imaging of brain activity to investigate walking and mobility decline in older adults (mind in motion study): hypothesis, theory, and methods. Front Aging Neurosci. 2020;11:11.
79. Ko LW, Stevenson C, Chang WC, Yu KH, Chi KC, Chen YJ, et al. Integrated gait triggered mixed reality and neurophysiological monitoring as a framework for next-generation ambulatory stroke rehabilitation. IEEE Trans Neural Syst Rehabil Eng. 2021;29:2435–44.
80. Stuart S, Belluscio V, Quinn JF, Mancini M. Pre-frontal cortical activity during walking and turning is reliable and differentiates across young, older adults and people with Parkinson's disease. Front Neurol. 2019;10
81. Clark DJ, Manini TM, Ferris DP, Hass CJ, Brumback BA, Cruz-Almeida Y, et al. Multimodal imaging of brain activity to investigate walking and mobility decline in older adults (mind in motion study): hypothesis, theory, and methods. Front Aging Neurosci. 2019;11:358.
82. Belli V, Orcioli-Silva D, Beretta VS, Vitório R, Zampier VC, Nóbrega-Sousa P, et al. Prefrontal cortical activity during preferred and fast walking in young and older adults: an fNIRS study. Neuroscience. 2021;473:81–9.
83. Nóbrega-Sousa P, Gobbi LTB, Orcioli-Silva D, Conceição NR, Beretta VS, Vitório R. Prefrontal cortex activity during walking: effects of aging and associations with gait and executive function. Neurorehabil Neural Repair. 2020;34(10):915–24.
84. Stuart S, Alcock L, Rochester L, Vitorio R, Pantall A. Monitoring multiple cortical regions during walking in young and older adults: dual-task response and comparison challenges. Int J Psychophysiol. 2019;135:63–72.
85. Reuter-Lorenz PA, Cappell KA. Neurocognitive aging and the compensation hypothesis. Curr Dir Psychol Sci. 2008;17(3):177–82.
86. Vitorio R, Stuart S, Gobbi LTB, Rochester L, Alcock L, Pantall A. Reduced gait variability and enhanced brain activity in older adults with auditory cues: a functional near-infrared spectroscopy study. Neurorehabil Neural Repair. 2018;32(11):976–87.
87. Orcioli-Silva D, Vitório R, Nóbrega-Sousa P, Beretta VS, Conceição NR, Oliveira AS, et al. Cortical activity underlying gait improvements achieved with dopaminergic medication during usual walking and obstacle avoidance in Parkinson disease. Neurorehabil Neural Repair. 2021;35(5):406–18.
88. Murman DL. The impact of age on cognition. Semin Hear. 2015;36(3):111–21.
89. Holtzer R, Izzetoglu M. Mild cognitive impairments attenuate prefrontal cortex activations during walking in older adults. Brain Sci. 2020;10(7):415.
90. Udina C, Avtzi S, Mota-Foix M, Rosso AL, Ars J, Kobayashi Frisk L, et al. Dual-task related frontal cerebral blood flow changes in older adults with mild cognitive impairment: a functional diffuse correlation spectroscopy study. Front Aging Neurosci. 2022;14:14.
91. Vitório R, Morris R, Das J, Walker R, Mancini M, Stuart S. Brain activity response to cues during gait in Parkinson's disease: a study protocol. PLoS One. 2022;17(11):e0275894.

92. Maidan I, Nieuwhof F, Bernad-Elazari H, Reelick MF, Bloem BR, Giladi N, et al. The role of the frontal lobe in complex walking among patients with Parkinson's disease and healthy older adults: an fNIRS study. Neurorehabil Neural Repair. 2016;30(10):963–71.
93. de Tommaso M, Ricci K, Montemurno A, Vecchio E, Invitto S. Walking-related dual-task interference in early-to-middle-stage Huntington's disease: an auditory event related potential study. Front Psychol. 2017;8:1292.
94. Hernandez ME, Holtzer R, Chaparro G, Jean K, Balto JM, Sandroff BM, et al. Brain activation changes during locomotion in middle-aged to older adults with multiple sclerosis. J Neurol Sci. 2016;370:277–83.
95. Lim SB, Yang C-l, Peters S, Liu-Ambrose T, Boyd LA, Eng JJ. Phase-dependent brain activation of the frontal and parietal regions during walking after stroke-an fNIRS study. Front Neurol. 2022;13:904722.
96. Ding H, Droby A, Anwar AR, Hausdorff JM, Nasseroleslami B, Mirelman A, et al. Treadmill training in Parkinson's disease: possible role of prefrontal modifications in the improved cortical-subcortical network function. Neural Regen Res. 2024;19(2):407–8.
97. Thumm PC, Maidan I, Brozgol M, Shustak S, Gazit E, Shema Shiratzki S, et al. Treadmill walking reduces pre-frontal activation in patients with Parkinson's disease. Gait Posture. 2018;62:384–7.
98. Huang C-Y, Chen Y-A, Wu R-M, Hwang I-S. Dual-task walking improvement with enhanced kinesthetic awareness in Parkinson's disease with mild gait impairment: EEG connectivity and clinical implication. Front Aging Neurosci. 2022;14:1041378.
99. Inbal M, Roni H, Irina G, Nir G, Roee H, Jeffrey MH, et al. Neural variability in the prefrontal cortex as a reflection of neural flexibility and stability in patients with Parkinson disease. Neurology. 2022;98(8):e839.
100. Maidan I, Fahoum F, Shustak S, Gazit E, Patashov D, Tchertov D, et al. Changes in event-related potentials during dual task walking in aging and Parkinson's disease. Clin Neurophysiol. 2019;130(2):224–30.
101. Possti D, Fahoum F, Sosnik R, Giladi N, Hausdorff JM, Mirelman A, et al. Changes in the EEG spectral power during dual-task walking with aging and Parkinson's disease: initial findings using Event-Related Spectral Perturbation analysis. J Neurol. 2021;268:161–8.
102. Assad M, Galperin I, Giladi N, Mirelman A, Hausdorff JM, Maidan I. Disease severity and prefrontal cortex activation during obstacle negotiation among patients with Parkinson's disease: is it all as expected? Parkinsonism Relat Disord. 2022;101:20–6.
103. Pelicioni PHS, Lord SR, Okubo Y, Menant JC. Cortical activation during gait adaptability in people with Parkinson's disease. Gait Posture. 2022;91:247–53.
104. Sharon T, Kurz I, Bernad-Elazari H, Shustak S, Galperin I, Giladi N, et al. Which obstacle attributes place additional demands on higher-level cognitive function in patients with Parkinson's disease? Parkinsonism Relat Disord. 2020;78:178–83.
105. Vitório R, Lirani-Silva E, Orcioli-Silva D, Beretta VS, Oliveira AS, Gobbi LTB. Electrocortical dynamics of usual walking and the planning to step over obstacles in Parkinson's disease. Sensors. 2023;23(10):4866.
106. Handojoseno AA, Shine JM, Nguyen TN, Tran Y, Lewis SJ, Nguyen HT, editors. The detection of Freezing of Gait in Parkinson's disease patients using EEG signals based on Wavelet decomposition. In 2012 Annual International Conference of the IEEE Engineering in Medicine and Biology Society; 2012. IEEE.
107. Asher EE, Plotnik M, Günther M, Moshel S, Levy O, Havlin S, et al. Connectivity of EEG synchronization networks increases for Parkinson's disease patients with freezing of gait. Commun Biol. 2021;4(1):1017.
108. Belluscio V, Stuart S, Bergamini E, Vannozzi G, Mancini M. The association between prefrontal cortex activity and turning behavior in people with and without freezing of gait. Neuroscience. 2019;416:168–76.
109. Cao Z, John AR, Chen H-T, Martens KE, Georgiades M, Gilat M, et al. Identification of EEG dynamics during freezing of gait and voluntary stopping in patients with Parkinson's disease. IEEE Trans Neural Syst Rehabil Eng. 2021;29:1774–83.

110. Handojoseno AA, Shine JM, Nguyen TN, Tran Y, Lewis SJ, Nguyen HT. Analysis and prediction of the freezing of gait using EEG brain dynamics. IEEE Trans Neural Syst Rehabil Eng. 2014;23(5):887–96.
111. John AR, Cao Z, Chen H-T, Martens KE, Georgiades M, Gilat M, et al. Predicting the onset of freezing of gait using EEG dynamics. Appl Sci. 2022;13(1):302.
112. Maidan I, Bernad-Elazari H, Gazit E, Giladi N, Hausdorff JM, Mirelman A. Changes in oxygenated hemoglobin link freezing of gait to frontal activation in patients with Parkinson disease: an fNIRS study of transient motor-cognitive failures. J Neurol. 2015;262(4):899–908.
113. Vitorio R, Stuart S, Mancini M. Executive control of walking in people with Parkinson's disease with freezing of gait. Neurorehabil Neural Repair. 2020;34(12):1138–49.
114. Waechter SM, Fearon C, McDonnell C, Gallego J, Quinlivan B, Killane I, et al., editors. The impact of dual tasking on cognitive performance in a Parkinson's disease cohort with and without freezing of gait: an EEG and behavioral based approach. In 2015 7th International IEEE/EMBS Conference on Neural Engineering (NER); 2015. IEEE.
115. Orcioli-Silva D, Vitório R, Beretta VS, da Conceição NR, Nóbrega-Sousa P, Oliveira AS, et al. Is cortical activation during walking different between Parkinson's disease motor subtypes? J Gerontol Series A. 2020;76(4):561–7.
116. Dagan M, Herman T, Bernad-Elazari H, Gazit E, Maidan I, Giladi N, et al. Dopaminergic therapy and prefrontal activation during walking in individuals with Parkinson's disease: does the levodopa overdose hypothesis extend to gait? J Neurol. 2021;268(2):658–68.
117. Orcioli-Silva D, Vitório R, Nóbrega-Sousa P, da Conceição NR, Beretta VS, Lirani-Silva E, et al. Levodopa facilitates prefrontal cortex activation during dual task walking in Parkinson disease. Neurorehabil Neural Repair. 2020;34(7):589–99.
118. Stuart S, Morris R, Giritharan A, Quinn J, Nutt JG, Mancini M. Prefrontal cortex activity and gait in Parkinson's disease with cholinergic and dopaminergic therapy. Mov Disord. 2020;35(11):2019–27.
119. Stuart S, Mancini M. Prefrontal cortical activation with open and closed-loop tactile cueing when walking and turning in Parkinson disease: a pilot study. J Neurol Phys Ther. 2020;44(2):121.
120. Günther M, Bartsch RP, Miron-Shahar Y, Hassin-Baer S, Inzelberg R, Kurths J, et al. Coupling between leg muscle activation and EEG during normal walking, intentional stops, and freezing of gait in Parkinson's disease. Front Physiol. 2019;10:870.
121. Tortelli R, Rodrigues FB, Wild EJ. The use of wearable/portable digital sensors in Huntington's disease: a systematic review. Parkinsonism Relat Disord. 2021;83:93–104.
122. Chaparro G, Balto JM, Sandroff BM, Holtzer R, Izzetoglu M, Motl RW, et al. Frontal brain activation changes due to dual-tasking under partial body weight support conditions in older adults with multiple sclerosis. J Neuroeng Rehabil. 2017;14(1):1–10.
123. De Sanctis P, Malcolm BR, Mabie PC, Francisco AA, Mowrey WB, Joshi S, et al. Mobile brain/body imaging of cognitive-motor impairment in multiple sclerosis: deriving EEG-based neuro-markers during a dual-task walking study. Clin Neurophysiol. 2020;131(5):1119–28.
124. Howell DR, Meehan WP III, Barber Foss KD, Reches A, Weiss M, Myer GD. Reduced dual-task gait speed is associated with visual Go/No-Go brain network activation in children and adolescents with concussion. Brain Inj. 2018;32(9):1129–34.
125. Karunakaran KK, Nisenson DM, Nolan KJ, editors. Alterations in cortical activity due to robotic gait training in traumatic brain injury. In 2020 42nd Annual International Conference of the IEEE Engineering in Medicine & Biology Society (EMBC); 2020. IEEE.
126. Chatterjee SA, Fox EJ, Daly JJ, Rose DK, Wu SS, Christou EA, et al. Interpreting prefrontal recruitment during walking after stroke: influence of individual differences in mobility and cognitive function. Front Hum Neurosci. 2019;13:194.
127. Hermand E, Compagnat M, Dupuy O, Salle J-Y, Daviet J-C, Perrochon A. Functional status is associated with prefrontal cortex activation in gait in subacute stroke patients: a functional near-infrared spectroscopy study. Front Neurol. 2020;11:11.

128. Lim SB, Louie DR, Peters S, Liu-Ambrose T, Boyd LA, Eng JJ. Brain activity during real-time walking and with walking interventions after stroke: a systematic review. J Neuroeng Rehabil. 2021;18(1):8.
129. Liu Y-C, Yang Y-R, Tsai Y-A, Wang R-Y, Lu C-F. Brain activation and gait alteration during cognitive and motor dual task walking in stroke—a functional near-infrared spectroscopy study. IEEE Trans Neural Syst Rehabil Eng. 2018;26(12):2416–23.
130. Compagnat M, Daviet JC, Hermand E, Billot M, Salle JY, Perrochon A. Impact of a dual task on the energy cost of walking in individuals with subacute phase stroke. Brain Inj. 2023;37(2):114–21.
131. Lee A, Kim H, Kim J, Choi D-S, Jung JH, Lee J, et al. Modulating effects of whole-body vibration on cortical activity and gait function in chronic stroke patients. Brain Neurorehabil. 2020;13(2)
132. Sui SX, Hendy AM, Teo W-P, Moran JT, Nuzum ND, Pasco JA. A review of the measurement of the neurology of gait in cognitive dysfunction or dementia, focusing on the application of fNIRS during Dual-Task Gait Assessment. Brain Sci. 2022;12(8):968.
133. Teo WP, Rantalainen T, Nuzum N, Valente L, Macpherson H. Altered prefrontal cortex responses in older adults with subjective memory complaints and dementia during dual-task gait: an fNIRS study. Eur J Neurosci. 2021;53(4):1324–33.
134. Baradaran Y, Rojas RF, Goecke R, Ghahramani M. A systematic review on functional near-infrared spectroscopy concurrent with quantitative balance assessment. IEEE Access. 2023;11:66641.
135. Almulla L, Al-Naib I, Ateeq IS, Althobaiti M. Observation and motor imagery balance tasks evaluation: an fNIRS feasibility study. PLoS One. 2022;17(3):e0265898.
136. Hernandez ME, O'Donnell E, Chaparro G, Holtzer R, Izzetoglu M, Sandroff BM, et al. Brain activation changes during balance-and attention-demanding tasks in middle-and older-aged adults with multiple sclerosis. Mot Control. 2019;23(4):498–517.
137. Huang C-Y, Chen L-C, Wu R-M, Hwang I-S. Effects of task prioritization on a postural-motor task in early-stage Parkinson's disease: EEG connectivity and clinical implication. GeroScience. 2022;44(4):2061–75.
138. Purcell NL, Goldman JG, Ouyang B, Bernard B, O'Keefe JA. The effects of dual-task cognitive interference and environmental challenges on balance in Huntington's disease. Mov Disord Clin Pract. 2019;6(3):202–12.
139. Bosch TJ, Groth C, Eldridge TA, Gnimpieba EZ, Baugh LA, Singh A. Altered cerebellar oscillations in Parkinson's disease patients during cognitive and motor tasks. Neuroscience. 2021;475:185–96.
140. Hansson EE, Beckman A, Håkansson A. Effect of vision, proprioception, and the position of the vestibular organ on postural sway. Acta Otolaryngol. 2010;130(12):1358–63.
141. Hinderaker M, Sylcott B, Williams K, Lin C-C. Aging affects the ability to process the optic flow stimulations: a functional near-infrared spectrometry study. J Mot Behav. 2020;52(4):466–73.
142. Karim H, Fuhrman SI, Sparto P, Furman J, Huppert T. Functional brain imaging of multi-sensory vestibular processing during computerized dynamic posturography using near-infrared spectroscopy. NeuroImage. 2013;74:318–25.
143. Lin C-C, Barker JW, Sparto PJ, Furman JM, Huppert TJ. Functional near-infrared spectroscopy (fNIRS) brain imaging of multi-sensory integration during computerized dynamic posturography in middle-aged and older adults. Exp Brain Res. 2017;235:1247–56.
144. Teo WP, Goodwill AM, Hendy AM, Muthalib M, Macpherson H. Sensory manipulation results in increased dorsolateral prefrontal cortex activation during static postural balance in sedentary older adults: an fNIRS study. Brain Behav. 2018;8(10):e01109.
145. Smith BA, Jacobs JV, Horak FB. Effects of magnitude and magnitude predictability of postural perturbations on preparatory cortical activity in older adults with and without Parkinson's disease. Exp Brain Res. 2012;222(4):455–70.
146. Varghese JP, McIlroy RE, Barnett-Cowan M. Perturbation-evoked potentials: significance and application in balance control research. Neurosci Biobehav Rev. 2017;83:267–80.

147. Basso Moro S, Bisconti S, Muthalib M, Spezialetti M, Cutini S, Ferrari M, et al. A semi-immersive virtual reality incremental swing balance task activates prefrontal cortex: a functional near-infrared spectroscopy study. NeuroImage. 2014;85(Pt 1):451–60.
148. Allexandre D, Hoxha A, Handiru VS, Saleh S, Selvan SE, Yue GH, editors. Altered cortical and postural response to balance perturbation in traumatic brain injury–an EEG pilot study. In 2019 41st Annual International Conference of the IEEE Engineering in Medicine and Biology Society (EMBC); 2019, 23–27 July 2019.
149. Ditz JC, Schwarz A, Müller-Putz GR. Perturbation-evoked potentials can be classified from single-trial EEG. J Neural Eng. 2020;17(3):036008.
150. Mierau A, Hülsdünker T, Strüder HK. Changes in cortical activity associated with adaptive behavior during repeated balance perturbation of unpredictable timing. Front Behav Neurosci. 2015;9
151. Payne AM, Ting LH. Worse balance is associated with larger perturbation-evoked cortical responses in healthy young adults. Gait Posture. 2020;80:324–30.
152. Payne AM, Ting LH. Balance perturbation-evoked cortical N1 responses are larger when stepping and not influenced by motor planning. J Neurophysiol. 2020;124(6):1875–84.
153. Solis-Escalante T, Stokkermans M, Cohen MX, Weerdesteyn V. Cortical responses to whole-body balance perturbations index perturbation magnitude and predict reactive stepping behavior. Eur J Neurosci. 2021;54(12):8120–38.
154. Palmer JA, Payne AM, Ting LH, Borich MR. Cortical engagement metrics during reactive balance are associated with distinct aspects of balance behavior in older adults. Front Aging Neurosci. 2021;13:13.
155. Mahoney JR, Holtzer R, Izzetoglu M, Zemon V, Verghese J, Allali G. The role of prefrontal cortex during postural control in Parkinsonian syndromes a functional near-infrared spectroscopy study. Brain Res. 2016;1633:126–38.
156. Miron-Shahar Y, Kantelhardt JW, Grinberg A, Hassin-Baer S, Blatt I, Inzelberg R, et al. Excessive phase synchronization in cortical activation during locomotion in persons with Parkinson's disease. Parkinsonism Relat Disord. 2019;65:210–6.
157. Helmich I, Coenen J, Henckert S, Pardalis E, Schupp S, Lausberg H. Reduced frontopolar brain activation characterizes concussed athletes with balance deficits. NeuroImage: Clin. 2020;25:102164.
158. Wang N, Liang J, Zhang H, Wan C, Liu S, Xu R, et al., editors. Correlation between Poststroke balance function and brain symmetry index in sitting and standing postures. In: 2021 43rd annual international conference of the IEEE Engineering in Medicine & Biology Society (EMBC); 2021, 1–5 Nov 2021.
159. Sathe A, Shenoy S, Sathe PK. Evaluation of cerebral cortex activation during balance tasks using fNIRS: a systematic review. Trend Sport Sci. 2021;28(2):93–107.
160. Agbangla NF, Audiffren M, Albinet CT. Use of near-infrared spectroscopy in the investigation of brain activation during cognitive aging: a systematic review of an emerging area of research. Ageing Res Rev. 2017;38:52–66.
161. Ansado J, Chasen C, Bouchard S, Northoff G. How brain imaging provides predictive biomarkers for therapeutic success in the context of virtual reality cognitive training. Neurosci Biobehav Rev. 2021;120:583–94.
162. Bishnoi A, Holtzer R, Hernandez ME. Brain activation changes while walking in adults with and without neurological disease: systematic review and meta-analysis of functional near-infrared spectroscopy studies. Brain Sci. 2021;11(3):291.
163. Lapanan K, Kantha P, Nantachai G, Hemrungrojn S, Maes M. The prefrontal cortex hemodynamic responses to dual-task paradigms in older adults: a systematic review and meta-analysis. Heliyon. 2023;9(7):e17812.
164. Li KZH, Bherer L, Mirelman A, Maidan I, Hausdorff JM. Cognitive involvement in balance, gait and dual-tasking in aging: a focused review from a neuroscience of aging perspective. Front Neurol. 2018;9:9.

165. Udina C, Avtzi S, Durduran T, Holtzer R, Rosso AL, Castellano-Tejedor C, et al. Functional near-infrared spectroscopy to study cerebral hemodynamics in older adults during cognitive and motor tasks: a review. Front Aging Neurosci. 2020;11:367.
166. Wang Q, Dai W, Xu S, Zhu S, Sui Y, Kan C, et al. Brain activation of the PFC during dual-task walking in stroke patients: a systematic review and meta-analysis of functional near-infrared spectroscopy studies. Front Neurosci. 2023;17
167. Wu Y, Dong Y, Tang Y, Wang W, Bo Y, Zhang C. Relationship between motor performance and cortical activity of older neurological disorder patients with dyskinesia using fNIRS: a systematic review. Front Physiol. 2023;14:1153469.
168. Yeung MK, Chan AS. A systematic review of the application of functional near-infrared spectroscopy to the study of cerebral hemodynamics in healthy aging. Neuropsychol Rev. 2021;31:139–66.
169. Maidan I, Nieuwhof F, Bernad-Elazari H, Bloem BR, Giladi N, Hausdorff JM, et al. Evidence for differential effects of 2 forms of exercise on prefrontal plasticity during walking in Parkinson's disease. Neurorehabil Neural Repair. 2018;32(3):200–8.
170. Merzagora AC, Foffani G, Panyavin I, Mordillo-Mateos L, Aguilar J, Onaral B, et al. Prefrontal hemodynamic changes produced by anodal direct current stimulation. NeuroImage. 2010;49(3):2304–10.
171. Polanía R, Nitsche MA, Paulus W. Modulating functional connectivity patterns and topological functional organization of the human brain with transcranial direct current stimulation. Hum Brain Mapp. 2011;32(8):1236–49.
172. Zheng X, Alsop DC, Schlaug G. Effects of transcranial direct current stimulation (tDCS) on human regional cerebral blood flow. NeuroImage. 2011;58(1):26–33.
173. Dagan M, Herman T, Harrison R, Zhou J, Giladi N, Ruffini G, et al. Multitarget transcranial direct current stimulation for freezing of gait in Parkinson's disease. Mov Disord. 2018;33(4):642–6.
174. Manenti R, Brambilla M, Rosini S, Orizio I, Ferrari C, Borroni B, et al. Time up and go task performance improves after transcranial direct current stimulation in patient affected by Parkinson's disease. Neurosci Lett. 2014;580:74–7.
175. Boggio PS, Ferrucci R, Rigonatti SP, Covre P, Nitsche M, Pascual-Leone A, et al. Effects of transcranial direct current stimulation on working memory in patients with Parkinson's disease. J Neurol Sci. 2006;249(1):31–8.
176. Nitsche MA, Paulus W. Excitability changes induced in the human motor cortex by weak transcranial direct current stimulation. J Physiol. 2000;527 Pt 3(Pt 3):633–9.

How Older Adults Can Avoid Falls via Proactive and Reactive Gait Adaptability: A Brief Introduction

3

Christopher McCrum and Elisabeth G. van der Hulst

Abstract

To understand and intervene in the problem of falls among older adults, we must consider in what ways falls can be avoided. In this chapter, we discuss how people can avoid obstacle-induced falls like trips and slips via proactive and reactive gait adaptation. We introduce each concept and detail how gait adaptation pre and post contact with obstacles can be implemented in order to avoid or reduce falls risk. We also discuss how ageing may affect proactive and reactive gait adaptation and adaptability, particularly in the context of sensory systems and movement execution. We conclude each section with some thoughts on interventions to improve these skills in older adults. Overall, both proactive and reactive gait adaptation to acute balance-threatening obstacles appear to be compromised with ageing. However, healthy older adults demonstrate the ability to improve in both aspects and this retained adaptability with ageing drives interest and research on these task-specific approaches to fall prevention.

Christopher McCrum and Elisabeth G. van der Hulst contributed equally.

C. McCrum (✉)
Department of Nutrition and Movement Sciences, NUTRIM School of Nutrition and Translational Research in Metabolism, Maastricht University Medical Centre, Maastricht, The Netherlands
e-mail: chris.mccrum@maastrichtuniversity.nl

E. G. van der Hulst
Department of Nutrition and Movement Sciences, NUTRIM School of Nutrition and Translational Research in Metabolism, Maastricht University Medical Centre, Maastricht, The Netherlands

REVAL Rehabilitation Research Center, Faculty of Rehabilitation Sciences, Hasselt University, Diepenbeek, Belgium

F. A. Barbieri et al. (eds.), *Locomotion and Posture in Older Adults*,
https://doi.org/10.1007/978-3-031-74123-4_3

Introduction

Walking is the most common activity preceding falls among older adults, as well as middle-aged and younger adults [1–11], and the association between walking and falls has been recognised for some time [12–14].

> Any observer who has watched an older person trying to board a bus which is just starting to move, will have noted the slow reflexes and the liability to fall which occur as the result of these changes. [13]

As this observation from Howell [13] indicates, it has been appreciated for some time that external, sudden changes in the immediate environment while ambulating pose a threat to older adults. While this was simply Howell's observation, one early systematic account of causes of falls among older adults supported the observation very soon afterwards. Sheldon [14], who reviewed the causes of 500 falls in 202 older individuals (50 years and older), reported stair walking, slipping, tripping and falling over unexpected objects to be among the most common causes of falls. Since then, trips and slips have often been reported to be the most common causes of falls among older adults [1, 6, 8, 9, 15], often related to uneven surfaces, trip hazards and slippery or wet surfaces [4, 16–18]. Trips and slips have also been reported to be the most common causes of falls leading to injuries [19–22]. Taken together, the above results generally indicate that mechanical disturbances during walking pose a significant threat to older adults in terms of risk of falling.

A fall due to a mechanical disturbance like a trip or a slip is the result of a change in the mechanical stability of the individual that they are unable to recover from. By mechanical stability, we refer to the relationship between the state of the centre of mass and the base of support. One reason why this may happen most often during walking is that both the position and velocity state of the centre of mass and the base of support are dynamic and not (almost) static, as is the case during standing. The centre of mass has a velocity during walking and the base of support is constantly changing and frequently small (i.e., one foot). As a result, we are mechanically unstable at many instants of the gait cycle, meaning that quite precise foot placement control and centre of mass regulation are needed to maintain forward walking without falling [23, 24] and this creates vulnerability to mechanical perturbations which would disrupt this delicate relationship. Note that this instantaneous mechanical stability of the body configuration (i.e., the state of the centre of mass—base of support relationship at each moment in time) is not necessarily reflective of the general fall risk or walking stability of an individual, depending on how these are defined [25]. Stability, consistency, or variability of various spatiotemporal aspects of the gait cycle during ongoing walking might provide insight into the overall gait pattern (or what some might refer to as global gait stability), but these are unique concepts both to each other and to the instantaneous mechanical stability of the body configuration during acute, specific, destabilising (or potentially destabilising) situations such as negotiation or contact with obstacles [26–29].

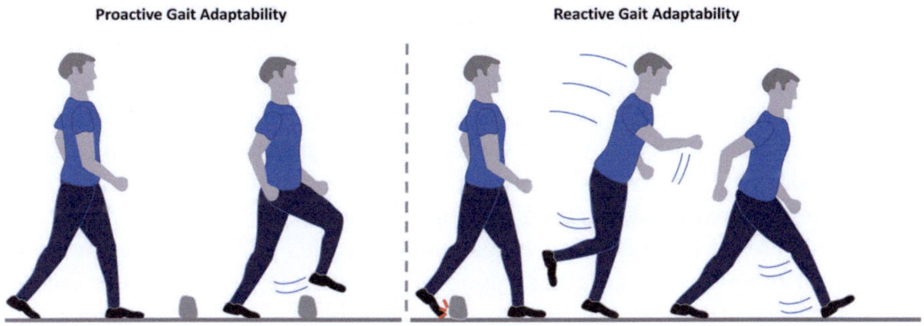

Fig. 3.1 Visual examples of a person demonstrating proactive and reactive gait adaptability

In this chapter, we will discuss proactive and reactive gait adaptability. Since these concepts do not necessarily have standardised definitions, it is important to define what we mean. Here, we adopt terminology used in Biology and Ecology, in which an adaptation refers to a change in the organism (or its behaviour) to meet the fleeting changes in its circumstances and adaptability refers to the capability to make adaptations [30]. By gait adaptation, we therefore simply mean any change or deviation in gait from its previous (presumably steady) state to cope with a change in the environment and by gait adaptability, we refer to the ability to adapt gait. In the context of avoiding or coping with perturbations, proactive adaptations occur before a potential perturbation occurs and reactive adaptations occur afterwards (Fig. 3.1). These can be observed at multiple 'levels', such as at a movement or global level by assessing spatiotemporal gait parameters or mechanical stability, but also at the level of neuromuscular control by assessing electromyography-derived parameters, for example. In the context of coping with mechanical perturbations, the former may be more directly relevant for determining the performance or ability of an individual during such challenging situations, whereas the latter may be used to help understand the underlying mechanisms for why an individual performs the way that they do. At least at the movement level, the literature to date quite convincingly shows that healthy adults, regardless of age, are capable of adapting to a huge variety of balance-challenging situations in a number of different ways, both proactively and reactively, and these findings have collectively driven interest in task-specific interventions for improving these skills in people with an increased risk of falls [31–40].

Proactive Gait Adaptability

Perception of Obstacles

When we consider a fall due to a mechanical disturbance, such as a trip or a slip, there are multiple key moments at which a person may have an opportunity to avoid, or reduce the impact, of the fall. The first of these is a window of time prior to contact with the potential mechanical disturbance in which the threat can be perceived early enough that the threat can be avoided. The ability to perceive such potential threats to stability while walking and pre-emptively adapt gait to either completely avoid, or reduce the impact of, the threat can collectively be termed proactive gait adaptability. Note that we focus here on perceiving and avoiding one specific obstacle. However, in situations such as slippery surfaces or uneven ground that represent a threatening situation generally, rather than one obstacle specifically, this may also result in proactive gait adaptations. As this description indicates, the first step of this process is the perception of the obstacle, for which the sensory systems, particularly the visual system, are responsible.

Various sensory systems contribute to balance control [41–44]. While proprioception and the vestibular system provide crucial information about body position and movement in space, they primarily come into play in gait adaptation to avoid falls upon physical contact with an obstacle. Of all the sensory systems, only the visual system can provide us with direct information about an obstacle in advance and is, therefore, essential for proactive gait adaptability. The visual system provides information about the size, location, shape and texture of obstacles, which is used to plan and adjust gait [45–47]. During normal straight walking, people spend most time looking in their current direction. But when there is an obstacle in their path, they naturally shift their gaze forward to focus on these features [48]. By fixating on the obstacles in advance, they gather essential information to effectively plan their foot placement and make appropriate adaptations to their walking pattern, if necessary [46]. How far individuals look ahead depends on the specific task and the complexity of the encountered hazards [49]. In general, it is about two steps beforehand [48], but other populations, such as people with Parkinson's disease, look longer at upcoming obstacles [50, 51].

However, the visual system typically declines with ageing and older adults therefore often experience impaired visual function, including declines in visual acuity, depth perception, and contrast sensitivity [42, 52–55]. Another sensory system that generally declines in function with age and shows an age-related increase in disorders is the vestibular system [56–61]. This has particular relevance for gathering visual information about upcoming obstacles due to the critical function of the vestibular-ocular reflex, which is responsible for stabilising the visual field on the retina during head movement [62]. The challenge of stable vision is compounded when declines in the musculoskeletal system result in increased difficulty in coordinating movement during walking, particularly in the head and trunk body segments. As a result of all of these age-related declines, the ability for accurate and timely detection of obstacles during walking can be negatively affected with age. It is therefore not surprising that both visual and vestibular function have been related to falls incidence [44, 63–71].

Negotiating Obstacles

Once information about an upcoming obstacle has been gathered and assessed, the next step of the process of proactive gait adaptation is selecting and executing a strategy for avoiding or mitigating the impact of said obstacle. There are multiple strategies to avoid upcoming obstacles. Patla et al. [72] suggested that these fall into one of three categories: stepping over the obstacle by increasing clearance or changing the trajectory of the limb; adapting the walking direction in order to go around or otherwise avoid the obstacle; or finally simply coming to a stop to avoid contact with the obstacle. Which strategy a person will select in order to avoid an obstacle depends on multiple factors. The decision of stepping over an obstacle instead of going around it has to do with the height of the obstacle. For example, Patla [46] indicated that when the obstacle height to lower leg length ratio is less than 1:1, the preferred strategy is to go over the obstacle, whereas if the obstacle is higher than this 1:1 ratio, people prefer to go around the obstacle to reduce the risk of a trip or fall. When stepping over the obstacle, alterations in movement are typically selected in a manner that reduce deviations in the centre of mass trajectory and that ensure sufficient toe clearance over the obstacle [73]. Three ways in which someone can spatially adjust their step to avoid an obstacle are by lengthening or shortening their step, or by stepping to the side. People typically prefer to shorten or lengthen the step instead of side stepping, presumably because they are already walking forwards and similar muscles used during gait can also be used to adjust the step length [74, 75], whereas stepping to the side would require a greater deviation from normal gait and would require more significantly altered muscle activation [76]. Chen et al. [77] and Patla et al. [75] indicated that when selecting to lengthen or shorten the step to cross an obstacle, forward progression, and therefore step lengthening is often preferred, since step shortening requires a decrease in the speed of the centre of mass to maintain stability, whereas lengthening your step does not, and in addition gives you more time to make any changes during swinging your limb. It is also worth mentioning that, in addition to the obstacle-related factors described, the strategy chosen may also depend on or be influenced by other factors relating to the environment and situation. For example, metabolic cost (safer strategies may cost more energy) or temporal constraints (such as a short available response time) may influence the selected obstacle avoidance strategy [74, 78, 79]. Daniels and Burn [78], for example, tested whether participants would choose an obstacle avoidance strategy that minimized energy cost. They forced participants to choose between two strategies based on obstacle length and depth, one of which would be the optimal strategy with minimal energy cost. They showed that participants were capable of choosing the most energy efficient strategy. However, safety and stability are usually also expected to be priorities [80, 81].

Regarding obstacle negotiation in older adults, studies have shown mixed results of strategies used by older adults, with both shorter and longer steps being used [82–87], potentially reflecting the various setups and protocols that have been used in these studies. As described above, older adults' sensorimotor function is typically reduced, and this creates a need to increase the time they have to gather sensory information from the environment and plan appropriate gait adaptations. A lower head angle during obstacle avoidance has been found for older adults, indicating more visual attention being directed to the obstacle [85]. Other behaviours that allow older adults more time to plan appropriate obstacle negotiations include walking with longer steps. This gives older adults more time per step to analyse the situation visually. They have more time to assess the obstacle and plan their movement trajectory, while keeping the walking speed equal [84, 87]. On the contrary, walking slower with shorter steps could also give older adults more preparation time [82, 85]. This comes with some risk though, since shorter steps can lead to an increased risk of contact with the obstacle, because the foot is placed closer to the obstacle [85, 88]. Muir et al. [85] indeed found that older adults are also more likely to hit an obstacle with their lead limb compared to younger adults.

Training Proactive Gait Adaptation

Training programs that focus on improving proactive gait adaptability have been shown to be effective in reducing fall risk [89]. There are several types of training that can be used to improve gait adaptability, including treadmill training with virtual obstacles [90] or physical obstacles [87], obstacle courses [91], and step training [92, 93]. All these studies used a wide variety of experimental setups, protocols and training durations, making it difficult to compare results across studies and draw conclusions about the timescale at which adaptations take place. A recent scoping review of 16 studies in older adults indeed reported huge variety in experimental setups, tasks and outcome measures [94]. The systematic review of Okubo et al. [89], which focused on intervention studies involving volitional step training, found that intervention duration ranged from 8 to 24 weeks, with 1 to 3 training sessions per week, again indicating huge variation in the literature. As a result, further research is needed to fully understand the most effective and generalisable components of proactive gait adaptability training for falls prevention.

Reactive Gait Adaptability

If we return to our key moments during an encounter with a mechanical obstacle in which a fall might be avoided, we can now consider the next key moment if proactive gait adaptation has not been sufficient to avoid the obstacle or reduce its impact. Now, a collision with an obstacle has occurred and the delicate relationship between the base of support and the centre of mass state has been disrupted. At this moment, sufficiently fast and effective responses are needed to restore this relationship and avoid a fall. In the course of a single, acute perturbation, we refer to this here as 'reactive gait recovery'. During repeated perturbations, such as those that might be applied during assessment or training, we refer to the change in the 'reactive gait recovery' with practice as 'adaptation of reactive gait recovery'. Both can be considered forms of reactive gait adaptability since in both cases, the reactive motor response to destabilisation is adapted, just on different timescales.

Reactive Gait Recovery

Reactive gait recovery following balance loss can be achieved in different ways depending on various factors such as the extent and direction of instability, the inherent reactive gait adaptability of the individual and the surrounding environment. Mechanically, Hof [95] demonstrated three mechanisms of standing balance control, namely, moving the centre of pressure under the feet, counter rotation of body segments about the centre of mass and applying an external force other than the ground reaction forces (for example, by grasping a handrail). In principle, similar solutions are available for reactive gait recovery, though due to the moving centre of mass, similar to unperturbed gait [23, 96, 97], foot placement by stepping as a means to move the centre of pressure appears to dominate during real falls, at least when nearby external support such as handrails are not available [98]. According to the earlier framework presented by Maki and McIlroy [99], which characterised balance recovery strategies in terms of the nature of support employed, stepping during reactive gait recovery (and grasping during reactive gait recovery) represent 'change-in-support' strategies. In order to successfully perform reactive gait recovery, a person must first detect the instability and/or perturbation and then select and perform an appropriate action. Unlike the situation described above for proactive gait adaptability, during reactive gait recovery, all sensory systems can provide information to allow detection of either contact with the mechanical perturbation or instability itself, though the contribution of each sensory system may vary with perturbation type and direction and perception of motion [100].

Regarding the effects of ageing on reactive gait recovery, it is frequently reported that older adults perform poorer than younger adults, reflecting their increased fall risk. Exactly what differs in their responses at the movement level varies depending upon the perturbation applied and the experimental context, but typically this is reflected in less stable recovery steps, longer recovery time or more recovery steps needed and, in some cases, more safety harness assistance [101–105]. One systematic review found lower muscle onset latencies in older versus younger adults during (mostly stance) perturbations [106], though to what extent this is due to delayed detection of instability or to delayed execution of reactive recovery is not clear.

Adaptability of Reactive Gait Recovery

Encouragingly, the literature just as consistently demonstrates that healthy older adults have preserved adaptability of reactive gait recovery, as the majority of studies analysing reactive gait recovery over multiple repeated perturbations observe significant improvement, often within single sessions [31, 32, 34, 39, 40, 102, 107–110]. Due to the wide variety in experimental setups and perturbations applied, it is difficult to come to clear conclusions, but it does seem that these improvements occur faster when the overall training dose is higher (either in terms of size or number of perturbations) [36, 111–115]. In terms of what contributes to adaptability of reactive gait recovery, the following have all been implicated, as described by McCrum et al. [36]: faster perturbation or instability detection and faster reactive gait recovery initiation [116, 117]; optimisation of motor programmes for stability recovery, including facilitation and suppression of functionally relevant and irrelevant reflexes and reactions, respectively [118–120]; and altered coordination in relevant, especially weight bearing, muscles to execute the appropriate reactive gait recovery actions [121–126]. In addition, it seems that intact sensory and neural function is required to at least some extent for successful adaptation, since patient populations with sensory or neural-related impairments tend to show reduced reactive gait recovery adaptability [111, 127–130].

Training Reactive Gait Recovery

Given the relative consistency with which adaptability of reactive gait recovery has been demonstrated, the last 20 years have seen much discussion and progress in applying repeated mechanical perturbations as a fall prevention measure [36, 89, 123, 131–141]. Despite this progress, however, research in large community and clinical trials is limited and a number of other knowledge gaps still exist that need to be addressed before widespread implementation is likely to be successful [36].

While it is clear that mechanical disturbances during walking are a major cause of falls, these can disturb gait in many different ways, positions and directions and can occur in many different environments. While we know that the literature often reports trips and slips during walking to be the most common cause [1, 6, 8, 9, 15], people self-reporting the situations that led to falls does not provide a great level of accuracy or detail into the numbers and various characteristics of the perturbations and environments that caused the falls, particularly when reported retrospectively [142, 143]. For experimental studies and training interventions, this creates uncertainty in how to best simulate these situations [139]. Part of the issue is that balance performance appears to be highly task specific [144–150] and improvement in one type of balance training or task does not necessarily translate to improvement in another task [151–155] and this task-specificity issue is not yet fully understood for mechanical gait perturbations tasks [36, 115, 156–161]. Another aspect that is not yet well understood is to what extent the ecological validity of the perturbations or tasks of the experimental and training protocols employing mechanical gait perturbations matters for translating the results to daily life. These gaps in our understanding should be kept in mind when interpreting the results of studies on proactive and reactive gait adaptability.

Conclusions

When encountering an obstacle during walking, older adults have a number of key moments in which the likelihood of a fall can be reduced. Proactive gait adaptations to avoid collision with a recognised obstacle and if not avoided, reactive gait adaptation to recovery stability are both ways in which falls can be avoided and each can be achieved in a multitude of ways. While both proactive and reactive gait adaptation to acute balance-threatening obstacles appear to be less effective with ageing, healthy older adults demonstrate the ability to improve in both aspects and this retained adaptability with ageing drives interest and research on these task-specific approaches to fall prevention.

References

1. Berg WP, Alessio HM, Mills EM, Tong C. Circumstances and consequences of falls in independent community-dwelling older adults. Age Ageing. 1997;26:261–8. https://doi.org/10.1093/ageing/26.4.261.
2. Hill K, Schwarz J, Flicker L, Carroll S. Falls among healthy, community-dwelling, older women: a prospective study of frequency, circumstances, consequences and prediction accuracy. Aust N Z J Public Health. 1999;23:41–8.
3. Kelsey JL, Procter-Gray E, Hannan MT, Li W. Heterogeneity of falls among older adults: implications for public health prevention. Am J Public Health. 2012;102:2149–56. https://doi.org/10.2105/AJPH.2012.300677.
4. Li W, Keegan TH, Sternfeld B, Sidney S, Quesenberry CP Jr, Kelsey JL. Outdoor falls among middle-aged and older adults: a neglected public health problem. Am J Public Health. 2006;96:1192–200. https://doi.org/10.2105/AJPH.2005.083055.
5. Muir SW, Berg K, Chesworth B, Speechley M. Use of the Berg Balance Scale for predicting multiple falls in community-dwelling elderly people: a prospective study. Phys Ther. 2008;88:449–59. https://doi.org/10.2522/ptj.20070251.
6. Niino N, Tsuzuku S, Ando F, Shimokata H. Frequencies and circumstances of falls in the National Institute for Longevity Sciences, Longitudinal Study of Aging (NILS-LSA). J Epidemiol. 2000;10:S90–4. https://doi.org/10.2188/jea.10.1sup_90.
7. Robinovitch SN, et al. Video capture of the circumstances of falls in elderly people residing in long-term care: an observational study. Lancet. 2013;381:47–54. https://doi.org/10.1016/s0140-6736(12)61263-x.
8. Talbot LA, Musiol RJ, Witham EK, Metter EJ. Falls in young, middle-aged and older community dwelling adults: perceived cause, environmental factors and injury. BMC Public Health. 2005;5:86. https://doi.org/10.1186/1471-2458-5-86.
9. Tinetti ME, Speechley M, Ginter SF. Risk factors for falls among elderly persons living in the community. N Engl J Med. 1988;319:1701–7. https://doi.org/10.1056/NEJM198812293192604.
10. van Schooten KS, Yang Y, Feldman F, Leung M, McKay H, Sims-Gould J, Robinovitch SN. The association between fall frequency, injury risk, and characteristics of falls in older residents of long-term care: do recurrent fallers fall more safely? J Gerontol A Biol Sci Med Sci. 2018;73:786–91. https://doi.org/10.1093/gerona/glx196.
11. Yang Y, van Schooten KS, Sims-Gould J, McKay HA, Feldman F, Robinovitch SN. Sex differences in the circumstances leading to falls: evidence from real-life falls captured on video in long-term care. J Am Med Dir Assoc. 2018;19:130–5. e131. https://doi.org/10.1016/j.jamda.2017.08.011.

12. Azar GJ, Lawton AH. Gait and stepping as factors in the frequent falls of elderly women. Gerontologist. 1964;4:83–4. https://doi.org/10.1093/geront/4.2_part_1.83.
13. Howell TH. Analysis of falls in old people. J Am Geriatr Soc. 1958;6:522–5.
14. Sheldon JH. On the natural history of falls in old age. Br Med J. 1960;2:1685–90. https://doi.org/10.1136/bmj.2.5214.1685.
15. Lord SR, Ward JA, Williams P, Anstey KJ. An epidemiological study of falls in older community-dwelling women: the Randwick falls and fractures study. Aust J Public Health. 1993;17:240–5. https://doi.org/10.1111/j.1753-6405.1993.tb00143.x.
16. Crenshaw JR, Bernhardt KA, Achenbach SJ, Atkinson EJ, Khosla S, Kaufman KR, Amin S. The circumstances, orientations, and impact locations of falls in community-dwelling older women. Arch Gerontol Geriatr. 2017;73:240–7. https://doi.org/10.1016/j.archger.2017.07.011.
17. Tinetti ME, Doucette JT, Claus EB. The contribution of predisposing and situational risk factors to serious fall injuries. J Am Geriatr Soc. 1995;43:1207–13. https://doi.org/10.1111/j.1532-5415.1995.tb07395.x.
18. Tinetti ME, Speechley M. Prevention of falls among the elderly. N Engl J Med. 1989;320:1055–9. https://doi.org/10.1056/NEJM198904203201606.
19. Buczak-Stec E, Gorynski P. Fall related hospital admissions among seniors in Poland in 2010. Przegl Epidemiol. 2013;67(57–62):141–4.
20. Gilasi HR, Soori H, Yazdani S, Taheri Tenjani P. Fall-related injuries in community-dwelling older adults in Qom Province, Iran, 2010–2012. Arch Trauma Res. 2015;4:e22925. https://doi.org/10.5812/atr.22925.
21. Roudsari BS, Ebel BE, Corso PS, Molinari NA, Koepsell TD. The acute medical care costs of fall-related injuries among the U.S. older adults. Injury. 2005;36:1316–22. https://doi.org/10.1016/j.injury.2005.05.024.
22. Timsina LR, Willetts JL, Brennan MJ, Marucci-Wellman H, Lombardi DA, Courtney TK, Verma SK. Circumstances of fall-related injuries by age and gender among community-dwelling adults in the United States. PLoS One. 2017;12:e0176561. https://doi.org/10.1371/journal.pone.0176561.
23. Bruijn SM, van Dieen JH. Control of human gait stability through foot placement. J R Soc Interface. 2018;15:20170816. https://doi.org/10.1098/rsif.2017.0816.
24. Hof AL, Gazendam MG, Sinke WE. The condition for dynamic stability. J Biomech. 2005;38:1–8. https://doi.org/10.1016/j.jbiomech.2004.03.025.
25. Curtze C, Buurke TJW, McCrum C. Notes on the margin of stability. J Biomech. 2024;166:112045. https://doi.org/10.1016/j.jbiomech.2024.112045.
26. Dingwell JB, Cusumano JP, Cavanagh PR, Sternad D. Local dynamic stability versus kinematic variability of continuous overground and treadmill walking. J Biomech Eng. 2001;123:27–32. https://doi.org/10.1115/1.1336798.
27. Granata KP, England SA. Reply to the letter to the editor. Gait Posture. 2007;26:329–30. https://doi.org/10.1016/j.gaitpost.2007.02.002.
28. Perry JA, Srinivasan M. Walking with wider steps changes foot placement control, increases kinematic variability and does not improve linear stability. R Soc Open Sci. 2017;4:160627. https://doi.org/10.1098/rsos.160627.
29. Stergiou N, Decker LM. Human movement variability, nonlinear dynamics, and pathology: is there a connection? Hum Mov Sci. 2011;30:869–88.
30. Gause GF. The relation of adaptability to adaptation. Q Rev Biol. 1942;17:99–114.
31. Bohm S, Mademli L, Mersmann F, Arampatzis A. Predictive and reactive locomotor adaptability in healthy elderly: a systematic review and meta-analysis. Sports Med. 2015;45:1759–77. https://doi.org/10.1007/s40279-015-0413-9.
32. Carty CP, Cronin NJ, Lichtwark GA, Mills PM, Barrett RS. Mechanisms of adaptation from a multiple to a single step recovery strategy following repeated exposure to forward loss of balance in older adults. PLoS One. 2012;7:e33591. https://doi.org/10.1371/journal.pone.0033591.

33. Dijkstra BW, Horak FB, Kamsma YP, Peterson DS. Older adults can improve compensatory stepping with repeated postural perturbations. Front Aging Neurosci. 2015;7:201. https://doi.org/10.3389/fnagi.2015.00201.
34. Grevendonk L, et al. Impact of aging and exercise on skeletal muscle mitochondrial capacity, energy metabolism, and physical function. Nat Commun. 2021;12:4773. https://doi.org/10.1038/s41467-021-24956-2.
35. McCrum C. Fall prevention in community-dwelling older adults. N Engl J Med. 2020;382:2579–80. https://doi.org/10.1056/NEJMc2005662.
36. McCrum C, Bhatt TS, Gerards MHG, Karamanidis K, Rogers MW, Lord SR, Okubo Y. Perturbation-based balance training: principles, mechanisms and implementation in clinical practice. Front Sports Act Living. 2022a;4:1015394. https://doi.org/10.3389/fspor.2022.1015394.
37. McCrum C, Epro G, Meijer K, Zijlstra W, Brüggemann GP, Karamanidis K. Locomotor stability and adaptation during perturbed walking across the adult female lifespan. J Biomech. 2016;49:1244–7. https://doi.org/10.1016/j.jbiomech.2016.02.051.
38. McCrum C, Karamanidis K, Willems P, Zijlstra W, Meijer K. Retention, savings and interlimb transfer of reactive gait adaptations in humans following unexpected perturbations. Commun Biol. 2018;1:230. https://doi.org/10.1038/s42003-018-0238-9.
39. Pavol MJ, Runtz EF, Pai YC. Young and older adults exhibit proactive and reactive adaptations to repeated slip exposure. J Gerontol A Biol Sci Med Sci. 2004;59:494–502. https://doi.org/10.1093/gerona/59.5.m494.
40. Wang YR, Wang SJ, Bolton R, Kaur T, Bhatt T. Effects of task-specific obstacle-induced trip-perturbation training: proactive and reactive adaptation to reduce fall-risk in community-dwelling older adults. Aging Clin Exp Res. 2020;32:893–905. https://doi.org/10.1007/s40520-019-01268-6.
41. Eysel-Gosepath K, McCrum C, Epro G, Bruggemann GP, Karamanidis K. Visual and proprioceptive contributions to postural control of upright stance in unilateral vestibulopathy. Somatosens Mot Res. 2016;33:72–8. https://doi.org/10.1080/08990220.2016.1178635.
42. Lord SR, Sherrington C, Menz HB, Close JCT. Falls in older people: risk factors and strategies for prevention. 2nd ed. New York: Cambridge University Press; 2011.
43. MacKinnon CD. Sensorimotor anatomy of gait, balance, and falls. Handb Clin Neurol. 2018;159:3–26. https://doi.org/10.1016/B978-0-444-63916-5.00001-X.
44. Maki BE, McIlroy WE. Postural control in the older adult. Clin Geriatr Med. 1996;12:635–58.
45. Patla AE. Age-related changes in visually guided locomotion over different terrains: major issues. In: Stelmach GE, Hömberg V, editors. Sensorimotor impairment in the elderly. Dordrecht: Springer; 1993. p. 231–52. https://doi.org/10.1007/978-94-011-1976-4_16.
46. Patla AE. Understanding the roles of vision in the control of human locomotion. Gait Posture. 1997;5:54–69. https://doi.org/10.1016/S0966-6362(96)01109-5.
47. Rietdyk S, Rhea CK. Control of adaptive locomotion: effect of visual obstruction and visual cues in the environment. Exp Brain Res. 2006;169:272–8. https://doi.org/10.1007/s00221-005-0345-y.
48. Patla AE, Vickers JN. How far ahead do we look when required to step on specific locations in the travel path during locomotion? Exp Brain Res. 2003;148:133–8. https://doi.org/10.1007/s00221-002-1246-y.
49. Marigold DS, Patla AE. Gaze fixation patterns for negotiating complex ground terrain. Neuroscience. 2007;144:302–13. https://doi.org/10.1016/j.neuroscience.2006.09.006.
50. Alcock L, Gaina B, Hausdorff JM, Lord S, Rochester L. Enhanced obstacle contrast to promote visual scanning in fallers with Parkinson's disease: role of executive function. Neuroscience. 2020;436:82–92.
51. Vitório R, Lirani-Silva E, Barbieri FA, Raile V, Stella F, Gobbi LT. Influence of visual feedback sampling on obstacle crossing behavior in people with Parkinson's disease. Gait Posture. 2013;38(2):330–4.
52. Lord SR, Delbaere K, Sturnieks DL. Aging. Handb Clin Neurol. 2018;159:157–71. https://doi.org/10.1016/B978-0-444-63916-5.00010-0.

53. Paraskevoudi N, Balci F, Vatakis A. "Walking" through the sensory, cognitive, and temporal degradations of healthy aging. Ann N Y Acad Sci. 2018; https://doi.org/10.1111/nyas.13734.
54. Schultz AB. Mobility impairment in the elderly: challenges for biomechanics research. J Biomech. 1992;25:519–28.
55. Whitney S, Morris LO. Multisensory impairment in older adults: evaluation and intervention. In: Calhoun KH, Eibling DE, Wax MK, Kost KM, editors. Geriatric otolaryngology. New York: Taylor & Francis Group; 2006. p. 109–23.
56. Agrawal Y, et al. Presbyvestibulopathy: diagnostic criteria consensus document of the classification committee of the Bárány Society. J Vestib Res. 2019;29:161–70. https://doi.org/10.3233/ves-190672.
57. Anson E, Jeka J. Perspectives on aging vestibular function. Front Neurol. 2015;6:269. https://doi.org/10.3389/fneur.2015.00269.
58. Arshad Q, Seemungal BM. Age-related vestibular loss: current understanding and future research directions. Front Neurol. 2016;7:231. https://doi.org/10.3389/fneur.2016.00231.
59. Iwasaki S, Yamasoba T. Dizziness and imbalance in the elderly: age-related decline in the vestibular system. Aging Dis. 2015;6:38–47. https://doi.org/10.14336/AD.2014.0128.
60. Ji L, Zhai S. Aging and the peripheral vestibular system. J Otol. 2018;13:138–40. https://doi.org/10.1016/j.joto.2018.11.006.
61. Zalewski CK. Aging of the human vestibular system. Semin Hear. 2015;36:175–96. https://doi.org/10.1055/s-0035-1555120.
62. Kingma H, van de Berg R. Chapter 1—Anatomy, physiology, and physics of the peripheral vestibular system. In: Joseph MF, Thomas L, editors. Handbook of clinical neurology, vol. 137. Elsevier; 2016. p. 1–16. https://doi.org/10.1016/B978-0-444-63437-5.00001-7.
63. Agrawal Y, Carey JP, Della Santina CC, Schubert MC, Minor LB. Disorders of balance and vestibular function in US adults: data from the National Health and Nutrition Examination Survey, 2001–2004. Arch Intern Med. 2009;169:938–44. https://doi.org/10.1001/archinternmed.2009.66.
64. Donovan J, De Silva L, Cox H, Palmer G, Semciw AI. Vestibular dysfunction in people who fall: a systematic review and meta-analysis of prevalence and associated factors. Clin Rehabil. 2023;37:1229–47. https://doi.org/10.1177/02692155231162423.
65. Ekvall Hansson E, Magnusson M. Vestibular asymmetry predicts falls among elderly patients with multi-sensory dizziness. BMC Geriatr. 2013;13:77. https://doi.org/10.1186/1471-2318-13-77.
66. Herssens N, How D, van de Berg R, McCrum C. Falls among people with bilateral vestibulopathy: a review of causes, incidence, injuries, and methods. JAMA Otolaryngol—Head Neck Surg. 2022;148:187–92. https://doi.org/10.1001/jamaoto.2021.3673.
67. Jack CI, Smith T, Neoh C, Lye M, McGalliard JN. Prevalence of low vision in elderly patients admitted to an acute geriatric unit in Liverpool: elderly people who fall are more likely to have low vision. Gerontology. 1995;41:280–5. https://doi.org/10.1159/000213695.
68. King MB. Falls. In: Halter JB, Ouslander JG, Tinetti ME, Studenski S, High KP, Asthana SA, editors. Hazzard's geriatric medicine and gerontology. 6th ed. New York: McGraw-Hill; 2009.
69. Lord SR, Sambrook PN, Gilbert C, Kelly PJ, Nguyen T, Webster IW, Eisman JA. Postural stability, falls and fractures in the elderly: results from the Dubbo Osteoporosis Epidemiology Study. Med J Aust. 1994a;160(684–685):688–91.
70. Lord SR, Ward JA, Williams P, Anstey KJ. Physiological factors associated with falls in older community-dwelling women. J Am Geriatr Soc. 1994b;42:1110–7.
71. Menant JC, St George RJ, Fitzpatrick RC, Lord SR. Perception of the postural vertical and falls in older people. Gerontology. 2012;58:497–503. https://doi.org/10.1159/000339295.
72. Patla AE, Prentice SD, Robinson C, Neufeld J. Visual control of locomotion: strategies for changing direction and for going over obstacles. J Exp Psychol Hum Percept Perform. 1991;17:603–34. https://doi.org/10.1037/0096-1523.17.3.603.
73. Weerdesteyn V, Hollands KL, Hollands MA. Gait adaptability. Handb Clin Neurol. 2018;159:135–46. https://doi.org/10.1016/b978-0-444-63916-5.00008-2.

74. Moraes R, Lewis MA, Patla AE. Strategies and determinants for selection of alternate foot placement during human locomotion: influence of spatial and temporal constraints. Exp Brain Res. 2004;159:1–13. https://doi.org/10.1007/s00221-004-1888-z.
75. Patla AE, Prentice SD, Rietdyk S, Allard F, Martin C. What guides the selection of alternate foot placement during locomotion in humans. Exp Brain Res. 1999;128:441–50. https://doi.org/10.1007/s002210050867.
76. Winter DA. The biomechanics and motor control of human gait. University of Waterloo Press; 1987.
77. Chen HC, Ashton-Miller JA, Alexander NB, Schultz AB. Effects of age and available response time on ability to step over an obstacle. J Gerontol. 1994;49:M227–33. https://doi.org/10.1093/geronj/49.5.m227.
78. Daniels KAJ, Burn JF. Human locomotion over obstacles reveals real-time prediction of energy expenditure for optimized decision-making. Proc Biol Sci. 2023;290:20230200. https://doi.org/10.1098/rspb.2023.0200.
79. Moraes R, Patla AE. Determinants guiding alternate foot placement selection and the behavioral responses are similar when avoiding a real or a virtual obstacle. Exp Brain Res. 2006;171:497–510. https://doi.org/10.1007/s00221-005-0297-2.
80. Chou LS, Draganich LF, Song SM. Minimum energy trajectories of the swing ankle when stepping over obstacles of different heights. J Biomech. 1997;30:115–20. https://doi.org/10.1016/s0021-9290(96)00111-x.
81. Jansen SE, Toet A, Werkhoven PJ. Human locomotion through a multiple obstacle environment: strategy changes as a result of visual field limitation. Exp Brain Res. 2011;212:449–56. https://doi.org/10.1007/s00221-011-2757-1.
82. Chen HC, Ashton-Miller JA, Alexander NB, Schultz AB. Stepping over obstacles: gait patterns of healthy young and old adults. J Gerontol. 1991;46:M196–203. https://doi.org/10.1093/geronj/46.6.m196.
83. Fonteyn EM, Heeren A, Engels JJ, Boer JJ, van de Warrenburg BP, Weerdesteyn V. Gait adaptability training improves obstacle avoidance and dynamic stability in patients with cerebellar degeneration. Gait Posture. 2014;40:247. https://doi.org/10.1016/j.gaitpost.2014.04.190.
84. Hoogkamer W, Potocanac Z, Duysens J. Quick foot placement adjustments during gait: direction matters. Exp Brain Res. 2015;233:3349–57. https://doi.org/10.1007/s00221-015-4401-y.
85. Muir BC, Haddad JM, Heijnen MJ, Rietdyk S. Proactive gait strategies to mitigate risk of obstacle contact are more prevalent with advancing age. Gait Posture. 2015;41:233–9. https://doi.org/10.1016/j.gaitpost.2014.10.005.
86. Raffegeau TE, Brinkerhoff SA, Kellaher GK, Baudendistel S, Terza MJ, Roper JA, Hass CJ. Changes to margins of stability from walking to obstacle crossing in older adults while walking fast and with a dual-task. Exp Gerontol. 2022;161:111710. https://doi.org/10.1016/j.exger.2022.111710.
87. Weerdesteyn V, Nienhuis B, Mulder T, Duysens J. Older women strongly prefer stride lengthening to shortening in avoiding obstacles. Exp Brain Res. 2005;161:39–46. https://doi.org/10.1007/s00221-004-2043-6.
88. Chou LS, Draganich LF. Placing the trailing foot closer to an obstacle reduces flexion of the hip, knee, and ankle to increase the risk of tripping. J Biomech. 1998;31:685–91. https://doi.org/10.1016/s0021-9290(98)00081-5.
89. Okubo Y, Schoene D, Lord SR. Step training improves reaction time, gait and balance and reduces falls in older people: a systematic review and meta-analysis. Br J Sports Med. 2017;51:586–93. https://doi.org/10.1136/bjsports-2015-095452.
90. Mirelman A, et al. Addition of a non-immersive virtual reality component to treadmill training to reduce fall risk in older adults (V-TIME): a randomised controlled trial. Lancet. 2016;388:1170–82. https://doi.org/10.1016/s0140-6736(16)31325-3.
91. Yamada M, et al. Complex obstacle negotiation exercise can prevent falls in community-dwelling elderly Japanese aged 75 years and older. Geriatr Gerontol Int. 2012;12:461–7. https://doi.org/10.1111/j.1447-0594.2011.00794.x.

92. Schoene D, Lord SR, Delbaere K, Severino C, Davies TA, Smith ST. A randomized controlled pilot study of home-based step training in older people using videogame technology. PLoS One. 2013;8:e57734. https://doi.org/10.1371/journal.pone.0057734.
93. Shigematsu R, Okura T, Nakagaichi M, Tanaka K, Sakai T, Kitazumi S, Rantanen T. Square-stepping exercise and fall risk factors in older adults: a single-blind, randomized controlled trial. J Gerontol A Biol Sci Med Sci. 2008;63:76–82. https://doi.org/10.1093/gerona/63.1.76.
94. Kim K, Vinent M, Deller L, Zijlstra W. A scoping review of voluntary gait adaptability tasks requiring cognitive demands in older adults. Phys Act Nutr. 2023;27:30–40. https://doi.org/10.20463/pan.2023.0004.
95. Hof AL. The equations of motion for a standing human reveal three mechanisms for balance. J Biomech. 2007;40:451–7. https://doi.org/10.1016/j.jbiomech.2005.12.016.
96. van den Bogaart M, Bruijn SM, Spildooren J, van Dieën JH, Meyns P. The effect of constraining mediolateral ankle moments and foot placement on the use of the counter-rotation mechanism during walking. J Biomech. 2022;136:111073. https://doi.org/10.1016/j.jbiomech.2022.111073.
97. van Leeuwen AM, van Dieën JH, Daffertshofer A, Bruijn SM. Active foot placement control ensures stable gait: effect of constraints on foot placement and ankle moments. PLoS One. 2020;15:e0242215. https://doi.org/10.1371/journal.pone.0242215.
98. Te B, Komisar V, Aguiar OM, Shishov N, Robinovitch SN. Compensatory stepping responses during real-life falls in older adults. Gait Posture. 2023;100:276–83. https://doi.org/10.1016/j.gaitpost.2023.01.005.
99. Maki BE, McIlroy WE. The role of limb movements in maintaining upright stance: the "change-in-support" strategy. Phys Ther. 1997;77:488–507. https://doi.org/10.1093/ptj/77.5.488.
100. Arena SL, Davis JL, Grant JW, Madigan ML. Tripping elicits earlier and larger deviations in linear head acceleration compared to slipping. PLoS One. 2016;11:e0165670. https://doi.org/10.1371/journal.pone.0165670.
101. Bierbaum S, Peper A, Karamanidis K, Arampatzis A. Adaptational responses in dynamic stability during disturbed walking in the elderly. J Biomech. 2010;43:2362–8. https://doi.org/10.1016/j.jbiomech.2010.04.025.
102. McCrum C, Karamanidis K, Grevendonk L, Zijlstra W, Meijer K. Older adults demonstrate interlimb transfer of reactive gait adaptations to repeated unpredictable gait perturbations. GeroScience. 2020;42:39–49. https://doi.org/10.1007/s11357-019-00130-x.
103. Pai YC, Bhatt T, Wang E, Espy D, Pavol MJ. Inoculation against falls: rapid adaptation by young and older adults to slips during daily activities. Arch Phys Med Rehabil. 2010;91:452–9. https://doi.org/10.1016/j.apmr.2009.10.032.
104. Pavol MJ, Runtz EF, Edwards BJ, Pai YC. Age influences the outcome of a slipping perturbation during initial but not repeated exposures. J Gerontol A Biol Sci Med Sci. 2002;57:M496–503. https://doi.org/10.1093/gerona/57.8.m496.
105. Süptitz F, Moreno Catala M, Brüggemann GP, Karamanidis K. Dynamic stability control during perturbed walking can be assessed by a reduced kinematic model across the adult female lifespan. Hum Mov Sci. 2013;32:1404–14. https://doi.org/10.1016/j.humov.2013.07.008.
106. Phu S, Sturnieks DL, Lord SR, Okubo Y. Impact of ageing, fall history and exercise on postural reflexes following unpredictable perturbations: a systematic review and meta-analyses. Mech Ageing Dev. 2022;203:111634. https://doi.org/10.1016/j.mad.2022.111634.
107. Epro G, Mierau A, McCrum C, Leyendecker M, Bruggemann GP, Karamanidis K. Retention of gait stability improvements over 1.5 years in older adults: effects of perturbation exposure and triceps surae neuromuscular exercise. J Neurophysiol. 2018b;119:2229–40. https://doi.org/10.1152/jn.00513.2017.
108. Gerards MHG, Meijer K, Karamanidis K, Grevendonk L, Hoeks J, Lenssen AF, McCrum C. Adaptability to balance perturbations during walking as a potential marker of falls history in older adults. Front Sports Act Living. 2021;3:682861. https://doi.org/10.3389/fspor.2021.682861.

109. McCrum C, et al. A pilot study on the feasibility and effectiveness of treadmill-based perturbations for assessing and improving walking stability in chronic obstructive pulmonary disease. Clin Biomech. 2022b;91:105538. https://doi.org/10.1016/j.clinbiomech.2021.105538.
110. Pai YC, Yang F, Bhatt T, Wang E. Learning from laboratory-induced falling: long-term motor retention among older adults. Age (Dordr). 2014b;36:9640. https://doi.org/10.1007/s11357-014-9640-5.
111. Karamanidis K, Epro G, McCrum C, König M. Improving trip- and slip-resisting skills in older people: perturbation dose matters. Exerc Sport Sci Rev. 2020;48:40–7. https://doi.org/10.1249/JES.0000000000000210.
112. König M, Epro G, Seeley J, Catala-Lehnen P, Potthast W, Karamanidis K. Retention of improvement in gait stability over 14 weeks due to trip-perturbation training is dependent on perturbation dose. J Biomech. 2019;84:243–6. https://doi.org/10.1016/j.jbiomech.2018.12.011.
113. Lee A, Bhatt T, Liu X, Wang Y, Pai YC. Can higher training practice dosage with treadmill slip-perturbation necessarily reduce risk of falls following overground slip? Gait Posture. 2018;61:387–92. https://doi.org/10.1016/j.gaitpost.2018.01.037.
114. Lee A, Bhatt T, Pai YC. Generalization of treadmill perturbation to overground slip during gait: effect of different perturbation distances on slip recovery. J Biomech. 2016;49:149–54. https://doi.org/10.1016/j.jbiomech.2015.11.021.
115. Liu X, Bhatt T, Pai YC. Intensity and generalization of treadmill slip training: high or low, progressive increase or decrease? J Biomech. 2016;49:135–40. https://doi.org/10.1016/j.jbiomech.2015.06.004.
116. Nashner LM. Balance adjustments of humans perturbed while walking. J Neurophysiol. 1980;44:650–64. https://doi.org/10.1152/jn.1980.44.4.650.
117. Parijat P, Lockhart TE. Effects of moveable platform training in preventing slip-induced falls in older adults. Ann Biomed Eng. 2012;40:1111–21. https://doi.org/10.1007/s10439-011-0477-0.
118. Dietz V, Quintern J, Sillem M. Stumbling reactions in man: significance of proprioceptive and pre-programmed mechanisms. J Physiol. 1987;386:149–63.
119. Haridas C, Zehr EP, Misiaszek JE. Adaptation of cutaneous stumble correction when tripping is part of the locomotor environment. J Neurophysiol. 2008;99:2789–97. https://doi.org/10.1152/jn.00487.2007.
120. Nashner LM. Adapting reflexes controlling the human posture. Exp Brain Res. 1976;26:59–72.
121. Eng JJ, Winter DA, Patla AE. Strategies for recovery from a trip in early and late swing during human walking. Exp Brain Res. 1994;102:339–49.
122. Epro G, McCrum C, Mierau A, Leyendecker M, Brüggemann GP, Karamanidis K. Effects of triceps surae muscle strength and tendon stiffness on the reactive dynamic stability and adaptability of older female adults during perturbed walking. J Appl Physiol. 2018a;124:1541–9. https://doi.org/10.1152/japplphysiol.00545.2017.
123. Pai YC, Bhatt TS. Repeated-slip training: an emerging paradigm for prevention of slip-related falls among older adults. Phys Ther. 2007;87:1478–91. https://doi.org/10.2522/ptj.20060326.
124. Pijnappels M, Bobbert MF, van Dieen JH. Contribution of the support limb in control of angular momentum after tripping. J Biomech. 2004;37:1811–8. https://doi.org/10.1016/j.jbiomech.2004.02.038.
125. Pijnappels M, Reeves ND, Maganaris CN, van Dieen JH. Tripping without falling; lower limb strength, a limitation for balance recovery and a target for training in the elderly. J Electromyogr Kinesiol. 2008;18:188–96. https://doi.org/10.1016/j.jelekin.2007.06.004.
126. Rogers MW, Mille ML. Balance perturbations. Handb Clin Neurol. 2018;159:85–105. https://doi.org/10.1016/b978-0-444-63916-5.00005-7.
127. Bhatt T, Dusane S, Patel P. Does severity of motor impairment affect reactive adaptation and fall-risk in chronic stroke survivors? J Neuroeng Rehabil. 2019;16:43. https://doi.org/10.1186/s12984-019-0510-3.
128. McCrum C, Eysel-Gosepath K, Epro G, Meijer K, Savelberg HH, Bruggemann GP, Karamanidis K. Deficient recovery response and adaptive feedback potential in dynamic gait

stability in unilateral peripheral vestibular disorder patients. Physiol Rep. 2014;2:e12222. https://doi.org/10.14814/phy2.12222.
129. Nevisipour M, Grabiner MD, Honeycutt CF. A single session of trip-specific training modifies trunk control following treadmill induced balance perturbations in stroke survivors. Gait Posture. 2019;70:222–8. https://doi.org/10.1016/j.gaitpost.2019.03.002.
130. Rand MK, Wunderlich DA, Martin PE, Stelmach GE, Bloedel JR. Adaptive changes in responses to repeated locomotor perturbations in cerebellar patients. Exp Brain Res. 1998;122:31–43. https://doi.org/10.1007/s002210050488.
131. Devasahayam AJ, et al. The effect of reactive balance training on falls in daily life: an updated systematic review and meta-analysis. Phys Ther. 2022;103 https://doi.org/10.1093/ptj/pzac154.
132. Gerards MHG, McCrum C, Mansfield A, Meijer K. Perturbation-based balance training for falls reduction among older adults: current evidence and implications for clinical practice. Geriatr Gerontol Int. 2017;17:2294–303. https://doi.org/10.1111/ggi.13082.
133. Grabiner MD, Crenshaw JR, Hurt CP, Rosenblatt NJ, Troy KL. Exercise-based fall prevention: can you be a bit more specific? Exerc Sport Sci Rev. 2014;42:161–8. https://doi.org/10.1249/JES.0000000000000023.
134. Grabiner MD, Donovan S, Bareither ML, Marone JR, Hamstra-Wright K, Gatts S, Troy KL. Trunk kinematics and fall risk of older adults: translating biomechanical results to the clinic. J Electromyogr Kinesiol. 2008;18:197–204. https://doi.org/10.1016/j.jelekin.2007.06.009.
135. Lurie JD, et al. Surface perturbation training to prevent falls in older adults: a highly pragmatic, randomized controlled trial. Phys Ther. 2020; https://doi.org/10.1093/ptj/pzaa023.
136. Lurie JD, Zagaria AB, Pidgeon DM, Forman JL, Spratt KF. Pilot comparative effectiveness study of surface perturbation treadmill training to prevent falls in older adults. BMC Geriatr. 2013;13:49. https://doi.org/10.1186/1471-2318-13-49.
137. Maki BE, et al. Preventing falls in older adults: new interventions to promote more effective change-in-support balance reactions. J Electromyogr Kinesiol. 2008;18:243–54. https://doi.org/10.1016/j.jelekin.2007.06.005.
138. Mansfield A, Wong JS, Bryce J, Knorr S, Patterson KK. Does perturbation-based balance training prevent falls? Systematic review and meta-analysis of preliminary randomized controlled trials. Phys Ther. 2015;95:700–9. https://doi.org/10.2522/ptj.20140090.
139. McCrum C, Gerards MHG, Karamanidis K, Zijlstra W, Meijer K. A systematic review of gait perturbation paradigms for improving reactive stepping responses and falls risk among healthy older adults. Eur Rev Aging Phys Act. 2017b;14:3. https://doi.org/10.1186/s11556-017-0173-7.
140. Pai YC, Bhatt T, Yang F, Wang E. Perturbation training can reduce community-dwelling older adults' annual fall risk: a randomized controlled trial. J Gerontol A Biol Sci Med Sci. 2014a;69:1586–94. https://doi.org/10.1093/gerona/glu087.
141. Rosenblatt NJ, Marone J, Grabiner MD. Preventing trip-related falls by community-dwelling adults: a prospective study. J Am Geriatr Soc. 2013;61:1629–31. https://doi.org/10.1111/jgs.12428.
142. Cummings SR, Nevitt MC, Kidd S. Forgetting falls. The limited accuracy of recall of falls in the elderly. J Am Geriatr Soc. 1988;36:613–6.
143. Griffin J, Lall R, Bruce J, Withers E, Finnegan S, Lamb SE, Pre FITSG. Comparison of alternative falls data collection methods in the Prevention of Falls Injury Trial (PreFIT). J Clin Epidemiol. 2019;106:32–40. https://doi.org/10.1016/j.jclinepi.2018.09.006.
144. Bhatt T, Espy D, Yang F, Pai YC. Dynamic gait stability, clinical correlates, and prognosis of falls among community-dwelling older adults. Arch Phys Med Rehabil. 2011;92:799–805. https://doi.org/10.1016/j.apmr.2010.12.032.
145. Kiss R, Schedler S, Muehlbauer T. Associations between types of balance performance in healthy individuals across the lifespan: a systematic review and meta-analysis. Front Physiol. 2018;9:1366. https://doi.org/10.3389/fphys.2018.01366.

146. Mackey DC, Robinovitch SN. Postural steadiness during quiet stance does not associate with ability to recover balance in older women. Clin Biomech. 2005;20:776–83. https://doi.org/10.1016/j.clinbiomech.2005.05.002.
147. McCrum C, Eysel-Gosepath K, Epro G, Meijer K, Savelberg HH, Bruggemann GP, Karamanidis K. Associations between bipedal stance stability and locomotor stability following a trip in unilateral vestibulopathy. J Appl Biomech. 2017a;33:112–7. https://doi.org/10.1123/jab.2016-0004.
148. Owings TM, Pavol MJ, Foley KT, Grabiner MD. Measures of postural stability are not predictors of recovery from large postural disturbances in healthy older adults. J Am Geriatr Soc. 2000;48:42–50.
149. Patla A, Frank J, Winter D. Assessment of balance control in the elderly: major issues. Physiother Can. 1990;42:89–97. https://doi.org/10.3138/ptc.42.2.089.
150. Ringhof S, Stein T. Biomechanical assessment of dynamic balance: specificity of different balance tests. Hum Mov Sci. 2018;58:140–7. https://doi.org/10.1016/j.humov.2018.02.004.
151. Aviles J, Allin LJ, Alexander NB, Van Mullekom J, Nussbaum MA, Madigan ML. Comparison of treadmill trip-like training versus Tai Chi to improve reactive balance among independent older adult residents of senior housing: a pilot controlled trial. J Gerontol A Biol Sci Med Sci. 2019;74:1497. https://doi.org/10.1093/gerona/glz018.
152. Chien JE, Hsu WL. Effects of dynamic perturbation-based training on balance control of community-dwelling older adults. Sci Rep. 2018;8:17231. https://doi.org/10.1038/s41598-018-35644-5.
153. Freyler K, Krause A, Gollhofer A, Ritzmann R. Specific stimuli induce specific adaptations: sensorimotor training vs reactive balance training. PLoS One. 2016;11:e0167557. https://doi.org/10.1371/journal.pone.0167557.
154. Krause A, et al. Neuromuscular and kinematic adaptation in response to reactive balance training—a randomized controlled study regarding fall prevention. Front Physiol. 2018;9:1075. https://doi.org/10.3389/fphys.2018.01075.
155. Kummel J, Kramer A, Giboin LS, Gruber M. Specificity of balance training in healthy individuals: a systematic review and meta-analysis. Sports Med. 2016;46:1261–71. https://doi.org/10.1007/s40279-016-0515-z.
156. Bhatt T, Wang Y, Wang S, Kannan L. Perturbation training for fall-risk reduction in healthy older adults: interference and generalization to opposing novel perturbations post intervention. Front Sports Act Living. 2021;3:697169. https://doi.org/10.3389/fspor.2021.697169.
157. Dusane S, Bhatt T. Mixed slip-trip perturbation training for improving reactive responses in people with chronic stroke. J Neurophysiol. 2020;124:20–31. https://doi.org/10.1152/jn.00671.2019.
158. Dusane S, Bhatt T. Effect of multisession progressive gait-slip training on fall-resisting skills of people with chronic stroke: examining motor adaptation in reactive stability. Brain Sci. 2021;11 https://doi.org/10.3390/brainsci11070894.
159. König M, Epro G, Seeley J, Potthast W, Karamanidis K. Retention and generalizability of balance recovery response adaptations from trip perturbations across the adult life span. J Neurophysiol. 2019;122:1884–93. https://doi.org/10.1152/jn.00380.2019.
160. König M, Santuz A, Epro G, Werth J, Arampatzis A, Karamanidis K. Differences in muscle synergies among recovery responses limit inter-task generalisation of stability performance. Hum Mov Sci. 2022;82:102937. https://doi.org/10.1016/j.humov.2022.102937.
161. Song PYH, Sturnieks DL, Davis MK, Lord SR, Okubo Y. Perturbation-based balance training using repeated trips on a walkway vs. belt accelerations on a treadmill: a cross-over randomised controlled trial in community-dwelling older adults. Front Sports Act Living. 2021;3:702320. https://doi.org/10.3389/fspor.2021.702320.

Effects of Aging on Gait and Posture

4

Natalia Madalena Rinaldi, Gabriela Vigorito Magalhães, and Anderson Rodrigues Delunardo

Abstract

The aging process is often characterized by changes in the musculoskeletal and sensory systems and central nervous system. These modifications due to the aging process result in postural control and mobility problems. As a consequence, the risk of falling increases and the daily life activities and mobility of older adults are negatively affected. Therefore, it is important to describe the effects of aging on mechanisms involved in postural control and gait. This chapter provides an overview of these factors, including the effects of the aging process on postural control and walking. Finally, a brief overview of posture and gait variables will be outlined to provide the best understanding of balance/gait deficits.

Introduction

According to the United Nations Department of Economic and Social Affairs (UN DESA), population aging is an irreversible trend. It is estimated that the older adult population (65+ years of age) will grow from 761 million in 2021 to 1.6 billion in 2050 [1]. With the consequent aging of the population, the economic, social, and management challenges of aging are also growing, which, among other objectives, include the search for healthy aging mediated by reducing functional loss and the

N. M. Rinaldi (✉)
Biomechanical Analysis of Movement Laboratory (Bio.Mov), Center of Physical Education and Sports, Federal University of Espírito Santo, Espírito Santo, Brazil
e-mail: natalia.rinaldi@ufes.br

G. V. Magalhães · A. R. Delunardo
Biomechanical Analysis of Movement Laboratory (Bio.Mov), Graduate Program in Physical Education, Federal University of Espírito Santo, Espírito Santo, Brazil

F. A. Barbieri et al. (eds.), *Locomotion and Posture in Older Adults*,
https://doi.org/10.1007/978-3-031-74123-4_4

number of accidents associated with progressive deleterious processes common to the geriatric population [1].

Aging is a natural and multifactorial process, accompanied by changes in human structure and capacity. Among these, the following can be highlighted: reduction in muscle mass [2]; significant alterations in the central and peripheral nervous system; ineffectiveness of neurocognitive abilities [3]; motor and sensory dysfunctions [4], as well as changes in the components of functional capacity, such as reduction in strength production capacity, flexibility, agility, and reaction time [2, 5]. These factors, caused by the aging process, affect postural control and gait.

Postural control is the ability to maintain the center of mass within the support base, an important aspect for performing daily activities [6, 7]. With advancing age, there is a decline in postural control performance, such as increased displacement and velocity of the center of pressure compared to young adults [8]. In addition, walking is one of the most performed activities during daily activities. The ability to walk safely and efficiently is an important predisposition in maintaining independence with the aging process [9]. Thus, the older population develops a more cautious gait, characterized by changes in spatio-temporal parameters (e.g., reduction in velocity and length and increase in step width [10]) and variables related to postural stability (e.g., center of pressure (COP) trajectory toward the medial direction, faster COP velocity in the initial contact of the foot with the ground, and slower velocity in the middle support phase of the gait cycle) [11].

Moreover, performing daily activities involves motor and cognitive demands, such as overcoming an obstacle. This is a challenging task for older adults compared to the free walking situation, since the displacement of the center of mass (CoM) is greater, more time in single support (one foot on the ground) is required, and an increased degree of contralateral flexion of the hip takes place [12]. Recently, Raffegeau et al. (2022) [13] found that older adults try to preserve postural stability while overcoming obstacles but may be unable to ensure safer limb elevation to overcome obstacles at faster velocities. Therefore, these changes in gait increase the risk of tripping over the obstacle, which contributes to falls, injuries, disability, and loss of functional independence, ultimately affecting the quality of life of older adults [14].

The objective of this chapter is to discuss the effects of aging on gait and postural control, focusing on the control mechanisms related to these two components. To achieve this objective, the chapter is divided into two topics: the first discusses gait changes in regular terrain and the second addresses the sensory and motor aspects related to postural control combined with other motor tasks due to the aging process.

Changes in Behavior of Spatio-temporal Parameters During Walking Through in Older Adults

Walking is a basic activity, but it is considered a complex task [15], especially when performed under challenging conditions, such as walking on narrow sidewalks and when there is need to overcome obstacles, which are associated with a higher risk of falls in the older population [16, 17]. Physiological, musculoskeletal, sensory [18], and postural control [19] changes due to aging interfere with the functional performance of older adults and cause changes in gait [20], such as increased gait variability; slower, shorter, and narrower steps [21, 22].

Gait variability is the step-by-step fluctuation of gait spatio-temporal variables [15], in which spatial variables tend to decrease and temporal variables to increase [23]. The increase in variability is often associated with postural instability, increased risk of falls [15], and worse gait performance [23], especially in the older population. Stability during gait is measured by the margin of stability (MoS), which occurs from the relationship of displacement and recovery of the extrapolated CoM (XCoM) with the base of support (BoS) [24], which tends to decrease with aging [13]. Postural instability during gait, as mentioned, is greater in the mediolateral direction in older adults [13, 25]. This happens because the CoM trajectory is directed to the lateral edge of the BoS when walking [25] and, by correlating directly to the width of the step [26], which tends to be decreased in older adults, results in lower mediolateral MoS [13].

Thus, worse gait performance due to aging is associated with slower walking velocity with longer time in double support, shorter step length and width with high variability [23, 27], with the most evident changes in step velocity and length [20]. These changes occur in the attempt to adopt a cautious gait pattern [23], although they increase even more the risk of falls.

The spatio-temporal variables commonly studied are gait velocity, step length, and step width. Therefore, the behavior of these variables during free walking in older adults will be discussed below.

Gait Velocity

Gait velocity is determined by the relationship between the length and time of each step, configuring the spatio-temporal characteristic of this variable [28], measured in meters per second (m/s). Velocity is a variable that describes a person's overall physical performance and ability to adapt to unexpected conditions while walking [15], such as the need for quick direction changes and obstacle avoidance. In addition, velocity is an important marker of functional independence, particularly in the older adult population [15], and is a predictive variable of CoM stability for the anteroposterior and mediolateral directions in BoS [29].

Aging causes decreased walking velocity [30], which is associated with functional decline [31], frailty and disability [32] of older adults, and predisposes to a higher risk of falling [30]. Gait velocities lower than 1 m/s have been used to characterize a high risk of falls in the older adult population [33, 34]. Reductions in velocity tend to occur due to changes in equilibrium, being a compensatory strategy used to increase MoS [10, 21] and reduce the work to control the CoM at the support base [35], resulting in a more cautious gait [36]. Furthermore, this reduction is associated with muscle weakness [22, 37] and lower power of the lower limbs [38], which reduce the ability to propel the body forward. It is suggested that the reduction in velocity can be attributed to the reduction of its spatial component, that is, step length [36], which also causes an increase in the time in double support. This adaptation is considered an attempt to make gait safer [22, 27, 37].

For healthy men and women, without significant physical limitations and/or neurological and musculoskeletal conditions until the age of approximately 40–45 years, an increase in walking velocity is identified [30, 37], being the peak velocity during life in this age group [37]. In contrast, older adults walk more slowly [22] and show a greater decline in velocity in older age groups [38]. For men in the age range of 50–65 years, it was found that they present similar walking velocity, but those aged over 71 years tend to walk more slowly, and a greater reduction in velocity was identified in older adults over 81 years of age [30, 37, 38]. For women, a downward trend was identified in gait velocity from the age of 50, with slower velocity at increasing age, mainly from 71 to 75 years of age or over [30, 37, 38]. In addition, they also have greater velocity variability [37], which increases the risk of falls.

Step Length

Step length is calculated as the anteroposterior distance from the heel of one limb to the opposite heel after one step [39]· This spatial variable predicts postural stability for the anteroposterior and mediolateral directions of the CoM in BoS during gait [29] and reflects gait quality and functional level, especially in the older adult population [15, 31].

During gait, older adults have shorter steps [22]. The reduced length is a kinematic alteration that occurs as a compensatory mechanism to preserve stability and avoid falls [30], showing that, as aging progresses, older adults tend to develop a cautious gait pattern [10]. Also, it becomes important to analyze step length, since it is a co-dependent variable[31] and directly related to the gait velocity [22], which is also decreased. Studies show that the decrease in step length further reduces walking velocity [22, 30], as well as increases the time of double support [22] and the risk of falls [30]. Therefore, adopting measures that increase step length may be effective to improve gait velocity and stability in the older adult population [20].

This reduction in step length with advancing age is evident from the age of 60 in women, with a reduction with advancing age, and in men between 71 and 75 years of age or over [30]. The same occurs for stride length, especially in women, in all age groups up to 80 years, with greater variability. This behavior occurs mainly due to the reduction in muscle strength [37]. Weakness in the hip extensors and plantiflexors muscles [40] is believed to reduce the ability to propel the body forward, as well as reduce the strength of the knee flexors, which lead to lower efficiency in the swing phase of the gait [41]. Thus, force changes can affect the step length and, consequently, gait velocity [37].

Step Width

Step width refers to the lateral distance from the midpoint of one foot to the midpoint of the other foot. It is related to stability in the mediolateral direction of the CoM in BoS during gait [29] and shows the adjustments made in this direction to maintain balance when walking [15]. When decreased, as occurs in aging to mitigate gait energy costs and control CoM [25], it provides a reduction in gait stability in the mediolateral direction [10] and reduces gait velocity [30].

With advancing age, there is a decrease in step width [27, 30, 31, 37, 42], especially above 70 years of age [30], being more evident in women [30, 31, 42]. This alteration also occurs due to the loss of muscle strength with the aging process and takes place as an attempt to increase stability during the task [42]. It is believed that a decline in gluteus medius muscle strength occurs from the age of 45, with an acceleration after the age of 70, and that this is associated with a reduction in step width [43]. Still, width is a variable associated with the height of the individual [31], that is, the taller the individual, the greater the width of the step tends to be. This fact also confirms the reduced width with advancing age, especially in women.

Associated with this, a greater variability of step width is identified in older adults when compared with young adults [21, 27], affecting the behavior of rhythm and dynamic balance or the support base [31]. Variation above 2.5 cm is considered an excessive variability of step width [20], being related to the risk of falls in older adults and being able to differentiate between those who fall and those who do not. This increase occurs because maintaining lateral stability during gait is a challenge for older adults due to the decline in sensorimotor functions and motor control [21] and the greater mediolateral oscillation of the CoM in BoS [25]. However, older adults with significant functional decline may have reduced variability. This is due to physical restrictions, movement deficits, and lower gait velocity [31], which makes gait even more unstable.

Changes in Behavior of Spatio-temporal Parameters of Gait of Older Adults When Overcoming an Obstacle

Gait in older adults is marked by slow, short, and narrow steps [21]. When associated with overcoming obstacles, such as stepping onto sidewalks and climbing stairs [44], the changes in locomotor pattern discussed earlier are even more evident [13]. These changes occur because these combined activities require greater interaction between the processing and execution areas of the nervous system, involving planning and correction of possible postural instabilities [42] that are influenced by aging.

When compared with young adults, older adults have lower velocity when walking with obstacle overcoming [45, 46]. This is because they need more time to process visual information during the swing phases and when overcoming an obstacle [47, 48]. Consequently, there is a reduction in the step length, which leads to greater proximity to the obstacle [45, 49]. There is also a reduction in step width and an increase in width variability [50]. These changes indicate a reduction in the control of the CoM in the mediolateral direction over the BoS during obstacle overcoming and indicate a greater chance of errors to control the CoM when positioning the foot after overcoming it [50]. Also, older adults decrease the elevation of the foot when overcoming the obstacle [46]. These adaptations occur in an attempt to avoid contact with the obstacle, but it causes the stability of the gait to be affected during overtaking [51] and increases the proximity to the obstacle, thus increasing the risk of tripping [46].

Young adults are prone to bumping into the obstacle while overtaking with the trailing limb, while older adults are prone to bumping and consequently tripping over the leading limb while overtaking [46]. This occurs because in young adults, during overtaking, the foot moves forward and up, which facilitates the increase in knee flexion to overcome the obstacle [49]. In addition, the CoM lies behind the support foot, which increases the time for planning on positioning of the second limb for a better support base [46]. For older adults, during overtaking, the foot moves forward and down [52] and, when tripping occurs, there is a need for greater force production to elevate the limb and position it properly [49]. In addition, there is a greater displacement of the CoM, which moves away from the limits of the MoS [49], further hindering the recovery of balance in the support base, since the MoS tends to be less adaptable during overtaking with the trailing limb [52]. The chances of contact with the leading limb by older adults during overcoming the obstacle also occur due to the reduction in step length [49], which allows greater approximation with obstacle and increases the musculoskeletal demands for balance recovery. As a result, older adults have a higher risk of falling, considering that the recovery of the leading limb after tripping is more difficult [49].

Moreover, the position of the obstacle in relation to the starting point seems to influence the behavior and positioning of the foot before and after overcoming the obstacle in older adults [53]. For both limbs, older adults decrease the horizontal distance of the foot from the obstacle before overtaking and after overtaking when the obstacle is in a position further away from the start of the gait [53]. This occurs because during walking there is an increase in the variability of foot positioning, which compromises the proper positioning of the foot in relation to the obstacle when it is away [53].

Changes in Behavior of Spatio-temporal Parameters of Dual-Task Walking in Older Adults

Performing several tasks at the same time is common in everyday life and requires high cognitive demand. This type of situation requires attention to be divided to properly complete all tasks [54], such as talking while walking [55]; walking on uneven and narrow surfaces [15]; performing the grasping movement while overcoming an obstacle [53], such as climbing steps and opening a door simultaneously.

The ability to perform a dual task is considered a clinical marker for identifying cognitive impairment [56], risk of falls [57], and the state of frailty in older adults [58]. While young adults generally adapt well to gait with a dual task and are able to allocate attention to both tasks, older adults may not have enough attention resources to focus on the gait associated with a task [19], especially if it is complex and requires additional cognitive resources [59]. This is due to the decline in sensory-motor coordination, in executive function due to aging [60], and because the cognitive task requires attentional resources that, consequently, are not available for gait control [55]. Yet, when engaged in dual tasks, older adults tend to prioritize the other task instead of the gait, especially if it is a cognitive task [54], which further increases the risk of falls when walking.

Older adults present worse performance than young adults when subjected to gait with cognitive tasks [61]; they require more neural resources to perform them simultaneously [62]. Dual-task walking is challenging for older adults, which reflects in slower walking velocity and lower MoS when compared with free walking. This velocity reduction occurs in an attempt to prioritize gait and maintain stability, especially in the mediolateral direction [26]. Also, the type of associated task influences the performance of the dual task and modulates the magnitude of gait decline in older adults, such as tasks related to word fluency, memory, countdown, and reaction time [54, 61], as well as grip movement when overcoming obstacle [53].

When walking with a dual task related to verbal fluency, such as mentioning the largest number of words related to a specific category, older adults generated fewer words and presented lower walking velocity [61] and greater step width [54] when compared with young adults. This occurs because there is a competition between the control of balance and the task of verbal fluency, which leads to a compensatory strategy of increasing the width of the base to protect the balance in the mediolateral direction [54] to avoid falling [55]. When subjected to memory tasks, such as recalling a list of previously spoken words, older adults tend to have a reduction in step velocity, width, and length compared to young adults [15]. This alteration occurs because aging causes an impairment of memory processing [63] and requires a greater need for attentional resources to perform this task, leading to impaired gait in an attempt to perform the cognitive task. These changes may indicate less stability during walking and a higher risk of falls [16], especially during common everyday activities, such as trying to remember a person's name, a street, or a phone number while walking.

When they perform the gait with the cognitive task of counting down, such as counting down the multiples of seven, older adults, compared to young adults, present greater task interference and cognitive cost, as well as lower gait velocity [61]. Furthermore, when this cognitive task is associated with more challenging gait, such as walking in places with curves, changes in spatio-temporal parameters are even more evident. Older adults have a reduction in gait velocity, cadence, and step length. They also present shorter time in single support, shorter length and greater width of the stride [55]. These findings show that when submitted to the dual task in a challenging condition, older adults present impairments in activity control, greater motor-cognitive demand, and greater instability [26, 55]. These changes are adaptations that occur in an attempt to maintain balance during walking and avoid falling [55]. Finally, when compared with young adults, older adults also present greater interference when walking with a reaction time task, such as abruptly stopping walking when hearing a noise. Older adults present worse performance during the task and reduction in walking velocity, with increasing difficulty in more complex tasks [61], for example, when the frequency of noise increases.

Older adults, when subjected to a motor task during walking, such as grasping objects, reduce the velocity of the CoM in the anteroposterior direction as they approach the obstacle. This behavior also occurs in older adults with a history of falls, who, during the grasping movement, reduce the velocity of the CoM to the point of interrupting the gait to accommodate the motor task [64]. Also, when subjected to overcoming obstacles with the grasping movement, older adults present lower gait velocity and step length, as well as greater width and duration [13]. These adopted behaviors show that the addition of a manual task influences gait in older adults and that they adopt a conservative strategy to perform both tasks, in an attempt to maintain balance and MoS [13]. Nevertheless, these modifications occur due to the sharing of visual attention between the two motor tasks, and the visual attention to the grasping movement may be able to impair the gait when overcoming an obstacle [53]. Thus, the manual task influences the locomotor parameters of the gait during overcoming of obstacles, an activity that is present in everyday life, such as the grip task when opening the door after climbing a ladder or reaching for something while overcoming a carpet at home.

The changes in spatio-temporal gait variables of older adults during walking through, obstacles avoidance, and dual-task walking are described in the diagram in Fig. 4.1.

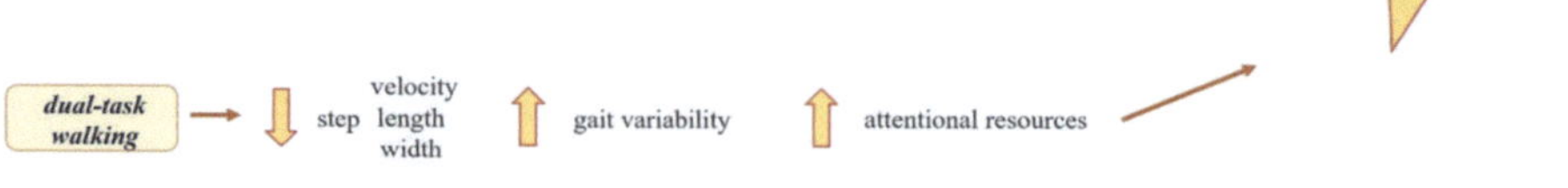

Fig. 4.1 Changes in spatio-temporal gait variables of older adults during walking through, obstacles avoidance, and dual-task walking

Effects of Aging on Postural Control

Postural control is a motor skill [65] based on a complex interaction of muscular and neural physiological mechanisms, including motor, cognitive, adaptive, anticipatory, and perceptual processes [66], having postural orientation and stability [67] as dual objective. Postural orientation can be considered the ability to maintain an appropriate relationship and/or alignment between body segments regarding sensory information on different surfaces, task characteristics, and environmental conditions [66, 67]. Postural stability, in turn, deals with control and the ability to maintain appropriate relationship of CoM and BoS, given by the relationship between the body and the support surface [66, 67].

From the interpretation of information from sensory feedback systems (visual, vestibular, and somatosensory), subsequent motor responses are performed to maintain posture [68] or else maintain the projected center of mass within the limits of stability [66], an area where oscillation is safe [69]. These motor responses, configured as different movement strategies, can be classically distinguished as ankle, hip, and step strategies [66], enunciated according to the characteristics of postural disturbance, individual expectations, goals, and previous experiences [70]. Older women, in the presence of inaccurate visual (closed eyes) and somatosensory (irregular environments) information depend more on the hip strategy for maintaining balance [71]. Moreover, in comparison to young adults, who tend to normally evoke ankle strategies to maintain posture, older adults tend to evoke more frequently the hip strategy, based on actions of flexing and extending the hip [27].

Postural control is essential for an individual to perform voluntary movements and react appropriately to external disturbances [27]. Conversely, the inefficiency of this skill is associated with reduced quality of life, of independence, risk of injury, and especially falls [68, 71], an unexpected and abrupt event associated with both loss of balance and failure in the mechanisms of postural control [8].

Although aging is a natural process, it is accompanied by structural changes and deleterious effects of physiological systems that lead to an increase in the incidence of falls in the geriatric population [68]. Having as one of its main causes the disorders in the components necessary to balance control [3], the fall happens when an individual fails to maintain a proper relationship of CoM and BoS and advances the limits of stability. Stability is altered by extrinsic and intrinsic factors, related, respectively, to the environment, surface type, and task requirements, as well as biomechanics and individual capacities, including those associated with the efficiency of postural control mechanisms [5, 14, 27]. In addition to the reduction in self-confidence and independence, falls increase mortality rates and non-fatal injuries in older adults [3]. Recurrent falls, in turn, increase the risk of fractures and negatively impact the development of daily activities, quality of life, and risk of death among the older adult population [67]. Moreover, the fear of falling, by leading older adults to restrict their activities and by increasing the demand for attention in locomotion and balance, aggravates the deleterious effects of aging [72].

Given this context, it is extremely important to understand the changes in postural control mechanisms associated with aging, to, among other objectives, seek ways for reducing the risk of falls in this population.

Assessment of Postural Control

The assessment of postural control is carried out by the implementation of tests and techniques, such as Posturography [73]. This test, carried out with individuals standing on force plates, examines spatial measures of CoM and center of pressure (COP), where greater movement is associated with instability, while lower movement, conversely, is associated with stability [74]. The COP analyzed in the force platforms is the distribution center of the total force applied to the support surface [66]; this is a measure that represents the sum of neuromuscular components acting at different joint levels [70].

Posturography can be performed under different conditions, such as with (eyes open) or without (eyes closed) visual feedback [75]. The analysis of the COP variables, generated in a Stabilogram, can reveal important information for risk analysis of falls in older adults, as well as the mechanisms involved in balance control [73]. Gadelha et al. (2018) [76], when analyzing average COP velocity (cumulative distance over the period of sampling) and COP displacement amplitude (difference between minimum COP values along the anteroposterior and mediolateral axis) of older adults in different stages of sarcopenia, found an association between COP variables and stages of sarcopenia. These authors found that more advanced stages of sarcopenia were associated with worse stabilometric results, such as increased COP displacement amplitude. Other variables, such as oscillation velocity, can be used to differentiate groups of different ages and verify the risk that falls in the older adult population [77].

In the literature, other metrics are also discussed in the assessment of postural control. The time-to-contact (TTC) measure—when considering spatial and temporal measurements regarding movements with respect to BoS (CoM approximation of the stability limit)—defines, in functional terms, the time that the system has to reverse any disturbance before the posture is threatened [74]. The entropy sample, fractal dimension, and Lyapunov exponent, which are nonlinear measures, consider the temporal components of the variation of COP displacements, allowing to quantify the regularity, adaptability, stability, and complexity of postural control [70]. Other forms of analysis of postural control also include tests such as the Sensory Organization Test (SOT) , where the variables of balance, movement strategies (ankle; hip), and sensory information are analyzed together [71]. Given the importance of understanding the effects of aging on dynamic stability [78], one may still cite MoS, configured as the minimum margin of the distance between an XCoM and the edge of the BoS, which should be positive for maintaining posture during gait [26].

Finally, with special importance to clinical practice, tests such as the Berg Balance Scale (BBS) and the Balance Evaluation System Test (BESTest) can be applied. The first is made up of balancing tasks such as standing in single-legged support [79], from which information is provided, based on the score achieved in the test, associated with the risk of falls [80]. BESTest, in turn, examines the deficits of balance maintenance by a series of tasks characterized in systems: biomechanical constraints, stability limits, anticipatory postural adjustments, postural responses, sensory orientation, and gait stability [81].

Effects of Aging on the Sensory Compensation System and Strategy

Sensory feedback in postural control is given by the integration of information from the visual, somatosensory, and vestibular systems [66]. The first provides information on the positioning and movement of the head in relation to objects, as well as serving as a reference for verticality [66]. Somatosensory feedback provides information about body position and movement [66]. The vestibular system provides information about the position and movement of the head in relation to gravity [66]. The postural control performance is negatively affected by manipulation and increased visual (eyes open vs. closed), somatosensory (stable vs. unstable surfaces), and cognitive challenges, especially in dual-task contexts [82]. Moreover, the increase in oscillation in conditions of greater complexity and difficulty, such as unstable surfaces (inaccurate somatosensory feedback) and conditions of deprivation of visual information [83], is more pronounced in older adults when compared with young people and adults [84]. This fact is associated with important changes in sensory feedback mechanisms in older adults, especially in the somatosensory system.

The decline of visual functions in older adults is associated with anatomical and functional changes. Functionally, the deleterious effects are present in visual acuity, contrast sensitivity, visual field size, depth perception, among others [85]. Interestingly, however, older adults rely more on visual feedback for balance control when compared with proprioceptive and vestibular feedback [85]. The occlusion of vision, in turn, can clearly reveal the deficiencies of the other feedback systems [8].

Proprioception, as part of the somatosensory system, with reduced effectiveness associated with the deleterious processes of aging, especially in people aged over 75 years, is essential for coordination of movements in maintaining balance [79], awareness of position, and joint movement [86]. Its functioning is based on the stimulation, coordination, and integration of signals from specific mechanoreceptors, such as muscle spindles, Golgi tendon organs, and Pacinian corpuscles, located in muscles, tendons, and joint capsules [86, 87]. Plantar mechanoreceptors, located in the sole of the human foot, sensitive to pressure, load, vibration, and stretch, are associated with the efficiency of postural control [88]. However, when aging takes place, these receptors present reduced sensitivity, which is associated with reduced balance [89]. Strategies such as stimuli by mechanical vibrations, electrical and non-electrical stimulation, such as the use of textured surfaces, have been effective in facilitating the sensory feedback of these mechanoreceptors [90].

Aging is associated with important structural and functional changes, including reductions in the responses of muscle spindles and nerve fibers, as well as important changes at the central level, with alterations in the integrity of brain white matter and gray matter, reductions in the number of dendrites in the motor cortex, decrease in the number of neurons and receptors, and various neurochemical modifications [86, 87]. Such changes contribute to the increased dependence on visual cues for stability control in the older adult population [86].

Older adults with vestibular disorders, despite presenting reduced stability limits when compared with healthy ones, are still able to maintain a posture similar to healthy older adults by using somatosensory and visual cues to compensate for inaccurate vestibular information [69].

Depending on the functional state, the task, and the context in which balance control is performed, in a strategic way, the central nervous system is able to reconsider the weight and importance of the sensory sources used in balance control [66], where the most reliable sensory sources are emphasized, while the least reliable ones are weakened [86]. The integrity of this strategy is important for maintaining the efficiency of balance control in different contexts [67].

To maintain balance, in relation to young adults, older adults have reduced ability to adapt to conditions where visual and somatosensory information is impaired [27]. This inefficiency is particularly visible when multiple sensory sources are inaccurate, such as in unstable surface conditions (inaccurate somatosensory information) and closed eyes (inaccurate visual information) [71]. When performing postural tasks, compared to young adults, older adults present different patterns in activated and recruited brain regions, based on differentiation and compensation models [90]. The first is associated with non-selective recruitment of brain regions as a consequence of the inefficiency of previously functional regions and the second is associated with compensation of the neurobiological decline of aging by cortical overactivation [91].

Finally, with the degeneration of sensory systems in older adults, as well as the neuromuscular system, including a reduction in functional motor units and diminished postural or muscular reflexes, measured by the time required for the onset of muscle activity in response to disturbances, efficiency is lost [92]. In their meta-analysis, Phu et al. (2022) [92] found that older adults have an average velocity of postural reflexes (63–164 ms) compared to young adults (77–181 ms), which reinforces their lower ability to perceive movements or external disturbances.

The changes in postural control of older adults are described in the diagram in Fig. 4.2.

Cognitive Demand and Dual Task

Aging is accompanied by structural and functional changes in the central nervous system, including changes in the volume of cortical gray matter, associated with the decline of cognitive functions such as memory and attention [93]. Cognitive decline in older adults is also associated with reduced performance in language skills,

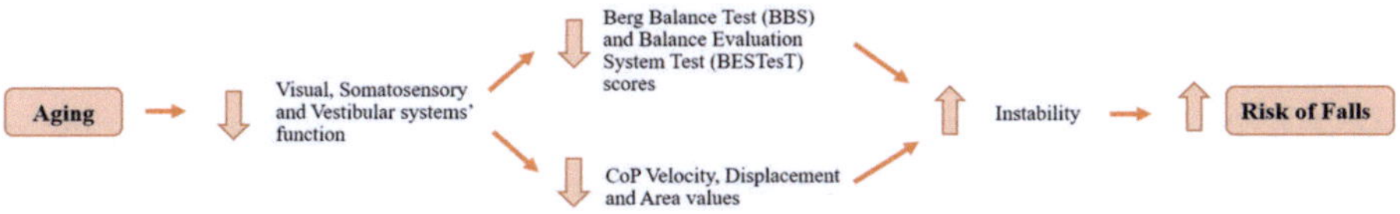

Fig. 4.2 Key changes in postural control of older adults in relation to COP variables and clinical tests

perception, planning and execution of tasks, as well as in maintaining balance, with greater oscillation accompanied by fear of falling and recurrence of falls [80].

With aging, postural control acquires an attentional character rather than an automatic one [94], thus requiring, especially from the geriatric population, the allocation of greater cognitive processing in the form of attention resources [14]. This phenomenon can also be aggravated by anxiety associated with fear of falling, which further increases the demands of attention for locomotion and balance [72].

The knowledge base regarding cognitive demand (attentional resources) in posture maintenance has been based on dual-task investigations [93]. These investigations have been used to examine the interactions between attentional resources and posture control [4], as well as the limitations of the nervous system in processing simultaneous information [95], by the simultaneous performance of a postural task and a cognitive or motor task [82]. Among the cognitive and motor tasks used, we can highlight the tasks of reaction time, discrimination, mental tracking, memory [95], in addition to verbal fluency and common tasks in daily activities associated with communication, such as listening [82].

As means of compensating, older adults tend to activate additional brain regions when performing a cognitive task when compared with younger adults [93]. However, the cognitive changes associated with aging impair the effective allocation of attentional resources [14], increase the cost of the task, and lead to a decline in performance, both of postural control (increased oscillation) and cognitive task when performed simultaneously [77]. This cost is further exacerbated by increasing the complexity of tasks, both for postural control, in conditions of inaccurate sensory information [77], and for cognitive tasks, in conditions of greater complexity and task load [82]. Since dual tasks portray conditions common to daily life [82], it is important to find ways to reduce these costs.

The practice of physical exercise has the potential to counterbalance the deleterious effects of aging [33]. Adherence to multicomponent training programs aimed at increasing performance in balance, coordination, cognitive ability, flexibility, and the ability to produce strength, as well as task-based and gait-based functional exercises [92, 96, 97], in addition to programs such as Tai Chi [92] and physical therapeutic exercises [98] is recommended. Complementary activities such as virtual reality games [98] have potential to reduce deleterious effects of aging while also contributing to the adoption of an active lifestyle.

Final Remarks

As described, older adults present changes in balance control characterized by an increased amplitude of COP displacement. These changes are even more evident when sensory information is manipulated (eyes open and irregular environments) since they depend more on the hip strategy to maintain balance. Moreover, the gait of older adults is characterized by slow steps with longer time in double support, which may be related to reduced stability. Thus, older adults adopt a cautious and conversational strategy when overcoming obstacles, such as reducing the control of the center of mass over the support base.

These changes in balance and locomotion control due to the aging process increase the risk of falls, consequently impairing the performance of daily activities.

References

1. United Nations, Department of Economic and Social Affairs. World Social Report 2023: leaving no one behind in an ageing world. 2023.; E23.IV2. Available from: https://desapublications.un.org/publications/world-social-report-2023-leaving-no-one-behind-ageing-world.
2. Maktouf W, Durand S, Boyas S, Pouliquen C, Beaune B. Combined effects of aging and obesity on postural control, muscle activity and maximal voluntary force of muscles mobilizing ankle joint. J Biomech. 2018;79:198–206.
3. Cuevas-Trisan R. Balance problems and fall risks in the elderly. Clin Geriatr Med. 2019;35(2):173–83.
4. Brustio PR, Rainoldi A, Petrigna L, Rabaglietti E, Pizzigalli L. Postural stability during dual- and triple-task conditions: the effect of different levels of physical fitness in older adults. Sci Sports. 2021;36(2):143–51.
5. Roman-Liu D. Age-related changes in the range and velocity of postural sway. Arch Gerontol Geriatr. 2018;77:68–80.
6. Rahal MA, Alonsoi AC, Andrusaitis FR, Rodrigues TS, Speciali DS, Greve JMD, et al. Analysis of static and dynamic balance in healthy elderly practitioners of Tai Chi Chuan versus ballroom dancing. Clinics. 2015;70(3):157–61.
7. Alonso AC, Mochizuki L, Silva Luna NM, Ayama S, Canonica AC, Greve JMDA. Relation between the sensory and anthropometric variables in the quiet standing postural control: is the inverted pendulum important for the static balance control? Biomed Res Int. 2015;2015:985312.
8. Brech GC, Bobbio TG, Cabral KN, Coutinho PM, Castro LR, Mochizuki L, et al. Changes in postural balance associated with a woman's aging process. Clinics. 2022;77:100041.
9. Callisaya ML, Blizzard L, Schmidt MD, McGinley JL, Srikanth VK. Ageing and gait variability–a population-based study of older people. Age Ageing. 2010;39(2):191–7.
10. Herssens N, Verbecque E, Hallemans A, Vereeck L, Rompaey VV, Saeys W. Do spatiotemporal parameters and gait variability differ across the lifespan of healthy adults? A systematic review. Gait Posture. 2018;64:181–90.
11. Mehdizadeh S, Van Ooteghem K, Gulka H, Nabavi H, Faieghi M, Taati B, et al. A systematic review of center of pressure measures to quantify gait changes in older adults. Exp Gerontol. 2021;143:111170.
12. Galna B, Lord S, Rochester L. Is gait variability reliable in older adults and Parkinson's disease? Towards an optimal testing protocol. Gait Posture. 2013;37:580–5.
13. Raffegeau TE, Brinkerhoff AS, Kellaher GK, Baudendistiel S, Terza MJ, Roper JA. Changes to margins of stability from walking to obstacle crossing in older adults while walking fast and during a dual-task. Exp Gerontol. 2022;161:111710.

14. Motealleh A, Sinaei E, Nouraddinifard E, Rezaei I. Comparison of postural control in older adults under different dual-task conditions: a cross-sectional study. J Bodyw Mov Ther. 2021;26:443–7.
15. Lindemann U. Spatiotemporal gait analysis of older persons in clinical practice and research. Z Gerontol Geriatr. 2020;53(2):171–8.
16. Hennah C, Ellis G, Doumas M. Dual-task walking in healthy aging: effects of narrow and wide walking paths. PLoS One. 2021;16(12):e0261647.
17. Lee S. Falls associated with indoor and outdoor environmental hazards among community-dwelling older adults between men and women. BMC Geriatr. 2021;21(1):1–12.
18. Wilkinson DJ, Piasecki M, Atherton PJ. The age-related loss of skeletal muscle mass and function: measurement and physiology of muscle fibre atrophy and muscle fibre loss in humans. Ageing Res Rev. 2018;47:123–32.
19. Woollacott M, Shumway-Cook A. Attention and the control of posture and gait: a review of an emerging area of research. Gait Posture. 2002;16(1):1–14.
20. Magnani PE, Junior RCF, Zanellato NFG, Genovez MB, Alvarenga IC, Abreu DCC. The influence of aging on the spatial and temporal variables of gait during usual and fast speed in older adults aged 60 to 102 years. Hum Mov Sci. 2019;68:102540.
21. Skiadopoulos A, Moore EE, Sayles HR, Schimid KK, Stergiou N. Step width variability as a discriminator of age-related gait changes. J Neuroeng Rehabil. 2020;17:2–13.
22. Winter DA, Patla AE, Frank JS, Walt SE. Biomechanical walking pattern changes in the fit and healthy elderly. Phys Ther. 1990;70(6):340–7.
23. Stotz A, Hamacher D, Zech A. Relationship between muscle strength and gait parameters in healthy older women and men. Int J Environ Res Public Health. 2023;20(7):5362.
24. Hof AL, Gazendam MG, Sinke WE. The condition for dynamic stability. J Biomech. 2005;38:1–8.
25. Bruijn SM, van Dieën JH. Control of human gait stability through foot placement. J R Soc Interface. 2018;15(143):20170816.
26. Yamaguchi T, Mesani K. Effects of age on dynamic balance measures and their correlation during walking across the adult lifespan. Sci Rep. 2022;12:14301.
27. Osoba MY, Rao AK, Agrawal SK, Lalwani AK. Balance and gait in the elderly: a contemporary review. Laryngoscope Investig Otolaryngol. 2019;4(1):143–53.
28. Baudendistel ST, Schmitt AC, Stone AE, Raffegeau TE, Roper JA, Hass CJ. Faster or longer steps: maintaining fast walking in older adults at risk for mobility disability. Gait Posture. 2021;89:86–91.
29. Lencioni T, Carpinella I, Rabuffetti M, Cattaneo D, Ferrarin M. Measures of dynamic balance during level walking in healthy adult subjects: relationship with age, anthropometry and spatio-temporal gait parameters. Proc Inst Mech Eng H. 2020;234(2):131–40.
30. Lau LK, Wee SL, Pang WJB, Chen KK, Jabbar KA, Yap PLK, et al. Reference values of gait velocity and gait spatiotemporal parameters for a South East Asian population: the Yishun study. Clin Interv Aging. 2020;15:1753–65.
31. Dapp U, Vinyard D, Golgert S, Krumpoch S, Freiberger E. Reference values of gait characteristics in community-dwelling older persons with different physical functional levels. BMC Geriatr. 2022;22:713.
32. Rabin LA, Smart CM, Crane PK, Amariglio RE, Bermen LM, Boada M, et al. Subjective cognitive decline in older adults: an overview of self-report measures used across 19 international research studies. J Alzheimers Dis. 2015;48(1):S63–86.
33. Verghese J, Holtzer R, Lipton RB, Wang C. Quantitative gait markers and incident fall risk in older adults. J Gerontol A Biol Sci Med Sci. 2009;64:896–901.
34. Kyrdalen IL, Thingstad P, Sandvik L, Ormstad H. Associations between gait velocity and well-known fall risk factors among community-dwelling older adults. Physiother Res Int. 2019;24(1):E1743.
35. Herssens N, van Criekinge T, Saeys W, Truijen S, Vereeck L, van Rompaey V, et al. An investigation of the spatio-temporal parameters of gait and margins of stability throughout adulthood. J R Soc Interface. 2020;17:20200194.

36. Mortaza N, Abu Osman NA, Mehdikhani N. Are the spatio-temporal parameters of gait capable of distinguishing a faller from a non-faller elderly? Eur J Phys Rehabil Med. 2014;50(6):677–91.
37. Jabbar KA, Seah WT, Lau LK, Pang BWJ, Ng DHM, Tan QLLT, et al. Fast gait spatiotemporal parameters in adults and association with muscle strength—the Yishun study. Gait Posture. 2021;85:217–23.
38. Kawai H, Taniguchi Y, Seino S, Sakurai R, Osuka Y, Obuchi S, et al. Reference values of gait parameters measured with a plantar pressure platform in community-dwelling older Japanese adults. Clin Interv Aging. 2019;14:1265.
39. Hollman JH, McDade EM, Petersen RC. Normative spatiotemporal gait parameters in older adults. Gait Posture. 2011;34(1):111–8.
40. Muehlbauer T, Granacher U, Borde R, Hortobagyi T. Non-discriminant relationships between leg muscle strength, mass and gait performance in healthy young and old adults. Gerontology. 2018;64(1):11–8.
41. Güner S, Haghari S, Inanıcı F, Alsancak S, Aytekın G. Knee muscle strength in multiple sclerosis: relationship with gait characteristics. J Phys Ther Sci. 2015;27(3):809–13.
42. Kawai H, Taniguchi Y, Seino S, Sakurai R, Osuka Y, Obuchi S, et al. Reference values of gait parameters measured with a plantar pressure platform in community-dwelling older Japanese adults. Clin Interv Aging. 2019;4:1265–76.
43. Kubinski SN, McQueen CA, Sittloh KA, Dean JC. Walking with wider steps increases stance phase gluteus medius activity. Gait Posture. 2015;41(1):130–5.
44. Chu NCW, Sturnieks DL, Lord SR, Menant JC. Visuospatial working memory and obstacle crossing in young and older people. Exp Brain Res. 2022;240(11):2871–83.
45. Yamagata M, Tateuchi H, Pataky T, Shimizu I, Ichihashi N. Relation between frontal plane center of mass position stability and foot elevation during obstacle crossing. J Biomech. 2021;116:110219.
46. Muir BC, Bodratti LA, Morris CE, Haddad JM, Emmerik REA, Rietdyk S. Gait characteristics during inadvertent obstacle contacts in young, middle- aged and older adults. Gait Posture. 2020;77:100–4.
47. Patla AE, Vickers J. How far ahead do we look when required to step on specific locations in the travel path during locomotion? Exp Brain Res. 2003;148:133–8.
48. Winter DA. The biomechanics and motor control of human gait: normal, elderly and pathological—. 2nd ed. Waterloo: Waterloo Biomechanics Press; 1991.
49. Chen H-CC, Ashton-Miller JA, Alexander NB, Schultz AB. Stepping over obstacles: gait patterns of healthy young and old adults. J Gerontol. 1991;46:M196–203.
50. Muir BC, Rietdyk S, Haddad JM, Heijnen MJH. Proactive gait strategies to mitigate risk of obstacle contact are more prevalent with advancing age. Gait Posture. 2015;41(1):233–9.
51. Pieruccini-Faria F, Sarquis-Adamson YS, Montero-Odasso M. Mild cognitive impairment affects obstacle negotiation in older adults: results from "gait and brain study". Gerontology. 2019;65(2):164–73.
52. Patla AE, Prentice SD, Gobbi LTB. Visual control of obstacle avoidance during locomotion: strategies in young children, young and older adults. Adv Psychol Res. 1996;114:257–77.
53. Rinaldi NM, Lim J, Hamill J, Van Emmerik R, Moraes R. Walking combined with reach-to-grasp while crossing obstacles at different distances. Gait Posture. 2018;65:1–7.
54. Fallahtafti F, Boron JB, Venema DM, Kim HJ, Yentes JM. Task specificity impacts dual-task interference in older adults. Aging Clin Exp Res. 2021;33(3):581–7.
55. Biazus-Sehn LF, Baptista RR, Mestriner RG, Loss BP, Aldabe D, Stigger FS. Influence of dual-tasking on straight ahead and curved walking in older adults. J Aging Phys Act. 2020;30(3):411–20.
56. Ehsani H, Mohler MJ, O'connor K, Zamrini E, Tirambulo C, Toosizadeh N. The association between cognition and dual-tasking among older adults: the effect of motor function type and cognition task difficulty. Clin Interv Aging. 2019;14:659–69.

57. Bayot M, Dujardin K, Dissaux L, Tard C, Defebvre L, Bonnet CT, et al. Can dual-task paradigms predict falls better than single task?—a systematic literature review. Neurophysiol Clin. 2020;50(6):401–40.
58. Rossi PG, De Andrade LP, Ansai JH, Farche ACS, Carnaz L, Dalpubel D, et al. Dual-task performance: influence of frailty, level of physical activity, and cognition. J Geriatr Phys Ther. 2019;42(3):E142E147.
59. Hennah C, Doumas M. Dual-task walking on real-world surfaces: adaptive changes in walking velocity, step width and step height in young and older adults. Exp Gerontol. 2023;177:112200.
60. Zukqwski LA, Iyigün G, Giuliani CA, Plummer P. Effect of the environment on gait and gaze behavior in older adult fallers compared to older adult non-fallers. PLoS One. 2021;15(3):e0230479.
61. Goh HT, Pearce M, Vas A. Task matters: an investigation on the effect of different secondary tasks on dual-task gait in older adults. BMC Geriatr. 2021;21(1):510.
62. Nobrega-Sousa P, Gobbi LTB, Orcioli-Silva D, Conceicao NRD, Beretta VS, Vitorio R. Prefrontal cortex activity during walking: effects of aging and associations with gait and executive function. Neurorehabil Neural Repair. 2020;34(10):915–24.
63. Castora-Binkley M, Peronto CL, Edwards JD, Small BJ. A longitudinal analysis of the influence of race on cognitive performance. J Gerontol B Psychol Sci Soc Sci. 2015;70(4):512–8.
64. Rinaldi NM, Moraes R. Older adults with history of falls are unable to perform walking and prehension movements simultaneously. Neuroscience. 2016;316:249–60.
65. Ivanenko Y, Gurfinkel VS. Human postural control. Front Neurosci. 2018;12
66. Shumway-Cook A, Woollacott M. Normal postural control. In: Motor control: Translating research into clinical practice. Baltimore: Lippincott Williams & Wilkins; 2007. p. 161–93.
67. Horak FB. Postural orientation and equilibrium: what do we need to know about neural control of balance to prevent falls? Age Ageing. 2006;35(suppl_2):ii7–11.
68. Rath R, Wade MG. The two faces of postural control in older adults: stability and function. EBioMedicine. 2017;21:5–6.
69. Gazzola JM, Caovilla HH, Doná F, Ganança MM, Ganança FF. A quantitative analysis of postural control in elderly patients with vestibular disorders using visual stimulation by virtual reality. Braz J Otorhinolaryngol. 2020;86(5):593–601.
70. Kędziorek J, Błażkiewicz M. Nonlinear measures to evaluate upright postural stability: a systematic review. Entropy. 2020;22(12)
71. Alcock L, O'Brien TD, Vanicek N. Association between somatosensory, visual and vestibular contributions to postural control, reactive balance capacity and healthy ageing in older women. Health Care Women Int. 2018;39(12):1366–80.
72. Sapmaz M, Mujdeci B. The effect of fear of falling on balance and dual task performance in the elderly. Exp Gerontol. 2021;147:111250.
73. Quijoux F, Nicolaï A, Chairi I, Bargiotas I, Ricard D, Yelnik A, et al. A review of center of pressure (COP) variables to quantify standing balance in elderly people: algorithms and open-access code*. Physiol Rep [Internet]. 2021;9(22):E15067.
74. Haddad JM, Gagnon JL, Hasson CJ, Van Emmerik REA, Hamill J. Evaluation of time-to-contact measures for assessing postural stability. J Appl Biomech. 2006;22(2):155–61.
75. Howcroft J, Lemaire ED, Kofman J, McIlroy WE. Elderly fall risk prediction using static posturography. PLoS One. 2017;12(2):E0172398.
76. Gadelha AB, Neri SGR, de Oliveira RJ, Bottaro M, de David AC, Vainshelboim B, et al. Severity of sarcopenia is associated with postural balance and risk of falls in community-dwelling older women. Exp Aging Res. 2018;44(3):258–69.
77. Tavares JT, Biasotto-Gonzalez DA, Boa Sorte Silva NC, Suzuki FS, Lucareli PRG, Politti F. Age-related changes in postural control in physically inactive older women. J Geriatr Phys Ther. 2019;42(3):E81.
78. Xu S, Yang Z, Wang D, Zhang S, Lu J, Lin J, et al. Enhanced assessment of human dynamic stability by eliminating the effect of body height: modeling and experiment study. Comput Methods Biomech Biomed Engin. 2023;26(9):1044–54.

79. Wang Q, Li L, Mao M, Sun W, Zhang C, Mao D, et al. The relationships of postural stability with muscle strength and proprioception are different among older adults over and under 75 years of age. J Exerc Sci Fit. 2022;20(4):328–34.
80. Tavares GMS, Pacheco BP, Gottlieb MGV, Müller DVK, Santos GM. Interaction between cognitive status, fear of falling, and balance in elderly persons. Clinics. 2020;75:E1612.
81. Horak FB, Wrisley DM, Frank J. The Balance Evaluation Systems Test (BESTest) to differentiate balance deficits. Phys Ther. 2009;89(5):484–98.
82. Carr S, Pichora-Fuller M, Li K, Campos J. Effects of age on listening and postural control during realistic multi-tasking conditions. Hum Mov Sci. 2020;73:102664.
83. Magalhães GV, Razuk M, Vieira LA, Rinaldi NM. Postural control performance of active and inactive older adults assessed through postural tasks with different levels of difficulty. Motriz: Revista de Educação Física. 2022;28:E10220015421.
84. Šarabon N, Kozinc Ž, Marković G. Effects of age, sex and task on postural sway during quiet stance. Gait Posture. 2022;92:60–4.
85. Saftari LN, Kwon OS. Ageing vision and falls: a review. J Physiol Anthropol. 2018;37(1):11.
86. Henry M, Baudry S. Age-related changes in leg proprioception: implications for postural control. J Neurophysiol. 2019;122(2):525–38.
87. Ferlinc A, Fabiani E, Velnar T, Gradisnik L. The importance and role of proprioception in the elderly: a short review. Materia Socio Medica. 2019;31:219.
88. Palazzo F, Nardi A, Lamouchideli N, Caronti A, Alashram A, Padua E, et al. The effect of age, sex and a firm-textured surface on postural control. Exp Brain Res. 2021;239:2181.
89. Andreato L, Oliveira D, Follmer B, Bertolini S. The influence of age and overweight or obesity on foot sensitivity and postural control: a systematic review. Australas J Ageing. 2020;39:39.
90. Viseux F, Lemaire A, Barbier F, Charpentier P, Leteneur S, Villeneuve P. How can the stimulation of plantar cutaneous receptors improve postural control? Review and clinical commentary. Neurophysiologie Clinique/Clin Neurophysiol. 2019;49:263–8.
91. Malcolm B, Foxe J, Joshi S, Verghese J, Mahoney J, Molholm S, et al. Aging-related changes in cortical mechanisms supporting postural control during base of support and optic flow manipulations. Eur J Neurosci. 2020;1–19:8139.
92. Phu S, Sturnieks D, Lord SR, Okubo Y. Impact of ageing, fall history and exercise on postural reflexes following unpredictable perturbations: a systematic review and meta-analyses. Mech Ageing Dev. 2022;203:E111634.
93. Li K, Bherer L, Mirelman A, Maidan I, Hausdorff J. Cognitive involvement in balance, gait and dual-tasking in aging: a focused review from a neuroscience of aging perspective. Front Neurol. 2018;9:913.
94. Dallaire M, Gagnon G, Fortin É, Nepton J, Severn AF, Côté S, et al. The impact of Parkinson's disease on postural control in older people and how sex can mediate these results: a systematic review. Geriatrics. 2021;6:105.
95. Pinho JP, Azevedo APS, Serrão JC, Forner-Cordero A, Amadio AC, Mezêncio B. Aging effects of haptic input on postural control under a dual-task paradigm. Exp Gerontol. 2022;168:E111928.
96. Thomas E, Battaglia G, Patti A, Brusa J, Leonardi V, Palma A, et al. Physical activity programs for balance and fall prevention in elderly: a systematic review. Medicine. 2019;98:E16218.
97. Dipietro L, Campbell WW, Buchner DM, Erickson KI, Powell KE, Bloodgood B, et al. Physical activity, injurious falls, and physical function in aging: an umbrella review. Med Sci Sports Exerc. 2019;51(6):1303.
98. Bacha JMR, Gomes GCV, de Freitas TB, Viveiro LAP, da Silva KG, Bueno GC, et al. Effects of kinect adventures games versus conventional physical therapy on postural control in elderly people: a randomized controlled trial. Games Health J. 2017;7(1):24–36.

Synergic Control of Action Stabilizing Vertical Posture

5

Sandra Maria Sbeghen Ferreira de Freitas,
Paulo Barbosa de Freitas,
and Janina Manzieri Prado-Rico

Abstract

The performance of voluntary movements requires the coordination of multiple elements, such as motor units, muscles, and joint motions. Humans have more motor elements than necessary to accomplish a given task, and the flexible interaction among those elements promoted the development of the motor abundance principle and the motor synergy hypothesis. The uncontrolled manifold (UCM) framework offers an analytical instrument to investigate this principle and hypothesis and provides insights into how the central nervous system controls and coordinates the motor elements to the task performance. In this chapter, we present the UCM approach, its core principles, and practical applications in the context of the synergic control of the upright posture. We also report how the UCM approach has been employed by researchers to answer hypothesis-driven questions pertaining to motor control in different populations. Lastly, we discuss the UCM approach as a promising tool for early detection of motor impairments and its potential as a valuable biomarker for neurological disorders.

S. M. S. F. de Freitas (✉)
Master and Doctoral Program in Physical Therapy, Universidade Cidade de São Paulo, São Paulo, Brazil
e-mail: sandra.freitas@unicid.edu.br

P. B. de Freitas
Interdisciplinary Graduate Program in Health Sciences, Universidade Cruzeiro do Sul, São Paulo, Brazil

J. M. Prado-Rico
Department of Neurology, The Pennsylvania State University College of Medicine and Milton S. Hershey Medical Center, Hershey, PA, USA

F. A. Barbieri et al. (eds.), *Locomotion and Posture in Older Adults*,
https://doi.org/10.1007/978-3-031-74123-4_5

Introduction

The production of voluntary movement, from the simplest to the most complex, relies on the control and coordinated actions of two or more motor elements at all levels of analysis (e.g., motor units, muscle activity, joint motion, or finger forces). For instance, performing a planar movement around the elbow toward a target requires the muscular contraction of the agonist muscle (e.g., triceps brachii) to generate force and torque, extend the elbow and reach the target. This muscle comprises hundreds of motor units that must coordinate their actions, activating and deactivating at certain moments with determined firing rates, to produce a specific force level. At a higher hierarchical level, this movement depends on the action of a primary muscle (e.g., triceps brachii) along with synergists (e.g., anconeus), stabilizers, and neutralizers. Furthermore, at the same level, antagonists (e.g., biceps brachialis) come into play to decelerate the movement as it approaches the target [1–3]. Similarly, we have more joints to control the upright standing posture [4] or walking [5], and more fingers to grasp an object [6] than necessary to perform these motor actions. Therefore, it can be assumed that there is redundancy in the human motor system, meaning that humans possess more motor elements than are required to achieve the goal of a given motor task [7].

In the field of motor control, the fact that the central nervous system (CNS) needs to control and coordinate numerous motor elements to produce a specific movement and achieve a determined goal has been interpreted as either a problem [7] or an advantage [9]. For a significant number of researchers (for a comprehensive review, see [10]), the redundancy in our motor system is viewed as a challenge that the CNS must address. This challenge was originally introduced by the Russian researcher Nicolai Bernstein, who coined it as the "degrees of freedom (DOFs) problem" [7, 8]. Some researchers recognize that the solution adopted by the CNS is to "freeze" the DOFs to limit or inhibit the action of one or more elements [10]. Others propose that the solution to the redundancy problem lies in optimization, which involves seeking a unique solution based on specific criteria for minimizing or maximizing certain parameters, such as minimizing energy expenditure, joint torque, or jerk (the third derivative of position), or maximizing movement smoothness (for a comprehensive review, see [11]).

A third group of researchers does not view motor redundancy as a problem but rather as a sophisticated and effective mechanism to simultaneously ensure both stability and flexibility in movement production [9, 12, 13]. In this view, relevant motor elements are controlled and coordinated to warrant the stability of one or more relevant performance variables associated with a specific movement. Consequently, success in performing a task or executing movements in an environment with constant variations in external forces and frequent changes in intrinsic body states depends on the CNS's ability to maintain the stability of important performance variables.

The term synergy is a key concept in explaining how multi-element coordination occurs in goal-directed movements. Some researchers define synergy as the process by which the CNS unites various elements (e.g., muscles, fingers, or joint angles), known as effectors, into smaller groups (coordinative structures) to reduce the number of degrees of freedom that need to be controlled by the system [14–16]. According to the motor abundance hypothesis, synergy can be defined as a neural organization responsible for controlling and coordinating the actions of multiple motor elements relevant to the performance of a specific motor task. This organization ensures that these elements *co-vary*, ultimately aiming to stabilize one or more performance variables [9, 17]. Therefore, the CNS attains movement control by creating combinations among effectors to achieve specific goals in a task, making this "coordinative structure" goal-and task-dependent. This neural organization not only makes the movements more effective (i.e., less variable) but also allows adaptation and adjustments of the movements to different situations and task conditions. Hence, two fundamental aspects of motor control are: (1) task performance *stability*, which refers to the ability of the CNS to control a task performance variable and restore it to a previous steady-state or trajectory after a small, transient perturbation, and (2) *agility*, which is the ability of the CNS to reduce stability (i.e., the strength of a synergy) to change posture and initiate a movement or change in the steady-state [18]. Understanding how stability and agility are reached through motor synergies is important, for instance, for designing rehabilitation programs for individuals with movement impairments or after recovering from injuries.

One way to determine whether the CNS generates motor synergy, according to the principle of motor abundance, is to examine the variability of the elemental variables (i.e., effectors) and the variability of one or more variables important for task performance. To accomplish this, an analytical approach developed by Scholz and Schöner and first published in 1999 [12], known as the Uncontrolled Manifold (UCM), has been employed. Since then, the UCM has been used to investigate the stability of actions in multi-element systems in both healthy individuals [12, 19–23] and those with neurological and orthopedic impairments (for a review, see [24]).

In this chapter, our goals are to: (1) present how the UCM analysis is performed and the outcomes calculated and (2) review the studies that employed the framework of the UCM hypothesis to comprehend the control and coordination of multiple elements in postural control.

Uncontrolled Manifold (UCM) Hypothesis

The framework of the UCM hypothesis posits that the CNS leverages the co-variation of elemental variables within a multi-dimensional space to reduce the variability (across trials, cycles, or time periods) of one or more crucial task goals, referred to as performance variables. In simpler terms, the UCM hypothesis suggests that during task execution, the CNS takes into account various elements that contribute to task performance, such as joint motion or muscle activation. These elemental variables are then organized by the CNS within a multi-dimensional space where they can interact. Through the manipulation of these variables, the CNS aims to enhance control or stability in task performance. This coordination enables the CNS to effectively reduce variability in task outcomes across different trials, cycles, or time periods. Ultimately, the goal is to optimize task performance by identifying movement patterns or coordination strategies that result in more consistent and accurate outcomes [12].

The UCM approach quantifies and distinguishes between the variability (measured by variance) of motor elements that tends to lead to errors in an important performance variable for the task, and the variability that reflects the use of flexible coordination patterns that maintain the stability of the salient performance variable [12, 13]. All the trial-to-trial variance of the motor elements are projected into the null space of the relationship between the elemental variables and performance variable. This variance is then divided into two components: the variance within the space that does not cause changes in the performance variable (the UCM subspace for that variable, V_{UCM}, "good" variance) and the variance within the space that is orthogonal to the UCM subspace, which does cause changes (i.e., error) in the performance variable (V_{ORT}, "bad" variance). Furthermore, a synergy index (ΔV) reflecting the difference between V_{UCM} and V_{ORT} is computed [25]. If the CNS aims to stabilize a specific performance variable and creates a synergy to control that particular task characteristic, the amount of V_{UCM}, normalized by the dimensionality of the corresponding spaces, will always be greater than the amount of V_{ORT}, also quantified by the dimensionality of its spaces. Conversely, if ΔV is negative, meaning that V_{ORT} is greater than V_{UCM}, it is concluded that the CNS is not actively involved in stabilizing that particular task performance variable [12, 13]. Therefore, ΔV is an outcome reflecting the level of stability of a determined performance variable.

Remaining upright while releasing a load requires individuals to change the body configuration and make adjustments in the postural synergy before performing an action to facilitate its execution [26]. In this task, it has been observed a drop in stability, indicated by a reduction in ΔV starting approximately 200 ms prior to the load release. The changes in the synergy control have been called as anticipatory synergy adjustments (ASAs). The outcomes used to describe ASA, reflecting agility, are the time of ASA initiation (*t*ASA) and the magnitude of the drop of ΔV ($\Delta\Delta V$). The *t*ASA is defined as the time when ΔV drops below its average steady-state value by more than two standard deviations until the movement initiation. The $\Delta\Delta V$ is the difference between ΔV in the steady state and ΔV at the movement initiation [27].

By getting familiar with the previously described UCM outcomes (V_{UCM}, V_{ORT}, ΔV, *t*ASA, and $\Delta\Delta V$), we can discuss, from the perspective of the UCM, the concept of synergy in postural tasks. Figure 5.1 depicts an example of a postural task involving rhythmic, whole-body voluntary movement with visual feedback of the center of pressure (COP) displayed on the computer monitor. During this task, the CNS adjusts the body posture by controlling the position of the center of mass (COM) relative to the base of support (the area between feet). For example, when standing upright, the CNS continuously adjusts the COM position to prevent falling. To achieve this, the CNS utilizes the co-variation of lower limb joint motions across cycles to stabilize the COM, a crucial performance variable, and maintain postural control [28–30]. Assuming that movements around the lower limb joints occur solely in the sagittal plane, there are three DOFs—one for each ankle, knee, and hip joint—that can be

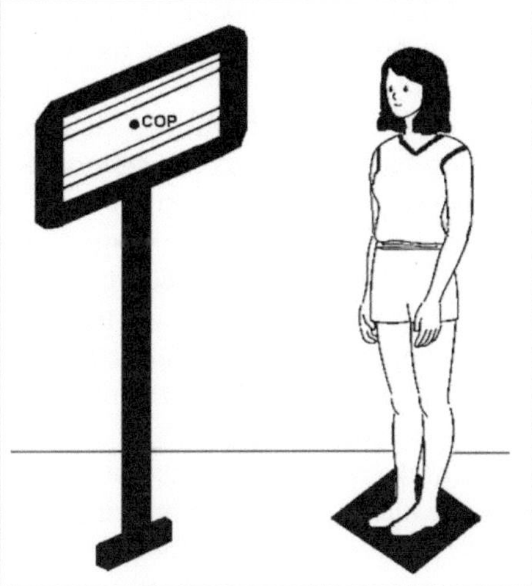

The mapping between small changes of the ankle, knee, and hip joint angles across trials and changes of the instantaneous COM position can be express as:

$$\begin{aligned}\Delta COM \approx\ & \Delta\alpha_A\ (c_S m_S L_{AK} + c_T m_T L_{KH} \\ & + c_{TR} m_{TR} L_{HCOM}) \\ & - \Delta\alpha_K\ (c_T m_T L_{KH} \\ & + c_{TR} m_{TR} L_{HCOM}) \\ & + \Delta\alpha_H\ (c_{TR} m_{TR} L_{HCOM})\end{aligned}$$

where m_S, m_T, and m_{TR} and c_S, c_T, and c_{TR} are the masses and positions of the COM of the shank, thigh, and trunk, respectively. L is the segment length defined between ankle and knee (AK), knee and hip (KH), and hip and COM position (HCOM).

Fig. 5.1 Participant's position (left side of the figure) for the whole-body movement in upright standing. Visual feedback of the COP is shown on the monitor screen as a black circle and participants need to move it up and down between targets. Changes of joint angles of lower limb (ankle, knee and hip) are geometrically related to changes of relevant performance variables, such as the COM position (right side of the figure)

used to achieve the task, while anterior–posterior COM position has only one DOF. Thus, we have three elemental variables (DOFs) to control a single performance variable, i.e., the anterior–posterior COM position. In each cycle of the whole-body movement, individuals may employ different combinations of the three joint motions, resulting in substantial variability (variance) within joint configurations that may not impact the performance variable (i.e., COM position). Conversely, specific combinations of joint motions across cycles may result in variability of the performance variable. Consequently, and as mentioned earlier, following the UCM approach, the overall variance in joint configurations can be decomposed into two distinct subspaces within joint space: the "good" joint variance (V_{UCM}), which has no bearing on performance and leads to an equivalent instantaneous anterior-posterior COM position; and the "bad" joint variance (V_{ORT}), which does impact performance, inducing variability in the COM position during upright stance.

Before going any further, we will present in a simplistic way how the UCM outcomes are calculated. The first step is to define the performance variable, the one we assume that is under direct control of the CNS, and the elemental variables, i.e., the effectors that are responsible for achieving the control of that specific performance variable. In our previous example, the performance variable is the instantaneous COM anterior–posterior position, and the elemental variables are the ankle, knee, and hip angles in the sagittal plane. The second and critical step in the UCM analysis is to establish the relationship between elemental variables and performance variable. In our example, this relationship should encompass the small changes in ankle, knee, and hip joint motions and their effects on the instantaneous COM position, a procedure known as estimating the Jacobian matrix. This estimation enables us to comprehend how variations in these joint angles influence the overall movement pattern of the body's COM.

The mapping between elemental and performance variables at the kinematic level, as illustrated in our example, for estimating Jacobian matrix is accomplished through a geometrical model (see Fig. 5.1). However, depending on the level of analysis or the specific performance variable under investigation, defining a geometrical model can be challenging and then other methods have been used. For example, in studies related to multi-muscle synergy, the assumption was that muscles did not operate independently [20, 30]. Consequently, groups of muscle activities (referred to as muscle modes or M-modes) were first defined as the elemental variables. The M-modes encompass coordinated activation patterns of multiple muscles. In the studies using the UCM approach, the M-modes collaborate to execute specific movements or tasks and are typically identified through principal component analysis (PCA) (for more details, refer to [20]). According to the principle of synergic control of movement applied to postural control, the CNS co-varies the magnitudes of the M-modes to stabilize a performance variable [20, 30], in this case, shifts in COP position. Hence, the establishment of the relationship (i.e., estimation the Jacobian matrix) between M-modes and specific performance variables (mainly the COP position) has been achieved through multiple linear regression (MLR) analysis. The coefficients obtained in this process were used to define the Jacobian matrix in the context of multi-muscle synergy studies. Since then, numerous studies, encompassing both healthy individuals [30–35] and those with or at risk of neurodegenerative diseases [36–38], have explored the utilization of M-modes and MLR analysis when assessing the postural stabilization during voluntary whole-body tasks and self-perturbation tasks (e.g., load-release tasks) during standing posture.

Research exploring the synergic control of maintaining an upright body position using the UCM approach has primarily focused on stabilizing either COM or COP position. These two task-related performance variables are well-documented in the literature as being under the regulation of the postural control system [4, 39]. While the COM is often observed as the main variable related to body position, COP position measurements, calculated from data acquired by force plates, offer greater reliability [28, 40]. Additionally, other variables, such as trunk orientation, may hold significance in postural stabilization [4]. Consequently, the choice of the performance variable can vary depending on the specific task's goals. Furthermore, it is important to acknowledge that the CNS may simultaneously control more than one performance variable to effectively execute the task [35].

As mentioned before, to apply the UCM approach effectively, it is crucial to establish an adequate relationship between elemental variables and performance variables (the Jacobian matrix). In kinematic synergy studies, many investigations have derived the Jacobian analytically by examining the connection between joint motion and COM position. However, the COP position is considered a significant performance variable in postural control research and is frequently used to assess the extent of postural sway during upright standing [28]. Previous kinematic synergy studies did not typically include COP position as a performance variable, primarily because establishing an analytical mapping between the two subspaces (joint motion and COP position) is not straightforward and, in some cases, can be exceedingly complex or even impossible. In an effort to address this challenge, Freitas and colleagues [40] undertook an approach where they mapped joint motion onto COP position changes using MLR analysis. Their findings indicated that COP position, similar to COM position (which yielded consistent results regardless of the method used to estimate the Jacobian), was indeed an important performance variable for addressing the synergic control of movement during upright standing tasks. This suggests that in cases where a formal geometric model is unavailable or overly complicated, the application of MLR analysis may be suitable for Jacobian matrix estimation, similar to that applied in multi-muscle synergy studies.

In the task depicted in Fig. 5.1, individuals are positioned on a force plate and engage in rhythmic body movements while receiving real-time visual feedback of the COP (black circle) displayed on a computer monitor. In this particular task, they were instructed to maintain stability by preventing excessive foot motion and avoiding falls, moving the COP between target zones delimited by two horizontal lines. Consequently, the successful execution of this task may necessitate the implicit or explicit control of both COM and COP, as per the task instructions. Furthermore, in such a task, an additional performance variable may require stabilization by the controller: the orientation of the trunk. The stability of the trunk plays a crucial role in supporting the head and ensuring clear vision of the computer monitor.

Consider a similar experimental setup as depicted in Fig. 5.1. However, instead of engaging in rhythmic body movements, individuals are asked to stand as still as possible while receiving visual feedback of the COP at the center of the computer monitor. In this context, their goal is to minimize postural sway, which is reflected by changes in COP position. According to the existing literature, during quiet upright standing, postural sway is primarily (if not exclusively) regulated by the ankle joint, known as the "ankle strategy." However, in certain situations that demand rapid responses, a combination of ankle and hip joint movements, referred to as the "hip strategy," may come into play [41–43]. Within the UCM framework, various flexible patterns of joint coordination are recognized for stabilizing body position. The flexibility of joint coordination exemplifies the principle of motor abundance. This principle involves leveraging a variety of potential multi-joint solutions. Specifically, rather than relying on the work of a single joint or on the combination of two, the system has at its disposal multiple joint combinations that can be employed to achieve postural stability [29, 36, 39]. Therefore, it is argued that the hip and ankle strategies represent only the extremes of a continuum encompassing numerous possible coordination patterns [44]. The postural control system can then select the most adequate solution to maintain the upright quiet stance or respond to internal or external perturbations.

Three hypothetical models have been proposed to elucidate the synergic movement control based on the structure of the two variance components (V_{UCM} and $V_{ORT,}$ as illustrated in Fig. 5.2) and ΔV during a quiet standing task [28, 39]. When the synergy index surpasses zero, it indicates that the stability of a particular significant performance variable is achieved through synergic control. The hypothetical models

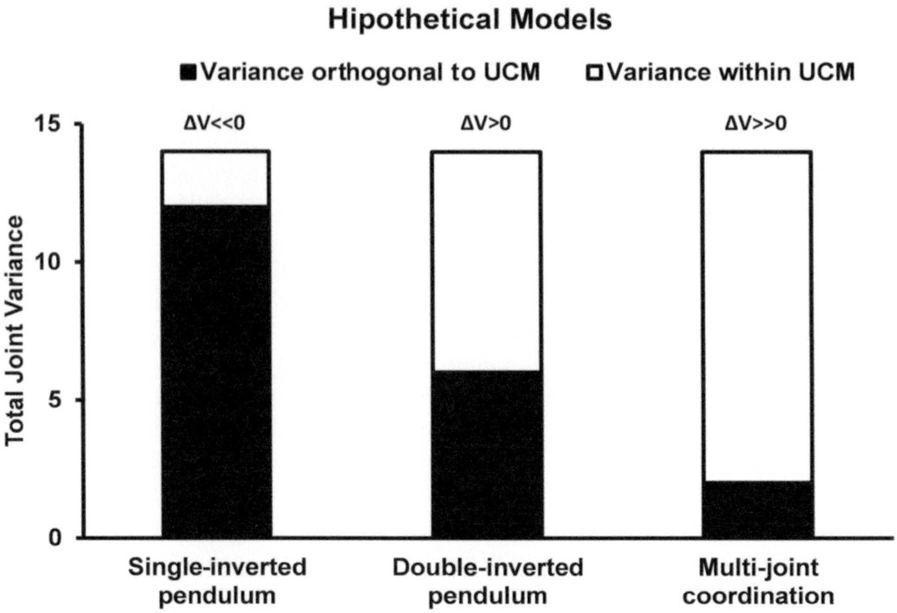

Fig. 5.2 Hypothetical models for changes on the variance components, orthogonal (V_{ORT}, black) and within (V_{UCM}, white) the UCM for single ("ankle" strategy), double-inverted ("hip" strategy) pendulum, and multi-joint coordination during quiet standing. The hipothetical ΔV (i.e., synergy index) is presented for each hypothetical model

operate under the assumption that the configuration of variance components varies depending on the chosen motor strategy for task execution. In the first hypothetical model, which corresponds to employing an ankle strategy to regulate postural sway (similar to a single-inverted pendulum), alterations in ankle motion would result in corresponding changes in COP position. Consequently, a larger V_{ORT} would be expected in comparison to V_{UCM}, as depicted in the left bar graph of Fig. 5.2 (where $\Delta V \ll 0$ because $V_{ORT} \gg V_{UCM}$). Alternatively, the adoption of a hip strategy (similar to a double-inverted pendulum; middle bar graph in Fig. 5.2) may reduce changes in COP position (where $\Delta V > 0$ because $V_{ORT} < V_{UCM}$), although not to the same extent as envisioned in the third hypothetical model (right bar graph in Fig. 5.2). The third model represents the utilization of motor abundance, where multi-joint angles exhibit co-variation, leading to an increased amount of variance within the UCM (which does not affect COP position) and a decreased amount of variance orthogonal to the UCM. If this scenario holds true, it becomes plausible to assert the existence of a synergic control mechanism in place to stabilize upright posture (where $\Delta V \gg 0$ because $V_{UCM} \gg V_{ORT}$).

Application of UCM Hypothesis to Postural Control

Since the seminal study by Scholz and Schöner published in 1999 [12], the UCM hypothesis has been applied to investigate the synergic control of various tasks in upright standing. Some of these tasks include self-induced posture perturbations [20, 30], voluntary movements involving the entire body [4], or even maintaining as still as possible (quiet upright posture; [29]). The initial studies on the synergic control of upright posture aimed to understand how a set of muscle actions (the M-modes) or joint motions varies across trials or over time to stabilize significant task-related variables. This synergic control of movement is crucial for maintaining postural stability in upright standing, such as COP [30] and COM [4, 29] position or trunk orientation [4]. It is important to note that stabilizing COP or COM position implies reducing their variability in comparison to situations that would lead to greater body instability, which would negatively affect balance.

The initial studies explore the utilization of multi-muscle synergies by individuals to perform various tasks while maintaining an upright stance [20, 30, 45]. These tasks included releasing a load with extended arms, executing rapid bilateral arm movements, or voluntarily adjusting their COP position based on visual feedback in front of them [30]. In those studies, three M-modes were identified from a group of 11 leg and trunk muscles and used in the UCM analysis, assuming that these M-modes were employed to stabilize the COP shift. The conclusion was drawn from the observation that the good M-mode variance (V_{UCM}) exceeded the bad variance (V_{ORT}); that is, ΔV was positive. It is important to note that this was only evident when the COP shift was in the same direction as the data used to establish the Jacobian matrix [30]. Overall, the studies concluded that fewer control variables (in this case, M-modes rather than individual muscle activities) co-vary to achieve a specific COP position and M-modes are scaled by the CNS in a manner that stabilizes specific COP positions while preserving their shift direction.

In the kinematic control level (i.e., joint motion space), a similar task used in the previous study (i.e., voluntary moving of the COP position displayed as visual feedback) was examined [4]. The authors hypothesized that kinematic synergies played a role in stabilizing two distinct task variables: trunk orientation and COM position [4]. In this study, kinematic synergies were assumed to be employed during cyclic voluntary movements while visual feedback was provided on a computer monitor, focusing either on the COP or a specific individual joint motion (i.e., hip, knee, or ankle). Additionally, two other task parameters were manipulated, reflecting the interplay between speed and accuracy: the range of motion and increased task difficulty. As the tasks involved cyclic movements, the UCM analysis was conducted between cycles (as opposed to between trials performed in prior studies). The joint angles of the hip, knee, and ankle were geometrically associated with both the COM position and trunk orientation. The UCM results indicated that the variance in hip, knee, and ankle joint motion was constrained to the UCM subspace (i.e., large V_{UCM}). This alignment was consistent with the stabilization of the two chosen task variables, regardless of variations in task parameters, such as amplitude, accuracy, or the type of visual feedback. Notably, the authors observed that ΔV remained consistent across different task parameters. However, they noted changes in the effects on two variance components: both V_{UCM} and V_{ORT} decreased with a reduced range of motion and increased task difficulty (i.e., smaller targets). These findings supported the notion of modulating elemental variables in joint motion level to stabilize two significant task-related variables. In light of these results, the authors concluded that the synergies employed during whole-body voluntary movements served dual purposes: maintaining the stability of sensory information flow (consistent with the hypothesis of trunk orientation stabilization) and ensuring postural stability (in line with the hypothesis of COM stabilization). Furthermore, these findings provided support to the idea that different motor synergies are employed to stabilize multiple task-related variables; thereby contributing to the successful execution of the task. Notably, this study also laid the groundwork for future research to identify other important task-related variables associated with whole-body voluntary movements, such as COP position [40].

Other studies have also explored the stabilization of the COP position but have consistently focused on assessing multi-muscle synergies [46, 47]. In one particular study, researchers investigated the role of multi-muscle synergies in stabilizing the COP position both before and during a voluntary shift [47]. Their findings revealed that multi-muscle synergies effectively stabilized the COP position in the anterior-posterior direction before the voluntary COP shift. However, intriguingly, this stabilization did not persist during the actual movement. The observed synergy structure appeared to diminish, likely due to decreased variance in the UCM space (V_{UCM}), increased variance in the orthogonal space (V_{ORT}), or a combination of both factors. Consequently, the synergy index approached or dipped below zero. This led the researchers to speculate that alterations in multi-muscle synergies were necessary to facilitate a rapid motor response, specifically the rapid COP shift in response to an imperative light signal [47].

It has been speculated that joint motion variability occurs even when individuals attempt to stand quietly, which is closely associated with the observable postural sway. Therefore, to investigate whether kinematic synergy plays a role in preserving the stability of the head [39, 48, 49], COM [29, 39, 48–51], and COP [28] position, researchers applied the UCM approach using a range of kinematic elemental variables, involving three to nine DOFs. In these studies, the investigators consistently observed that the task of quiet standing was achieved through coordinated variations in joint motion strategically employed to stabilize the critical postural control variables. Furthermore, when visual information was absent (i.e., in participants with closed eyes), changes in joint motion increased, but their variance was predominantly constrained within the UCM subspace, thus minimally impacting the COM position, for example [29]. Once again, these findings strongly suggested that synergies can be adapted by the CNS to effectively stabilize important performance variables due to task instruction.

Changes in the synergic control of the quiet standing task were also observed when individuals engaged in either a motor [33, 50, 52–55] or cognitive [51, 56] dual-task. When performing a secondary motor task involving holding a tray with or without a ball and moving it between targets while standing, the joint motion variance increased, primarily within the UCM subspace [50]. This increase did not significantly affect the synergy structure, indicating that the CNS capitalizes on the joint motion variance to maintain the COM position. Conversely, when a cognitive task was carried out during quiet standing, there was a reduction in the COP changes accompanied by decreased joint motion variance that could otherwise lead to COP alterations (V_{ORT}) [51, 56]. Furthermore, this scaled-down reduction in V_{ORT} due to the performance of the secondary task did not disrupt the structure of kinematic synergy. Instead, it allowed more flexibility in maintaining an upright stance while concurrently executing the cognitive task, particularly when considering a greater number of DOFs in the model [56]. In summary, it can be argued that the execution of a secondary task, whether motor or cognitive, affects the total joint motion variance but leaves the synergy structure intact. Consequently, the CNS effectively utilizes the available DOFs to stabilize the COM position while simultaneously handling other tasks. Tomita and colleagues [52, 57] also proposed a prioritization of COM position stabilization during the performance of reaching a target with the index finger while standing. This prioritization was particularly evident in less stable conditions of the base of support [52]. They made this observation when applying the UCM approach at the kinematic level with a whole-body model comprising 49 DOFs, comparing the variance components (V_{UCM} and V_{ORT}) and the synergy index between two performance variables: the stability of the fingertip position and the COM position. Their findings revealed that synergic control was consistently maintained for the COM position throughout the movement trajectory, but not for the index fingertip position [52]. The latter exhibited reduced control during the deceleration phase of the movement. This effect on the fingertip position was more pronounced under unstable conditions, suggesting that this phase necessitates increased compensatory control (and, subsequently, greater neural resources) to successfully achieve the target while preserving postural stability.

Synergic control during upright standing, operating at multiple levels including muscle and kinematics, plays a critical role in maintaining the position of the body's COM. At the muscle torque level, this control is closely associated with stabilizing the movements of the COM [58]. When individuals maintain a quiet, upright posture, their muscles are activated in response to neural commands, generating torques at various joints to ensure postural stability. Consequently, it is reasonable to consider that synergic control at the muscle torque level is primarily linked to the neural mechanisms responsible for stabilizing posture. The single-inverted pendulum model or ankle strategy has established that upright standing is primarily regulated through ankle joint torques [41, 42]. However, the double-inverted pendulum model (the hip strategy) involves the coordination of torques around both the ankle and hip joints to control balance. The work by Park and colleagues [58], employing the UCM approach, showed that the coordination among torques at the ankle, knee, and hip joints contributes to the stabilization of COM movements. These findings lend support to the idea that multiple joints can cooperate to maintain upright standing, extending beyond the traditional focus on just the ankle or hip joints. Nevertheless, it's important to note that the study by Park and colleagues only assessed three joint motions and torques. Future research with a more comprehensive examination of

DOFs would be needed to explore the potential involvement of additional proximal joints in the synergic control of muscle torques during upright standing.

Clinical Application of the UCM Approach

The majority of research on synergic control of upright posture has focused on healthy, young individuals. However, there have been some studies conducted on individuals with balance issues, including older adults [28, 59], those with Parkinson's disease (PD) [36, 38, 60, 61], cerebellar ataxia [62], and stroke survivors [57] (for a comprehensive review, refer to [24]). The application of the UCM approach offers a distinct advantage when examining synergic control in individuals with balance problems. It allows for a direct link between the variability in elemental space (regardless of the level) and the impaired crucial task-related variables during upright standing. These findings not only reveal the extent of elemental variability in specific situations but also how these elements interact to achieve a particular goal with reduced variability, thereby preserving stability.

In the case of older adults, the synergy structure for maintaining a quiet standing posture is generally preserved. However, it may exhibit less flexibility (lower V_{UCM}) when compared to young adults [28, 59]. Furthermore, this flexibility can be influenced by changes in sensory conditions, such as alterations in visual information (e.g., with or without real-time visual feedback) [28].

Deficits in the synergic control of movement in PD have been associated with a decrease in the stability of actions measured by the ΔV, during the steady-state phase of a postural task [26, 38]. These patients also present impairment in agility [26], which involves preparing for quick actions and is measured using the *t*ASA and $\Delta\Delta V$ described before [18, 26, 38, 60]. Postural instability is considered one of the most clinically significant features of PD. While postural deficits are typically seen in more advanced stages of the Hoehn and Yahr scale (H&Y, [63]), certain aspects of postural control exhibit changes even in the early stages of the disease (H&Y stages I and II). Patients with PD at H&Y stages I-II, who do not yet exhibit clinical postural instability, have been found to show reduced V_{UCM} in the M-modes when compared to healthy individuals [60]. Additionally, they exhibit lower synergy index but have a similar level of variance in M-modes related to changes in the COP position [36, 60]. Collectively, these findings suggest that individuals in the early stages of PD may struggle to leverage motor abundance when performing tasks such as releasing a load while standing.

In patients undergoing levodopa treatment, the impact of dopamine-replacement therapy has shown a positive effect on multi-muscle synergies preceding self-triggered postural perturbations, as observed in studies by Falaki and colleagues [26] and Freitas and collaborators [38]. Individuals with Parkinson's disease (PD) in the on-drug state have improved multi-muscle synergy organization, showing higher steady state synergy index values and longer ASA than individuals in the off-drug state [26]. Interestingly, even levodopa-naïve PD patients exhibited an immediate impact on their synergy index after taking their first dose of levodopa at the beginning of their treatment [38]. These findings suggest that PD patients exhibit increased behavioral flexibility and enhanced feedforward control of movement following levodopa replacement therapy.

Complementing dopamine-replacement therapy, deep brain stimulation (DBS) has been recognized as an effective treatment for motor symptoms, especially in advanced stages of PD [64]. In PD patients with DBS implants, there was an observed improvement in ASA indices during the DBS-on state while performing postural tasks [65]. This suggests that DBS treatment may offer benefits in modifying synergies in preparation for rapid actions, such as potentially mitigating freezing of gait (FOG), a significant and disabling motor symptom in PD. It is important to emphasize that deficits in ASA have been considered potential contributors to FOG [18, 60]. In a recent study focusing on multi-muscle synergies during step initiation, a crucial component of gait, PD patients exhibited smaller ASA indices compared to age-matched controls. This observation supports the hypothesis that impaired feedforward control may be a contributing factor to FOG [61]. This could be an area of interest for future studies.

The UMC approach has emerged as a highly sensitive tool, offering potential value as an early biomarker for PD and the early detection of postural instability during the disease's initial stages [38]. Moreover, this approach has demonstrated its capability to identify preclinical motor deficits in individuals who are asymptomatic but at risk of developing neurodegenerative conditions, as highlighted in previous studies [37, 66]. In particular, chronic exposure to welding fumes, which can include overexposure to substances like manganese, has been linked to neurobehavioral impairments [67, 68]. Investigations involving asymptomatic welders have uncovered significant alterations in the synergic control of hand movements and multi-muscle synergies during postural tasks [37, 66]. These findings have shown strong correlations with MRI-detected changes in brain structures such as the basal ganglia and cerebellum-related structures [37, 66]. Together, the UCM analysis outcomes appear to hold great promise as an approach for assessing motor deficits in preclinical stages. This promising avenue could lead to early prevention strategies and future therapeutic interventions, providing valuable insights into the management of neurodegenerative diseases.

Indeed, these studies have significantly contributed to our deepened understanding of synergic control in individuals dealing with balance problems caused by aging or neurological diseases (for further insights, refer to [18]). However, it is important that only a limited number of investigations has explored other populations with diverse health conditions. For instance, studies have examined synergic control during upright standing in individuals coping with chronic non-specific low back pain, comparing them to pain-free controls [69], as well as individuals with motor-incomplete spinal cord injuries [70]. This becomes particularly intriguing when considering that both of these groups may encounter balance challenges. Nevertheless, there remains a crucial need for more comprehensive research to explore whether the synergic control employed to stabilize task-related variables is consistently preserved across a broader spectrum of individuals dealing with balance problems.

While certain health conditions can alter the synergic control of upright posture, research has shown that engaging in balance training, such as standing on an unstable surface (for example, a board with a narrow beam), actually enhance synergic control [32]. Interestingly, the practice of dance has also been found to improve multi-muscle synergies used by older adults to stabilize their COP position during perturbed upright standing [71]. Similar outcomes demonstrating improved synergic control through practice have been reported in tasks involving fine motor skills, even at the level of the finger forces [72, 73]. Overall, these findings suggest that synergies can be enhanced through regular practice, resulting in a reduction in variability associated with changes in task-related variables and an increase in the flexibility of combining elemental variables. These insights hold clinical significance, particularly for individuals dealing with balance issues, including older adults both with and without PD. To expand our understanding further, future studies should explore how the synergic control of upright standing evolves in individuals with impaired postural stability following the practice of balance tasks, as well as other forms of exercise and sports activities.

Final Considerations

Synergic control, as described here, represents how the CNS efficiently utilizes the wide array of available motor elements, such as muscle activity, joint motions, and torques, to stabilize important performance variables while performing specific movements. The UCM hypothesis has emerged as a valuable tool for investigating the utilization of motor abundance, particularly in tasks related to maintaining an upright standing posture. Synergic control becomes evident when individuals are required to respond to external perturbations, make adjustments to their posture due to self-induced perturbations, engage in whole-body voluntary movements, or simply maintain a stable and quiet posture. The synergy indices, as measured using the UCM approach, exhibit variations depending on the specific task and are scaled with respect to certain task parameters. This underscores the UCM approach's capability to detect subtle alterations in the synergic control of upright posture. Individuals dealing with balance impairments resulting from aging or neurological disorders often display reduced synergy indices. However, it is noteworthy that these indices can potentially be improved through targeted training, specific tasks, various physical exercises, or participation in sports. This observation holds significant relevance and should be a focal point for future studies, as the findings have the potential to inform and shape future therapeutic interventions.

References

1. Marsden CD, Obeso JA, Rothwell JC. The function of the antagonist muscle during fast limb movements in man. J Physiol. 1983;335:1–13.

2. Gottlieb GL, Corcos DM, Agarwal GC. Organizing principles for single-joint movements. I. A speed-insensitive strategy. J Neurophysiol. 1989;62:342–57.
3. Gottlieb GL, Song QL, Almeida GL, Hong DA, Corcos D. Directional control of planar human arm movement. J Neurophysiol. 1997;78:2985–98.
4. Freitas SMSF, Duarte M, Latash ML. Two kinematic synergies in voluntary whole-body movements during standing. J Neurophysiol. 2006;95:636–45.
5. Krishnan V, Rosenblatt NJ, Latash ML, Grabiner MD. The effects of age on stabilization of the mediolateral trajectory of the swing foot. Gait Posture. 2013;38:923–8.
6. Zatsiorsky VM, Latash ML. Multifinger prehension: an overview. J Mot Behav. 2008;40:446–75.
7. Bernstein N. The co-ordination and regulation of movements. London: Pergamon Press; 1967.
8. Latash ML, editor. Bernstein's construction of movements: the original text and commentaries; 2020. https://doi.org/10.4324/9780367816797.
9. Latash ML. The bliss (not the problem) of motor abundance (not redundancy). Exp Brain Res. 2012;217:1–5.
10. Guimarães AN, Ugrinowitsch H, Dascal JB, Porto AB, Okazaki VHA. Freezing degrees of freedom during motor learning: a systematic review. Mot Control. 2020;24:457–71.
11. Todorov E. Optimality principles in sensorimotor control. Nat Neurosci. 2004;7:907–15.
12. Scholz JP, Schöner G. The uncontrolled manifold concept: identifying control variables for a functional task. Exp Brain Res. 1999;126:289–306.
13. Scholz JP, Schöner G. Use of the Uncontrolled Manifold (UCM) approach to understand motor variability, motor equivalence, and self-motion. In: Levin MF, editor. Progress in motor control. New York: Springer; 2014. p. 91–100.
14. d'Avella A, Saltiel P, Bizzi E. Combinations of muscle synergies in the construction of a natural motor behavior. Nat Neurosci. 2003;6:300–8.
15. Ting LH, Macpherson JM. Ratio of shear to load ground-reaction force may underlie the directional tuning of the automatic postural response to rotation and translation. J Neurophysiol. 2004;92:808–23.
16. Ivanenko YP, Grasso R, Macellari V, Lacquaniti F. Control of foot trajectory in human locomotion: role of ground contact forces in simulated reduced gravity. J Neurophysiol. 2002;87:3070–89.
17. Latash ML, Scholz JP, Schoner G. Toward a new theory of motor synergies. Mot Control. 2007;11:276–308.
18. Latash ML, Huang X. Neural control of movement stability: lessons from studies of neurological patients. Neuroscience. 2015;301:39–48.
19. Scholz JP, Danion F, Latash ML, Schoner G. Understanding finger coordination through analysis of the structure of force variability. Biol Cybern. 2002;86:29–39.
20. Krishnamoorthy V, Latash ML, Scholz JP, Zatsiorsky VM. Muscle synergies during shifts of the center of pressure by standing persons. Exp Brain Res. 2003;152:281–92.
21. de Freitas PB, Freitas SMSF, Lewis MM, Huang X, Latash ML. Individual preferences in motor coordination seen across the two hands: relations to movement stability and optimality. Exp Brain Res. 2019;237:1–13.
22. Shim JK, Park J, Zatsiorsky VM, Latash ML. Adjustments of prehension synergies in response to self-triggered and experimenter-triggered load and torque perturbations. Exp Brain Res. 2006;175:641–53.
23. Yamagata M, Tateuchi H, Shimizu I, Ichihashi N. The effects of fall history on kinematic synergy during walking. J Biomech. 2019;82:204–10.
24. Vaz DV, Pinto VA, Junior RRS, Mattos DJS, Mitra S. Coordination in adults with neurological impairment—a systematic review of uncontrolled manifold studies. Gait Posture. 2019;69:66–78.
25. Park J, Singh T, Zatsiorsky VM, Latash ML. Optimality vs. variability: effect of fatigue in multi-finger redundant tasks. Exp Brain Res. 2012;216:591–607.

26. Falaki A, Huang X, Lewis MM, Latash ML. Dopaminergic modulation of multi-muscle synergies in postural tasks performed by patients with Parkinson's disease. J Electromyogr Kinesiol. 2017;33:20–6.
27. Latash ML. Towards physics of neural processes and behavior. Neurosci Biobehav Rev. 2016;69:136–46.
28. Freitas SMSF, Duarte M. Joint coordination in young and older adults during quiet stance: effect of visual feedback of the center of pressure. Gait Posture. 2012;35:83–7.
29. Krishnamoorthy V, Yang J-F, Scholz JP. Joint coordination during quiet stance: effects of vision. Exp Brain Res. 2005;164:1–17.
30. Krishnamoorthy V, Latash ML, Scholz JP, Zatsiorsky VM. Muscle modes during shifts of the center of pressure by standing persons: effect of instability and additional support. Exp Brain Res. 2004;157:18–31.
31. Danna-Dos-Santos A, Slomka K, Zatsiorsky VM, Latash ML. Muscle modes and synergies during voluntary body sway. Exp Brain Res. 2007;179:533–50.
32. Asaka T, Wang Y, Fukushima J, Latash ML. Learning effects on muscle modes and multi-mode postural synergies. Exp Brain Res. 2008;184:323–38.
33. Krishnan V, Aruin AS, Latash ML. Two stages and three components of the postural preparation to action. Exp Brain Res. 2011;212:47–63.
34. Klous M, Mikulic P, Latash ML. Two aspects of feedforward postural control: anticipatory postural adjustments and anticipatory synergy adjustments. J Neurophysiol. 2011;105:2275–88.
35. Klous M, Danna-dos-Santos A, Latash ML. Multi-muscle synergies in a dual postural task: evidence for the principle of superposition. Exp Brain Res. 2010;202:457–71.
36. Falaki A, Huang X, Lewis MM, Latash ML. Motor equivalence and structure of variance: multi-muscle postural synergies in Parkinson's disease. Exp Brain Res. 2017;235:2243–58.
37. de Freitas PB, Freitas SMSF, Prado-Rico JM, Lewis MM, Du G, Yanosky JD, Huang X, Latash ML. Synergic control in asymptomatic welders during multi-finger force exertion and load releasing while standing. Neurotoxicology. 2022;93:324–36.
38. Freitas SMSF, de Freitas PB, Falaki A, Corson T, Lewis MM, Huang X, Latash ML. Synergic control of action in levodopa-naïve Parkinson's disease patients: II. Multi-muscle synergies stabilizing vertical posture. Exp Brain Res. 2020;238:2931–45.
39. Hsu W-L, Scholz JP, Schöner G, Jeka JJ, Kiemel T. Control and estimation of posture during quiet stance depends on multi-joint coordination. J Neurophysiol. 2007;97:3024–35.
40. Freitas SMSF, Scholz JP, Latash ML. Analyses of joint variance related to voluntary whole-body movements performed in standing. J Neurosci Methods. 2010;188:89–96.
41. Winter DA, Prince F, Frank JS, Powell C, Zabjek KF. Unified theory regarding A/P and M/L balance in quiet stance. J Neurophysiol. 1996;75:2334–43.
42. Gatev P, Thomas S, Kepple T, Hallett M. Feedforward ankle strategy of balance during quiet stance in adults. J Physiol. 1999;514(Pt 3):915–28.
43. de Freitas PB, Freitas SMSF, Duarte M, Latash ML, Zatsiorsky VM. Effects of joint immobilization on standing balance. Hum Mov Sci. 2009;28:515–28.
44. Reimann H, Schöner G. A multi-joint model of quiet, upright stance accounts for the "uncontrolled manifold" structure of joint variance. Biol Cybern. 2017;111:389–403.
45. Krishnamoorthy V, Goodman S, Zatsiorsky V, Latash ML. Muscle synergies during shifts of the center of pressure by standing persons: identification of muscle modes. Biol Cybern. 2003;89:152–61.
46. Nardini AG, Freitas SMSF, Falaki A, Latash ML. Preparation to a quick whole-body action: control with referent body orientation and multi-muscle synergies. Exp Brain Res. 2019;237:1361–74.
47. Wang Y, Asaka T, Zatsiorsky VM, Latash ML. Muscle synergies during voluntary body sway: combining across-trials and within-a-trial analyses. Exp Brain Res. 2006;174:679–93.
48. Verrel J, Pradon D, Vuillerme N. Persistence of motor-equivalent postural fluctuations during bipedal quiet standing. PLoS One. 2012;7:e48312.

49. Scholz JP, Park E, Jeka JJ, Schöner G, Kiemel T. How visual information links to multi-joint coordination during quiet standing. Exp Brain Res. 2012;222:229–39.
50. Hsu W-L, Scholz JP. Motor abundance supports multitasking while standing. Hum Mov Sci. 2012;31:844–62.
51. Hagio K, Obata H, Nakazawa K. Effects on postural kinematics of performing a cognitive task during upright standing. Percept Mot Skills. 2020;127:639–50.
52. Tomita Y, Iizuka T, Turpin NA. Effects of postural instability on the coordination between posture and arm reaching. Hum Mov Sci. 2023;89:103088.
53. Wang Y, Zatsiorsky VM, Latash ML. Muscle synergies involved in shifting the center of pressure while making a first step. Exp Brain Res. 2005;167:196–210.
54. Wang Y, Zatsiorsky VM, Latash ML. Muscle synergies involved in preparation to a step made under the self-paced and reaction time instructions. Clin Neurophysiol. 2006;117:41–56.
55. Hsu W-L. Adaptive postural control for joint immobilization during multitask performance. PLoS One. 2014;9:e108667.
56. Azimi R, Abdoli B, Sanjari MA, Khosrowabadi R. Variability of postural coordination in dual-task paradigm. J Mot Behav. 2023:1–8.
57. Tomita Y, Turpin NA, Piscitelli D, Feldman AG, Levin MF. Stability of reaching during standing in stroke. J Neurophysiol. 2020;123:1756–65.
58. Park E, Reimann H, Schöner G. Coordination of muscle torques stabilizes upright standing posture: an UCM analysis. Exp Brain Res. 2016;234:1757–67.
59. Hsu W-L, Lin K-H, Yang R-S, Cheng C-H. Use of motor abundance in old adults in the regulation of a narrow-based stance. Eur J Appl Physiol. 2014;114:261–71.
60. Falaki A, Huang X, Lewis MM, Latash ML. Impaired synergic control of posture in Parkinson's patients without postural instability. Gait Posture. 2016;44:209–15.
61. Falaki A, Cuadra C, Lewis MM, Prado-Rico JM, Huang X, Latash ML. Multi-muscle synergies in preparation for gait initiation in Parkinson's disease. Clin Neurophysiol. 2023;154:12–24.
62. Monaco V, Aprigliano F, Lofrumento M, Martelli D, Micera S, Agrawal S. Uncontrolled manifold analysis of the effects of a perturbation-based training on the organization of leg joint variance in cerebellar ataxia. Exp Brain Res. 2021;239:501–13.
63. Hoehn MM, Yahr MD. Parkinsonism: onset, progression and mortality. Neurology. 1967;17:427–42.
64. Fox SH, Katzenschlager R, Lim S-Y, Barton B, de Bie RMA, Seppi K, Coelho M, Sampaio C, Movement Disorder Society Evidence-Based Medicine Committee. International Parkinson and movement disorder society evidence-based medicine review: update on treatments for the motor symptoms of Parkinson's disease. Mov Disord. 2018;33:1248–66.
65. Falaki A, Jo HJ, Lewis MM, O'Connell B, De Jesus S, McInerney J, Huang X, Latash ML. Systemic effects of deep brain stimulation on synergic control in Parkinson's disease. Clin Neurophysiol. 2018;129:1320–32.
66. Lewis MM, Lee E-Y, Jo HJ, Du G, Park J, Flynn MR, Kong L, Latash ML, Huang X. Synergy as a new and sensitive marker of basal ganglia dysfunction: a study of asymptomatic welders. Neurotoxicology. 2016;56:76–85.
67. Sanchez-Ramos J, Reimer D, Zesiewicz T, Sullivan K, Nausieda PA. Quantitative analysis of tremors in welders. Int J Environ Res Public Health. 2011;8:1478–90.
68. Cersosimo MG, Koller WC. The diagnosis of manganese-induced parkinsonism. Neurotoxicology. 2006;27:340–6.
69. McCaskey MA, Wirth B, Schuster-Amft C, de Bruin ED. Dynamic multi-segmental postural control in patients with chronic non-specific low back pain compared to pain-free controls: a cross-sectional study. PLoS One. 2018;13:e0194512.
70. Lee JW, Chan K, Unger J, Yoo J, Musselman KE, Masani K. Interjoint coordination between the ankle and hip joints during quiet standing in individuals with motor incomplete spinal cord injury. J Neurophysiol. 2021;125:1681–9.

71. Wang Y, Watanabe K, Asaka T. Effect of dance on multi-muscle synergies in older adults: a cross-sectional study. BMC Geriatr. 2019;19:340.
72. Olafsdottir HB, Zatsiorsky VM, Latash ML. The effects of strength training on finger strength and hand dexterity in healthy elderly individuals. J Appl Physiol (1985). 2008;105:1166–78.
73. Wu Y-H, Pazin N, Zatsiorsky VM, Latash ML. Improving finger coordination in young and elderly persons. Exp Brain Res. 2013;226:273–83.

Balance Control in Older Adults

6

Jaap H. van Dieën and Mirjam Pijnappels

Abstract

To avoid falls during everyday movements, we need to maintain balance, i.e., control the position of our body's center of mass relative to our base of support. The balance control system comprises sensory subsystems, their afferent nerves, an extensive brain network, its efferent nerves, and the motor system. Physiological aging of each of these subsystems may limit the ability to control balance in standing and walking. To test the balance control in older adults, methods based on questionnaires, functional tests of posture and movement are available. More advanced methods may quantify the ability to control or regain balance or the performance of specific subsystems.

Introduction

The basic activities that humans perform seemingly automatically, like standing and walking, require active control of balance to prevent falls. Unfortunately, aging has detrimental effects on balance control and this can lead to falls, which cause a serious threat to the individuals involved and a burden on society. At least, 25% of individuals aged 65 years and over falls at least once per year and half of these individuals fall even more frequently [1]. About 5% of these falls result in serious injuries such as head injuries, and hip or wrist fractures. According to the World Health Organization, annual fall rates resulting in emergency department visits range between 6 and 9 per 10,000 people aged over 60, of which 50% leads to hospital admission. The number of injuries caused by falls is projected to be 100% higher in the year 2030 due to the aging of the world's population. Consequently,

J. H. van Dieën (✉) · M. Pijnappels
Department of Human Movement Sciences, Vrije Universiteit Amsterdam, Amsterdam Movement Sciences, Amsterdam, The Netherlands
e-mail: j.van.dieen@vu.nl

F. A. Barbieri et al. (eds.), *Locomotion and Posture in Older Adults*,
https://doi.org/10.1007/978-3-031-74123-4_6

the direct medical costs related to falls will increase over the next 15 years by 170% [2]. In addition to physical injuries and the related loss of independence, falls often cause fear of falling [3] and avoidance of physical activity [4], with negative effects for health, independence, and quality of life.

Most falls occur during everyday movements like standing, walking, and transitioning, for example, from sitting on a chair to standing upright [5]. Falls are often caused by the physical status of the individual, but also by environmental factors. Fit and healthy older adults, for example, often fall during activities outdoors due to major balance perturbations (e.g., tripping over irregular pavement), while more fragile older adults more often fall indoors due to minor perturbations, sometimes even without clear external cause [6].

What does it take to adequately control balance during everyday movement tasks and what are the effects of aging on balance control and how can we assess these effects? In this chapter, we try to answer these questions by giving a description of the balance control system and its function in standing and walking. In addition, we address the age-related anatomical and physiological processes that affect this system and the consequences thereof for balance in standing and walking. Finally, we provide an overview of commonly used clinical tests as well as more novel and advanced methods for assessment of balance (impairments).

The Balance Control System

Balance control can be defined as the control of the body's center of mass (COM) relative to the base of support (BOS). In a static situation, such as in upright stance on one or two legs, the COM has to be kept over the BOS. When, in a dynamic situation, the COM is positioned outside the BOS, it has to be brought back over the BOS, or the BOS must be enlarged or moved to attain the same situation (Fig. 6.1). To change the position of the COM, two strategies can be used [7]. Muscles around the ankle joint can create a joint torque to accelerate the body around the ankles in the desired direction. Alternatively, movements of proximal body parts can cause a change in total amount of rotation (angular momentum) of the body, which can accelerate the body COM in the desired direction. An example of the latter is the swaying of the arms to maintain balance on the edge of a cliff. Finally, also the BOS can be moved or enlarged by stepping or by grabbing for hand support.

Given our vertical posture, gravity exerts a continuous perturbing effect, which tends to move the COM out of the BOS. Because the stiffness of lower limb joints and the muscle spanning these joints is insufficient to counteract this effect, even unperturbed upright stance requires active balance control [8]. This is reflected in the continuous movement of the COM during standing, called postural sway (Fig. 6.2). To activate muscles appropriately to move the COM in the desired direction and over the desired range, the nervous system requires information on the current position and velocity of the COM. This information is also indispensable to correctly adjust the BOS if needed. Sensory information thus plays an important role in balance control. The sensory modalities involved, the central nervous system

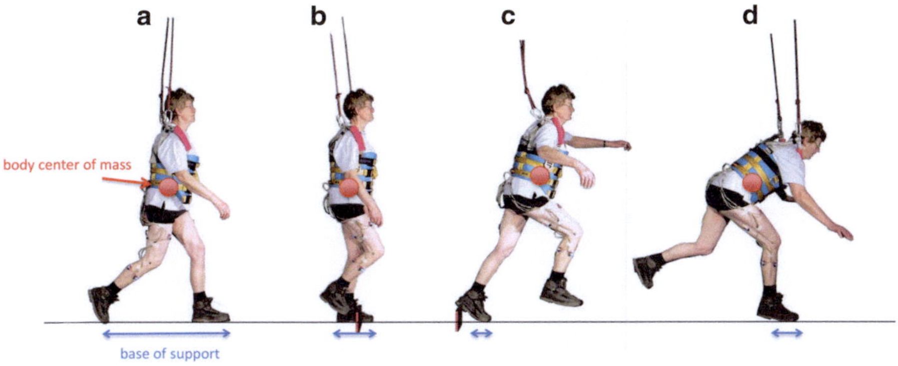

Fig. 6.1 Illustration of the essentials of balance control by means of the situations before and after a balance perturbation during gait (tripping). To control balance, the body COM (the location of the point around which the body mass is distributed) has to be maintained above the BOS, formed by the feet (and sometimes by other body parts in contact with the world, such as the hand on a cane). (**a**) The BOS in fore-aft direction is formed by both feet and the COM is located above it. (**b**) The BOS is formed by the left foot only and the COM has a forward velocity. The swing leg, which would normally be placed forward to displace the BOS, is blocked by an obstacle, due to which balance is perturbed, i.e., the COM travels beyond the BOS. (**c**) During balance recovery, the forward rotation can be decelerated by generating fast and large muscle force and moments in the stance leg, especially around the left ankle. (**d**) The blocked leg is placed over the obstacle with a large and fast step to displace the BOS for enough forward to regain balance

(CNS) and the muscles thus form a feedback system. The sensory system measures the current status; the CNS decides on actions needed to maintain or regain balance and based on this activates muscles; the muscles perform the required mechanical actions and the result is measured again by the sensory system. In addition to feedback, anticipation plays an important role in balance control; sensory information is used to predict future perturbations and anticipatory action can be taken to attenuate or even avoid a perturbation. The balance control system is summarized in Table 6.1 and Fig. 6.3 and more extensively described in the subsequent sections.

The Sensory System

The vestibular, the visual, and the proprioceptive and exteroceptive somatosensory systems all contribute to balance control. Adequate functioning of these systems and their connections with the CNS is crucial.

The vestibular system is localized in the head, behind the ears, and senses linear and angular accelerations of the head. Because gravity is basically a linear acceleration, it also provides information on the orientation of the head relative to the vertical. Afferent connections run mainly to the cerebellum, either directly or via the vestibular nuclei, which also connect to the thalamus and motor neurons of eye muscles and skeletal muscles, providing the means for very fast feedback. The importance of the vestibular system for maintenance of vertical postures can be

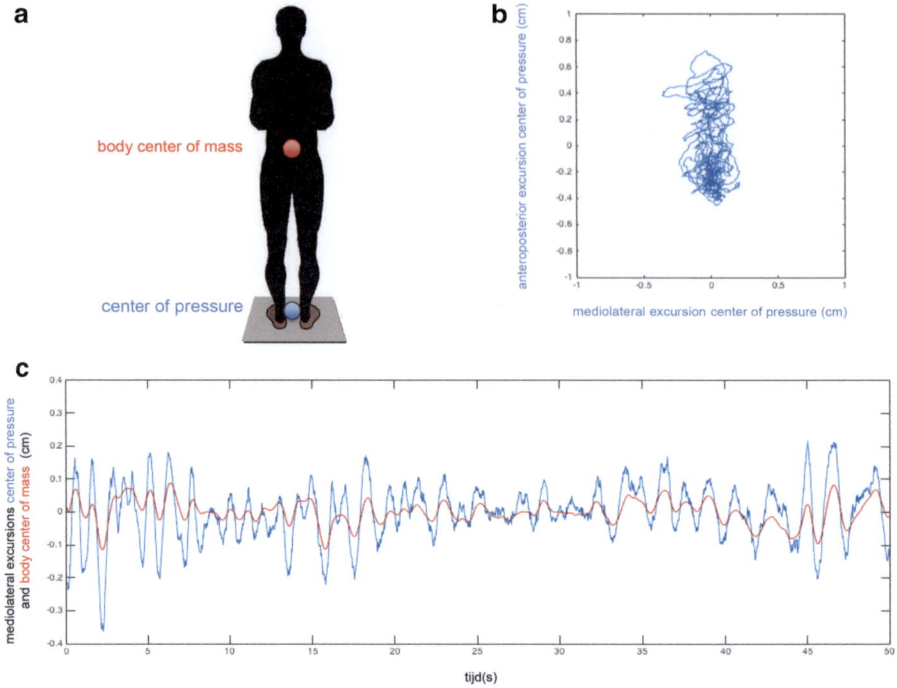

Fig. 6.2 Balance control in standing. (**a**) In upright stance the COM is located approximately in the center of the BOS; small movements of the COM and of the point of application of the ground reaction force are present continuously. (**b**) The fore-aft and sideward movements of the COM of the ground reaction force within the BOS illustrate the seemingly random movements within a relatively small part of the BOS. (**c**) The sideward movements of the COM (red) and BOS (blue) as a function of time illustrate that the movements of these points are related but not equal. For an explanation of their mutual relation see for example [72]. Although the position of the COM has to be controlled to maintain balance, the point of application of the ground reaction force is easier to measure and consequently it is often used to assess balance control

demonstrated by artificial stimulation. A weak current stimulation between the mastoid processes during standing causes an illusion of sway toward the side of the cathode and elicits sway in the opposite direction [9]. A substantial percentage of adults over 70 years of age show impaired vestibular function. Anatomically, a loss of sensors in the vestibular organs is apparent and this coincides with lower amplitudes of responses elicited by vestibular stimulation. Although it is well established that vestibular disorders increase fall risk, it is not yet clear whether reduced vestibular function in healthy older adults also has this effect [10].

The visual system converts light patterns on the retina into an image of the environment, including an estimate of the vertical [11]. Consequently, an environment that provides inconsistent or incorrect clues on the orientation of the vertical, like a building with diagonal window frames, is often experienced as unpleasant. Self-movement causes changes of the light pattern on the retina, which thus provides information on the linear and angular movements of the head. The optical nerve

Table 6.1 Balance control system: most important subsystems, functions, and effects of aging

Balance control system	Subsystems	Function in balance control	Effects of aging
Sensory system	Vestibular system	Senses linear and angular acceleration of the head and the gravitational acceleration	Loss of sensors; decreased amplitude of vestibular reflexes
	Visual system	Senses linear/angular acceleration of the head, vertical and horizontal references, and potential balance threats in the environment	Loss of sensors; reduced acuity, contrast sensitivity, depth perception, adaptation to low lighting and varying distance to objects in environment
	Proprioceptive somatosensory system (muscle spindles, tendon organs, joint, and skin receptor)	Senses posture and movement of body segments relative to each other	Loss of number and sensitivity of sensors; reduced joint position sense
	Exteroceptive somatosensory system (receptors in foot soles and hands)	Senses tactile information and forces exerted on environment via feet and hands	Loss of sensors; reduced sensitivity foot soles
Central nervous system	Spinal cord and brainstem	Spinal reflexes and automated balance responses	Loss of white matter (myelin sheets and myelinized nerve fibers); slowing down of transmission of sensory information
	Sensory nuclei, (pre-) motor, frontal and prefrontal cortex	Anticipation to self-generated and external perturbations; inhibition of planned activities	Loss of white (myelin sheets and myelinized nerve fibers) and gray matter (nerve cells); impaired sensory integration and inhibition
	Cerebellum	Sensorimotor integration	Loss of gray matter (nerve cells); impaired coordination
Motor system	Motor units	Force regulation	Loss of motor units; reduced precision
	Muscles	Force production	Loss of (mainly type II) muscle fibers; reduced muscle strength and power
	Tendons	Force transmission from muscle to skeleton	Reduced stiffness; slower force transmission

connects the retina to the thalamus and the mid-brain and it is assumed that the latter connections are particularly important for balance control. The importance of visual information for balance control becomes immediately apparent from the increase in postural sway when one closes the eyes [12] or when a large part of the environment within the field of view is moving [13]. Visual information is also essential for

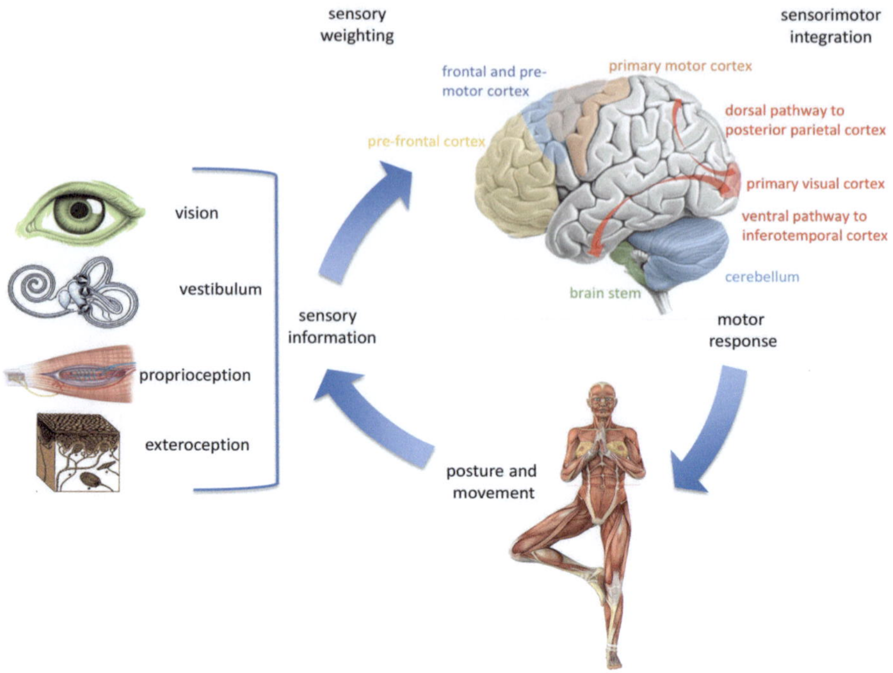

Fig. 6.3 The most important elements of the balance control feedback loop. The sensory system, consisting of the visual, vestibular, proprioceptive, and exteroceptive systems, provides information to the central nervous system. The most relevant brain areas for balance control are indicated, except for the thalamus which is not visible due to its central location. The central nervous system weights and integrates information from the different sensory modalities and generates motor responses to activate the muscles to adapt posture or movement to maintain balance

anticipation to potential balance threats. From the fifth decade onward, changes in the eyes lead to a reduction in visual acuity, contrast sensitivity and depth perception and to a reduced ability to adjust to poor lightning and varying distance to objects in the environment. Especially the reductions in depth perception and contrast sensitivity are correlated to increased fall risk in daily life [10], as is the use of multifocal glasses, which hampers perception of objects in close proximity of the feet [14].

The proprioceptive somatosensory system is distributed over the whole body and comprises muscle spindles, Golgi tendon organs, joint and skin receptors [15]. This system provides information on the orientation and movement of body segments relative to each other, for which the muscle spindles are the main source of information. The muscle spindles encode changes in muscle length and the speed thereof and are at the spinal level directly connected to the motor neurons of the homonymous muscles and via interneurons to nearby heteronymous muscles. In addition, ascending pathways relay this information to the cerebellum and thalamus. Muscle spindles can be stimulated with mechanical vibrations between 50 and 100 Hz. Studies using this type of stimulation have shown that muscle spindles in leg, trunk and neck muscles are important for balance control [16] and specifically the quality of proprioceptive information from ankle muscles appears important as this is strongly correlated to the ability to stand on one leg [17]. Compared to standing, balance control during walking is much less affected by proprioception [16], but vibration of the gluteus medius muscle during gait does have some effect on balance control in the frontal plane [18]. With aging, the number of muscle spindles as well as the sensitivity of remaining spindles decrease. This is reflected in a reduced acuity in perception of the posture and movements of joints. Reductions in acuity of posture and movement perception of the knee, ankle and big toe have been shown to be related to postural sway, to a reduced ability to stand on one leg and to the risk of falling in daily life [19].

The exteroceptive somatosensory system comprises a range of receptors in the soles of the feet that can provide information on the forces acting on the feet based on the resulting strain of the skin. The importance of these receptors for balance control is illustrated, among other factors, by the increase in postural sway that can be elicited by electrical stimulation of the foot soles [20]. Tactile information from other body parts, such as the hands through contact with an external object, even if that does not offer mechanical support, also contributes to balance control [21]. With aging, the number and the sensitivity of skin receptors in the foot soles decreases. Consequently, the threshold to perceive changes in pressure on the foot sole increases and the acuity for two-point discrimination decreases. These sensory losses are correlated to postural sway and fall risk [19].

Afferent nerve connections from the sensory system to the CNS loose nerve fibers and remaining nerve fibers lose their myelin sheaths. This leads to a reduction in nerve conduction and hence slowing down of balance feedback responses [19].

The Central Nervous System

At the lowest level of the CNS, in the spinal cord, proprioceptive and exteroceptive signals are integrated to produce motor responses in case of balance perturbations. The spinal reflexes are mainly organized locally, i.e., they mainly involve muscles around the perturbed joint and they are aimed at correcting posture or movement of that joint. These reflexes are not always functional from a balance control perspective and they may even be counterproductive [22].

Balance control requires integrated responses of muscles around several joints simultaneously. The brainstem can generate these automated responses and animal experiments have shown that these remain intact even when all connections with higher brain centers have been disrupted. Yet higher centers of the brain are involved in more complex balance responses, if only because they are based on integration of information from several sensory modalities, as described above. This is important for two reasons. First, estimates of balance can be based on weighted information from different modalities, because their reliability is not perfect and does vary over time. Using a weighted sum of the estimates from single sources provides a robust estimate and the flexibility of weighting allows adaptation to, for example, environmental conditions. Second, integration of information is necessary because, for example, the meaning of signals from the vestibular or visual systems depends on the orientation of the head relative to the rest of the body, for which only proprioceptive information is available. The cerebellum appears to play a key role in adjustment of the motor activity aimed at maintaining and restoring balance on the basis of sensory information regarding the state of the body and the environment [23]. Patients with cerebellar disorders therefore show severe balance problems and they are characterized by compensatory behavior, such as a wide stance to enlarge the BOS.

Predictable balance perturbations can be avoided or attenuated by anticipatory actions. For example, when a planned movement like picking up an object will perturb balance, anticipatory muscle activity or movement of the body acting in the direction opposite of the perturbation is initiated [24]. In such anticipatory actions, the cortex and specifically the premotor cortex plays an important role [25]. Similar anticipatory actions can be observed when an external but predictable balance perturbation occurs. When an obstacle that may perturb balance is seen during walking, it may be avoided by adjusting limb trajectory [26]. Such tasks involve visual processing via multiple cortical pathways [27, 28]. Also, memory plays a role, since, for example, visual information on obstacle dimensions is no longer available when stepping over an obstacle with the trailing leg. Prefrontal areas are, in all likelihood, involved in the planning of such adjustments in motor behavior and in inhibiting the initially planned activity. However, since reactions to suddenly appearing obstacles are markedly faster than voluntary reactions, it seems likely that sub-cortical areas of the brain initiate the responses, while higher centers further modify them [29].

The role of the cortex in responding to balance perturbations is debated, but there is evidence to suggest that premotor and primary motor cortices play a role in the pre-selection of postural responses based on information available prior to the perturbation and in adjusting responses later in time [30]. Also, balance control in unperturbed gait is related to cortical activity in the left premotor area [31]. All in all, a very extensive network appears active in balance control, with key roles for the cerebellum, premotor and motor areas as well as the prefrontal cortex. From this perspective, it comes as no surprise that cortical lesions after stroke and Alzheimer's disease, or even simultaneously performing a demanding cognitive task, can seriously impair balance control and increase the risk of falls.

With aging, the brain loses neurons and neural connections. These losses vary across brain areas, with the most prominent and least prominent losses in prefrontal areas and the cerebellum [32]. These losses affect the integration of sensory information for balance control. Consequently, older adults are more sensitive to sensory perturbations, such as those caused by artificial stimulation, but also real-life perturbations, such as that caused by movement of objects that occupy a large part of the visual field. Also, older adults need more time to adjust when the reliability of one of the sources of sensory information changes [10, 33]. Possibly this is caused by a reduced ability to inhibit incoming information due to degeneration of the prefrontal cortex, but fear of losing balance may be an alternative cause [34]. These age-related brain changes are related to reduced balance control, limitations of mobility and an increased fall risk [35].

The Motor System

Muscles and tendons comprise the most important components of the motor part of the balance control system. To correct large balance perturbations, fast and forceful contractions of muscles in legs [36], trunk [37], and even arms [38] are required, while balance control in unperturbed stance requires only moderate but accurate force production. The calf muscles and the hip abductor muscles play key roles in control of balance during bipedal stance in, respectively, the sagittal and frontal planes [39]. The latter muscles and in addition the hip adductor and ankle evertor and invertor muscles are also key in the control of unipedal stance [40] and these muscle groups appear to play an important role in balance control during gait [41–44]. Muscle strength depends on the number of parallel muscle fibers and consequently on the cross-sectional area of the muscle. The rate at which these forces are transferred to the skeleton and hence at which movements can be controlled, largely depends on tendon stiffness. Finally, the accuracy of muscle for production depends mainly on the number of motor units per muscle.

The physiological cross-sectional area of muscles decreases between 20 and 80 years of age, due to a loss of predominantly the fast type II muscle fibers. Muscle strength is maintained more or less up to 50 years of age but gradually declines after that by about 50% at age 80. The strength of hip abductors is correlated to the time that older adults are able to stand on one leg [40] and the strength of the knee extensor muscles is correlated to the stability of gait [45]. In addition, strength and cross-sectional area of trunk muscles were reported to be negatively correlated to postural sway and fall risk [46]. These associations suggest that muscle strength can be a limiting factor in dealing with minor balance perturbations that occur during standing and walking.

The rate at which muscles can increase force and the power that muscles can produce, i.e., the product of muscle force and shortening velocity, also decrease with age [47]. This is due to changes in the contractile properties of muscle fibers, but also to a decreased stiffness of muscle tendons [48]. The age-related loss of muscle power is about twice as large as the loss in muscle strength and consequently older adults are limited particularly in performing fast dynamic movement tasks [10]. Balance recovery responses are a clear example of this. Older adults are far less often successful in regaining their balance after tripping over an obstacle than young adults and this holds especially for older adults with weak and slow muscles [49].

The age-related loss of the number of motor units per muscle, which is most pronounced in distal muscles, and the increase in variability of motor unit firing reduce the precision with which older adults can produce muscle force [50]. It has been shown that older adults with a history of falls are less precise in producing muscle forces than their healthier counterparts [51].

Conclusion

Age-related physiological changes of all the sensory subsystems and their afferent nerves, of parts of the CNS, and of muscles and tendons can all limit the ability to control balance. The functional decline of parts of the balance control system and its effect on balance control can be compensated by other parts of the system and can vary widely between individuals.

Balance Control in Standing

In standing, the BOS is formed by one or both feet. When standing upright the COM will be at about 1 m above the support surface, which implies that body sway over a small angle can cause a substantial gravitational moment. Active control of balance is required to counteract these gravitational moments. In the subsequent sections, we will describe how balance is controlled in unperturbed, quiet standing and how balance is corrected after external perturbations. In addition, we describe how balance control in standing is usually assessed and how it changes with aging, with an emphasis on the factors that limit balance control in these situations.

Unperturbed Stance

In standing upright, we sway continuously and the COM moves apparently randomly over the BOS (Fig. 6.2). The continuous COM movement is a consequence of the disturbing effects of gravity and of muscle activity. The magnitude of postural sway is often used as a measure of the quality of balance control. In two-legged stance, the COM moves over a small and central part of the BOS. Balance control is more challenged when the BOS is reduced, by placing the feet close together, in tandem stance, or by standing on one leg. If instructed to do so, we can usually decrease the amount of postural sway, which implies that we do not normally attempt to minimize it, possibly because this costs energy [52], but there is also evidence to suggest that we produce a certain amount of postural sway to gather sensory information on balance [53].

Older adults generally show a larger postural sway than young adults, especially in the mediolateral direction [54] and their sway amplitude increases more when they close their eyes [55]. Consequently, many older adults are incapable of standing in tandem stance with their eyes closed. However, the increase in sway is also larger in older adults than in young adults when proprioception is perturbed [33]. More generally, it thus seems that older adults are less able to compensate for perturbations of one of the sensory modalities that contribute to postural control. Surprisingly sometimes, postural sway in upright stance is smaller in older than in young adults, possibly because young adults can afford not to control their balance very tightly, as standing does not challenge them. This explanation is supported by the finding that young adults decreased their sway more than older adults when asked to lean maximally forward or backward [56].

The quality of balance control in standing can be limited by age-related sensory impairments, as described in Sect. 6.2 of this chapter, but also by changes in the CNS. Experiments in which subjects perform cognitive dual tasks, for example, counting down from 100 with 7s, show that either balance or the cognitive task is more affected by simultaneous performance in older than in young adults. This is possibly related to the fact that the cortex is more involved in balance control in older adults [35]. Cortical involvement appears to be determined by the relative difficulty of the task, hence the higher cortical activity in older adults is probably compensatory [57]. However, impaired brain function can limit balance control. This is shown by the effect of orthostatic hypotension on balance, where insufficient regulation of blood pressure, which is common among older adults, causes insufficient oxygen supply to the brain. The speed at which blood pressure is regulated after transitioning from sit to stance in older adults is associated with the time that balance can be maintained in tandem stance with eyes closed [58]. Also an association between cognitive abilities and balance control in stance has been found [59]. Finally, the motor system can limit balance control. The time that older adults can maintain balance in various standing postures is associated with muscle strength [60] and lower precision of muscle force production is associated with larger postural sway [61].

External Perturbation of Standing Balance

If a mechanical perturbation causes or threatens the body COM to move outside the BOS, reactive balance control is needed. Reactive balance control is usually tested by sudden and unexpected translations or rotations of a platform that the person stands on. Generally, older adults show larger postural sway after such perturbations than young adults [62, 63] and they produce higher joint moments to regain balance [62]. Also, older adults and especially adults with balance problems more often make a step, using displacement of the BOS to regain balance [64, 65].

Balance perturbations cause early spinal reflexes and later responses generated by higher centers of the CNS. The early responses can be delayed in older adults by around 5 ms relative to young adults, probably due to lower nerve conduction velocity. Delays of about 20 ms are found for the later responses and this is attributed to slower information processing in the brain [35]. The magnitude of postural sway after perturbations is associated with thresholds of sensors in foot soles [63] as well as with delays of early and late responses [35]. In addition, the magnitude of sway and the necessity to make a step after perturbations are associated with muscle strength of ankle and trunk muscles [63, 66], in line with the relation between trunk muscle strength and fall risk as described above. The effect of muscle strength on perturbation responses is striking, since older adults were shown to produce higher joint moments than young adults and because these moments were well below maximum levels predicted based on muscles strength [62]. Possibly, the rate at which muscle force and hence joint moments can be developed is the true limiting factor, as this is in turn associated with muscle strength.

Conclusion

The degree to which older adults can constrain postural sway to a small part of the BOS and the ability to remain standing when the BOS is reduced are limited by age-related changes in the sensory system, the CNS and the motor system. The ability to regain standing balance without stepping appears to be limited mainly by the rate at which muscle activation can be increased and at which the muscles can produce force, which are determined by changes in the peripheral and central nervous system, as well as the muscles themselves.

Balance Control in Gait

In this section, we will describe how balance is controlled, how perturbations are avoided and how balance is regained during gait. Methods to assess balance control will be discussed and an overview is given of the changes that occur with aging as well as of the factors that limit balance control during gait in healthy older adults.

Unperturbed Gait

During gait, the body COM has a forward velocity and consequently the BOS must be displaced to prevent falling. The properties of the human body greatly simplify the control in the fore-aft direction when walking at constant velocity. The inertia of the legs and the velocity of the body make the leg swing forward just enough to obtain the correct new BOS to maintain balance and gait velocity. Obviously, this is a simplification of reality and active control is necessary to deal with variations in the environment and control of balance in the mediolateral direction is even more challenging [67].

Several measures to characterize balance control during gait have been developed and many of these are based on the notion that the movements in unperturbed gait are expected to be regular (i.e., subsequent steps should resemble each other) and that the movement should be stable (i.e., small perturbations of gait are quickly corrected). Many different parameters quantify the (ir-)regularity or (in-)stability of gait [68]; it is, however, beyond the scope of this chapter to describe these in detail, suffices to state that larger irregularity (or variability) and lower stability are related to age [69], fall history [70] and fall risk [71].

As in standing, the position of the COM relative to the edges of the BOS provides a measure of the margin of safety in balance control. For gait, the velocity of the COM has to be taken into account [72]. The so-obtained dynamic margin of safety ("margin of stability") is frequently used to assess mediolateral balance.

Older adults walk with wider steps than young adults and although this is seen as a compensation to increase the BOS, this is associated with an increase in the amplitude and velocity of sideward movement of the body COM and when environmental conditions dictate a smaller step width this leads to a reduced safety margin [73]. In addition, the variability of this safety margin is larger in older than young adults and this further increases the probability of balance loss. This is likely a consequence of the fact that foot placement is less well coordinated to the ongoing movement of the COM in older than in young adults, presumably as a consequence of impaired proprioception [74].

Although it is well established that balance control in gait is dependent on sensory information and affected by larger parts of the CNS (see Sect. 6.2), little is known about the interactions and the limiting factors in these systems regarding balance control in gait. It is known that muscle strength is related to gait stability [45] and regularity [75]. Also, it has been found that reduced mediolateral margins of safety are related to degenerative changes in the brain, indicating that individuals with impaired connectivity between sub-cortical and prefrontal brain areas do not adequately compensate for their impaired balance control by regulating step width [76].

Avoidance of Balance Perturbations during Gait

In daily life gait, we encounter all sorts of potential balance perturbations that we should try to avoid, or when we fail to do so, we must try to regain balance in order to prevent falling. Tripping is reported to be the most common cause of falls among healthy older adults both indoors and outdoors [77]. In this paragraph and the next, we will concentrate on avoiding balance perturbations and recovering from balance perturbations, with tripping as a point in case.

When an obstacle blocks the planned path of the swing leg, it is avoided by either elevating the swing leg higher and lengthening its step or by shortening the step by placing the leg in front of the obstacle to cross it with the other leg first. In young adults, the choice between these strategies appears to be made such that the deviation relative to the initially planned step is minimal [78]. Older adults, however, appear to prefer lengthening their step [79]. This preference may reduce the probability of losing balance, as it avoids that the leg is placed underneath or even behind the body COM [80]. However, it may also be a consequence of older adults not being able to react quick enough to perform the short step strategy [81].

Obviously, visual information is crucial for adequate obstacle avoidance. The length of the ultimate step before the obstacle and the path of the leg over the obstacle are adjusted to position, height, and other properties of the obstacle [82]. Young adults gather the information needed to do so in the few meters before reaching the obstacle. The duration of visual fixation of the obstacle depends on obstacle height, suggesting that detailed information is gathered [83]. This implies that visual acuity and contrast sensitivity at a few meters distance, but also short-term memory, are important for successful avoidance and may explain why wearing multifocal glasses increases fall risk (Sect. 6.2).

When older adults cross an obstacle, they do so with smaller toe clearance than young adults [84]. They are also less successful in avoiding obstacles when these are first seen when they are already close. Interestingly, this effect is much smaller than one would expect based on age effects in reaction time tests [81]. The importance of cognitive processes for obstacle avoidance is evident from the fact that cognitive impairments [85] and dual task performance [86] reduce the probability of success at this task.

Perturbations of Balance in Gait

If an obstacle cannot be avoided, a collision of the swing leg with the obstacle will cause a trip; the forward placement of the leg is hampered and, if one does not react adequately, a forward rotation of the body, further accelerated by gravity, ends in a fall. Balance recovery requires that one decelerates the forward rotation and places one leg over the obstacle to obtain an adequate BOS and to continue walking (Fig. 6.1). Two types of recovery reactions have been described [87]; if the leg is blocked early in the swing phase, it is quickly elevated over the obstacle and placed behind the obstacle, if the leg is blocked late in the swing phase, it is placed on the floor in front of the obstacle and subsequently the other leg steps over the obstacle first. In both cases, the stance leg during the trip has an important contribution to deceleration of the forward rotation by a fast and forceful forward directed push-off. At about 80 ms after impact with the obstacle, functional changes in muscle activity are observed in both legs, probably triggered by somatosensory information from the skin or distal joints and muscles of the blocked leg [88]. Changes in movements of the head occur too late for visual and vestibular inputs to contribute to the generation of these early responses.

Older adults are clearly less successful in performing balance recovery reactions after tripping than young adults. They decelerate the forward rotation less and place their recovery leg less far over the obstacle [89] and fall more often than young adults [77]. The reaction time after tripping as measured from changes in muscle activity does not appear to be the limiting factor as it is only marginally different between young and older adults and not different between older adults who fall and do not fall after these perturbations [36]. In simulations of the recovery reaction, in which people are released from a forward leaning position, the velocity of the forward movement of the recovery leg appears to be the limiting factor for successful recovery. A lower rate of the increase in neural drive to the leg muscles appears to underlie this lower movement speed [90]. Successful recovery after tripping is actually also determined by the degree to which one is able to decelerate the forward movement of the trunk [91]. Muscles in the stance leg and trunk are responsible for decelerating the forward rotation of the body before a leg is placed over the obstacle [92, 93]. This requires fast adaptations of leg muscle activity and a maximal activity of the calf muscles. The joint torques produced by these muscles are adapted more slowly in older than in young adults and this is at least in part due to a slower increase in neural drive to these muscles [89]. Older adults with a lower leg muscle strength and a lower maximum rate of joint torque development around knee and ankle joints fall more often after being tripped than their stronger and faster peers [49].

Conclusion

The quality of balance control and the ability to avoid obstacles during gait both decline with age. It is, as of yet, not clear what the limiting factors are. Muscle strength is associated with the quality of balance control during gait, but this may not reflect causality. Cognitive impairment appears to play a role, although its importance remains to be determined. The ability to regain balance after a perturbation of gait also declines with age and this is caused by a reduced ability to generate fast changes in muscle force, probably due to changes in the CNS as well as in the muscles and muscle tendons themselves (see also Sect. 6.2).

Assessment of Balance Control

A variety of methods to assess balance in older adults has been proposed, ranging from questionnaires to extensive test batteries. These methods are often used to establish (causes of) balance problems to target interventions and to assess the effects of interventions. The most common clinical tests assess static balance in standing or dynamic balance during functional movements such as stepping and walking. In general, these clinical tests measure the success or failure to maintain balance during a certain task or the quality of the performance of a balance task. In contrast, physiological tests assess the potential impairments underlying balance problems [94]. In this section, we discuss subjective methods, static, dynamic, and functional balance tests and we present tests aimed at assessing balance recovery and establishing the underlying causes of balance problems. The information described below is summarized in Table 6.2.

Subjective Assessment of Balance Problems

Assessment of balance control usually starts with asking question, for example, on fall history. Having fallen in the preceding year is a strong predictor future falls (e.g., 71) and hence an important indication of balance problems. In addition, individuals may report to experience balance problems or fear of falling. Such indicators of balance problems can be assessed systematically with questionnaires on fear of falling or balance confidence [111]. Fear of falling, defined as the concern that one may fall during daily activities, can be measured with Falls Efficacy Scale-international (FES-i), a 16-items questionnaire [95], or its shortened 7-items version

Table 6.2 Overview of tests of the balance control system

Type of measurement	Test	Way of testing	Score
Subjective tests	Fall history	Have you fallen in the last 12 months? If so, how often?	Dichotomous score (yes/no) or number of falls
	Falls Efficacy Scale-international (FES-i) [95]	16 items questionnaire on fear of falling during several activities	Ordinal score 16–64; high score = high fear
	Activities-specific Balance Confidence (ABC) scale [96]	16 items questionnaire on confidence in performance of several activities without losing balance or falling	Ordinal score per item 0–100; high score = high confidence
Static balance tests	(Semi)tandem stance	Maintain for 10 s, can be combined with closing eyes, unstable support surface, dual task; stopwatch	Dichotomous score (yes/no) or duration; shorter duration = worse balance
	Instrumented (semi)tandem stance	Maintain for 10 s, can be combined with closing eyes, unstable support surface, dual task; force plate, camera system, or inertial measurement unit	Quantitative score (displacement/speed/acceleration body center of mass or center of pressure); faster, larger sway = worse balance
Dynamic balance tests	Limits of Stability (LOS) test	Self-induced maximal movement in eight directions without stepping; force plate (e.g., NeuroCom; Biodex Balance System)	Quantitative score; smaller/slower displacement = worse balance
	MEdioLateral Balance Assessment (MELBA) test [97]	Self-induced mediolateral weight shifts; force plate or camera system	Quantitative score; lower frequency/speed = impaired balance
Functional balance tests	Performance Oriented Mobility Assessment (POMA of Tinetti) [98]	Balance evaluation (13 balance tasks, scored 0–16) and mobility evaluation (6 gait tasks, scored 0–12)	Ordinal score 0–28; lower score = worse balance/mobility; score <19 high fall risk
	Berg Balance Scale (BBS) [99]	14 items, scored with 5-point scale	Ordinal score 0–56; lower score = worse balance; score <43 high fall risk
	Timed Up and Go test (TUG) [100]	Time to get up from chair, walk 3 m, turn around, walk back and sit down; stopwatch	Continuous score (total time); longer time = worse balance/mobility
	Short Physical Performance Battery (SPPB) [101]	Five items (gait, three balance tests, repeated sit-to-stand)	Ordinal score 0–12; lower score = worse balance/mobility

Test of balance recovery	Standing balance perturbations [102, 103]	Platform translation/rotation or upper body push/pull in standing; instrumented platform	Dichotomous score (yes/no stepping response) or quantitative score; stronger perturbation of standing or gait = worse balance
	Gait perturbations [104–107]	Platform translation/rotation or upper body push/pull in walking; instrumented treadmill	Quantitative scores based on spatiotemporal gait variables, margins of stability, trunk kinematics
		Belt accelerations/deceleration; treadmill	Quantitative scores based on spatiotemporal gait variables, margins of stability, trunk kinematics
Subsystem tests	Physiological Profile Assessment (PPA) [108] www.neura.edu.au/fbrg	15 items (3 vision, 3 proprioception, 3 muscle strength, 2 reaction time, 4 postural sway) or short version with 5 items (1 per domain)	1 score for fall risk based on z-scores reference group
	Balance Evaluation Systems Test (BESTest) [109] http://www.bestest.us	27 items (5 biomechanical, 3 balance, 5 transitions, 5 reactive, 3 sensory, 7 gait) or short version with 14 items	Ordinal score 0–108 (short version 0–28); lower score = worse balance/mobility
	Sensory organization test (SOT) [110]	Postural sway in six conditions: Eyes open/closed, rigid/unstable support surface, fixed/moving visual surround (e.g., NeuroCom)	Quantitative score based on sway per condition and weighted average total score

[112]. High fear of falling is associated with worse balance performance in standing and in gait [111]. As an alternative to these questionnaires, the icon-FES uses images of activities and asks the individual to indicate whether these would elicit fear of falling [113]. The Activities-specific Balance Confidence (ABC) scale is a commonly used 16-items questionnaire [96] to measure balance confidence, the inverse of fear of falling, which as such has a more positive connotation. It reflects one's confidence in the ability to maintain balance during daily activities. For gait specifically the 10-item "Gait Efficacy Scale" can be used [114].

Static Balance Tests

Widely used method for static balance testing are based on assessment of the ability to maintain balance over a constrained BOS, for example, with the feet close together or in tandem stance for a certain period of time. The 10-s (semi-) tandem stance is probably the most used. The inability to perform this test is indicative of impaired balance control [115]. To make such tests more challenging and to specifically address, the role of the proprioceptive system, the visual system, or of cognitive processing, the same tests can be performed with closed eyes, on a compliant surface, or with a cognitive dual task.

Tests of static balance can be enhanced by measuring postural sway with a camera system or inertial sensors measuring the movement of body segments, from which the movements of the COM can be estimated. This so-called posturography allows measurement of the amplitude, velocity or acceleration of movements of the COM in fore-aft and sideward directions. This postural sway is also often estimated from movements of the point of application of the ground reaction force (or center of pressure) (Fig. 6.2), measured with a force plate or cheaper alternatives such as the Wii Balance Board [116]. At low movement speed, the center of pressure gives a good approximation of the movements of the body COM, but at higher speeds, the difference between the amplitude of the COM and the center of pressure increases. The quality of balance control as measured this way decreases with age (see Sect. 6.3), but the predictive value thereof for fall risk is not clear yet [117]. The interpretation of these measures is thus still open to discussion.

Dynamic Balance Tests

Dynamic posturography tests the responses to self-imposed or externally imposed balance perturbations. A commonly used clinical approach to measure balance under self-induced perturbations is the limits of stability (LOS) test, which measures the maximum range of motion that one can make by leaning the body in a specified direction without stepping [118]. A recent method, called MEdioLateral Balance Assessment (MELBA), tests the ability to follow a moving target by making sideward movements of the COM at incremental speed. This test has been shown to be reliable, sensitive to differences between young and older adults and indicative of balance problems during gait on a treadmill and in daily life [97]. In addition, the test results are correlated to strength of the hip abductor muscles [119]. Another promising and simple test measures the distance that one can walk over narrow beams of decreasing width [120–124].

Functional Balance Tests

The most commonly used functional, clinical balance tests are the Tinetti balance test, or Performance Oriented Mobility Assessment (POMA) [98], the Berg Balance Scale (BBS) [99], the Timed Up and Go test (TUG) [100], and the Short Physical Performance Battery (SPPB) [101]. These tests measure the ability to maintain balance in tasks such as getting up from a chair, standing and walking. These tests are simple and cheap and have been shown to have good reliability within and between observers [94]. However, other aspects of physical capacity also determine the outcomes and balance problems are identified only when these are already quite severe [115]. Relatively fit, community-dwelling older adults are often able to use compensatory strategies masking impairments of their balance control system during such tests [115], leading to ceiling effects and making these tests less suitable for early detection of balance problems [94].

The outcomes of clinical, functional balance tests are often interpreted in relation to fall risk. However, their predictive value for falls is rather limited. The TUG is for example often used to assess fall risk, but in fact does not differentiate older fallers from non-fallers [125]. Also for the other tests, there is no or only very limited evidence for a predictive value with respect to fall risk [94]. These tools are indicative of increased risk only in populations that they were developed for. In addition, the outcomes are not very sensitive to change, for example changes due to interventions to prevent falls [126].

Currently, instrumented versions of functional balance tests are developed and used. Sensors are employed during the tests to obtain more objective and precise results and a higher sensitivity to subtle balance impairments. Accelerometers and gyroscopes provide detailed information on timing and execution of movements in functional tasks such as walking [70] and getting up from a chair [127]. The outcomes are promising indicators of balance problems and fall risk, but also for these measures solid evidence is lacking [128]. Accelerometers and gyroscopes can also be used in daily life. Recent studies have shown that information on the stability of walking [71] and standing up from a chair [129] acquired from acceleration data obtained in daily life may have added value for the prediction of fall risk, but external validation of these findings is needed and the clinical value still needs to be demonstrated.

Testing Balance Recovery

Falls are ultimately the result of the inability to regain balance after a perturbation and this may argue for specifically testing reactive balance control or balance recovery. Waist pulls and platform translations and rotations have been used to measure the ability to regain balance after perturbations of standing [102, 130–132]. The necessity to make a step, especially after sideward or backward perturbations of standing balance is a strong predictor of future falls [130, 131]. A drawback of these tests is that standardized perturbations do not necessarily exceed the capacity of the individual, causing ceiling effects. More advanced instruments that not only standardize the perturbation intensity, but also allow to gradually increase it, are needed to bypass this problem [66, 107]. Such instruments are usually expensive and their added value in the clinical context is still being studied.

Most falls occur during walking and balance recovery mechanisms may be different between walking and standing. Therefore, similar mechanical perturbations have also been used in a research context to assess balance recovery during walking. Such studies used custom-made devices to push or pull at the trunk or pelvis level [104–107], and recently the design for a device to produce controlled perturbations was made publicly available [133]. More suitable for clinical application though, may be perturbations through surface translations, which can be applied in multiple directions by treadmills embedded in a moveable platform [134, 135]. Anteroposterior perturbations can be applied with less sophisticated instruments, by accelerating or decelerating the treadmill belt [135]. To develop clinically applicable assessment tools based on such technology, more reliable and sensitive outcome measures that adequately quantify balance recovery and that require minimal instrumentation need to be developed [136, 137].

Testing the Balance Control System

Tests of the balance control system aim at establishing the specific nature and/or causes of balance problems, to allow tailored interventions. The Physiological Profile Assessment (PPA) is an extensive test battery that addresses visual, vestibular, and proprioceptive functions as well as leg muscle strength, reaction time, and static and dynamic posturography [108]. The items were selected based on their importance for balance control and the PPA has good predictive value for falls [108]. The Balance Evaluation Systems Test (BESTest) comprises a number of items from previously developed functional tests (such as the TUG and LOS) and aims to assess specific domains of balance control, such as stability in reaching and walking, anticipatory and reactive control and also some determinants of balance control such as muscle strength, [109]. Although not specifically developed to this end, the BESTest has good predictive value for fall risk [138].

Sensory manipulations are often used to establish specific causes of balance problems. A commonly used test is the sensory organization test (SOT), which comprises a movable force plate and a moveable environment to impose visual perturbations. Using six specific conditions with eyes open or closed, the differences in postural sway between conditions provide information on the relative contributions of the visual, proprioceptive, and vestibular systems to balance control. In addition, the results provide information on the ability to compensate for unreliable sensory information from the modalities involved [139].

More advanced tests to assess the contributions of different subsystems to balance control are under development, for example, for standing balance [140], or for balance in treadmill walking [110]. These methods combine sensory and mechanical perturbations to provide a detailed identification of the balance control system. The ability to maintain balance during gait in complex environments, which challenges cognitive function can be tested with tools such as the "interactive walkway," which uses Kinect sensors and projections of obstacles or targets on the floor [141].

Conclusion

No single test is sufficient to fully characterize static or dynamic balance control and to predict falls [142]. Dependent on the clinical question at hand, a combination of tests will be needed. It is striking that anticipatory control, such as when avoiding obstacles receives limited attention in clinical balance testing, while this might be an important determinant of fall risk. Furthermore, clinical tests, by necessity, standardize and simplify the complexity of balance threatening conditions that one may be exposed to in daily life. Although dynamic tests can provide information on reactive control of balance, these are usually applied in standing postures and not during dynamic activities such as walking. It is still unclear to what extent such simplifications threaten the validity of the outcomes. From this perspective, the development of balance assessment based on ambulatory measurements in daily life seems a promising approach to obtain a more complete picture.

References

1. Lord SR, Sherrington C, Menz HB. Falls in older people: risk factors and strategies for prevention. 2nd ed. Cambridge: Cambridge University Press; 2001.
2. WHO. WHO global report on falls prevention in older age. Geneva: WHO Press; 2007.
3. Weijer RHA, Hoozemans MJM, Meijer OG, van Dieën JH, Pijnappels M. The short- and long-term temporal relation between falls and concern about falling in older adults without a recent history of falling. PLoS One. 2021;16:e0253374.
4. Delbaere K, Crombez G, Vanderstraeten G, Willems T, Cambier D. Fear-related avoidance of activities, falls and physical frailty. A prospective community-based cohort study. Age Ageing. 2004;33(4):368–73.
5. Robinovitch SN, Feldman F, Yang Y, Schonnop R, Leung PM, Sarraf T, et al. Video capture of the circumstances of falls in elderly people residing in long-term care: an observational study. Lancet. 2013;381(9860):47–54.
6. Kelsey JL, Berry SD, Procter-Gray E, Quach L, Nguyen US, Li W, et al. Indoor and outdoor falls in older adults are different: the maintenance of balance, independent living, intellect, and Zest in the Elderly of Boston Study. J Am Geriatr Soc. 2010;58(11):2135–41.

7. Hof AL. The equations of motion for a standing human reveal three mechanisms for balance. J Biomech. 2007;40:451–7.
8. Loram ID, Lakie M. Direct measurement of human ankle stiffness during quiet standing: the intrinsic mechanical stiffness is insufficient for stability. J Physiol. 2002;545:1041–53.
9. Iles JF, Baderin R, Tanner R, Simon A. Human standing and walking: comparison of the effects of stimulation of the vestibular system. Exp Brain Res. 2007;178(2):151–66.
10. Sturnieks DL, St George R, Lord SR. Balance disorders in the elderly. Neurophysiol Clin. 2008;38(6):467–78.
11. St George RJ, Fitzpatrick RC. The sense of self-motion, orientation and balance explored by vestibular stimulation. J Physiol. 2011;589:807–13.
12. Paulus WM, Straube A, Brandt T. Visual stabilization of posture. Physiological stimulus characteristics and clinical aspects. Brain. 1984;107(Pt 4):1143–63.
13. Redfern M, Yardley L, Bronstein A. Visual influences on balance. J Anxiety Disord. 2001;15:81–94.
14. Lord SR, Dayhew J, Howland A. Multifocal glasses impair edge-contrast sensitivity and depth perception and increase the risk of falls in older people. J Am Geriatr Soc. 2002;50(11):1760–6.
15. Proske U, Gandevia SC. The proprioceptive senses: their roles in signaling body shape, body position and movement, and muscle force. Physiol Rev. 2012;92(4):1651–97.
16. Courtine G, De Nunzio AM, Schmid M, Beretta MV, Schieppati M. Stance- and locomotion-dependent processing of vibration-induced proprioceptive inflow from multiple muscles in humans. J Neurophysiol. 2007;97(1):772–9.
17. Son J, Ashton-Miller JA, Richardson JK. Frontal plane ankle proprioceptive thresholds and unipedal balance. Muscle Nerve. 2009;39(2):150–7.
18. Roden-Reynolds DC, Walker MH, Wasserman CR, Dean JC. Hip proprioceptive feedback influences the control of mediolateral stability during human walking. J Neurophysiol. 2015;114(4):2220–9.
19. Shaffer SW, Harrison AL. Aging of the somatosensory system: a translational perspective. Phys Ther. 2007;87(2):193–207.
20. Cofre Lizama LE, Pijnappels M, Verschueren S, Reeves NP, van Dieën JH. Can explicit visual feedback of postural sway efface the effects of sensory manipulations on mediolateral balance performance? J Neurophysiol. 2016;115:907–14.
21. Jeka JJ. Light touch contact as a balance aid. Phys Ther. 1997;77(5):476–87.
22. Welch TD, Ting LH. Mechanisms of motor adaptation in reactive balance control. PLoS One. 2014;9(5):e96440.
23. Manzoni D. The cerebellum may implement the appropriate coupling of sensory inputs and motor responses: evidence from vestibular physiology. Cerebellum. 2005;4(3):178–88.
24. van Dieen J, de Looze M. Directionality of anticipatory activation of trunk muscles in a lifting task depends on load knowledge. Exp Brain Res. 1999;128(3):397–404.
25. Jacobs JV, Lou JS, Kraakevik JA, Horak FB. The supplementary motor area contributes to the timing of the anticipatory postural adjustment during step initiation in participants with and without Parkinson's disease. Neuroscience. 2009;164(2):877–85.
26. Moraes R, Lewis MA, Patla AE. Strategies and determinants for selection of alternate foot placement during human locomotion: influence of spatial and temporal constraints. Exp Brain Res. 2004;159(1):1–13.
27. Hesse C, Lane AR, Aimola L, Schenk T. Pathways involved in human conscious vision contribute to obstacle-avoidance behaviour. Eur J Neurosci. 2012;36(3):2383–90.
28. Patla AE, Goodale MA. Obstacle avoidance during locomotion is unaffected in a patient with visual form agnosia. Neuroreport. 1996;8:165–8.
29. Weerdesteyn V, Nienhuis B, Hampsink B, Duysens J. Gait adjustments in response to an obstacle are faster than voluntary reactions. Hum Mov Sci. 2004;23(3–4):351–63.
30. Jacobs JV, Horak FB. Cortical control of postural responses. J Neural Transm (Vienna). 2007;114(10):1339–48.

31. Bruijn SM, van Dieën JH, Daffertshofer A. Beta activity in the premotor cortex is increased during stabilized as compared to normal walking. Front Hum Neurosci. 2015;9:593.
32. Sullivan EV, Deshmukh A, Desmond JE, Lim KO, Pfefferbaum A. Cerebellar volume decline in normal aging, alcoholism, and Korsakoff's syndrome: relation to ataxia. Neuropsychology. 2000;14(3):341–52.
33. Wiesmeier IK, Dalin D, Maurer C. Elderly use proprioception rather than visual and vestibular cues for postural motor control. Front Aging Neurosci. 2015;7:97.
34. Eikema DJ, Hatzitaki V, Tzovaras D, Papaxanthis C. Age-dependent modulation of sensory reweighting for controlling posture in a dynamic virtual environment. Age (Dordr). 2012;34(6):1381–92.
35. Papegaaij S, Taube W, Baudry S, Otten E, Hortobagyi T. Aging causes a reorganization of cortical and spinal control of posture. Front Aging Neurosci. 2014;6:28.
36. Pijnappels M, Bobbert MF, van Dieen JH. Control of support limb muscles in recovery after tripping in young and older subjects. Exp Brain Res. 2005;160(3):326–33.
37. van der Burg JC, Pijnappels M, van Dieen JH. Out-of-plane trunk movements and trunk muscle activity after a trip during walking. Exp Brain Res. 2005;165(3):407–12.
38. Pijnappels M, Kingma I, Wezenberg D, Reurink G, van Dieen JH. Armed against falls: the contribution of arm movements to balance recovery after tripping. Exp Brain Res. 2010;201(4):689–99.
39. Winter DA, Prince F, Frank JS, Powell C, Zabjek KF. Unified theory regarding A/P and M/L balance in quiet stance. J Neurophysiol. 1996;75(6):2334–43.
40. Allet L, Kim H, Ashton-Miller J, De Mott T, Richardson JK. Frontal plane hip and ankle sensorimotor function, not age, predicts unipedal stance time. Muscle Nerve. 2012;45(4):578–85.
41. Kim M, Collins SH. Once-per-step control of ankle-foot prosthesis push-off work reduces effort associated with balance during walking. J Neuroeng Rehabil. 2015;12:43.
42. Rankin BL, Buffo SK, Dean JC. A neuromechanical strategy for mediolateral foot placement in walking humans. J Neurophysiol. 2014;112(2):374–83.
43. van Leeuwen AM, van Dieën JH, Daffertshofer A, Bruijn SM. Active foot placement control ensures stable gait: effect of constraints on foot placement and ankle moments. PLoS One. 2020;15:e0242215.
44. van Leeuwen AM, van Dieën JH, Daffertshofer A, Bruijn SM. Ankle muscles drive mediolateral center of pressure control to ensure stable steady state gait. Sci Rep. 2021;11:21481.
45. Toebes MJ, Hoozemans MJM, Dekker J, van Dieen JH. Associations between measures of gait stability, leg strength and fear of falling. Gait Posture. 2015;41:76–80.
46. Granacher U, Gollhofer A, Hortobagyi T, Kressig RW, Muehlbauer T. The importance of trunk muscle strength for balance, functional performance, and fall prevention in seniors: a systematic review. Sports Med. 2013;43(7):627–41.
47. Thelen DG, Schultz AB, Alexander NB, Ashton-Miller JA. Effects of age on rapid ankle torque development. J Gerontol Ser A Biol Sci Med Sci. 1996;51(5):M226–32.
48. Reeves ND, Narici MV, Maganaris CN. Myotendinous plasticity to ageing and resistance exercise in humans. Exp Physiol. 2006;91(3):483–98.
49. Pijnappels M, van der Burg PJ, Reeves ND, van Dieen JH. Identification of elderly fallers by muscle strength measures. Eur J Appl Physiol. 2008;102(5):585–92.
50. Enoka RM, Christou EA, Hunter SK, Kornatz KW, Semmler JG, Taylor AM, et al. Mechanisms that contribute to differences in motor performance between young and old adults. J Electromyogr Kinesiol. 2003;13(1):1–12.
51. Carville SF, Perry MC, Rutherford OM, Smith IC, Newham DJ. Steadiness of quadriceps contractions in young and older adults with and without a history of falling. Eur J Appl Physiol. 2007;100(5):527–33.
52. Houdijk H, Brown S, van Dieen JH. The relation between postural sway magnitude and metabolic energy cost during upright standing on a compliant surface. J Appl Physiol. 2015;119:696–703.
53. Carpenter MG, Murnaghan CD, Inglis JT. Shifting the balance: evidence of an exploratory role for postural sway. Neuroscience. 2010;171(1):196–204.

54. Pasma JH, Bijlsma AY, van der Bij MD, Arendzen JH, Meskers CG, Maier AB. Age-related differences in quality of standing balance using a composite score. Gerontology. 2014;60(4):306–14.
55. Choy NL, Brauer S, Nitz J. Changes in postural stability in women aged 20 to 80 years. J Gerontol A Biol Sci Med Sci. 2003;58(6):525–30.
56. van Wegen EEH, van Emmerik REA, Riccio GE. Postural orientation: age-related changes in variability and time-to-boundary. Hum Mov Sci. 2002;21(1):61–84.
57. Papegaaij S, Taube W, van Keeken HG, Otten E, Baudry S, Hortobagyi T. Postural challenge affects motor cortical activity in young and old adults. Exp Gerontol. 2016;73:78–85.
58. Pasma JH, Bijlsma AYJ, Klip JM, Stijntjes M, Blauw GJ, Muller M, et al. Blood pressure associates with standing balance in elderly outpatients. PLoS One. 2014;9:e106808.
59. Stijntjes M, Pasma JH, van Vuuren M, Blauw GJ, Meskers CG, Maier AB. Low cognitive status is associated with a lower ability to maintain standing balance in elderly outpatients. Gerontology. 2015;61(2):124–30.
60. Bijlsma AY, Pasma JH, Lambers D, Stijntjes M, Blauw GJ, Meskers CG, et al. Muscle strength rather than muscle mass is associated with standing balance in elderly outpatients. J Am Med Dir Assoc. 2013;14:493–8.
61. Kouzaki M, Shinohara M. Steadiness in plantar flexor muscles and its relation to postural sway in young and elderly adults. Muscle Nerve. 2010;42(1):78–87.
62. Gu M-J, Schultz AB, Shepard NT, Alexander NB. Postural control in young and elderly adults when stance is perturbed: dynamics. J Biomech. 1996;29(3):319–29.
63. Wu G. The relation between age-related changes in neuromusculoskeletal system and dynamic postural responses to balance disturbance. J Gerontol A Biol Sci Med Sci. 1998;53(4):M320–6.
64. Schulz BW, Ashton-Miller JA, Alexander NB. Compensatory stepping in response to waist pulls in balance-impaired and unimpaired women. Gait Posture. 2005;22(3):198–209.
65. McIlroy WE, Maki BE. Changes in early automatic postural responses associated with the prior-planning and execution of a compensatory step. Brain Res. 1993;631(2):203–11.
66. Rijken NH, van Engelen BG, de Rooy JW, Geurts AC, Weerdesteyn V. Trunk muscle involvement is most critical for the loss of balance control in patients with facioscapulohumeral muscular dystrophy. Clin Biomech (Bristol, Avon). 2014;29(8):855–60.
67. Kuo AD. Stabilization of lateral motion in passive dynamic walking. Int J Robot Res. 1999;18(9):917–30.
68. Bruijn SM, Meijer OG, Beek PJ, van Dieen JH. Assessing the stability of human locomotion: a review of current measures. J R Soc Interface. 2013;10(83):20120999.
69. Hamacher D, Singh NB, Van Dieen JH, Heller MO, Taylor WR. Kinematic measures for assessing gait stability in elderly individuals: a systematic review. J R Soc Interface. 2011;8(65):1682–98.
70. Toebes MJ, Hoozemans MJ, Furrer R, Dekker J, van Dieen JH. Local dynamic stability and variability of gait are associated with fall history in elderly subjects. Gait Posture. 2012;36(3):527–31.
71. van Schooten KS, Pijnappels M, Rispens SM, Elders P, Lips P, van Dieen JH. Ambulatory fall-risk assessment: amount and quality of daily-life gait predict falls in older adults. J Gerontol A Biol Sci Med Sci. 2015;70:608–15.
72. Hof AL, Gazendam MGJ, Sinke WE. The condition for dynamic stability. J Biomech. 2005;38(1):1–8.
73. Arvin M, Mazaheri M, Pijinappels M, Hoozemans MJM, Burger BJ, Verschueren SM, et al. Effects of narrow base gait on mediolateral balance control in young and older adults. J Biomech. 2016;43:1264–7.
74. Arvin M, Hoozemans M, Pijnappels M, Duysens J, Verschueren SM, van Dieën JH. Where to step? Contributions of stance leg muscle spindle afference to planning of mediolateral foot placement for balance control in young and older adults. Front Physiol. 2018;9(1134)
75. Kang HG, Dingwell JB. Separating the effects of age and walking speed on gait variability. Gait Posture. 2008;27(4):572–7.

76. Bruijn SM, Van Impe A, Duysens J, Swinnen SP. White matter microstructural organization and gait stability in older adults. Front Aging Neurosci. 2014;6:6.
77. van Dieën JH, Pijnappels M, Bobbert MF. Age-related intrinsic limitations in preventing a trip and regaining balance after a trip. Saf Sci. 2005;43(7):437–53.
78. Patla AE, Prentice SD, Rietdyk S, Allard F, Martin C. What guides the selection of alternate foot placement during locomotion in humans. Exp Brain Res. 1999;128(4):441–50.
79. Weerdesteyn V, Nienhuis B, Mulder T, Duysens J. Older women strongly prefer stride lengthening to shortening in avoiding obstacles. Exp Brain Res. 2005;161(1):39–46.
80. Moraes R, Allard F, Patla AE. Validating determinants for an alternate foot placement selection algorithm during human locomotion in cluttered terrain. J Neurophysiol. 2007;98:1928–40.
81. Chen HC, Ashton-Miller JA, Alexander NB, Schultz AB. Effects of age and available response time on ability to step over an obstacle. J Gerontol. 1994;49(5):M227–33.
82. Patla AE, Rietdyk S, Martin C, Prentice S. Locomotor patterns of the leading and the trailing limbs as solid and fragile obstacles are stepped over: some insights into the role of vision during locomotion. J Mot Behav. 1996;28:35–47.
83. Patla AE, Vickers JN. Where and when do we look as we approach and step over an obstacle in the travel path? Neuroreport. 1997;8:3661–5.
84. McFadyen BJ, Prince F. Avoidance and accommodation of surface height changes by healthy, community-dwelling, young, and elderly men. J Gerontol. 2002;57:B166–B74.
85. Persad CC, Giordani B, Chen HC, Ashton-Miller JA, Alexander NB, Wilson CS, et al. Neuropsychological predictors of complex obstacle avoidance in healthy older adults. J Gerontol B Psychol Sci Soc Sci. 1995;50(5):272–7.
86. Chen HC, Schultz AB, Ashton-Miller JA, Giordani B, Alexander NB, Guire KE. Stepping over obstacles: dividing attention impairs performance of old more than young adults. J Gerontol Ser A Biol Sci Med Sci. 1996;51(3):M116–22.
87. Eng JJ, Winter DA, Patla AE. Strategies for recovery from a trip in early and late swing during human walking. Exp Brain Res. 1994;102:339–49.
88. Pijnappels M, Bobbert MF, van Dieen JH. How early reactions in the support limb contribute to balance recovery after tripping. J Biomech. 2005;38(3):627–34.
89. Pijnappels M, Bobbert MF, van Dieen JH. Push-off reactions in recovery after tripping discriminate young subjects, older non-fallers and older fallers. Gait Posture. 2005;21(4):388–94.
90. Thelen DG, Muriuki M, James J, Schultz AB, Ashton-Miller JA, Alexander NB. Muscle activities used by young and old adults when stepping to regain balance during a forward fall. J Electromyogr Kinesiol. 2000;10(2):93–101.
91. Pavol MJ, Owings TM, Foley KT, Grabiner MD. Mechanisms leading to a fall from an induced trip in healthy older adults. J Gerontol A Biol Sci Med Sci. 2001;56(7):M428–37.
92. Pijnappels M, Bobbert MF, van Dieen JH. Contribution of the support limb in control of angular momentum after tripping. J Biomech. 2004;37(12):1811–8.
93. van der Burg JC, Pijnappels M, van Dieen JH. The influence of artificially increased trunk stiffness on the balance recovery after a trip. Gait Posture. 2007;26(2):272–8.
94. Mancini M, Horak FB. The relevance of clinical balance assessment tools to differentiate balance deficits. Eur J Phys Rehabil Med. 2010;46(2):239–48.
95. Yardley L, Beyer N, Hauer K, Kempen G, Piot-Ziegler C, Todd C. Development and initial validation of the Falls Efficacy Scale-International (FES-I). Age Ageing. 2005;34(6):614–9.
96. Powell LE, Myers AM. The Activities-specific Balance Confidence (ABC) Scale. J Gerontol Ser A Biol Med Sci. 1995;50A(1):M28–34.
97. Cofre Lizama LE, Pijnappels M, Rispens SM, Reeves NP, Verschueren SM, van Dieen JH. Mediolateral balance and gait stability in older adults. Gait Posture. 2015;42:79–84.
98. Tinetti ME. Performance-oriented assessment of mobility problems in elderly patients. J Am Geriatr Soc. 1986;34(2):119–26.
99. Berg K, Wood-Dauphinee S, Williams JI, Gayton D. Measuring balance in the elderly: preliminary development of an instrument. Physiother Can. 1989;41(6):304–11.
100. Podsiadlo D, Richardson S. The timed "Up & Go": a test of basic functional mobility for frail elderly persons. J Am Geriatr Soc. 1991;39(2):142–8.

101. Guralnik JM, Simonsick EM, Ferrucci L, Glynn RJ, Berkman LF, Blazer DG, et al. A short physical performance battery assessing lower extremity function: association with self-reported disability and prediction of mortality and nursing home admission. J Gerontol. 1994;49(2):M85–94.
102. Weerdesteyn V, Laing AC, Robinovitch SN. The body configuration at step contact critically determines the successfulness of balance recovery in response to large backward perturbations. Gait Posture. 2012;35(3):462–6.
103. Fujimoto M, Bair WN, Rogers MW. Center of pressure control for balance maintenance during lateral waist-pull perturbations in older adults. J Biomech. 2015;48(6):963–8.
104. Toebes MJ, Hoozemans MJM, Dekker J, van Dieen JH. Effects of unilateral leg muscle fatigue on balance control in perturbed and unperturbed gait in healthy elderly. Gait Posture. 2014;40:215–9.
105. Vlutters M, van Asseldonk EHF, van der Kooij H. Lower extremity joint-level responses to pelvis perturbation during human walking. Sci Rep. 2018;8(1):14621.
106. Bruijn SM, Meijer OG, Beek PJ, van Dieën JH. The effects of arm swing on human gait stability. Exp Biol. 2010;213:3945–52.
107. Rabago CA, Dingwell JB, Wilken JM. Reliability and minimum detectable change of temporal-spatial, kinematic, and dynamic stability measures during perturbed gait. PLoS One. 2015;10(11):e0142083.
108. Lord SR, Menz HB, Tiedemann A. A physiological profile approach to falls risk assessment and prevention. Phys Ther. 2003;83(3):237–52.
109. Horak FB, Wrisley DM, Frank J. The Balance Evaluation Systems Test (BESTest) to differentiate balance deficits. Phys Ther. 2009;89(5):484–98.
110. Chien JH, Eikema DJ, Mukherjee M, Stergiou N. Locomotor sensory organization test: a novel paradigm for the assessment of sensory contributions in gait. Ann Biomed Eng. 2014;42(12):2512–23.
111. Schepens S, Sen A, Painter JA, Murphy SL. Relationship between fall-related efficacy and activity engagement in community-dwelling older adults: a meta-analytic review. Am J Occup Ther. 2012;66(2):137–48.
112. Kempen GI, Yardley L, van Haastregt JC, Zijlstra GA, Beyer N, Hauer K, et al. The Short FES-I: a shortened version of the falls efficacy scale-international to assess fear of falling. Age Ageing. 2008;37(1):45–50.
113. Delbaere K, Smith ST, Lord SR. Development and initial validation of the Iconographical Falls Efficacy Scale. J Gerontol A Biol Sci Med Sci. 2011;66(6):674–80.
114. Weijer RHA, Hoozemans MJM, van Dieen JH, Pijnappels M. Construct validity and reliability of the modified Gait Efficacy Scale for older adults. Disabil Rehabil. 2020;44:2464.
115. Pasma JH, Engelhart D, Schouten AC, van der Kooij H, Maier AB, Meskers CG. Impaired standing balance: the clinical need for closing the loop. Neuroscience. 2014;267:157–65.
116. Huurnink A, Fransz DP, Kingma I, van Dieen JH. Comparison of a laboratory grade force platform with a Nintendo Wii Balance Board on measurement of postural control in single-leg stance balance tasks. J Biomech. 2013;46(7):1392–5.
117. Pajala S, Era P, Koskenvuo M, Kaprio J, Tormakangas T, Rantanen T. Force platform balance measures as predictors of indoor and outdoor falls in community-dwelling women aged 63-76 years. J Gerontol A Biol Sci Med Sci. 2008;63(2):171–8.
118. Blaszczyk JW, Lowe DL, Hansen PD. Ranges of postural stability and their changes in the elderly. Gait Posture. 1994;2(1):11–7.
119. Arvin M, van Dieën JH, Faber GS, Pijnappels M, Hoozemans MJM, Verschueren SM. Hip abductor neuromuscular capacity: a limiting factor in mediolateral balance control in older adults? Clin Biomech. 2016;37:27–33.
120. Sawers A, Ting LH. Beam walking can detect differences in walking balance proficiency across a range of sensorimotor abilities. Gait Posture. 2015;41(2):619–23.
121. Sawers A, Hafner B. Validation of the Narrowing Beam Walking Test in lower limb prosthesis users. Arch Phys Med Rehabil. 2018;99(8):1491–8 e1.

122. Sawers A, Hafner BJ. Narrowing beam-walking is a clinically feasible approach for assessing balance ability in lower-limb prosthesis users. J Rehabil Med. 2018;50(5):457–64.
123. Sawers A, Hafner BJ. Using clinical balance tests to assess fall risk among established unilateral lower limb prosthesis users: cutoff scores and associated validity indices. PM R. 2020;12(1):16–25.
124. Sawers A, Hafner BJ. Performance-based balance tests, combined with the number of falls recalled in the past year, predicts the incidence of future falls in established unilateral transtibial prosthesis users. PM R. 2022;14(4):434–44.
125. Barry E, Galvin R, Keogh C, Horgan F, Fahey T. Is the Timed Up and Go test a useful predictor of risk of falls in community dwelling older adults: a systematic review and meta-analysis. BMC Geriatr. 2014;14:14.
126. Freiberger E, de Vreede P, Schoene D, Rydwik E, Mueller V, Frändin K, et al. Performance-based physical function in older community-dwelling persons: a systematic review of instruments. Age Ageing. 2012;41(6):712–21.
127. Regterschot GR, Zhang W, Baldus H, Stevens M, Zijlstra W. Sensor-based monitoring of sit-to-stand performance is indicative of objective and self-reported aspects of functional status in older adults. Gait Posture. 2015;41(4):935–40.
128. Shany T, Wang K, Liu Y, Lovell NH, Redmond SJ. Review: are we stumbling in our quest to find the best predictor? Over-optimism in sensor-based models for predicting falls in older adults. Healthc Technol Lett. 2015;2(4):79–88.
129. Iluz T, Weiss A, Gazit E, Tankus A, Brozgol M, Dorfman M, et al. Can a body-fixed sensor reduce Heisenberg's uncertainty when it comes to the evaluation of mobility? Effects of aging and fall risk on transitions in daily living. J Gerontol A Biol Sci Med Sci. 2016;71(11):1459–65.
130. Hilliard MJ, Martinez KM, Janssen I, Edwards B, Mille M-L, Zhang Y, et al. Lateral balance factors predict future falls in community-living older adults. Arch Phys Med Rehabil. 2008;89(9):1708–13.
131. Sturnieks DL, Menant J, Delbaere K, Vanrenterghem J, Rogers MW, Fitzpatrick RC, et al. Force-controlled balance perturbations associated with falls in older people: a prospective cohort study. PLoS One. 2013;8(8):e70981.
132. Alizadehsaravi L, Koster R, Muijres W, Maas H, Bruijn SM, van Dieën JH. The underlying mechanisms of improved balance after one and ten sessions of balance training in older adults. Hum Mov Sci. 2022;81:102910.
133. Tan GR, Raitor M, Collins SH. Bump'em: an open-source, bump-emulation system for studying human balance and gait. In: IEEE International Conference on Robotics and Automation (ICRA). Paris: IEEE; 2020. p. 9093–9.
134. Roeles S, Rowe PJ, Bruijn SM, Childs CR, Tarfali GD, Steenbrink F, et al. Gait stability in response to platform, belt, and sensory perturbations in young and older adults. Med Biol Eng Comput. 2018;56:2325.
135. Rieger M, Papegaaij S, Pijnappels M, Steenbrink F, van Dieën JH. Transfer and retention effects of gait training with anterior-posterior perturbations to postural responses after medio-lateral gait perturbations in older adults. Clin Biomech. 2020;75:104988.
136. Rieger M, Papegaaij S, Steenbrink F, Pijinappels M, van Dieën JH. Development of a balance recovery performance measure for gait perturbation training based on the center of pressure. Front Sports Act Living. 2021;3:617430.
137. Taylor Z, Walsh GS, Hawkins H, Inacio M, Esser P. Perturbations during gait: a systematic review of methodologies and outcomes. Sensors (Basel). 2022;22(15)
138. Yingyongyudha A, Saengsirisuwan V, Panichaporn W, Boonsinsukh R. The Mini-Balance Evaluation Systems Test (Mini-BESTest) demonstrates higher accuracy in identifying older adult participants with history of falls than do the BESTest, Berg Balance Scale, or Timed Up and Go Test. J Geriatr Phys Ther. 2015;39:64.
139. Peterka RJ. Sensorimotor integration in human postural control. J Neurophysiol. 2002;88(3):1097–118.

140. Pasma JH, Engelhart D, Maier AB, Schouten AC, van der Kooij H, Meskers CG. Changes in sensory reweighting of proprioceptive information during standing balance with age and disease. J Neurophysiol. 2015;114(6):3220–33.
141. Geerse DJ, Coolen BH, Roerdink M. Kinematic validation of a multi-Kinect v2 instrumented 10-meter walkway for quantitative gait assessments. PLoS One. 2015;10(10):e0139913.
142. Kingma H, Gauchard GC, de Waele C, van Nechel C, Bisdorff A, Yelnik A, et al. Stocktaking on the development of posturography for clinical use. J Vestib Res. 2011;21(3):117–25.

Part II

Walking

Gait Stability and Aging

7

Luis Mochizuki and Sandra Aliberti

Abstract

Stability is an important concept in biomechanics. It means that a mechanical system in equilibrium should resist changing its motion properties after an external perturbation. Gait is one of the most common ways of locomotion in humans. Walking is a motor action achieved by the interaction of the nervous system, muscles, joints, and bones with the environment and its external forces. Moreover, unhealthy conditions can change how older people walk when they cause motor impairments. Therefore, it is important to comprehend how individuals deal with an external perturbation to maintain their walking pattern, i.e., how to control the body to keep it stable during walking. The aim of this chapter is to describe the tools based on the dynamical systems approach that are built to evaluate the stability during gait with a focus on aging. Concepts of dynamical systems in gait analysis, the main concerns when applying those tools, and how the most common biomechanical variables applied to gait analysis should be prepared for that purpose.

Introduction

In 1901, Ferrier [1] stated that the stretching of the foot is a physiological mechanism that neutralizes body vibration during walking, increases foot contact with the ground, and increases body stability to support the body weight. Different biomechanisms are available to stabilize the body during walking. Moreover, the analysis of

L. Mochizuki (✉)
School of Arts, Sciences and Humanities, University of São Paulo, São Paulo, Brazil
e-mail: mochi@usp.br

S. Aliberti
Paulista University, São Paulo, Brazil

F. A. Barbieri et al. (eds.), *Locomotion and Posture in Older Adults*,
https://doi.org/10.1007/978-3-031-74123-4_7

stability during walking or running has been increasing in the last half-century. We did a search at PUBMED database, and since the 1970s, there has been an exponential growth in the number of papers involving these subjects (stability AND gait OR walking OR running) (Fig. 7.1). The aim of this chapter is to describe the tools to evaluate the stability of walking; the main concerns to applying those tools and concepts of dynamical systems in gait analysis and how the most common biomechanical variables applied to gait analysis should be prepared for that.

Stability can be understood from different points of view. For mechanics, stability is a condition that classifies the body's equilibrium as stable and unstable. Stable equilibrium occurs when any external perturbation does not change its final potential energy. For mechanics, direction stability deals with the perpendicular forces applied to the body that are moving along a path. For fluid mechanics, stability deals with the effects of turbulence on the motion of the body. In mathematics, stability is the analysis of partial equations and dynamical systems and its tendency to converge or diverge. In motor control, stability is usually associated with balance and equilibrium. Maintaining the upright standing balance demands stabilizing the projection of the position of the center of mass (COM) inside of the limits of the basis

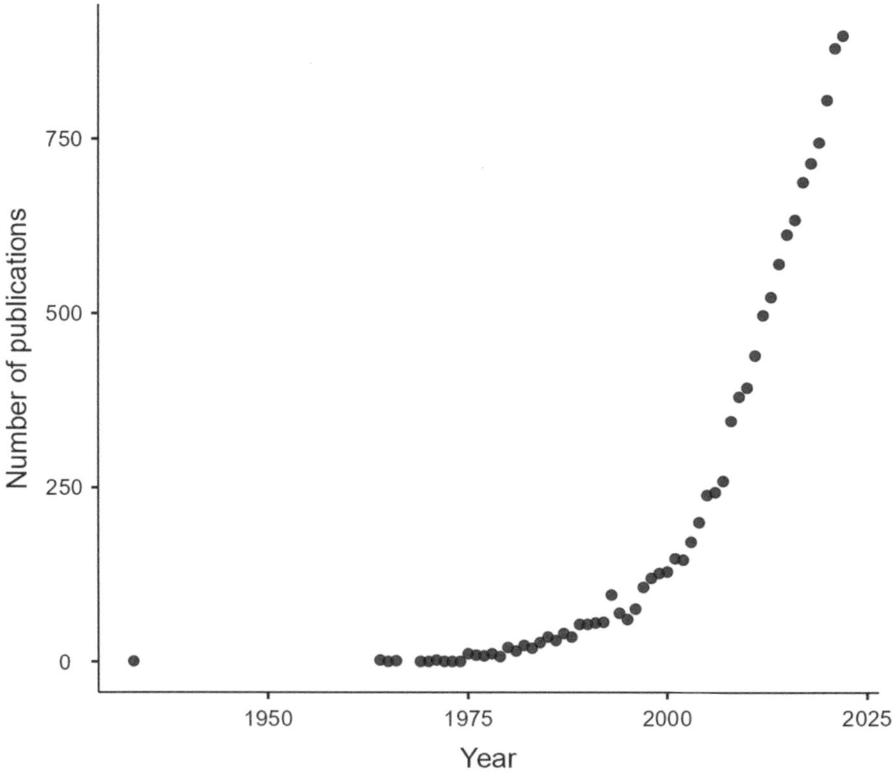

Fig. 7.1 Number of articles indexed in PUBMED using the query [(GAIT or WALKING or RUNNING) and DYNAMICS]

of support. For motor control, stability is not only associated with balance. It is associated with maintaining a certain body position during a motor action in every necessary situation. The most common situation is the standing position. Other examples are maintaining shoulder position while doing hand activities or hip position while walking. The ability to hold a stable joint position during a motor action is important for performance and to decrease the risk of injuries.

A dynamical system can be evaluated by the behavior of its trajectories under small perturbations of its initial conditions. The sensibility to small changes in the initial conditions defines if a dynamical system can be fully predicted or it has specific conditions on which its behavior becomes complicated. The apparent randomness of a system results from the lack of accurate knowledge of the initial conditions [2], while intrinsic randomness is related to intrinsic and complex relations within the dynamical system [2]. There are different examples of dynamical systems in nature, but we shall focus on those related to motor behavior.

Walking can be modeled and studied as a dynamical system [3]. Therefore, walking can be described, analyzed, and predicted. The time series of stride intervals during walking presents allometric properties [4], which suggests that its fluctuations exhibit a long-range correlation and are not related to short-range correlation nor any random processes. Stride frequency or gait cadence results from the interaction between the internal system and the external forces and constraints. The combination of ground reaction forces, stance time, stride frequency, and length changes gait velocity. What is the source of such intrinsic variability?

Walking is a motor action achieved by the interaction of the nervous system, muscles, joints, and bones with the environment and its external forces. Moreover, unhealthy conditions are prone to change how people walk. On the other hand, evaluating how someone walks gives valuable information about their health status. The coordination between the body's structures under distinct types of stress might lead to affect how they are coupled. To explore the natural restraint of the anatomical structures, different couplings between joints are tested during motor development and learning. Therefore, it is important to comprehend how individuals deal with an external perturbation to maintain their walking pattern, i.e., how to control the body to keep it stable during walking.

The Tools to Evaluate the Stability of Walking

Physiological systems are open systems (they change energy or mass with the environment), nonlinear, and their periodicity is triggered by external and internal factors. Mathematical concepts to analyze the nonlinear behavior of dynamical systems are available for the analysis of physiological systems. Most nonlinear tools are designed for low-dimension deterministic chaos. It means that such dynamical systems are determinist (predictable) and sensitive to initial conditions (chaotic behavior). But the dimension of physiological systems is not a priori known. Besides, the nature of randomness in physiological systems is hard to understand because it can come from any interaction with the world.

What variables should we use to apply dynamical system tools to evaluate the dynamics of walking? Descriptive variables obtained from gait analysis are usually used in the dynamical systems approach, such as stride-to-stride distance, joint angles or body position, and body acceleration. Time series of those variables are commonly used to calculate the Lyapunov exponents, the dynamical systems metric related to stability.

Aleksandr Mikhailovich Lyapunov was born on 6 June 1857 at Yaroslavl, Russia [5]. In 1880, he graduated in mathematics at Saint Petersburg University, where he was very influenced by Professor P.L. Chebyshev. In Moscow, in 1892, he defended his doctoral thesis "The general problem of the stability of motion" and one member of his doctoral thesis's committee members was N.E. Zhukovski (the father of Russian aviation). In his thesis, Lyapunov discussed the fact that the motion of a particle can be stable in relation to one variable, but it can be unstable in relation to another variable. Besides, he suggested that, given a function $x(t)$, there is a critical number which is the characteristic number of this function. This characteristic number or Lyapunov exponent (LyE) has been used to analyze if two points $x_1(t)$ and $x_2(t)$, in the state space of a dynamical system that is initially very close, remain together in time. This notion of motion stability can be measured with LyE; therefore, it can be used to understand chaotic motion. Chaos relates to aperiodic dynamics in deterministic equations in which there is a sensitivity to initial conditions [6]. In a chaotic motion [5], long-term prediction is seriously affected because those two points move apart as time increases.

Stability can be measured with LyE and recurrence quantification analysis (RQA). In this chapter, we will focus on local dynamic behavior by LyE. LyE measures the sensitivity of a dynamical system to small perturbations. The short-term and long-term maximum LyEs are, respectively, related to the structure of the gait and complementary gait information [3]. First, entropy and variability can be found in articles as measures of stability. Second, it is not unusual to find LyE as a measure of variability or combined with entropy. Entropy determines the complexity of a system. Variability relates to how variable is the behavior/response of a system. Thus, entropy and variability are not truly measures of stability, but they access concepts that might be connected to stability [7]. From RQA, it is possible to measure repeatability (absolute agreement among repetitions, how often a dynamical system shows a similar behavior by percent recurrence), predictability (how predictable is a dynamical system by percent determinism), complexity (entropy), and stationarity (how stationary is a dynamical system in time by trend). Repeatability and predictability are measures associated with stability.

The dynamical system's approach to understanding local dynamical stability calculates LyE to generate gait information. Bruijn et al. [8] compared different approaches to measure gait stability (the maximum LyE, the maximum Floquet multiplier, variability measures, long-range correlations, extrapolated COM, stabilizing and destabilizing forces, foot placement estimator, gait sensitivity norm, and maximum allowable—perturbation); they have shown the maximum LyE has a construct validity to explain stability, more specifically, the short maximum LyE is a valid predictor of the probability of falling (predictive validity). Review [9] found

LyE is the most common nonlinear dynamical measure to distinguish the gait kinematics of healthy older adults and older adults at risk of falling. The studies we will present are based on motion capture data and on accelerometers that were attached to the lower limb. Oscillations due to different gait phases are analyzed under the dynamical systems approach.

Emmerik et al. [7] suggest stability should be defined based on the constraints of the task. Stability in shorter and longer time scales are captured by different approaches (respectively, LyE and the state space analysis based on maximal Floquet multipliers) that might show opposite results.

Stability, Development, and Aging

There are concerns about the use of LyE or local dynamical stability. Should we use local dynamical stability to understand the changes in walking across ages? Local dynamical stability changes due to aging. Toddlers, young, and older adults do not have similar local dynamical stability during walking [10]; however, those changes might not be observed when directional components of acceleration are used to calculate LyE. Bisi et al. [10] compared walking in toddlers and young and older adults. These authors applied short-term LyE and RQA to compare strides among participants. Short-term LyE was calculated from all combined three orthogonal trunk acceleration components and RQA were able to discern between strides from toddlers and young adults, and from young adults and older adults. Besides, stability does not have a monotonic relation to aging. Terrier and Reynard [11] compared LyE calculated from participants aged from 20 to 69 years old. They walked on a treadmill for 5 min wearing a 3D accelerometer on the trunk. The authors found a quadratic association between age and gait instability in the mediolateral direction. Gait instability begins to increase at an accelerated rate as early as age 40–50. Consequently, local dynamical stability might be used to compare the effects of aging in walking.

Walking on a treadmill and overground does not have the same stability [9]. Bizovska et al. [12], Ihlen et al. [13], and Hamacher et al. [14] showed that overground walking presented higher LyE across ages. Reviews [3, 9] also showed LyE is lower in older people than younger adults.

Another comparison across ages was performed with amputees. To identify how amputees control the pelvis when they have walked under different conditions, Howcroft et al. [15] evaluated unilateral transtibial amputees of different ages, but they found similar behaviors across ages. Unilateral transtibial amputees aged from 40 to 90 years old have similar pelvis stability when they have done level ground walking and simulated uneven ground walking. Howcroft et al. [16] evaluated those amputees walking with inertial sensors on the pelvis during level and uneven conditions. The maximum LyE was similar for those two conditions.

Stability in walking can be also associated with the risk of falling. Young and old adults do not have the same consequences after an accidental fall. Older adults have higher mortality after a fall than young adults and they are prone to have more health conditions related to falls. Therefore, the risk of falling in older adults is a public health problem. The presence of risk factors (loss of muscle power and strength, balance diseases, visual problems, and others) is used to define the risk of falling. Functional tests have been also designed to determine the risk of falling in older adults. Although it is quite known which are the risk factors and functional tests, both fail to prevent falls. Therefore, researchers are still looking for variables or tests to clearly find the ones that are more associated with the risk of falling. Lockhart and Liu [16] designed an experiment to evaluate whether the largest LyE is sensitive enough to differentiate people prone to accidental falls. Healthy young and older adults, and fall-prone older adults walked on a treadmill for 1 min and the kinematics of the trunk and foot were recorded for further analysis. Maximum LyE was the highest for the fall-prone older adults' group.

Another study about falls in the elderly evaluated how older adults recover from a fall on a slippery surface. About 100 older adults participated in a gait-slip experiment. Yang and Pai [17] asked to older adults to walk on a pathway with a sliding device. The trajectory of whole-body COM was measured and used to calculate the LyE. Short- and long-term LyE were not different between fallers and those who did not fall; although, LyE presented more sensitivity to detect falls than specificity to detect recoveries from falling.

To understand the risk of falling, studies have compared the stability during walking of fallers and non-fallers [16] and how older adults recover stability when they were walking under an unexpected slippery condition [17]. Although LyE could differentiate fallers and non-fallers, this metric was not sensible enough to discriminate when older adults slept. Another risk of falling is performing a dual task. Howcroft et al. [18] proposed that older participants should walk saying words starting with A, F, or S in random order. These authors showed that such a cognitive load did not affect the maximum LyE calculated from pelvis acceleration. Those three studies suggest that stability measured with LyE does not have a simple association with the risk of falling. Although LyE can discriminate between fallers and non-fallers, when older people perform a dual task, the changes due to the task do not affect stability. It is important to emphasize that participants performed the same task during those studies, which was walking. Even though older adults present more difficulties in performing more dangerous or complex tasks, they have preserved the same level of stability compared to walking in safe conditions.

Lyapunov exponents are sensitive to find changes in gait stability not only due to falls. Unstable walking behaviors might be observable when someone rumbles or clumbles while walking. Claudication can be induced by peripheral arterial disease (PAD). Myers et al. [19] compared older people with PAD and matched healthy controls when they were walking on a treadmill. PAD participants had higher largest LyE compared to the control group. Another health condition that changes gait patterns is orthopedical conditions. Such conditions induce pain or lead to physical constraints in joint movements. Osteoarthritis is one example of such condition. Alkjaer et al. [20] showed that older women with osteoarthritis and matched controls have similar stability in joint kinematics. Alkjaer et al. [20] evaluated the ankle and knee kinematics for 6-minute walking test on a treadmill and used those data to calculate the largest LyE. Those women with osteoarthritis presented similar knee and ankle largest LyE compared with matched controls. To avoid pain, it is common to observe that people change how to move. This pain avoidance was studied by Hamacher et al. [21] using visual feedback. Visual feedback was applied to change gait patterns to avoid pain in parts of the body. Hamacher et al. [21] applied this approach to 60-year-old women. Those authors found that visual feedback of frontal plane pelvis and trunk movements have increased the largest LyE.

Stability and Gait Speed

When researchers design an experimental protocol for gait analysis, one typical concern is walking speed. Two main branches appear: studies with self-selected walking speed and studies with fixed walking speed. Any walking speed can be achieved by a combination of stride length and stride frequency. For fast running, athletes usually do not change stride frequency but increase stride length [20]. Russel and Haworth [22] compared LyE calculated during preferred walking stride frequency (PSF), and higher and lower stride frequencies in young adults. The authors found that local dynamic stability was maximal at the PSF, becoming less stable for higher and lower stride frequencies.

England and Granata [23] examined gait instability in relation to walking velocity. When the data from every stride were time-normalized to one hundred data points per stride, these authors found that LyE was linearly associated with walking velocity. Temporal variation per stride introduces a more quadratic trend. Smaller LyE represents a more stable system. England and Granata [23] found every lower limb joint was more stable at lower velocities.

Sampling Frequency and Stability

Mehdizadeh [24] summarized the methodological approaches to quantifying LyE in young and older adults during normal walking. He has extracted important methodological information about how LyE was calculated (sampling rate, body segments, and joints, number of strides/steps, variable type, filtering, time-normalizing, state space dimension, time delay, and LyE algorithm) and compared (walking surface, data recording method, and walking speed).

To calculate the LyE, phase space portraits are necessary to identify the nearest neighbors. An important requirement to calculate local dynamical stability is the minimum number of data points. As a rule, it is necessary 10^d, where d is the data dimension [25]. To achieve such a requirement, it is important to use the adequate sampling frequency and collect data for time enough to have enough data. England and Granata [23] investigated the effect of halving the number of data samples per stride. They compared results from data that were re-sampled at 3000 samples per 30 strides versus results from the same walking trials that were re-sampling at 1500 samples per 30 strides; both resample rates retained the stride-to-stride temporal variation of the original kinematic data. Although shorter data set lengths reduced the mean value of λMax by 17.2%.

Riva et al. [26] measured variability and stability (standard deviation, coefficient of variation, poincaré plots, maximum Floquet multipliers, short-term LyE, recurrence quantification analysis, multiscale entropy, harmonic ratio, and index of harmonicity) with stride duration and trunk acceleration data during walking. Those authors verified the effect of sampling frequency and directional changes in walking (young adults should walk for 6 min along a 30 m pathway) on variability and stability measures. They found that multiscale entropy, short-term LyE, and recurrence quantification analysis were not affected by directional changes nor by sampling frequency (100 and 200 Hz).

Riva et al. [27] calculated the short-term/long-term LyE and RQA in ten young adults. Participants walked in a straight line at a self-selected speed on a 250-m-long dead-end road (about 180 strides). The acceleration of the trunk and shank were measured. The authors have studied the minimum number of strides required to use those measures. Ten strides were enough for LyE and RQA to depict walking behaviors.

Reynard and Terrier [28] calculated the local dynamical stability (LDS) using LyE in walking tests, and they found: (1) the intra-session repeatability of gait LDS was about 0.50 for long-term LDS and 0.85 for short-term LDS, the intersession repeatability was around 0.6 for both short and long-term LDS; (2) Long-term LDS estimated from short-duration measurements (35 strides) exhibited low repeatability, while that of short- term LDS was around 0.75; (3) Long-term LDS exhibited discrepancy between the predicted repeatability and the actual repeatability, while it was not the case for short-term LDS; (4) Considering both intra correlation coefficient and standard error mean, short-term LDS measured over one step tended to have better intra-and inter-session reliability than short-term LDS measured over one stride. Therefore, the authors have recommended normalizing sample length before computing LDS to thwart the trend to higher LDS estimates with longer measurements. For long-term LDS, it is highly recommended to record long-duration walking tests with a treadmill; its use should be restricted to group-level assessment with a sufficient sample size to lower type II error risk. For short-term LDS, it is recommended to use λ 0.5; it may be sufficient to detect moderate changes (around 20%) at the individual level. However, due to the lower inter-session repeatability, one should aggregate measures taken on different days to better approximate the true LDS.

Although filtering removes information within the data, Mehdizadeh (2018) [24] showed the LyE values calculated with and without filtering were in the same range, suggesting filtering the signal before calculating LyE does not have a deteriorating effect on the LyE value.

Algorithms to Calculate the Lyapunov Exponent

Local dynamic stability or largest (maximum) LyE depicts how rate-close trajectories converge or diverge infinitesimally within an n-dimensional phase space [29]. Mostly, two algorithms are applied to calculate the largest LyE: Wolf [30] and Rosenstein [31] algorithms.

Wolf et al. [30] presented a technique to calculate the non-negative LyE from finite amounts of experimental data, but this technique is limited to systems where a well-defined one-dimensional (l-D) map can be recovered. This approach is based on a spectral estimation of LyE. Wolf et al. [30] remind us that is necessary to attend to three factors to calculate LyE: the number of points necessary to provide an adequate number of replacement points (between 10^d and 30^d, where d is the embedded dimension), the number of orbits to probe stretching (but not folding) within the attractor (10–100), and the number of data points per orbit that allow for proper attractor reconstruction with delay coordinates ($d \times 10^{d-1}$ to $d \times 100^{d-1}$).

Rosenstein et al. [31] proposed another technique to calculate the largest LyE, claiming its reliability for small data sets. Those authors have used the method of delays to develop a fast and easily implemented algorithm. The matrix of reconstructed trajectories of the data is used to reconstruct the dynamics of the system. Then, Rosenstein's algorithm locates the nearest neighbor of each point on the trajectory. The authors have used time series as short as only 100–1000 data points successfully.

It is important to emphasize that the more accurate LyE is observable with larger data sets [29]. One thing that must be avoided, for the necessary data length, is to indiscriminately increase the sampling rate. Despite a higher sampling rate does augment the length of a time series, it does not necessarily increase information. A parsimonious relation between information and sampling frequency exists (Nyquist frequency) and must be considered to decide the adequate sampling frequency.

Conclusion

Gait stability can suggest whether an older adult shows a stable and unstable gait pattern. Dynamical systems approach offers the frame and proper concepts to define stability, variability, and coordination. Many parameters based on dynamical systems or variability are used to study gait stability in older people. Definitions of those parameters tell that different issues might be accessed during gait stability studies that do not have a relation to stability. Important concerns about sampling, minimum number of strides, data normalization, and reliability were presented. LyE can be used to compare persons of different ages.

References

1. Ferrier JF. The stretching of the foot during walking. Comptes Rendus des Seances de la Societe de Biologie et de ses Filiales. 1901;53:721–2.
2. Hamill J, van Emmerik RE, Heiderscheit BC, Li L. A dynamical systems approach to lower extremity running injuries. Clin Biomech (Bristol, Avon). 1999;14(5):297–308.
3. Bera MN, Acin A, Kus M, et al. Randomness in quantum mechanics: philosophy, physics and technology. Rep Prog Phys. 2017;80:124001.
4. Hausdorff JM, Peng CK, Ladin Z, Wei JY, Goldberger AL. Is walking a random walk? Evidence for long-range correlations in stride interval of human gait. J Appl Physiol. 1995;78(l):349–58.
5. Parks PC. A. M. Lyapunov's stability theory—100 years on. IMA J Math Control Inform. 1992;9:275–303.
6. Glass L. Synchronization and rhythmic processes in physiology. Nature. 2001;410:277–84.
7. van Emmerik REA, Ducharme SW, Amado AC, Hamill J. Comparing dynamical systems concepts and techniques for biomechanical analysis. J Sport Health Sci. 2016;5(1):3–13.
8. Bruijn SM, Meijer OG, Beek PJ, van Dieen JH. Assessing the stability of human locomotion: a review of current measures. J R Soc Interface. 2013;10:20120999.
9. Amirpourabasi A, Lamb SE, Chow JY, Williams GKR. Nonlinear dynamic measures of walking in healthy older adults: a systematic scoping review. Sensors. 2022;22:4408.
10. Bisi MC, Riva F, Stagni R. Measures of gait stability: performance on adults and toddlers at the beginning of independent walking. J Neuro Eng Rehab. 2014;11:131–9.
11. Terrier P, Reynard F. Effect of age on the variability and stability of gait: a cross-sectional treadmill study in healthy individuals between 20 and 69 years of age. Gait Posture. 2015;41:170–4.
12. Bizovska L, Svoboda Z, Kubonova E, Vuillerme N, Hirjakova Z, Janura M. The differences between overground and treadmill walking in nonlinear, entropy-based and frequency variables derived from accelerometers in young and older women: preliminary report. Acta Bioeng Biomech. 2018;20:93–100.
13. Ihlen EAF, Weiss A, Beck Y, Helbostad JL, Hausdorff JM. A comparison study of local dynamic stability measures of daily life walking in older adult community-dwelling fallers and non-fallers. J Biomech. 2016;49(9):1498–503.
14. Hamacher D, Hamacher D, Rehfeld K, Schega L. Motor-cognitive dual-task training improves local dynamic stability of normal walking in older individuals. Clin Biomech. 2016;32:138–41.
15. Howcroft J, Lemaire ED, Kofman J, Kendell C. Understanding dynamic stability from pelvis accelerometer data and the relationship to balance and mobility in transtibial amputees. Gait Posture. 2015;41(3):808–12.
16. Lockhart TE, Liu J. Differentiating fall-prone and healthy adults using local dynamic stability. Ergonomics. 2008;51(12):1860–72.
17. Yang F, Pai YC. Can stability really predict an impending slip-related fall among older adults? J Biomech. 2014;47(16):3876–81.
18. Howcroft JD, Lemaire ED, Kofman J, McIlroy WE. Analysis of dual-task elderly gait using wearable plantar-pressure insoles and accelerometer. Conf Proc IEEE Eng Med Biol Soc. 2014;2014:5003–6.
19. Myers SA, Johanning JM, Stergiou N, Celis RI, Robinson L, Pipinos II. Gait paring dynamical systems concepts disease. J Vasc Surg. 2009;49(4):924–31.
20. Alkjaer T, Raffalt PC, Dalsgaard H, Simonsen EB, Petersen NC, Bliddal H, Henriksen M. Gait variability and motor control in people with knee osteoarthritis. Gait Posture. 2015;42(4):479–84.
21. Hamacher D, Hamacher D, Schega L. Does visual augmented feedback reduce local dynamic stability while walking? Gait Posture. 2015;42(4):415–8.
22. Russell DM, Haworth JL. Walking at the preferred stride frequency maximizes local dynamic stability of knee motion. J Biomech. 2014;47:102–8.
23. England SA, Granata KP. The influence of gait speed on local dynamic stability of walking. Gait Posture. 2007;25(2):172–8.

24. Mehdizadeh S. The largest Lyapunov exponent of gait in young and elderly individuals: a systematic review. Gait Posture. 2018;60:241–50.
25. Rossler OE. Continuous chaos—four prototype equations. Ann NY Acad Sci. 1979;316:376–92.
26. Riva F, Grimpampi E, Mazzà C, Stagni R. Are gait variability and stability measures influenced by directional changes? Bio Medical Engineering OnLine. 2014;13:56–65.
27. Riva F, Bisi MC, Stagni R. Gait variability and stability measures: minimum number of strides and within-session reliability. Comput Biol Med. 2014;50:9–13.
28. Reynard F, Terrier P. Local dynamic stability of treadmill walking: intrasession and week-to-week repeatability. J Biomec. 2014;47:74–80.
29. Cignetti F, Decker LM, Stergiou N. Sensitivity of the Wolf's and Rosenstein's algorithms to evaluate local dynamic stability from small gait data sets. Ann Biomed Eng. 2012;40:1122.
30. Wolf A, Swift JB, Swinney HL, Vastano JA. Determining lyapunov exponentts from a time series. Physica D. 1985;16:285–317.
31. Rosenstein MT, Collins JJ, De Luca CJ. A practical method for calculating largest Lyapunov exponents from small data sets. Physica D. 1993;65:117–34.

Visual Control of Adaptive Locomotion and Changes Due to Ageing

8

Mark Hollands, Kristen Hollands, and Shirley Rietdyk

Abstract

This chapter will review current theories of how adults use vision to guide adaptations to the basic locomotor rhythm in order to cope with environmental demands e.g. to step over an obstacle in our path, or to guide the foot to specific safe areas in the terrain, or to cope with the challenges to balance posed by descending stairs. A finding common to different gait adaptations is that they are usually, by necessity, programmed in advance to ensure stability and maximize efficiency. Thus visual cues are predominantly sampled and used in a feedforward or anticipatory manner to make gait adjustments. Recent evidence suggests that older adults, particularly those characterised as being at higher risk of tripping and falling, show changes in visuomotor control during adaptive locomotion and that the resulting changes to visual behaviour may be causally related to lower limb movement inaccuracies, compromised balance control and associated increased falls risk. The putative neural and biomechanical mechanisms underlying these changes will be discussed alongside the potential applications of current knowledge to falls prevention and rehabilitation in older adult populations.

M. Hollands (✉)
School of Sport and Exercise Sciences, Liverpool John Moores University, Liverpool, UK
e-mail: M.A.Hollands@ljmu.ac.uk

K. Hollands
School of Allied Health Professions, MacKay Building, Keele University,
Keele, Staffordshire, UK
e-mail: k.sorensen@keele.ac.uk

S. Rietdyk
Department of Health and Kinesiology, Purdue University, West Lafayette, IN, USA
e-mail: srietdyk@purdue.edu

F. A. Barbieri et al. (eds.), *Locomotion and Posture in Older Adults*,
https://doi.org/10.1007/978-3-031-74123-4_8

Introduction

In the United Kingdom, around 30% of adults over the age of 65 living in the community fall each year. Furthermore, falls are the main cause of disability and the leading cause of death from injury among people aged over 75 in the United Kingdom. Older adults who survive a fall often suffer ongoing problems such as injury and infection, increasing risk for loss of mobility, depression, anxiety and an increased mortality risk. The associated healthcare costs of older adult falls in Britain alone are estimated at around £1 billion per year [1]. Therefore, understanding the mechanisms underlying falls in older adults has become an important target in ageing research, with the aim to develop effective prevention strategies.

The majority of falls result from slips or trips [2, 3] which represent a failure to place the feet appropriately to meet environmental demands, usually specified by visual information describing the locations of features such as: stair tread edges, the location and dimensions of obstacles and safe areas in the terrain. Within this chapter we will summarize our current understanding of how vision is used to guide three common walking tasks: (1) stepping onto targets, (2) ascending and descending stairs and (3) crossing obstacles. Throughout the chapter we will also review the literature demonstrating that there are age-related differences in the visual control of these common walking tasks and explore the putative neural and physiological mechanisms underlying age-related decline in function. A final aim is to discuss the relevance of these findings to the problems of falls in older adults and offer suggestions for possible interventions to restore or compensate for age-related dysfunction in the visual control of walking.

Visually Guided Target Stepping

This section aims to summarize our current understanding of how visual information is used to guide accurate lower limb movements to specific locations on the ground during walking and will provide evidence that compromised eye movement control or maladaptive gaze strategies contribute to gait deficits in patient and older adult populations. Other objectives are to explore the mechanisms underlying suboptimal gaze and stepping behaviour and to suggest potential intervention strategies to improve eye and stepping coordination and reduce falls risk. Since much of our understanding of visual control of limb movements and the role of eye movements is based on investigations of the upper limb, this review will begin with a brief overview of the eye–hand coordination literature before considering the similarities and differences in eye-foot coordination.

The majority of every day visually guided limb movements (e.g. reaching to pick up a cup of tea) are characterized by an initial saccadic eye movement to the target of interest [4] which usually results in the image of the target landing on the fovea; the most sensitive part of the retina. This behaviour is often termed visual fixation. Usually, only a single fixation is made for any single action, and gaze is often redirected away from the object before the limb reaches it [4]. Although there are very few studies that describe gaze behaviour during everyday activities, sport science literature has consistently described how the duration of the final fixation of a target (e.g. a basketball hoop or a corner of a soccer goal) prior to movement initiation, is causally related to the accuracy of the action. Joan Vickers carried out much of the seminal work in this area and coined the term 'quiet eye duration' to describe this parameter [5]. It has been demonstrated that skilled athletes show significantly longer quiet eye durations than less-skilled athletes, successful actions are preceded by longer quiet eye durations than unsuccessful actions, and that training individuals to increase quiet eye duration has a positive impact on accuracy [6–10]. In combination, these studies demonstrate that visually fixating a target is beneficial for producing accurate visually guided actions and that movement accuracy is dependent on optimal timing of eye movements to fixate targets.

Although, the specific roles of visual fixation are not fully understood, it is likely that the main function of directing gaze at a target is to provide information about the position of the target with respect to the body which is used by the motor system (or systems) controlling the limb to plan and execute the required amplitude and direction of movement in an open-loop or ballistic manner [4]. It is important to note, however, that pointing the eyes at a target provides not only visual information about target properties (e.g. direction and distance) but also has the potential to provide non-visual information such as eye muscle proprioception and efference copy of eye movement commands which signal eye direction with respect to the head [11]. This information may provide additional cues as to where the target is located with respect to the limb being controlled. Support for this notion can be found in primate neurophysiological studies. There are single neurones in the posterior parietal cortex of monkeys that are most active when the monkeys fixate targets at a specific combination of depth and eccentricity (e.g. one neurone may be preferentially active when eyes are directed 15° to the left and 10 cm in front of the head, a different neurone may be preferentially active when eyes are directed at a target laying straight ahead at a distance of 5 cm) [12]. These findings clearly demonstrate that signals derived from eye position can describe the location of the target being fixated in three-dimensional space. Although there is not yet any direct evidence of similar neural mechanisms in humans there is evidence from behavioural studies that pointing the eyes at target locations is useful even when they are not visible [13] and that final hand location when stepping and reaching to invisible targets is geometrically related to the direction in which gaze is aligned [14]. If the hypothesis is correct that pointing the eyes at a target provides a combination of visual and non-visual information that can tell the CNS where the target is in 3D space, then this might help explain the large extent to which eye and hand movements are coordinated by the CNS during reaching and pointing. For example, the latency of both eye and hand movements to look and point at targets varies greatly depending on the context in which the target is presented [15]. However, the relative timing between the eye and hand movement initiation is relatively invariant suggesting that the instructions to move them are generated synchronously. It has also been shown that when looking at, and reaching to, targets that disappear at movement onset, if the eyes start at a more eccentric location that the hand, and so move a larger distance, the hand tends to overshoot the target [16]. Conversely, it has been shown that eye kinematics are influenced by hand movement characteristics [17, 18]. There are many more examples of studies which provide evidence that eye and hand motor systems interact to produce coordinated movements when looking and pointing to targets. However, there are surprisingly few studies which have studied the coordination of eye and foot movements during walking tasks.

Hollands et al. (1995) were the first to document where and when individuals look during locomotion in a study of the timing relationships between participants' eye and stepping movements as they walked along a pathway of irregularly placed stepping targets [19]. The results showed that participants invariably fixated a target just prior to initiating a step towards it and that there was a close timing relationship between eye and foot movement initiation similar to that seen in eye–hand coordination studies. The same authors subsequently demonstrated that eye-stepping coordination was also seen when targets were temporarily rendered invisible [20]. Despite delays in step initiation resulting from the temporary removal and subsequent reinstatement of visual information, the mean interval between the start of the eye movement and the start of the swing towards a target did not vary significantly. These findings support the notion that eye and stepping movements are not programmed independently but rather are planned simultaneously as part of a coordinated eye-stepping movement similar to well-documented eye–hand coordination evident during reaches to targets. Although it is important to know when vision is sampled, this does not tell us how it is used to guide limb movements e.g. for planning the stepping trajectory in an open loop control manner or for online guidance of the limb onto the target via a closed loop control process. Hollands and Marple-Horvat (1996) showed that intermittently removing vision of stepping targets at different gait phases only affected behaviour when the limb was in stance phase (i.e. did not affect the limb in swing phase) and only when vision was unavailable during late stance [21]. Other studies have subsequently confirmed that removing vision during the stance phase of the targeting foot results in increased variability and reduced accuracy of subsequent foot placement, whereas removing vision during the ongoing swing phase has no effect [22]. These studies suggest that vision of a target is normally used in an open loop or feedforward way prior to movement initiation and is not usually needed to guide the foot onto a target. There is evidence that this behaviour represents an energy efficient biomechanical strategy resulting in pre-programmed ballistic limb movements [22–24]. However, other studies have shown that it is possible for young adults to make online adjustments to stepping trajectories as late as mid-swing phase in order to track a target that moves [25, 26] and that removing vision of the lower limb relative to a target results in reduced stepping accuracy [27]. Therefore the strategy of fixating a stepping target prior to step initiation and maintaining gaze on a target until late swing allows for optimal use of visual information to both plan and guide ongoing stepping actions. It should be noted that other studies have subsequently shown that the extent to which participants look ahead at stepping targets is dependent on the characteristics of the targets e.g. individuals tend to look two steps ahead when walking on regularly placed targets [28] but tend to look three steps in advance when walking on irregularly placed targets surrounded by differently coloured distractor targets [29]. Bonnen et al. (2021) showed that the angle of gaze relative to straight ahead increases systematically (i.e. gaze is directed increasingly closer to the feet) when walkers traverse terrain ranging from: (a) flat pavement, (b) a flat, packed earth trail containing very few obstacles, (c) an earth trail including small embedded rocks and small surface irregularities, and (d) a trail with large embedded rocks and larger surface irregularities [30]. In combination, these studies show that the extent to which walkers look ahead is dependent on the complexity or precision of the task. Despite this context- dependent variability in the relative timing of eye and stepping movements, in most situations, gaze is directed sequentially to future footfall target at some time point in advance of initiation of the step onto the target [24] suggesting that directing gaze to a location on the ground ahead is useful to the motor control system responsible for programming a step to that location. If this hypothesis is correct, then individuals who have problems making accurate eye movements should show problems in performing target stepping tasks.

The importance of making accurate eye movements in the control of accurate step generation was demonstrated in a study of cerebellar patients who exhibit both eye movement problems (including saccadic dysmetria resulting in the need for multiple saccades to fixate a target) and walking deficits (ataxic gait, including stepping inaccuracies) [31]. The authors compared stepping performance according to the extent of saccadic inaccuracy (i.e. whether patients made one, two, three or more than three saccades to fixate a target during a particular step) and found significant delays in step initiation which increased with the extent of eye movement inaccuracies. A similar approach was presented by Di Fabio et al. (2008) who studied the step climbing ability of progressive supranuclear palsy patients (PSP), a patient group who have problems generating vertical eye movements. The authors scored the patients on the extent of their oculomotor dysfunction and showed that those patients with the most severe eye movement symptoms showed diminished trailing limb step clearances putting them at an increased risk of tripping on the stair edge [32]. The results of these studies suggest that problems making eye movements may be causally linked to problems making stepping movements and raise the possibility that interventions aimed at improving eye movement function may have a positive effect on functional mobility. Indeed preliminary evidence suggests that eye movement training has a positive effect on performance in both cerebellar [33] and PSP patients [34]. These clinical studies show that stepping inaccuracies in patients with gait disorders may be caused, at least in part, by a reduced ability to fixate environmental features at appropriate times in the action sequence. Could the increased incidence of trips and falls in older adults also be partially explained by age-related changes in eye movements?

Chapman and Hollands (2006) [35] studied the gaze and stepping characteristics of older adults asked to make different combinations of target and obstacle stepping and compared their data to that collected from young adults. The older adults were separated into two groups, based on their performance in various clinical tests of functional mobility, representing those individuals deemed to have a low risk of falling and those deemed to have a higher risk of falling. Comparisons between the three groups showed that on average, the high-risk group looked away earlier from the current target than the other groups but only in the more complex tasks requiring additional future obstacles or targets (see Fig. 8.1) [35, 36]. The extent of premature redirection of gaze correlated with increased target stepping errors. A causal link between early gaze transfer and stepping inaccuracies was demonstrated in a further experiment that showed that simply instructing participants to maintain target fixation until after the foot had landed resulted in increased stepping accuracy [37].

However, this advice may not be appropriate in real-world contexts, and therefore in order to address this problem we need to know what is causing older adults to look away early.

Young et al. (2012a, 2012b) provided evidence that anxiety about upcoming obstacles is one factor that causes high-risk older adults to look away prematurely from targets [38] and that this anxiety can result from experiencing actual falls [39]. It is well-established that anxiety and fear of falling are significant predictors of falls prevalence [40]. These findings suggest that stepping inaccuracies resulting from anxiety-induced changes to gaze behaviour may offer a mechanistic partial explanation for the link between anxiety and falls risk. Interventions aimed at increasing self-confidence and reducing anxiety may well lead to improvements in gaze and stepping behaviour. Indeed, a recent proof-of-concept laboratory study showed that simply asking older adults to spend 10 s previewing a route containing obstacles prior to walking led to increased self-confidence, optimized gaze behaviour and associated improvements in stepping performance [41].

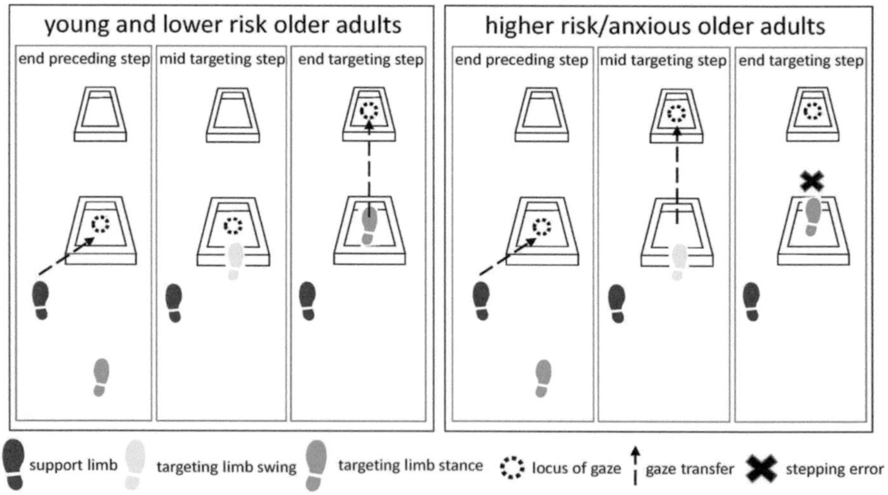

Fig. 8.1 The schematic to show the differences in gaze behaviour between higher risk/anxious older adults (HROA) and young/lower risk older adults (LROA) during a multiple stepping target task. The left panel shows that young and LROA generally fixate a target area prior to step initiation and maintain gaze on the target until after the targeting foot has landed. In contrast HROA (right panel) tend to transfer gaze away from the first stepping target (to look at the next target in the sequence) during the swing phase of the targeting limb resulting in a foot placement error

Other evidence suggests that age-related decline in cognitive function and the ability to appropriately switch attention between environmental hazards may underlie maladaptive gaze behaviour [42]. There is a large body of evidence demonstrating a link between cognitive decline and general falls risk in older adults and also between anxiety and cognitive decline [40]. A number of target stepping experiments have shown age- related decline in stepping performance is associated with cognitive function [43–46] and that delays in the timing and accuracy of step adjustments are related to, or predictive of, falls risk [38].

Finally, laboratory studies have shown age- and falls-risk related differences in visuomotor ability. High-risk older adults need to view stepping targets for longer than younger adults and low-risk older adults in order to make medial-lateral stepping adjustments [35] presumably because it takes longer to generate coordinated eye and stepping actions [25, 47]. Both Nonnekes et al.(2010) [48] and Young and Hollands (2012) [49] have proposed that delays in, possibly subcortical, visuomotor processing with aging may be responsible for disruption to timing and magnitude of stepping adjustments to visual cues in these populations.

In combination these findings suggest that maladaptive gaze behaviour, which contributes towards stepping inaccuracies and increased falls risk, results from age-related changes to a number of inter-related CNS functions. Interventions aimed at addressing this problem should therefore target each of these factors. Encouragingly, a recent randomized control trial studying the effects of multiple target stepping exercises, in

combination with a multi-component exercise programme, led to improved scores on functional mobility tests, increased target stepping accuracy, improved gaze behaviour and reduced fall rates in community dwelling older adults compared to a control group experiencing comparable exercise intensity [50]. Although the specific mechanisms that drove the improvement in walking and associated reduction in falls risk could not be fully elucidated it is possible that exercises aimed at improving visually guided stepping actions will prove effective in improving cognitive, visuomotor and physical function and reducing falls risk. One visually guided walking task that is particularly hazardous for older adults is stair walking. The next section will summarize our current understanding of the roles of vision in stair negotiation and the implications of visual decline on the problem of stair-falls in older adults.

Visual Control of Stair Walking

Falling on stairs is the leading cause of accidental death in older adults accounting for 60% of fall-related deaths [51]. Falls occur most often during stair descent [52–54] and often result from a trip on a stair edge or tread surface [52, 55] which need to be visually identified by the walker. Accordingly, as with other visually guided tasks requiring precise foot placement it is likely that appropriate direction of gaze to relevant environmental features at appropriate times is crucial for safe stair negotiation. Anecdotal evidence that supports the notion that gaze direction is important for safe stair walking comes from security video footage showing that falls are more likely to occur when an individual does not appear to look down prior to walking up or down stairs [56]. Zietz and Hollands (2009) studied gaze behaviour of both younger and older adults walking up and down the middle eight stairs of a 12-step staircase [57]. They found that both groups spent the majority of the time during both stair ascent and descent looking at the edges of stairs with an average time lead of around two to four steps. Interestingly, unlike gaze behaviour observed during target stepping described earlier in this chapter, participants did not generally look towards future foot placement locations on the stairs but rather gaze was constrained to the central portion of the stairway suggesting that gaze may serve another function than identifying locations on the steps to guide foot placement. Den otter et al. (2011) provided further evidence for this hypothesis by showing that 28–34% of treads were never fixated during stair walking and when participants travelled two stairs per step rather than one they still commonly (>35% of occasions) fixated stair treads they did not subsequently step on [58]. These studies raise the possibility that stair edges may provide visual cues that maximize perception of self-motion (derived from optic flow) to aid in balance maintenance in addition to the spatial properties of the stairs.

Zietz et al. (2011) studied the stepping characteristics and posture of older adults descending stairs under combinations of ambient light levels and stair edge contrast conditions in order to further elucidate the roles of vision describing tread edges in controlling stair walking [59]. They found that low levels of ambient lighting resulted in detrimental changes to stepping characteristics and increased tread edge contrast led to greater postural stability during stepping in the older adult groups. Other studies have confirmed that stair illumination levels and the visual properties of the stair covering influence confidence and walking characteristics of young and older adults [60, 61]. Thomas et al. (2020) [60] showed that illuminating an experimental staircase with low-power light bulbs led to lower self-confidence, a more cautious gait strategy and increased foot clearance variability with step edges compared to illumination with high-power LED bulbs. In a separate study, the same research group showed that a patterned stair surface resulted in reduced walking stability and lower confidence and found that a plain décor with edge highlighters provide optimal conditions for safe walking [61].

It is noteworthy that the role of vision when negotiating stairs seems to differ markedly from that during over ground target stepping as evidenced by the differences in gaze behaviour and effects of manipulating vision on stepping and balance characteristics. One possible reason for this difference is the predictability of the required step adjustments under comparison. Staircases usually have uniform stair dimensions and therefore the role of vision in describing their spatial properties will be understandably reduced compared to a task that required large and variable changes in step characteristics to achieve. Also, stair walking, and in particular stair descent, places much greater demands on postural and balance control than level walking, therefore it is possible that visual cues that aid the control of balance are preferentially attended. Arguably the greatest challenge to balance associated with stair walking occurs during the transitions from floor to stairs and vice versa.

Studying the visual control of such transitions is important since the three steps at the bottom and at the top of stairs are reported as the most common location for missteps and stair accidents [53, 62–64].

Miyasike-daSilva et al. (2010) studied the gaze behaviour of young adults ascending and descending stairs and included analysis of behaviour during the stair transitions [65]. Contrary to their predictions, they did not find that participants made additional or longer fixations during transition steps than during mid-steps and concluded that participants may rely more on peripheral than foveal vision to guide step transitions. This finding is consistent with the results from other studies showing that occluding the lower visual field during walking leads to various compensatory changes to head posture and gait parameters [66, 67] and that bifocal spectacles that distort the lower visual field have negative effects on stair walking characteristics [68] and increase falls risk [69]. The observed gaze strategy of maintaining a relatively constant angle between gaze and staircase may be advantageous to participants by not only simplifying the extraction of pertinent information from retinal flow fields for maintaining heading and guiding balance but also for providing peripheral vision of the lower limbs and stairs. Since visual information is crucial for safe stair walking both for identifying step edges and for controlling balance, what then are the implications for the increased prevalence of falls on stairs in older adults?

The visual system undergoes specific age-related changes which affect an individual's ability to see relevant stair features. For example, the ability of the pupil to dilate under low to moderate levels of illumination is greatly reduced with increasing age, resulting in limitations to the amount of light reaching the retina [70]. Indeed, it has been shown experimentally that reducing the levels of ambient lighting results in older adults exhibiting greater variability and average reduction in the size of the clearance between the toe and the stair during a step [59, 60]. There is also evidence that restricted visual conditions adversely affect the control of locomotion in transitions between floor level and stairs [60, 71]. Age-related changes in contrast sensitivity, which are pronounced at low levels of lighting, may hinder the detection of stair edges and transition regions. Visually identifying the tread edge is particularly problematic for older adults when the ambient illumination is low, the step covering is patterned or if they are visually impaired resulting in decreased stability, more cautious stepping, reduced foot clearance with the step and increased foot clearance variability [53, 60, 72–76]. Reduced foot/heel clearances over the tread-edge, greater clearance variability and misjudgements in foot placement when descending steps or stairs are factors that are all reported to increase falls risk [75, 77]. As mentioned above, multifocal eye glasses that correct eyesight problems experienced by the majority of older adults distort the lower peripheral visual field resulting in impaired step negotiation and accuracy of foot placement when stepping on to a raised surface or negotiating an obstacle course [78–80]. Finally, Zietz and Hollands (2009) identified significant differences in the length of time older adults fixated the stairs prior to stepping and a reduced variability in the extent to which older adults looked ahead [57]. These differences in looking strategies might be a by-product of age-related changes to visuomotor control. However, the authors did not measure body kinematics and so could not directly relate differences in gaze behaviour to stepping or balance performance. Nevertheless, this study suggests that visual information describing the tread edges is important for safe stair walking, and that there are age-related differences in when this information is sampled which might contribute towards altered stepping and balance control and associated increased falls risk.

Encouragingly, most of the age-related problems listed above can be easily addressed by manipulating environmental conditions e.g. ensuring stairwells are adequately illuminated and that tread edges are highlighted appropriately. Advice can be given when eye glasses are prescribed as to when it is appropriate to wear multi-focal lenses. It is also possible that the observed age-related differences in gaze behaviour may contribute to stepping inaccuracies and instability in older adults walking on stairs and, if so, may be amenable to intervention, but further studies of frail older adults are needed in order to establish that link. Finally, Elliott et al. (2009) showed that it is possible to manipulate the perceived height of a step using a simple visual illusion (a striped pattern on the stair riser) [81] leading to the adoption of a safer stepping strategy in terms of greater foot clearance over a step edge. The positive effects of similar visual illusions on stair walking safety and self-confidence have been demonstrated in several subsequent studies [61, 82–85] including one that used augmented reality to provide the illusion [86]. These studies provide important proof-of-concept for designing optimal environments/conditions to ameliorate age-related changes to stepping and balance resulting from visual and other sensory decline.

Visual Control of Obstacle Crossing

Stepping over obstacles, such as door thresholds and broken sidewalks, is a common requirement of community mobility [73]. The observation that trips account for up to 53% of falls in older adults [2, 3] indicates that older adults are not very successful at avoiding obstacles in their everyday lives. Since trips occur when the forward motion of the swing limb is obstructed by contacting the obstacle, this review focuses on stepping over an obstacle as opposed to circumventing a vertical obstacle. This lack of success could result from a number of age-related factors, including a compromised ability to visually detect the obstacle height and position, reduced ability to lift the limb adequately to clear the obstacle, and/or an inability to recover balance after the foot contacts the obstacle. For a systematic review of reactive responses to trips in older adults, the reader is referred to Galna et al. [87]. This reactive mechanism should be considered the ‘back up’ defence when the proactive mechanism fails [88]; avoiding the trip in the first place is the more effective means of ensuring stability. Thus, this section provides an overview of the literature regarding visual control of stepping over stationary, visible obstacles.

When walking up to a stationary obstacle, young participants visually sampled the obstacle, with obstacle fixations occurring for about 20% of the approach phase [89]. The frequency of obstacle fixations increased as a function of obstacle height

[89], reflecting increased visual attention on obstacles which have a higher risk of tripping [90]. The information gained from obstacle fixations is used to control movement in a feed-forward mode, rather than on-line, as young adults fixated on the obstacle during approach, but not during crossing [89]. Pontecorvo et al. [91] have demonstrated that obstacle fixations are related to success in crossing the obstacle in young adults. When stepping over stationary obstacles in the lab, participants inadvertently contact the obstacle in 1–2% of trials [92, 93]. While these trials are typically discarded, Heijnen et al. [92] demonstrated that these failures provide important insight into the behaviours that result in a trip and possible fall. Using this methodology, it was found that young participants who never contacted the obstacle had longer and more frequent fixations on the obstacle than those who contacted the obstacle at least twice during data collection (approximately 1.5 h duration) [91].

Changes in locomotor performance were also observed in young adults during modification of visual information of the foot relative to the obstacle (termed exproprioception), and when visible characteristics of the obstacle (termed exteroception) were reduced. When exproprioception is reduced with lower visual field occlusion goggles, young adults demonstrate increased toe clearance, toe clearance variability, foot placement farther away from the obstacle and increased contacts [90, 94, 95]. The increased variability indicates that the limb trajectory is modified in an on-line manner as the limb crosses the obstacle. Since participants do not foveate the obstacle during crossing [89], the participants are relying on peripheral visual cues during obstacle crossing for this on-line control. However, Rietdyk and Rhea [94] demonstrated that increased visual cues in the environment can guide foot placement when foot-obstacle exproprioception is obstructed. This group also demonstrated that when exteroceptive information was systematically reduced by decreasing the visual characteristics of the obstacle, obstacle contact rates increased [90]. In particular, when the interface of the ground and the bottom edge of the obstacle was not visible, such as observed when an obstacle is created with a dowel suspended across two vertical supports, contact rates were higher than when the bottom edge of the obstacle was clearly demarcated [90]. It is likely that the visibility of the obstacle–ground interface improves knowledge of obstacle position, leading to optimal foot placement around an obstacle, which in turn decreases contact risk as discussed below. Thus, it is clear that young adults use visual information in both a feedforward and on-line manner to ensure successful clearance of an obstacle.

Gaze behaviour in older adults during obstacle approach and crossing has been examined concurrently with various manipulations, such as dual tasking or responding to a limb-selection cue during approach [47, 96]. Older fallers looked away from the obstacle sooner than older non-fallers in a dual task condition; this early transfer of gaze was accompanied by increased foot placement variability [47]. When older adults were presented with a limb-selection cue during obstacle approach, relatively longer saccade/foot lift latency and prolonged gaze fixation time were observed relative to young adults [96]. Thus, differences in gaze behaviour are observed both as a function of age and fall risk. However, a direct comparison of gaze behaviour between young and older adults without various instructions or manipulations has not been examined when stepping over obstacles in the walkway. Muir et al. [97]

used head angle to infer gaze behaviour, and found that older adults (65–79 years) had a lower head angle than young adults during the approach phase, consistent with increased visual fixation on the obstacle. Reduced visual acuity did not drive this behaviour as all participants had corrected-to-normal vision. Rather, these changes likely reflect factors such as compromised visuomotor transformation or other vision factors, such as depth perception [98]. Next, we describe the age-related changes in gait behaviour that inform visual control of locomotion.

When older adults walk over a clear walkway or step over obstacles, they demonstrate slower gait speed and shorter step lengths than young adults, likely due to increased caution (e.g. [93, 97, 99, 100]). However, the slower speed would also provide more time to gather visual information, which would facilitate control of locomotion. The interpretation that the slower gait speed allows the older adult more time to gather visual information is consistent with the lower head angle observed when older adults approach the obstacle (Fig. 8.2) [97]. The observation that adults older than 80 years walked slower and looked down more than adults aged 65–79 years indicates that these strategies become more prevalent with advancing age [97]. While slower speed appears to be an appropriate strategy to maintain stability and optimize visual information, the shorter step length increases the

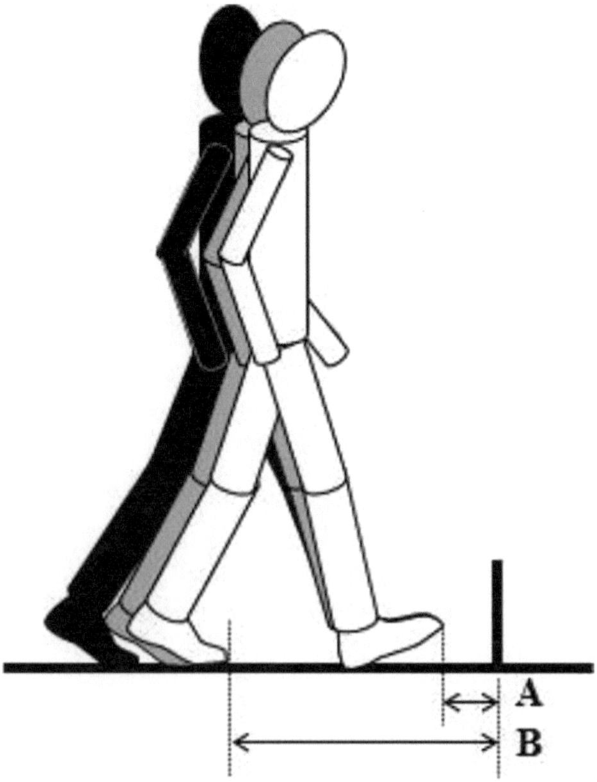

Fig. 8.2 Representative body positions for young (20–25 years, *black figure*), older (65–79 years, *grey figure*), and oldest adults (80–91 years, *white figure*). The head angle is tilted down more with advancing age, consistent with increased foveation on the obstacle during approach. The step length and lead approach distance (**b**) are progressively shorter with advancing age. However, trail foot placement before obstacle (**a**) was not different as a function of age. (Results from [93, 97, 99])

likelihood of contacting an obstacle during obstructed gait [99]. Thus, it is important to examine how older adults manage this contact risk.

The shorter step length when crossing obstacles results in closer foot placement to the obstacle before and/or after crossing, increasing the risk of obstacle contact [99]. To ensure safe placement of the foot, both young and older adults visually fixate on the landing area after the obstacle [89, 96]. This observation is further supported by the higher frequency of fixations on the landing area by young participants who never contacted the obstacle when compared to participants who inadvertently contacted the obstacle at least twice [91]. A remarkably consistent behaviour in the foot placement before the obstacle has been observed [93, 97, 99] (Fig. 8.2). Despite the change in step length, it is clear that the same foot placement in the ultimate step is selected. Thus, healthy aging older adults have maintained the ability to transform the visual information of obstacle position to an appropriate placement of the trail foot (second foot to cross the obstacle). This visuomotor transformation is likely facilitated by looking down more (Fig. 8.2) [97]. Trail foot placement is critical because a closer foot placement corresponds to a greater risk of obstacle contact with the trail limb in young adults [92, 101]. Thus, there is converging evidence that indicates that healthy older adults have adequate visuomotor transformation to maintain an invariant trail foot placement, in order to reduce the likelihood of obstacle contact with the trail limb.

A consistent trail foot placement coupled with a shorter step length necessitates that the lead foot is placed closer to the obstacle after the obstacle is cleared. This closer foot placement leads to increased likelihood of contact with the rear region of the foot during lead limb crossing. Indeed, this has been observed experimentally by examining the inadvertent obstacle contacts. Only older adults contacted the obstacle in Chen et al. [99], and all participants were described as having stepped on the obstacle—consistent with inadequate distance between the heel of the lead limb and the obstacle at crossing. Further, older adults had higher proportion of lead limb contacts than young adults [97, 102, 103]. The majority of inadvertent contacts occur with the trail limb for young adults with either full vision or lower visual field obstruction [90, 94, 95, 104–107]. More frequent trail limb contacts are attributed to the fact that the trail limb is not visible during crossing, so on-line visual control is not available. Conversely, lead limb contacts were more frequent when vision was distorted or fully obstructed [107–109]. Thus, the higher proportion of lead limb contacts in older adults may reflect impairment of the on-line visual guidance of the lead limb trajectory. Higher proportion of lead limb contacts in older adults are relevant because balance recovery from lead limb trips is more difficult due to the centre of mass (COM) motion relative to the base of support (BOS) [97, 103].

It is traditionally assumed that lower foot clearances are associated with increased trip risk, so foot clearances are typically quantified in adaptive locomotor research. Heijnen and Rietdyk [110] provided preliminary evidence that supports this intuitive assumption: Falls in the real world are related to lower foot clearances when crossing an obstacle in the lab in young adults [110]. However, age-related changes in clearance during obstacle crossing include increased clearance [111], decreased clearance [112, 113], and no significant change in clearance [93, 97, 99, 114]. Since obstacles and lab environments are different across studies, and clearance measures are sensitive to visible obstacle characteristics [90] and visual structure in environment [94], as described earlier, foot clearance may not provide a reliable indicator of age-related changes unless different labs adopt uniform obstacles and lab environments. Conversely, foot placement relative to the obstacle is a key parameter associated with trip-risk (Fig. 8.1) [92, 99, 101, 102, 109]. Similarly, on a clear walkway, foot placement is an efficient and important mechanism to maintain the relationship between the COM motion and the BOS [115]. Maintaining the COM-motion-to-foot-placement is considered a body-centric constraint, while placing the foot appropriately around an obstacle is considered an environmental constraint. When young adults approach and step over an obstacle, they proactively manage both constraints by shifting their priority from the body-centric constraint to the environmental constraint (the obstacle), presumably due to the larger threat to balance from the risk of tripping [116]. The shifting priority likely arises from supraspinal visual information from the obstacle [116]. Older adults were also able to manage both constraints, but, relative to young adults, demonstrated greater prioritization of foot placement around the obstacle, likely at the cost of step length consistency [117]. Future research should delineate how gaze strategies are associated with shifting priorities as a function of age.

Finally, we examine the relationship between vision and obstacle contact rates. Older adults contact more obstacles under the following conditions: wearing multifocal lenses [80, 108] and when provided visual samples of 16 ms duration at a rate of three samples per second during the approach (using liquid crystal goggles) [118]. Further, the depth perception of older adults was a significant determinant of obstacle contacts [98].

The findings reported here lead to a series of potential intervention strategies. First, older adults should be assessed for depth perception, and should be encouraged to wear single-distance lenses when walking (as opposed to multi-focal lenses). Second, optimal gaze behaviour for reducing trip and fall risk should be confirmed for older adults, and interventions that promote this gaze behaviour should be empirically tested. Therapeutic interventions to promote safe obstacle crossing should consider not only limb elevation, but also optimal foot placement. The environment can also be modified to optimize safe clearance of fixed obstacles. For example, kerbs should be painted with high contrast paint to increase the visibility of the location of the rising edge, which may reduce trip risk. We have had older adults indicate that the sidewalk kerbs with a curved rising edge, as opposed to a vertical rising edge, are especially problematic. This is likely due to the inability to determine the ideal foot placement before and after the rising edge, as there isn't a clear demarcation of the position of the rising edge. Further, adding visual structure around obstacles may be helpful, such as using a high contrast paint colour around doorways with a threshold.

Conclusions

This chapter has reviewed our current understanding of the visual control of three common adaptations to the basic locomotor pattern to avoid obstacles and guide the feet to safe locations in the environment. Although the review has highlighted variations in the types of visual and non-visual information used to guide balance and stepping movements in different contexts, it is clear that appropriate alignment of the eyes with respect to environmental features at particular points in the gait cycle are important for both programming and guiding safe and efficient stepping adjustments. The chapter has also reviewed evidence that age-related changes in gaze behaviour due to visual, visuomotor and cognitive decline have been causally linked to increased falls risk in older adults and, therefore, it is clear that these impairments should be targeted when designing intervention strategies aimed at reducing falls risk. Encouragingly, there is a growing body of evidence to suggest that interventions aimed at improving eye and stepping coordination, whether through training or through built-environment design, have a positive effect on stepping control and reducing falls risk. However, further work is still needed to fully understand the mechanisms underlying age-related changes in visual and sensorimotor processing so that effective interventions can be designed and implemented.

References

1. Scuffham P, Chaplin S, Legood R. Incidence and costs of unintentional falls in older people in the United Kingdom. J Epidemiol Community Health. 2003;57(9):740–4.
2. Berg WP, Alessio HM, Mills EM, Tong C. Circumstances and consequences of falls in independent community-dwelling older adults. Age Ageing. 1997;26(4):261–8.
3. Blake A, Morgan K, Bendall M, Dallosso H, Ebrahim S, Arie T, et al. Falls by elderly people at home: prevalence and associated factors. Age Ageing. 1988;17(6):365–72.
4. Land MF, Hayhoe M. In what ways do eye movements contribute to everyday activities? Vis Res. 2001;41(25–26):3559–65.
5. Vickers JN. Visual control when aiming at a far target. J Exp Psychol Hum Percept Perform. 1996;22(2):342–54.
6. Martell SG, Vickers JN. Gaze characteristics of elite and near-elite athletes in ice hockey defensive tactics. Hum Mov Sci. 2004;22(6):689–712.
7. Vickers JN. Gaze control in putting. Perception. 1992;21(1):117–32.
8. Vickers JN, Causer J, Vanhooren D. The role of quiet eye timing and location in the basketball three-point shot: a new research paradigm. Front Psychol. 2019;10:2424.
9. Vickers JN, Vandervies B, Kohut C, Ryley B. Quiet eye training improves accuracy in basketball field goal shooting. Prog Brain Res. 2017;234:1–12.
10. Wilson MR, Miles CA, Vine SJ, Vickers JN. Quiet eye distinguishes children of high and low motor coordination abilities. Med Sci Sports Exerc. 2013;45(6):1144–51.
11. Balslev D, Himmelbach M, Karnath HO, Borchers S, Odoj B. Eye proprioception used for visual localization only if in conflict with the oculomotor plan. J Neurosci. 2012;32(25):8569–73.
12. Hadjidimitrakis K, Breveglieri R, Placenti G, Bosco A, Sabatini SP, Fattori P. Fix your eyes in the space you could reach: neurons in the macaque medial parietal cortex prefer gaze positions in peripersonal space. PLoS One. 2011;6(8):e23335.

13. Enright JT. The non-visual impact of eye orientation on eye-hand coordination. Vis Res. 1995;35(11):1611–8.
14. Flanders M, Daghestani L, Berthoz A. Reaching beyond reach. Exp Brain Res. 1999;126(1):19–30.
15. Sailer U, Eggert T, Ditterich J, Straube A. Spatial and temporal aspects of eye-hand coordination across different tasks. Exp Brain Res. 2000;134(2):163–73.
16. van Donkelaar P. Eye-hand interactions during goal-directed pointing movements. Neuroreport. 1997;8(9–10):2139–42.
17. van Donkelaar P, Siu KC, Walterschied J. Saccadic output is influenced by limb kinetics during eye-hand coordination. J Mot Behav. 2004;36(3):245–52.
18. Engel KC, Soechting JE. Interactions between ocular motor and manual responses during two-dimensional tracking. Prog Brain Res. 2003;142:141–53.
19. Hollands MA, Marplehorvat DE, Henkes S, Rowan AK. Human eye-movements during visually guided stepping. J Mot Behav. 1995;27(2):155–63.
20. Hollands MA, Marple-Horvat DE. Coordination of eye and leg movements during visually guided stepping. J Mot Behav. 2001;33(2):205–16.
21. Hollands MA, MarpleHorvat DE. Visually guided stepping under conditions of step cycle-related denial of visual information. Exp Brain Res. 1996;109(2):343–56.
22. Matthis JS, Barton SL, Fajen BR. The biomechanics of walking shape the use of visual information during locomotion over complex terrain. J Vis. 2015;15(3):10.
23. Matthis JS, Fajen BR. Visual control of foot placement when walking over complex terrain. J Exp Psychol Hum Percept Perform. 2014;40(1):106–15.
24. Matthis JS, Yates JL, Hayhoe MM. Gaze and the control of foot placement when walking in natural terrain. Curr Biol. 2018;28(8):1224–33 e5.
25. Young WR, Hollands MA. Evidence for age-related decline in visuomotor function and reactive stepping adjustments. Gait Posture. 2012;36(3):477–81.
26. Reynolds RF, Day BL. Visual guidance of the human foot during a step. J Physiol. 2005;569(Pt 2):677–84.
27. Rietdyk S, Drifmeyer JE. The rough-terrain problem: accurate foot targeting as a function of visual information regarding target location. J Mot Behav. 2010;42(1):37–48.
28. Patla AE, Vickers JN. How far ahead do we look when required to step on specific locations in the travel path during locomotion? Exp Brain Res. 2003;148(1):133–8.
29. Yamada M, Higuchi T, Mori S, Uemura K, Nagai K, Aoyama T, et al. Maladaptive turning and gaze behavior induces impaired stepping on multiple footfall targets during gait in older individuals who are at high risk of falling. Arch Gerontol Geriatr. 2012;54(2):e102–8.
30. Bonnen K, Matthis JS, Gibaldi A, Banks MS, Levi DM, Hayhoe M. Binocular vision and the control of foot placement during walking in natural terrain. Sci Rep. 2021;11(1):20881.
31. Crowdy KA, Hollands MA, Ferguson IT, Marple-Horvat DE. Evidence for interactive locomotor and oculomotor deficits in cerebellar patients during visually guided stepping. Exp Brain Res. 2000;135(4):437–54.
32. Di Fabio RP, Zampieri C, Tuite P. Gaze control and foot kinematics during stair climbing: characteristics leading to fall risk in progressive supranuclear palsy. Phys Ther. 2008;88(2):240–50.
33. Crowdy KA, Kaur-Mann D, Cooper HL, Mansfield AG, Offord JL, Marple-Horvat DE. Rehearsal by eye movement improves visuomotor performance in cerebellar patients. Exp Brain Res. 2002;146(2):244–7.
34. Zampieri C, Di Fabio RP. Balance and eye movement training to improve gait in people with progressive supranuclear palsy: quasi-randomized clinical trial. Phys Ther. 2008;88(12):1460–73.
35. Chapman GJ, Hollands MA. Age-related differences in stepping performance during step cycle-related removal of vision. Exp Brain Res. 2006;174(4):613–21.
36. Chapman GJ, Hollands MA. Evidence for a link between changes to gaze behaviour and risk of falling in older adults during adaptive locomotion. Gait Posture. 2006;24(3):288–94.

37. Young WR, Hollands MA. Can telling older adults where to look reduce falls? Evidence for a causal link between inappropriate visual sampling and suboptimal stepping performance. Exp Brain Res. 2010;204(1):103–13.
38. Young WR, Wing AM, Hollands MA. Influences of state anxiety on gaze behavior and stepping accuracy in older adults during adaptive locomotion. J Gerontol B-Psychol. 2012;67(1):43–51.
39. Young WR, Hollands MA. Newly acquired fear of falling leads to altered eye movement patterns and reduced stepping safety: a case study. PLoS One. 2012;7(11):e49765.
40. Yogev-Seligmann G, Hausdorff JM, Giladi N. The role of executive function and attention in gait. Mov Disord. 2008;23(3):329–42. quiz 472
41. Curzon-Jones BT, Hollands MA. Route previewing results in altered gaze behaviour, increased self-confidence and improved stepping safety in both young and older adults during adaptive locomotion. Exp Brain Res. 2018;236(4):1077–89.
42. Stanley J, Hollands M. A novel video-based paradigm to study the mechanisms underlying age- and falls risk-related differences in gaze behaviour during walking. Ophthal Physl Opt. 2014;34(4):459–69.
43. Yamada M, Higuchi T, Tanaka B, Nagai K, Uemura K, Aoyama T, et al. Measurements of stepping accuracy in a multitarget stepping task as a potential indicator of fall risk in elderly individuals. J Gerontol A-Biol. 2011;66(9):994–1000.
44. Mazaheri M, Roerdink M, Bood RJ, Duysens J, Beek PJ, Peper CE. Attentional costs of visually guided walking: effects of age, executive function and stepping-task demands. Gait Posture. 2014;40(1):182–6.
45. Peper CE, Oorthuizen JK, Roerdink M. Attentional demands of cued walking in healthy young and elderly adults. Gait Posture. 2012;36(3):378–82.
46. Lindemann U, Klenk J, Becker C, Moe-Nilssen R. Assessment of adaptive walking performance. Med Eng Phys. 2013;35(2):217–20.
47. Yamada M, Tanaka H, Mori S, Nagai K, Uemura K, Tanaka B, et al. Fallers choose an early transfer gaze strategy during obstacle avoidance in dual-task condition. Aging Clin Exp Res. 2011;23(4):316–9.
48. Nonnekes JH, Talelli P, de Niet M, Reynolds RF, Weerdesteyn V, Day BL. Deficits underlying impaired visually triggered step adjustments in mildly affected stroke patients. Neurorehabil Neural Repair. 2010;24(4):393–400.
49. Young WR, Wing AM, Hollands MA. Influences of state anxiety on gaze behavior and stepping accuracy in older adults during adaptive locomotion. J Gerontol B Psychol Sci Soc Sci. 2012;67(1):43–51.
50. Yamada M, Higuchi T, Nishiguchi S, Yoshimura K, Kajiwara Y, Aoyama T. Multitarget stepping program in combination with a standardized multicomponent exercise program can prevent falls in community-dwelling older adults: a randomized, controlled trial. J Am Geriatr Soc. 2013;61(10):1669–75.
51. Dowswell T, Towner E, Cryer C, Jarvis S, Edwards P, et al. In: Industry. UDoTa, editor. Accidental falls: fatalities and injuries. An examination of the data sources and review of literature on preventative strategies. London: Department of Trade and Industry; 1999.
52. Cohen HH, Templer J, Archea J. An analysis of occupational stair accident patterns. J Saf Res. 1985;16:171.
53. Templer J. The staircase: studies of hazards falls and safer design. Cambridge: MIT Press; 1992.
54. Svanstrom L. Falls on stairs: an epidemiological accident study. Scand J Soc Med. 1974;2(3):113–20.
55. Cohen HH. A field study of stair descent. Ergon Des. 2000;(Spring):11–5.
56. Archea J. Guidelines for stair safety. Washington, DC: National Bureau of Standards; 1979.
57. Zietz D, Hollands M. Gaze behavior of young and older adults during stair walking. J Mot Behav. 2009;41(4):357–65.
58. Den Otter AR, Hoogwerf M, Van Der Woude LH. The role of tread fixations in the visual control of stair walking. Gait Posture. 2011;34(2):169–73.

59. Zietz D, Johannsen L, Hollands M. Stepping characteristics and Centre of Mass control during stair descent: effects of age, fall risk and visual factors. Gait Posture. 2011;34(2):279–84.
60. Thomas NM, Skervin T, Foster RJ, O'Brien TD, Carpenter MG, Maganaris CN, et al. Optimal lighting levels for stair safety: influence of lightbulb type and brightness on confidence, dynamic balance and stepping characteristics. Exp Gerontol. 2020;132:110839.
61. Thomas NM, Skervin TK, Foster RJ, Parr JV, Carpenter MG, O'Brien TD, et al. Influence of step-surface visual properties on confidence, anxiety, dynamic stability, and gaze behaviour in young and older adults. Hum Mov Sci. 2021;77:102774.
62. Sheldon JH. On the natural history of falls in old age. Br Med J. 1960;2(5214):1685–90.
63. Wild D, Nayak US, Isaacs B. Description, classification and prevention of falls in old people at home. Rheumatol Rehabil. 1981;20(3):153–9.
64. Cho H, Arnold AJ, Cui C, Yang Z, Becker T, Kulkarni A, et al. Risky behavior during stair descent for young adults: differences in men versus women. PLoS One. 2023;18(7):e0288438.
65. Miyasike-daSilva V, Allard F, McIlroy WE. Where do we look when we walk on stairs? Gaze behaviour on stairs, transitions, and handrails. Exp Brain Res. 2011;209(1):73–83.
66. Timmis MA, Bennett SJ, Buckley JG. Visuomotor control of step descent: evidence of specialised role of the lower visual field. Exp Brain Res. 2009;195(2):219–27.
67. Marigold DS. Role of peripheral visual cues in online visual guidance of locomotion. Exerc Sport Sci Rev. 2008;36(3):145–51.
68. Timmis MA, Johnson L, Elliott DB, Buckley JG. Use of single-vision distance spectacles improves landing control during step descent in well-adapted multifocal lens-wearers. Invest Ophthalmol Vis Sci. 2010;51(8):3903–8.
69. Lord SR, Dayhew J, Howland A. Multifocal glasses impair edge-contrast sensitivity and depth perception and increase the risk of falls in older people. J Am Geriatr Soc. 2002;50(11):1760–6.
70. Owsley C. Aging and vision. Vis Res. 2011;51(13):1610–22.
71. Cavanagh PRH, J.S. What is the role of vision during stair descent? In: Jeffrey AOD, Harvey LO, editors. Visual perception: the influence of H W Leibowitz decade of behaviour. Washington, DC: American Psychological Association; 2003. p. 213–42.
72. Buckley JG, Heasley K, Scally A, Elliott DB. The effects of blurring vision on medio-lateral balance during stepping up or down to a new level in the elderly. Gait Posture. 2005;22(2):146–53.
73. Buckley JG, Heasley KJ, Twigg P, Elliott DB. The effects of blurred vision on the mechanics of landing during stepping down by the elderly. Gait Posture. 2005;21(1):65–71.
74. Buckley JG, MacLellan MJ, Tucker MW, Scally AJ, Bennett SJ. Visual guidance of landing behaviour when stepping down to a new level. Exp Brain Res. 2008;184(2):223–32.
75. Hamel KA, Okita N, Higginson JS, Cavanagh PR. Foot clearance during stair descent: effects of age and illumination. Gait Posture. 2005;21(2):135–40.
76. Thomas JS, Schmidt EM, Hambrecht FT. Facility of motor unit control during tasks defined directly in terms of unit behaviors. Exp Neurol. 1978;59(3):384–97.
77. Simoneau GG, Cavanagh PR, Ulbrecht JS, Leibowitz HW, Tyrrell RA. The influence of visual factors on fall-related kinematic variables during stair descent by older women. J Gerontol. 1991;46(6):M188–95.
78. Johnson L, Buckley JG, Harley C, Elliott DB. Use of single-vision eyeglasses improves stepping precision and safety when elderly habitual multifocal wearers negotiate a raised surface. J Am Geriatr Soc. 2008;56(1):178–80.
79. Johnson L, Buckley JG, Scally AJ, Elliott DB. Multifocal spectacles increase variability in toe clearance and risk of tripping in the elderly. Invest Ophth Vis Sci. 2007;48(4):1466–71.
80. Menant JC, St George RJ, Sandery B, Fitzpatrick RC, Lord SR. Older people contact more obstacles when wearing multifocal glasses and performing a secondary visual task. J Am Geriatr Soc. 2009;57(10):1833–8.
81. Elliott DB, Vale A, Whitaker D, Buckley JG. Does my step look big in this? A visual illusion leads to safer stepping behaviour. PLoS One. 2009;4(2):e4577.

82. Foster RJ, Hotchkiss J, Buckley JG, Elliott DB. Safety on stairs: influence of a tread edge highlighter and its position. Exp Gerontol. 2014;55:152–8.
83. Foster RJ, Whitaker D, Scally AJ, Buckley JG, Elliott DB. What you see is what you step: the horizontal-vertical illusion increases toe clearance in older adults during stair ascent. Invest Ophthalmol Vis Sci. 2015;56(5):2950–7.
84. Skervin TK, Thomas NM, Schofield AJ, Hollands MA, Maganaris CN, Foster RJ. The next step in optimising the stair horizontal-vertical illusion: does a perception-action link exist in older adults? Exp Gerontol. 2021;149:111309.
85. Skervin TK, Thomas NM, Schofield AJ, Hollands MA, Maganaris CN, O'Brien TD, et al. Using a stair horizontal-vertical illusion to increase foot clearance over an inconsistently taller stair-riser. PLoS One. 2021;16(9):e0257159.
86. Miura S, Fukumoto R, Okamura N, Fujie MG, Sugano S. Visual illusion created by a striped pattern through augmented reality for the prevention of tumbling on stairs. IEEE Trans Vis Comput Graph. 2023:30.
87. Galna B, Peters A, Murphy AT, Morris ME. Obstacle crossing deficits in older adults: a systematic review. Gait Posture. 2009;30(3):270–5.
88. Patla AE. Understanding the roles of vision in the control of human locomotion. Gait Posture. 1997;5(1):54–69.
89. Patla AE, Vickers JN. Where and when do we look as we approach and step over an obstacle in the travel path? Neuroreport. 1997;8(17):3661–5.
90. Rietdyk S, Rhea CK. The effect of the visual characteristics of obstacles on risk of tripping and gait parameters during locomotion. Ophthalmic Physiol Opt. 2011;31(3):302–10.
91. Pontecorvo SM, Heijnen MJH, Muir BC, Rietdyk S. Relationship between gaze behavior and failure to cross a stationary, visible obstacle. In 2015 International Society for Posture and Gait Research World Congress, Seville, Spain; 2015.
92. Heijnen MJH, Muir BC, Rietdyk S. Factors leading to obstacle contact during adaptive locomotion. Exp Brain Res. 2012;223(2):219–31.
93. Lowrey CR, Watson A, Vallis LA. Age-related changes in avoidance strategies when negotiating single and multiple obstacles. Exp Brain Res. 2007;182(3):289–99.
94. Rietdyk S, Rhea CK. Control of adaptive locomotion: effect of visual obstruction and visual cues in the environment. Exp Brain Res. 2006;169(2):272–8.
95. Rhea CK, Rietdyk S. Visual exteroceptive information provided during obstacle crossing did not modify the lower limb trajectory. Neurosci Lett. 2007;418(1):60–5.
96. Di Fabio RP, Greany JF, Zampieri C. Saccade-stepping interactions revise the motor plan for obstacle avoidance. J Mot Behav. 2003;35(4):383–97.
97. Muir BC, Haddad JM, Heijnen MJ, Rietdyk S. Proactive gait strategies to mitigate risk of obstacle contact are more prevalent with advancing age. Gait Posture. 2015;41(1):233–9.
98. Menant JC, St George RJ, Fitzpatrick RC, Lord SR. Impaired depth perception and restricted pitch head movement increase obstacle contacts when dual-tasking in older people. J Gerontol A Biol Sci Med Sci. 2010;65(7):751–7.
99. Chen HC, Ashton-Miller JA, Alexander NB, Schultz AB. Stepping over obstacles: gait patterns of healthy young and old adults. J Gerontol. 1991;46(6):M196–203.
100. Winter DA. Biomechanics and motor control of human gait: normal, elderly and pathological. 2nd ed. Waterloo: University of Waterloo Press; 1991.
101. Chou LS, Draganich LF. Placing the trailing foot closer to an obstacle reduces flexion of the hip, knee, and ankle to increase the risk of tripping. J Biomech. 1998;31(8):685–91.
102. Muir BC, Bodratti LA, Morris CE, Haddad JM, van Emmerik REA, Rietdyk S. Gait characteristics during inadvertent obstacle contacts in young, middle-aged and older adults. Gait Posture. 2020;77:100–4.
103. Becker T, Rietdyk S. Inadvertent obstacle contacts when older adults step over obstacles: effect of sex, self-reported fatigue, gait parameters, and prescription medications. Braz J Mot Behav. 2022;16(5):385–99.
104. Heijnen MJH, Muir BC, Rietdyk S. Interpolation techniques to reduce error in measurement of toe clearance during obstacle avoidance. J Biomech. 2012;45(1):196–8.

105. Berard JR, Vallis LA. Characteristics of single and double obstacle avoidance strategies: a comparison between adults and children. Exp Brain Res. 2006;175(1):21–31.
106. Rhea CK, Rietdyk S. Influence of an unexpected perturbation on adaptive gait behavior. Gait Posture. 2011;34(3):439–41.
107. Mohagheghi AA, Moraes R, Patla AE. The effects of distant and on-line visual information on the control of approach phase and step over an obstacle during locomotion. Exp Brain Res. 2004;155(4):459–68.
108. Johnson L, Buckley JG, Scally AJ, Elliott DB. Multifocal spectacles increase variability in toe clearance and risk of tripping in the elderly. Invest Ophthalmol Vis Sci. 2007;48(4):1466–71.
109. Patla AE, Greig M. Any way you look at it, successful obstacle negotiation needs visually guided on-line foot placement regulation during the approach phase. Neurosci Lett. 2006;397(1–2):110–4.
110. Heijnen MJH, Rietdyk S, editors. Falls in the real world are related to obstacle crossing behaviors in a lab setting for young adults. In 2015 International Society for Posture and Gait Research World Congress, Seville, Spain; 2015.
111. Lu T-W, Chen H-L, Chen S-C. Comparisons of the lower limb kinematics between young and older adults when crossing obstacles of different heights. Gait Posture. 2006;23(4):471–9.
112. McFadyen BJ, Prince F. Avoidance and accommodation of surface height changes by healthy, community-dwelling, young, and elderly men. J Gerontol A Biol Sci Med Sci. 2002;57(4):B166–74.
113. Soma M, Masuda T, Shimamura R, Abiko T, Uematu H, Kawama K. Influence of a dual-task on toe clearance of the young and elderly while stepping over an obstacle. J Phys Ther Sci. 2010;22(1):75–9.
114. Barbieri FA, dos Santos PC, Vitorio R, van Dieen JH, Gobbi LT. Effect of muscle fatigue and physical activity level in motor control of the gait of young adults. Gait Posture. 2013;38(4):702–7.
115. Reimann H, Fettrow T, Jeka JJ. Strategies for the control of balance during locomotion. Kinesiol Rev. 2018;7:18–25.
116. Kulkarni A, Cui C, Rietdyk S, Ambike S. Between a walk and a hard place: how stepping patterns change while navigating environmental obstacles. Mot Control. 2023;27(1):20–34.
117. Kulkarni A, Cho H, Rietdyk S, Ambike S. Step length synergy is weaker in older adults during obstacle crossing. J Biomech. 2021;118:110311.
118. Vitorio R, Lirani-Silva E, Barbieri FA, Raile V, Stella F, Gobbi LT. Influence of visual feedback sampling on obstacle crossing behavior in people with Parkinson's disease. Gait Posture. 2013;38(2):330–4.

Cognition, Gait Disorders, and Fall Risk in Older Individuals

9

Manuel Montero-Odasso and Frederico Pieruccini-Faria

Abstract

Clinicians and researchers have commonly performed gait assessments and cognitive assessments separately when evaluating older adults. However, evidence from clinical practice, epidemiological studies, and clinical trials shows that gait and cognition are interrelated in older adults. Quantifiable alterations in gait among older adults are associated with a higher risk of falls, dementia, and disability. At the same time, emerging evidence indicates that early disturbances in cognitive processes, such as attention, executive function, and working memory are associated with slower gait and gait instability.These cognitive disturbances assist in the prediction of future mobility loss, falls, and progression to dementia. This chapter reviews the importance of the gait–cognition inter relationship in aging and presents evidence that gait performance mirrors cognitive function and provides insights about how brain and gait control contribute to fall risk in older adults. To this end, the benefits of dual-task gait assessments (e.g., walking while performing a cognitive-demanding task) as a marker of fall risk are presented.

M. Montero-Odasso (✉)
Gait and Brain Lab, Parkwood Institute, Lawson Health Research Institute, London, ON, Canada

Department of Medicine, Division of Geriatric, Schulich School of Medicine and Dentistry, University of Western Ontario, London, ON, Canada

Department of Epidemiology and Biostatistics, Schulich School of Medicine & Dentistry, University of Western Ontario, London, ON, Canada
e-mail: mmontero@uwo.ca

F. Pieruccini-Faria
Gait and Brain Lab, Parkwood Institute, Lawson Health Research Institute, London, ON, Canada

Department of Medicine, Division of Geriatric, Schulich School of Medicine and Dentistry, University of Western Ontario, London, ON, Canada

F. A. Barbieri et al. (eds.), *Locomotion and Posture in Older Adults*,
https://doi.org/10.1007/978-3-031-74123-4_9

Finally, evidence from an emerging therapeutic approach for reducing the risk of falls by improving certain aspects of cognition, through both non-pharmacological and pharmacological treatments is presented. Disentangling the relationship between early gait disturbances and early cognitive changes may be helpful for identifying older adults at higher risk of experiencing mobility decline and falls.

Introduction

Are Falls in Older Adults a Manifestation of Brain Failure?

Professor Bernard Isaacs postulated more than 40 years ago that attributing falls in older adults to muscular-skeletal-articular and sensory impairments and their effect on balance was over simplistic. Rather, a failure of our sophisticated brain mechanism for motor and balance control may play a critical role in triggering falls [1, 2].

Cognitive impairment and falls have a well-established relationship [3]. Dementia and falls often co-exist in older adults, with gait impairments being more prevalent in patients with cognitive impairment and dementia. Falls are a common geriatric syndrome affecting about a third of older adults each year, and a better understanding of the relationship between cognitive function and gait impairments may help clinicians and researchers develop interventions and preventive measures to delay the transition.

Falls syndrome is a major cause of morbidity among older adults, especially for those with cognitive problems. For instance, older adults with moderate to severe cognitive impairment have a higher risk of falls, with an annual incidence of around 60–80%, which is twice the rate of that in cognitively normal older adults [5]. The consequences of falls in this population are severe ; fallers with cognitive problems are approximately five times more likely to be admitted to institutional care than cognitively impaired people who do not fall [6]. They are also at high risk of major fall-related injuries, including fractures, head injuries, and mortality. In addition to the indirect costs and caregiver burden due to falls syndrome, the direct costs of emergency, acute, rehabilitation, and long-term care are substantial and challenge sustainability in several healthcare systems [7].

The precise mechanisms underlying the increased fall risk in cognitively impaired older adults are not completely understood; however, several studies have shown that impaired cognitive abilities reduce attentional resource allocation, compromise postural and gait stability [8]. Similarly, executive function, a set of cognitive processes, including attention, inhibitory control, working memory, and cognitive flexibility, is an essential cognitive resource required for normal walking. Impairments in executive function are associated with both dementia syndromes and fall risk [9]. One specific early change in gait performance seen among older adults with mild-to-moderate dementia is a decrease in gait speed [4]. The inter-relationship between cognitive and gait dysfunction has also been found in otherwise healthy older adults or those with subtle cognitive deficits that are not yet advanced enough to be identified using global measures of cognitive status. These findings challenge our understanding and definition of what is currently considered clinically relevant cognitive impairment. For instance, even among healthy older adults with "normal" cognition, low performance in executive function was prospectively associated with falls, as assessed using cut-off scores on global clinical tests of mental status, such as the Mini Mental Status Exam [11]. Mechanistically, the relationship between cognitive deficits and gait disturbances has been attributed to specific brain networks, such as the prefronto-parietal and cingulate areas that are selectively affected by diseases that accompany, but are not necessarily caused by, aging [10].

A systematic review and meta-analysis of 27 prospective cohort studies with at least 1 year of follow-up among healthy, community-dwelling older adults found that executive dysfunction was associated with a 40% increased risk of any fall, and falls associated with serious injury [12]. Similarly, early mobility decline, assessed as slowing of gait, has been found to co-exist with, or even precede the onset of clinically detectable cognitive decline in older adults [13]. This slowing of gait may begin up to 12 years before the clinical presentation of cognitive changes in older adults who later develop mild cognitive impairment syndrome (MCI), a transitional state between normal aging and early dementia [14, 15]. Longitudinal studies have also shown that older adults with MCI have a higher prevalence of gait impairments and a higher risk of falling compared to cognitively normal older adults [16, 17]. Gait decline in MCI is linked with impaired gait parameters that require higher-level brain control, including speed and variability (i.e., step-to-step fluctuations in time and distance), both of which are indexes of instability [18]. Thus, older adults with MCI represent a population at risk, not only for future dementia, but also for falls and should be specifically targeted for interventions to reduce fall risk.

Until recently, falls and dementia were studied and assessed as distinct geriatric syndromes (Fig. 9.1). This may have led to a gap in our understanding of the cognitive–motor interactions that affect the pathways to future falls and falls-related disability in older adults. This gap may also explain why cognition has received little attention with regard to intervention strategies for falls prevention. New evidence supports these two geriatric syndromes as interrelated outcomes associated with aging. Figure 9.1b shows the emerging view and conceptual framework to understand the inter-relationship in the concurrent decline of cognition and mobility in aging.

Cognition and Gait Instability

Although walking has long been considered a primarily automatic motor task, emerging evidence suggests that this view is too simplistic [19]. Walking in the real world requires paying attention to various environmental features and the ability to recover from postural perturbations to avoid stumbles or falls. Therefore, it is not

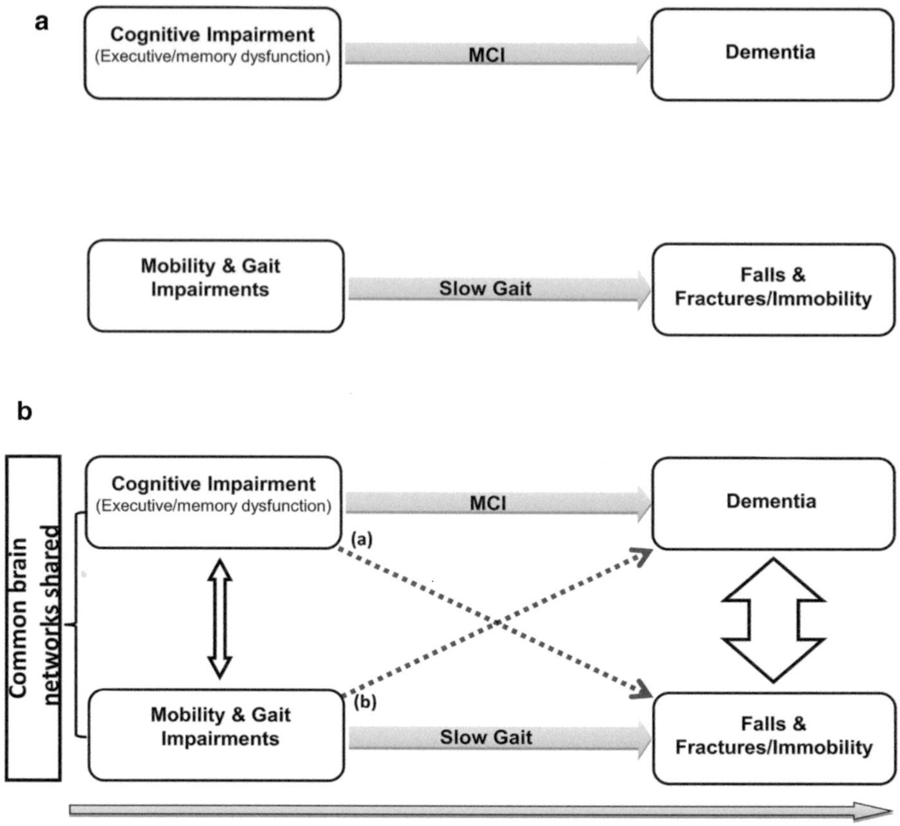

Fig. 9.1 (**a**) Traditional view of the parallel decline of gait and cognitive function with aging. Gait performance and cognitive function deteriorate with aging yielding two geriatric entities: falls and dementia. (**b**) Alternative, emerging view. Cognition predicts mobility decline and falls, on the one hand, and, on the other hand, mobility decline and slow gait predict cognitive deterioration. These phenomena occur in a concurrent manner. (Modified from Montero-Odasso et al. [3])

surprising that deficits in attention and executive function processes are independently associated with risk of postural instability, impairment in activities of daily living, and future falls [9].

The mechanistic evidence about the observed relationship between mobility and cognition is supported by brain imaging studies. Functional magnetic resonance imaging (fMRI) and near-infrared spectroscopy (NIRS) studies have demonstrated significant associations between basal ganglia, prefrontal motor regions, and gait during walking, specifically while simultaneously performing a cognitively demanding task, known as dual-tasking [11]. These studies suggest that shared cortical brain networks regulate complex thinking, memory, and gait control and that abnormalities accumulating throughout these specific brain networks as people age could lead to mobility decline. For instance, diffusion tension imaging studies (DTI), an imaging technique used to describe and detect white matter tracts connecting different cortical and sub-cortical regions, have shown that lower integrity of prefrontal-subcortical networks, including prefrontal cortex, basal ganglia, and medial temporal lobe, is related to slower gait and increased fall risk [9–11]. Moreover, lower white matter integrity in subcortical–cortical regions in functional older individuals with history of stroke was associated with poorer dual-task gait performance, but not poorer gait speed performance [20]. Overall, damaged connectivity between networks can negatively impact cognitive–motor interactions while navigating complex environments.

Cognition and Obstacle Negotiation

Falls triggered by obstacles are highly prevalent among older adults, accounting for nearly 40% of their falls [21]. Falls involving inappropriate obstacle negotiations are the fourth most common cause of falls in community-dwelling older adults [22]. These falls often result from trips, stumbles, incorrect balance transfers, and missteps [21, 22]. Cognition plays an important role in gait performance regulation to avoid obstacle contacts through the allocation of attentional resources for planning and risk assessment [23, 24]. Studies have demonstrated that older individuals with MCI make fewer anticipatory footstep adjustments under increased cognitive load (e.g., walking and talking) compared to cognitively preserved individuals [25]. This walking behavior may increase the risk of a collision since it may affect foot-obstacle clearances. These risky obstacle negotiation behaviors in individuals with MCI were associated with poorer cognition [25, 26] and reduced gray matter volume in frontotemporal regions [27], which are important for decision-making and visuospatial cognition. In individuals with history of falls, stepping performance while approaching the obstacle was significantly more variable/inconsistent compared with older individuals without history of falls, thus suggesting more instability during an obstacle negotiation [28]. Difficulties in allocating cognitive resources to maintain gait stability while approaching the obstacle may explain this walking behavior since obstacle negotiation could be seen as a concurrent mental task [24]. Together, these studies suggest that cognition can be crucial to negotiating balance hazards during navigation through gait performance regulation. Frontotemporal degeneration can be detrimental to obstacle negotiation capabilities, thus representing a potential target for noninvasive brain stimulation interventions aimed at falls prevention (Fig. 9.2).

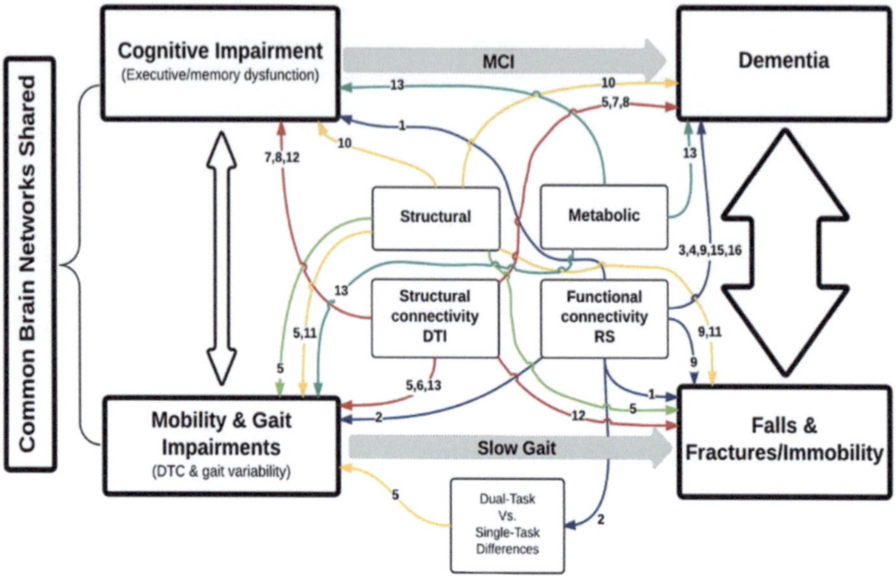

Fig. 9.2 Synthetizis from brain imaging evidence supporting the mechanistic relationship between cognitive decline, gait decline, future falls and progression to dementia syndromes in the conceptual framework described above in this chapter's topic

Mechanism and Pathophysiology of Falls

Basis of Posture Control

The human upright position is naturally unstable, with a narrow base of support and a high center of body mass. To maintain this delicate equilibrium while walking or standing, the human body has a harmonious modulation and coordination of the trunk and ankle flexibility. This equilibrium modulation is challenged by motor impairments, either muscle weakness, slowness, or poor coordination, that increase the risk of falling during physiological perturbations (e.g., body sway during standing or walking) or after an extrinsic destabilizing factor (e.g., during tripping). The rapid succession of strategies aimed at preserving body stability after a perturbation includes first the "ankle strategy" for small perturbations and later the "hip strategy" for larger perturbations. The ankle strategy is a motor plan characterized by the relaxation of trunk muscles and stiffening of the ankle joint, and the hip strategy relaxes the hip muscles and stiffens the leg muscles with the head moving out of phase and the hip moving to maintain the center of body mass over the base of support [29–32]. When the perturbation is more severe and the ankle and hip strategies are not efficient enough, a third motor plan is the "stepping strategy," during which the ankle joint is released and the subject performs one or more steps to enlarge the base of support. If these motor acts fail to preserve stability, the upper limbs play a major role in performing rescue strategies (e.g., holding on some support) or

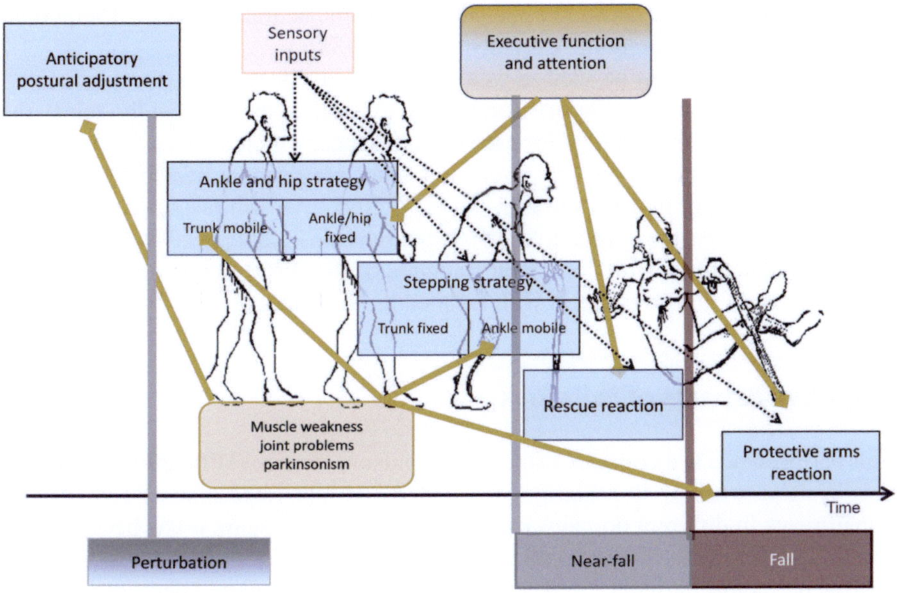

Fig. 9.3 Schematization of the rapid succession of strategies aimed at preserving body stability after a single perturbation. Note the role of cognitive function in the three rescue strategies [33]

protective reactions to limit the traumatic consequence of falling. This model helps to explain the pathophysiological link between trunk inflexibility, worsened by rigidity or fear of falling, instability (i.e., ankle strategy), and the mechanistical link between gait disorders and falling (i.e., "stepping strategy").

Figure 9.3 depicts the emerging role of cortical cognitive resources, attention, and executive functions, in each of these strategies [34]. An adequate flow of information through visual, vestibular, and somatosensory afferents is required, paired with attentional and executive resources to effectively adapt to the environment and to the type of perturbation by rapidly switching from one strategy to the other [34, 35].

The motor determinants of falls are characterized by a disorder of either the base of support or the center of body mass [29]. Parkinson's disease (PD) is a useful human model to study disorders related to the base of support. Patients with PD manifest disorders of both, the base of support and the center of body mass and, therefore, fall much more frequently than age-matched control individuals. Additional aging processes not strictly confined to the dopaminergic systems play a major role in the pathogenesis of the axial motor impairment. In recent years, mild Parkinsonian signs have been recognized in older subjects without PD. These patients present features recognized as risk factors for falling, including involvement of gait and postural stability as well as executive cognitive function. These mild Parkinsonian signs in older individuals without PD have been related to brain vascular lesions mainly involving the frontal regions [36], which support the hypothesis that cortical control of gait shares the same neural networks of important frontal lobe function including executive function [36].

Postural stability can be viewed as a strategy in itself. As such, the central nervous system adapting to the environmental constrains should rapidly select the appropriate stabilizing strategy for each circumstance, which evolves from postural perturbation, including a protective reaction when a fall cannot be avoided. Seniors with a higher rate of injuries show an impaired protective arm response during falling. The relevance of the protective arm response is also highlighted by the observation that older fallers with combined fractures of the distal radius and hip have a better prognosis than their peers with isolated hip fractures [37].

Cognitive Aspects of Falls Risk

Gait performance is a complex task that depends on the normal functioning of multiple systems working in a highly coordinated and integrated manner [38, 39]. As impairments in different domains can alter this delicate system, it has been hypothesized that different chronic conditions and risk factors for falls, such as visual or hearing problems, muscular weakness, osteoarthritis, or peripheral neuropathy, could be evidenced through gait performance [39]. Therefore, gait performance can be seen as a common pathway affected by different factors that can cause the falls syndrome. This fact may explain why gait problems are among the highest predictive risk factors for falls in older adults [38–41]. Walking requires paying attention to various environmental features and recovering from postural perturbations to avoid stumbles or falls. Therefore, it is not surprising that deficits in attention and executive function processes are independently associated with the risk of gait and postural instability, impairment in activities of daily living, and future falls [9].

The research on dual-task gait, i.e., the ability to perform a secondary task simultaneous to walking, increased exponentially after a seminal study has shown that the incapacity to maintain a conversation while walking ("stop walking when talking") was a strong predictor of future falls in cognitively impaired older adults [42]. Patients with a neurological overt disease, such as stroke, PD or mild cognitive impairment (MCI), and dementia, present a marked deterioration during dual-tasking [17, 43, 44]. This evidence helps to understand why patients with cognitive impairments and dementia syndromes are vulnerable to dual-task challenges and why falls are so prevalent in this group of patients. Daily life activities involve many attention-demanding events, which explains the high occurrence of falling while performing a secondary attentional-demanding task. Current evidence supports that dual-task gait and balance abilities worsen due to the impairment of attentional-related cognitive resources, including executive function. Even during standing, postural sway increases when a cognitive task is performed, suggesting that constant dynamic control of postural adjustments during standing also requires certain levels of cognitive attentional resources.

Even among cognitively healthy older adults, low performance in attention and executive function was prospectively associated with falls [11]. A systematic review and meta-analysis found that executive dysfunction was associated with a 1.44-fold increased risk for any fall and falls associated with serious injury [12].

Finally, evidence for the role of attention and cognition in postural control is also provided by the fact that psychotropic drugs, such as benzodiazepines and neuroleptics, that impair cognition affect postural control, reaction times, and increase the risk of falls [45]. Conversely, cognitive enhancers, including donepezil, which are usually used for the treatment of dementia, have been found to significantly reduce falls rather than near-falls in patients with PD, thus indicating that the drug did not improve stability, but rather cognitive resources that regulate postural and gait stabilities. Similarly, cognitive enhancers have been shown to improve gait and mobility in people with Alzheimer's disease (AD) [46, 47].

Dual-Task Gait Assessments

As explained above, dual-task gait performance is a sensitive measure of the role of cognitive deficits in gross motor performance, gait stability and navigation, and falls risk. Specifically, dual-task gait performance isolates the role of attention and executive function deficits in the regulation of brain gait control [3, 17, 43]. Emerging evidence is sustaining that "dual-task gait" can help to identify risk of falls in an individual without previous falls [3]. During the dual-task, the subject performs an attention-demanding task while walking to assess any modifications, compared to the reference, single-task condition, in either the cognitive or the walking subtasks [8]. The underlying hypothesis is that two simultaneously performed tasks interfere and compete for brain cortical resources [9]. Therefore, dual-task gait can act as a stress test to the brain to detect impeding mobility problems and risk of falls. Gait changes during dual-tasking (also known as dual-task costs) [48], such as slowing of gait, are interpreted as the increased cost of involvement of cortical attention processes while walking. The role of dual-task costs as a marker of future falls over simple gait assessments has been evaluated with mixed results in the literature due to the heterogeneity of studies, small sample sizes, limited prospective fall ascertainment, and the lack of standardization in dual-task procedures [49]. Although clinically meaningful, cut-off values of dual-task costs are still controversial and other unanswered questions remain. A growing body of evidence supports the potential clinical utility of this paradigm for fall prediction since it provides a valid and sensitive means of assessing motor–cognitive interactions and fall risk. Based on recent studies, a dual-task cost higher than 20% may denote individuals at higher risk of falls when they sustain a gait speed of 95 cm/s or faster, highlighting its sensitivity and predictive ability in older adults who have a relatively normal gait speed [50].

Gait Variability and Risk of Falls

Gait is a complex motor behavior with many measurable facets. This growing field of research provides an interesting window for the study of the regulation of locomotor and cognitive control. Gait speed is easily measured and provides valuable information about physical and medical status in the complete functional spectrum of older people [40, 51]. Another way to quantify gait instability that has garnered much attention in the literature recently is gait variability.

Changes in gait speed and variability are not mutually exclusive; however, they provide different information [52–54]. For example, Herman et al. [11] reported that gait variability during dual-tasking predicted future falls among community-living older adults during 2 years of follow-up, while gait speed did not. The variability of several spatial–temporal gait parameters has been studied, with stride-to-stride fluctuations in gait cycle timing (e.g., stride time) being the most widely reported [55]. In brief, it has been suggested that stride time reflects one of the final pathways of the outcomes regulated by the central nervous system. Stride time variability is becoming a relevant marker of gait stability, both in research and clinical settings, and can be measured easily and robustly [55]. The general assumption is that there is an inverse association between stride time variability and gait stability. Low stride time variability reflects automatic processes that require minimal higher cortical input and is associated with efficient and safe gait patterns [55]. Walking is one of the most "hard wired" human movements; the normal fluctuations in stride time variability are usually below 3% among healthy adults [55, 56]. However, higher gait variability has been described in older adults with frailty [57], PD [58], and AD [44, 59] and is prospectively associated with a high risk of future falls and mobility decline [60, 61]. Interestingly, increased stride time gait variability has been shown to predict future falls in community-dwelling older adults [11, 18, 62], even when gait speed failed to demonstrate an association with falls. Evidence has shown that gait variability not only serves as a clinically relevant approach in the evaluation of mobility but it may also be responsive to fall prevention interventions [55, 56].

Variability in stride time and stride length is related to the control of the rhythmic stepping mechanism and should, therefore, be considered as markers of adaptability to the walking environment [27, 63]. Sheridan et al. [59] reported that high gait variability during usual/unobstructed conditions could be a sensitive marker of dysfunction in the frontal cortical control of walking in subjects with moderate AD and executive dysfunction. Hausdorff et al. [19] showed that the degree of executive function efficiency was correlated to the degree of stride time variability. Notably, individuals with MCI [18] with 10% increase in gait variability performance during the follow-up presented an increased risk of an injurious fall compared to those who stayed below 10% increase in gait variability. These and other studies have shown that an interplay between gait variability, cognitive dysfunction, in particular executive function and attention, and the risk of falls exists.

Novel Therapeutically Approaches

Learning from Cognitively Impaired Populations

Deficits in cognitive function and mobility co-exist in older adults, even in the early stages of aging. Older people with MCI may have impairments in either memory (amnestic) or non-memory (non-amnestic) domains [19], as well as impairments in fine and complex motor skills, equilibrium, and limb coordination. Quantitative testing has revealed gait dysfunction in subjects with both the amnestic and non-amnestic MCI subtypes compared to healthy controls [16]. Neurological gaits, such as hemi-paretic and frontal or Parkinsonian gaits, were almost twice as common in amnestic MCI as in normal controls in this study. Additionally, subjects with MCI and gait abnormalities (defined as either having a slow gait or a neurological gait) were more disabled than subjects with MCI without gait abnormalities [16].

Low performance in three related cognitive domains (i.e., attention, executive function, and working memory) was associated with slowing of gait speed, specifically under dual-task conditions, suggesting that these specific cognitive domains are relevant for maintaining a normal gait pattern in the presence of a cognitive load [17]. It has been proven that increased variability of time-related gait parameters was significantly different under dual-task testing in older adults with MCI compared to age-matched normal controls but less affected in people with mild AD [44]. The same group compared the effect of dual-task of different complexity between cognitively normal controls and older adults with MCI [43]. A significant dual-task cognitive status interaction was found for gait variability but not for gait speed, further demonstrating that gait variability may be especially sensitive to dual-tasking and to the complexity of the task given. These findings suggest that cognitive control of gait performance is impaired in people with MCI and in the early clinical stages of dementia. Interestingly, these disturbances were not evident during the single-task test condition. This finding highlights the ability of tests that challenge brain function to reveal subtle or early gait problems. In summary, several studies have shown that gait is altered in people with early cognitive problems, most prominently under dual-task conditions. These findings may provide an explanation for the high risk of falls in people with MCI and executive dysfunction [15, 36–39, 64].

Algorithm for Screening At-Risk Individuals

In clinical practice, the identification of individuals at risk of future falls is highly important for prescriptions of appropriate interventions and prognosis accuracy. Gait is an uncostly simplified tool that can help clinicians and researchers to better estimate the risk of future falls in combination with other tests.

We propose using the risk scarification algorithm of the World Falls Guidelines initiative [65], that has two entry points (Fig. 9.4): first, opportunistic case finding or case finding during a health visit or through the use of "e-health records," and second, when older adults present to healthcare services as a result of a fall or related injury. Opportunistic case finding is necessary as older adults may not present following a fall and may be reluctant to report falls [5, 66–68]. Further, recollection of the occurrence or date of previous falls is unreliable [69], particularly concerning the exact timing in months. So, the one-year timing is a pragmatic compromise between accuracy of recollection and the natural history of falls risk factor progression [70]. Opportunistic case finding starts with the single question "Have you fallen in last 12 months." This single question is highly

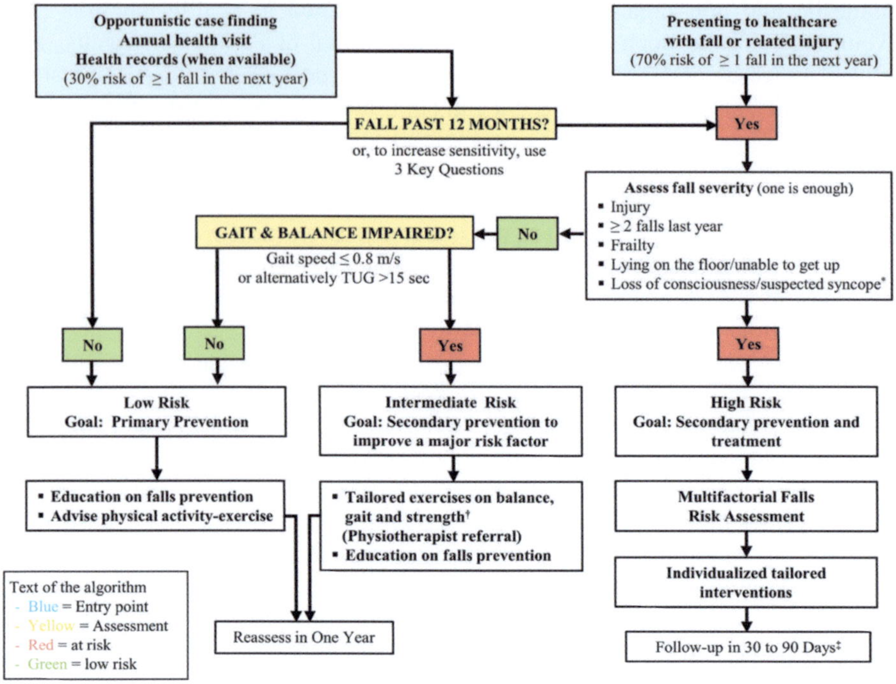

Fig. 9.4 Proposed approach and algorithm to stratify and manage falls in older adults

specific to predict future falls [71, 72] but with low sensitivity, as it takes no account of common risk factors and, consequently, results in higher false negatives. Tools that assess more than one fall risk factor, such as the "three key questions" (3KQ) [41], have a higher sensitivity; therefore, if resources are available, we conditionally recommend the addition of the following 3KQ: (i) Have you fallen in the past year, (ii) Do you feel unsteady when standing or walking? (iii) Do you have worries about falling? Additionally, the Stay Independent self-risk assessment, which contains 12 self-questions, as proposed by the Centers for Disease Control and Prevention (CDC)'s STEADI toolkit, can also be used in order to increase sensitivity to detect future risk [73, 74]. Age distribution of the older adult population when selecting a fall risk screening tool is important since sensitivity of the single question "Have you fallen in the past 12 months?" increases from 43% in those between 65 and 74 years old to 67% in those over 85 years old. Gait or balance disturbances should be assessed following a positive answer to history of falls or any of the three key questions [71].

There are several tests for assessing gait and balance impairment. For risk stratification, we recommended to use gait speed, with a cut-off value of <0.8 m/s for its predictive ability and simplicity [75]. Resources with simple instructions on how to measure gait speed can be found at www.worldfallsguidelines/resources. Alternatively, Timed Up and Go (TUG) test can be used, with a cut-off value of

>15 s, although evidence for fall risk stratification is mixed. There is evidence that TUG has falls predictive ability in lower functioning adults [75].

An older adult who does not have a history of falling, or who has a single non-severe fall and has no gait or balance problems, is deemed as being at low risk. Since low risk does not mean "no risk at all," we recommend primary prevention for these older adults. This "low risk" group should be reassessed annually. Older adults who had a single non-severe fall but with gait and or balance problems should be considered as being at "intermediate risk" and would benefit from a strength and balance exercise intervention since evidence shows that this type of exercise is effective in reducing falls risk [76]. Finally, those at "high risk" include older adults with a fall with one or more of the following characteristics: (i) accompanying injury, (ii) multiple falls (≥2 falls) in the previous 12 months, (iii) known frailty, (iv) inability to get up after the fall without help for at least an hour, and (v) accompanied by (suspected) transient loss of consciousness. With regard to frailty for risk stratification, this can be either previously identified frailty or a positive screening using a validated instrument. Commonly used frailty assessment instruments include the Frailty phenotype (FP) [77] and the Clinical Frailty Scale (CFS) [78].

Strategies to Prevent Falls and Enhance Mobility Targeting Cognition

Fall prevention trials in cognitively normal older adult populations have demonstrated, with varying degrees of success, that both multifactorial (e.g., review of medications, strength and balance training, visual and hearing correction, and environmental modifications) and single interventions (e.g., resistance exercises or progressive balance training) can be effective in preventing falls. In contrast, intervention studies targeting fall prevention in people with cognitive problems have been inconsistent or have only had modest success [79]. Older adults with cognitive problems, while at high risk for falls, represent a group who may be less responsive to the interventions that are effective among subjects that are cognitively intact. In other words, the benefits of single and multifactorial interventions for fall prevention do not translate successfully from cognitively normal older adults to those with dementia and are understudied [79, 80]. There are several potential explanations for the lack of benefit of fall prevention programs in the cognitively impaired population, including different underlying mechanisms for falls in those with cognitive problems and failure to address cognitive deficits adequately. Although much is known about the multifactorial nature of falls in cognitively normal individuals, the emerging knowledge about the nature and inter-relationship of risk factors in those with cognitive problems can help to understand how cognitive control of balance and gait can trigger falls in cognitive healthy individuals.

Current preliminary evidence from interventional studies supports that targeting cognition may reduce falls. Improving certain aspects of cognition, as a complementary intervention, can help to prevent falls in older adults. The following two sections review recent studies addressing the role of improving cognition to improve mobility and reduce falls in older adults.

Non-pharmacological Approaches

Cognitive remediation interventions have been shown to improve attention and executive function as well as memory in older adults without dementia. Table 9.1 summarizes recent studies that have specifically evaluated the effects of interventions to improve cognition on gait and fall risk. Verghese et al. [81] conducted a pilot study on 24 older adults who were randomly assigned to either a computerized cognitive remediation intervention or a wait-list. The ten participants who completed the cognitive remediation showed improvement in gait speed during normal walking and walking while talking (dual-task) compared to baseline (Fig. 9.5a). While the initial findings of this pilot trial need confirmation in larger-scale trials, they indicate that a non-pharmacological cognitive intervention can positively modify gait performance, especially during dual-task testing.

Silsupadol et al. [82] conducted an intriguing but small study among 21 older adults with balance and gait impairment. Participants were randomly assigned to one of the three interventions: single-task (active control), fixed-prioritization dual-task training, and dual-task training with variable-prioritization. Improvements in balance and gait speed were found in all groups after training (Fig. 9.5b). However, when a cognitive, dual-task was added during testing, only participants who received dual-task training exhibited significant improvements in gait speed ($p < 0.001$). Furthermore, the group that trained with variable-priority instructions demonstrated a dual-task training effect that was retained after 12 weeks of follow-up [82]. These results suggest that varying focus during training between the cognitive and motor tasks apparently had more benefits than training that required constant focus of attention on both tasks.

Schwenk et al. [83] conducted a randomized controlled trial (RCT) that evaluated the efficacy of a 12-week dual-task training program in 61 seniors with dementia. The intervention group received dual-task training, using progressively more complex activities, such as walking while throwing and catching a ball or walking while performing mental arithmetic, during a two-hour exercise session carried out twice a week. The control group received low-intensity exercise for 1 h once per week over the same period of follow-up. After the 12 weeks of training, the intervention group performed significantly better on gait in a complex dual-task condition ("walking while doing serial 3 subtractions") compared with the control group. Despite some limitations, including that the training in the intervention group included repeated exposures to the same dual-task test conditions that served as the main outcomes, this study shows RCT evidence [84] that dual-task training improves gait in people with mild-to-moderate dementia.

Finally, Mirelman et al. [85] reported an improvement in gait using a program of treadmill training enhanced with virtual reality in patients with PD. After 6 weeks of training, gait speed, stride time, and stride length significantly improved in usual and dual-tasking conditions as well as during over-ground obstacle negotiation (Fig. 9.5c). In addition, gait variability decreased (i.e., improved) under dual-task conditions [85]. Moreover, the improvements in dual-task walking were much larger than that seen in a previous study that followed an almost identical treadmill training program, without the virtual reality component. This finding suggests that a complex

Table 9.1 Cognitive training interventions for balance, gait, and fall risk

Study (year)	Study design	Type of intervention	Duration of training intervention	Participants	Summary of findings
Older adults without neurodegenerative disorders					
You et al. (2009) [101]	RCT	Dual-task CGI: simultaneous motor (walking 30 m) and cognitive (memory recall) task ($n = 8$), whereas the control group ($n = 5$) received a placebo treatment (walking while listening to simple music)	18 sessions, 30 min per session over 6 weeks	13 older adults (mean age: 68.3 ± 6.5 years) with a history of falls	Working memory performance under the dual-task condition improved ($p < 0.05$), but significant changes in gait speed and stability were not observed
Silsupadol et al. (2009) [82]	RCT	Participants were randomly assigned to one of three interventions: single-task training ($n = 7$), dual-task training with fixed-priority instructions ($n = 8$), and dual-task training with variable-priority instructions ($n = 6$)	12 sessions; 45-min individualized sessions, 3 times a week for 4 weeks	21 older adults (aged 65 years and older) with balance impairment	Improvement in balance and gait speed was found in all groups. Only the DT training with variable-priority instructions group demonstrated a DT training effect at the second week maintained at 12-week follow-up
Verghese et al. (2010) [84]	RCT	Computerized "Mindfit" program ($n = 10$). Each training session included a mixture of 21 visual, auditory, and cross-modality tasks compared with wait-list ($n = 10$)	24 sessions; 45–60 min/session, 3 times a week for 8 weeks, compared with wait-list controls	Sedentary older adults (mean age: 77.4 ± 7.0 years, MMSE: 29 ± 0.3) at training, and wait-list (mean age: 79.9 ± 7.5 years; MMSE: 29.1 ± 0.4)	Gait speed improved during normal walking ($p < 0.05$) and "walking while talking" ($p = 0.002$) only in study group. Speed of processing improved significantly in the training group ($p = 0.03$)

(continued)

Table 9.1 (continued)

Study (year)	Study design	Type of intervention	Duration of training intervention	Participants	Summary of findings
Van het Reve et al. (2014) [86]	RCT	Strength-balance (SB, $n = 98$) or strength-balance-cognitive (SBC, $n = 84$) training	2 times/week; 40-min SB. SBC received cognitive training, 3 times/week for 12 weeks	182 participants (aged ≥65 years) living in autonomous residences for the older	SBC group improved fast gait speed ($p = 0.04$), dual-task gait cost ($p = 0.03$), executive function (TMT B, $p = 0.001$), and fall rate ($p = 0.001$)
Falbo et al. (2016) [87]		Physical single task (ST) training ($n = 16$) and physical-cognitive dual-task (DT) training ($n = 20$)	12 weeks; 1 h twice Weekly in group-based exercise classes	36 healthy active individuals (age: 72.3 ± 5.8 years)	Gait performance increased in both groups, but executive function increased only in DT group
Smith-Ray et al. (2015) [102]	RCT	Computer-based cognitive training intervention ($n = 27$) or measurement-only control ($n = 24$)	10 weeks; 3 times per week, for 60 min per session	51 participants (age: 82 ± 6 years) from independent living facilities	Intervention group performed better than controls on the TUG
van Ooijen et al. (2016) [89]	RCT	Inpatient adaptability treadmill (AT) training, conventional treadmill (CT) training, or usual physical therapy (UPT)	30 sessions (40 min each); 5 per week for 6 weeks	70 participants with a fall-related hip-fracture (aged ≥65 years)	Subgroup of participants with executive dysfunction, improved walking, adaptability, and fear of falling
Parkinson's disease (PD)					
Yogev-Seligmann et al. [103]	Open-label, pilot	A 4-week program of one-on-one training included walking while performing several distinct cognitive tasks	12 sessions; three times a week for 4 weeks	Seven patients with PD (mean age: 63.8 ± 8.4 years)	Gait speed and gait variability during DT significantly improved. Untrained DT also improved and was retained 1 month after the end of the training

(continued)

Table 9.1 (continued)

Study (year)	Study design	Type of intervention	Duration of training intervention	Participants	Summary of findings
Mirelman et al. (2010) [85]	Repeated measures design	TT with virtual obstacles. The VR simulation required obstacle negotiation in two planes while continuing to walk on the treadmill. Comparison was made to a historical active control group who followed similar protocol of TT but without VR	18 sessions (three per week for 6 weeks)	20 participants with PD (mean age: 67.1 ± 6.5 years) moderately impaired but were able to walk unassisted for at least 5 min	Improvements in gait speed and stride length in usual walking. However, dual-tasking, gait speed ($p = 0.003$), and stride length ($p < 0.001$) were significantly higher after training with TT + VR compared with TT alone Dual-task gait variability decreased, and Trail Making Test improved after TT + VR training
Dementia					
Schwenk et al. (2010) [83]	RCT	Intervention group ($n = 20$) underwent dual-task-based exercise training (motor: throwing or catching a ball and cognitive: arithmetic tasks, repeating names of animals). The control group ($n = 29$) performed low-intensity exercise	24 sessions over 12 weeks, 1 h twice a week	49 participants (mean age: 81.9 ± 7.5 years) with confirmed mild-to-moderate dementia (MMSE 17–26: 21.4 ± 2.9)	DT training significantly improved gait velocity under dual-task ($p < 0.001$), cadence ($p = 0.007$), stride length ($p = 0.001$), single support ($p = 0.003$) under complex three-step backward calculation conditions compared with the control but not under the less challenging DT two-step forward calculation conditions

Adapted from Montero-Odasso et al. [3]

Note: *CGI* cognitive-gait intervention, *DT* dual-tasking, *MMSE* mini mental state examination, *RCT* randomized controlled trial, *TT* treadmill training, *VR* Virtual reality

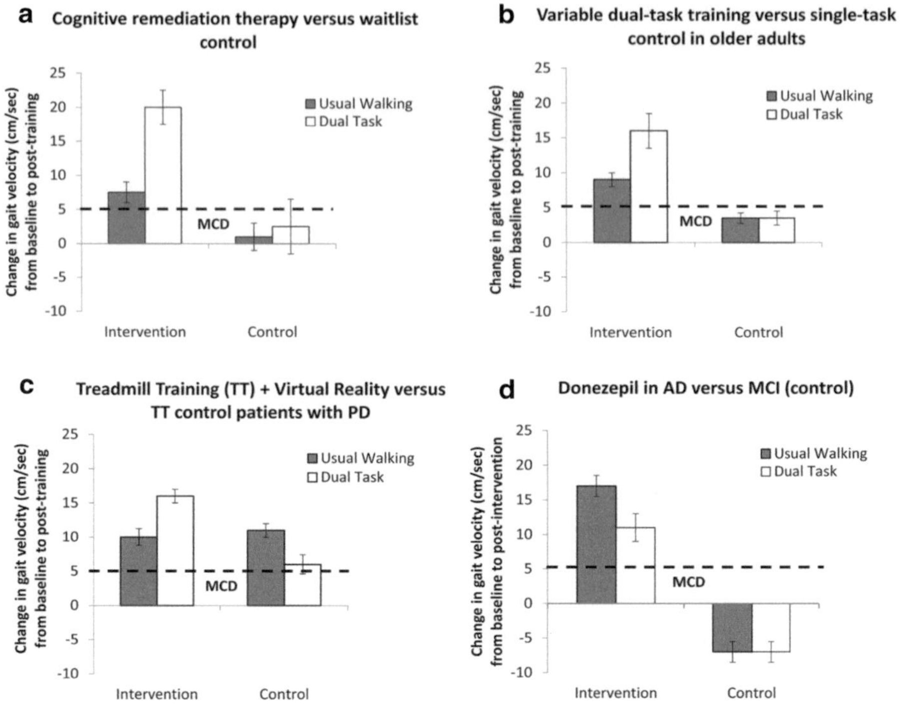

Fig. 9.5 Summary effects of four different forms of cognitive therapy on usual-walking gait speed and dual-tasking gait speed. Values shown change with respect to baseline. (Adapted from Montero-Odasso et al. [3])
Note: 5 cm/s has been identified as the minimal clinical meaningful difference (MCD) and 10 cm/s as a substantial difference. (**a**) Effects of 8 weeks of computerized cognitive remediation training (while seated) in sedentary older adults, compared with wait-list controls. Data from Silsupadol et al. [81]. (**b**) Effects of dual-task training during walking on gait speed in older adults with balance impairment, compared with subjects who only practiced walking. Data from Silsupadol [82]. (**c**) Effects of 6 weeks of TT augmented with VR among patients with PD, compared with an active control comparison of 6 weeks of TT alone. Usual-walking gait speed increased in both the TT alone and TT + VR groups; however, DT gait speed only improved among the patients who participated in TT + VR. Data from Silsupadol et al. and Mirelman et al. 2011 [81, 85]. (**d**) Effects of 4 months of donepezil use on gait speed in patients with Alzheimer's disease and compared with control patients with mild cognitive impairment. AD Alzheimer's disease, DT dual-tasking, MCD minimal clinically significant difference, MCI mild cognitive impairment, PD Parkinson's disease, TT Treadmill training, VR Virtual reality

motor–cognitive training may be more effective at improving dual-tasking and functional gait, compared to a program that focuses exclusively on motor function.

van het Reve et al. [86], through an RCT, demonstrated that strength-balance activity associated with cognitive tasks is more effective to improve dual-task gait and falls rate (decrease) than only strength-balance alone. Similarly, another RCT by Falbo et al. [87] found that physical activity associated with cognitive training is more effective to improve gait and executive function. Smith-ray et al. [88] demonstrated that a computer base cognitive training was effective to improve balance and gait speed in older individuals. Van Oijen et al. [89] demonstrated that walking on treadmill with more walking task complexities was more effective to decrease falls than conventional treadmill training to decrease falls rates in older adults with history of hip fractures. These results suggest that adding cognitive complexities to interventions may have greater potential to improve gait and decrease the fall risk in older adults.

Large-scale RCT trials are needed to generate critical evidence-based results before this approach can be widely recommended.

Pharmacological Approaches

Pharmacological interventions targeting attention and executive function have also improved gait performance in older adults [90, 91]. Table 9.2 summarizes studies that specifically evaluate the effects of cognitive pharmacological interventions to improve gait and fall risk in older individuals. Methylphenidate (MPH) has long been used to improve attention in children with attention deficit hyperactivity disorder; however, its potential to modify motor function is less known. In a pilot study, Auriel et al. [90] evaluated the effect of a single dose (20 mg) of MPH on cognitive function, gait performance, and markers of fall risk in 21 patients with PD who were receiving L-DOPA. A single dose of MPH was associated with a significant improvement in attention, executive function, gait speed, stride time variability, and the Timed Up and Go Test, i.e., validated markers of abnormal gait and fall risk. Ben-Itzhak et al. [91] tested the effect of MPH in 26 community-living older adults without dementia using a randomized, double-blind, crossover design. MPH improved executive function, gait speed, and reduced gait variability in this sample of older adults as well [91]. Additionally, a single dose of MPH reduced the detrimental effect of dual-task testing on gait variability. These initial findings suggest that MPH, and potentially other drugs designed to enhance attention, may have a role as a therapeutic option for reducing fall risk in older adults.

Cognitive function and the brain control of gait also share several neurotransmitters that may serve as additional potential targets for pharmacological interventions. Dopamine deficits have been associated with fall risk in patients with PD; levodopa typically improves many gait features in patients with this neurological disease. Interestingly, however, a recent study that assessed the role of dopamine neurotransmission in fall risk [92] demonstrated that dopaminergic denervation is apparently not associated with falls in older adults with PD. Conversely, the neurotransmitter acetylcholine has shown to have an important role in cognitive function and in controlling gait and balance [93]. Specific regions within the brain with cholinergic tracts include the hippocampus, nucleus basalis of Meynert, basal ganglia, thalamus, and the pedunculopontine nucleus. The thalamic cholinergic activity, which derives mainly from terminals of brainstem pedunculopontine nucleus neurons, plays a central role in the generation of the elementary movement patterns and gait and balance control [94]. The cholinergic system is also an important and specific controller of selective attention, likely an important factor in the dual-task decrement in walking that occurs in cognitively impaired adults. Therefore, correcting

Table 9.2 Cognitive pharmacotherapy for balance, gait, and fall risk

Study (year)	Study design	Type of intervention	Duration of intervention	Participants	Summary of findings
Subjective cognitive impairment (SCI)					
Ben-Itzhak et al. (2008) [91]	RCT, double-blind, placebo-controlled	Before and 2 h after taking 20 mg MPH or a placebo	2 h	26 older adults without dementia with subjective memory complaints (mean age: 73.8 ± 1.2 years, mean MMSE: 27.8 ± 1.4)	MPH improved Timed Up and Go ($p = 0.004$), stride time variability ($p = 0.03$), and EF ($p = 0.03$); effects not observed after treatment with the placebo
MCI					
Montero-Odasso et al. (2018) [100]	RCT, double-blind, placebo-controlled	First month with 5 mg/day of donepezil and next 5 months with 10 mg/day	6 months	60 patients with MCI (age: 75.3 ± 7 years; MMSE: 27.5 ± 2; MoCA: 23.6 ± 2.5)	Gait speed improved only under dual-task conditions, and there was a reduction in falls, albeit not significant
PD					
Auriel et al. (2006) [90]	Open-label, before–after design	Before and 2 h after taking a single dose of 20 mg of MPH	2 h	21 patients with PD who receive L-DOPA (mean age: 70.2 ± 9.2 years, MMSE: 28.8 ± 1.7)	Improvement in attention ($p = 0.025$), EF index showed only a trend ($p = 0.09$). Improvements in Timed Up and Go ($p = 0.001$), gait speed ($p = 0.005$), and stride time variability ($p = 0.013$)
Henderson et al. (2015) [98]	RCT, phase II	Rivastigmine titrated from 3 mg/day (or equivalent as placebo) and incremented every 4 weeks to a maximum of 12 mg per day at week 13 onward	8 months	130 patients with mild PD (mean age: 71.9 ± 4.8 years; 1.2; MoCA: 25 ± 1.4); half in the intervention groups and half in the placebo group	Intervention group (rivastigmine) was associated with a small but significant improvement in gait speed (greatest effect) and dual-task gait speed. Stride time variability decreased (improved) during follow-up but differences were not significant

Chung et al. (2010) [97]	Randomized, crossover, double-blind	Donepezil vs placebo. In each drug phase, subjects were instructed to take 5 mg/day of donepezil or placebo for 3 weeks and to increase to 10 mg/day for the remaining 3 weeks	6 weeks, 3 weeks washout, 6 weeks of placebo	23 patients with PD who reported falling or nearly falling (mean age: 68.3 ± 10.8 years; MMSE: 27.6 ± 4.5)	Less falls with donepezil than placebo ($p = 0.049$). Subjects with the most falls at baseline tended to show the largest improvements. No differences in Activities of Balance Confidence Scale, Berg Balance Scale, UPDRS III, or MMSE scores
AD					
Montero-Odasso et al. (2009) [17]	Open-label study with controls	5 mg/day of donepezil for 1 month and another 3 months with 10 mg/day MCI group with no treatment	4 months	Six patients with mild AD (mean age: 79.9 ± 4.8 years; MMSE: 22.3 ± 1.2; MoCA: 15 ± 1.4) compared with eight patients with MCI (mean age: 75.6 ± 6.2 years; MMSE: 27.9 ± 1.7; MoCA: 22.9 ± 1.7)	AD patients increased their gait speed ($p = 0.045$) and dual-task gait speed ($p = 0.047$) after 1 month. Stride time variability decreased (improved) during follow-up. Changes were maintained for 4 months. MCI (control) group declined in gait speed and variability
Assal et al. (2008) [96]	Before–after design	Galantamine mean dose of 17.8 ± 3.5 mg/day	6 months	Nine patients with mild-to-moderate AD (mean age: 77.9 ± 2.1 years; mean MMSE: 26.4 ± 5.2) compared with 18 no-treatment control subjects without dementia (mean age: 78.1 ± 1.0 years; mean MMSE: 29.4 ± 0.8)	Stride time was shorter under dual-tasking after treatment ($p = 0.01$). There was no change in the controls

(continued)

Table 9.2 (continued)

Study (year)	Study design	Type of intervention	Duration of intervention	Participants	Summary of findings
Beauchet et al. (2011) [99]	Before–after design	Memantine mean dose of 20 mg/day, titrated in 5 mg increments over 4 weeks	4.4– 8 months	17 patients with AD (mean age 83.8 ± 5.8 years; 52.9% women; MMSE: 14.5 ± 4.2) and 32 age- and gender-matched control patients with AD without any anti-dementia drug (mean age 80.0 ± 6.6 years; 56.3% women; MMSE: 23.2 ± 5.3)	Stride time variability decreased (improved) during follow-up in the memantine group (6.3 ± 6.1 vs 3.6 ± 1.3, $P = 0.038$)
Montero-Odasso et al. (2015) [47]	Phase II trial	5 mg/day of donepezil for 1 month and 5 months with 10 mg/day	5 months	43 patients with mild AD (mean age: 76.9 ± 8 years; MMSE: 24.63 ± 2; MoCA: 18.5 ± 4)	Gait velocity improved from 108.4 ± 18.6 to 113.3 ± 19.5 cm/s, $p = 0.01$; dual-task gait velocity from 80.6 ± 23.0 to 85.3 ± 22.3 cm/s, $p = 0.03$. Stride time variability showed a not statistically significant improvement. Trail Making Tests A ($p = 0.030$), B ($p = 0.001$), and B-A ($p = 0.042$) improved after intervention
Beauchet et al. (2011) [99]	Before–after design	Memantine mean dose of 20 mg/day, titrated in 5 mg increments over 4 weeks	4.4–8 months	17 patients with AD (mean age 83.8 ± 5.8 years; 52.9% women; MMSE: 14.5 ± 4.2) and 32 age- and gender-matched control patients with AD without any anti-dementia drug (mean age 80.0 ± 6.6 years; 56.3% women; MMSE: 23.2 ± 5.3)	Stride time variability decreased (improved) during follow-up in the memantine group (6.3 ± 6.1 vs 3.6 ± 1.3, $P = 0.038$)

Modified and updated from Montero-Odasso et al. [3]

Note: *AD* Alzheimer's disease, *EF* executive function, *MCI* mild cognitive impairment, *MMSE* mini mental state examination, *MoCA* montreal cognitive assessment, *MPH* methylphenidate, *PD* Parkinson's disease, *UPDRS* unified Parkinson's disease rating scale the cholinergic loss in dementia may improve attention and subsequently gait performance.

Cholinesterase inhibitors (ChEI), e.g., donepezil, galantamine, and rivastigmine, are the currently approved symptomatic treatments for AD and vascular dementia. The molecular mechanism of action for ChEI is achieved by increasing cortical and hippocampal acetylcholine, regulators of memory, and synaptic plasticity [95]. However, the mechanisms of clinical improvements in function in patients with dementia are not thoroughly understood. Possible explanations may relate to the cognitive action of the drug and to subtle improvements in motor function. For instance, there may be cognitive-related and non-cognitive-related enhancement mechanisms by which ChEIs might improve gait performance and potentially reduce fall risk [93]. Improving executive function and attention may affect gait control and cholinergic enhancement of the pedunculopontine nucleus may improve stride-to-stride variability. Both of these mechanisms have the theoretical potential to reduce the occurrence of falls. Whether by a direct effect or mediated through cognition, motor function improvement would consequently serve to stabilize mobility, reduce falls, and delay functional decline.

A few studies have evaluated the effect of ChEI in motor performance in older adults. These are generally pilot investigations or phase II trials, but they are, nonetheless, worthy of consideration given their novelty and potential importance to our understanding of therapeutic possibilities. Two pilot studies evaluated the effect of ChEI on gait performance [46, 96]. Assal et al. [96] tested the effect of galantamine on gait in nine participants with moderate AD. Their gait was compared with ten controls without dementia. Controls suffered a significant dual-task decrement in stride time, though there was no decrement among the participants with AD on galantamine. This finding suggests a galantamine-associated enhancement of the ability to adapt gait patterns to tasks that require attention. Montero-Odasso et al. [46] assessed the effect of donepezil over 4 months of treatment on gait speed and gait variability in six individuals with AD (Fig. 9.5d). Increases in gait speed and a reduction in gait variability were seen at 1 month following treatment with the 5 mg of donepezil. These benefits were further improved after 4 months of treatment when the full dose of 10 mg was achieved, suggesting a dose–response pattern. The control group, composed of eight individuals with MCI, experienced an expected reduction of gait speed and an increase in gait variability over time [46].

A Phase II clinical trial involving 53 participants with mild AD found that after 4 months of treatment, mean gait velocity and dual-task gait velocity significantly improved in the range of 5–8 cm/s. Changes in stride time variability were in the expected direction, although not statistically significant. Participants also showed significant improvements in Trail Making Tests parts A, B, and B-A [47]. These results suggest that cognitive enhancement through cholinergic stimulation can be effective to improve both cognitive and gait performances in more complex situations.

A randomized crossover study involving 23 older participants with PD, conducted by Chung et al., observed that fall frequency was almost 50% lower when the patients were on donepezil than when they were taking a placebo [97]. A recent

RCT conducted by Henderson in 2015 enrolled 130 PD patients and randomly assigned them to rivastigmine (3–12 mg/day) versus placebo group. After 8 months of treatment, participants assigned to rivastigmine (55 assessed) had improved step time variability for normal walking (odds ratio = 0.72, 95% CI 0·58–0·88; $p = 0{\cdot}002$) and the simple dual-task (odds ratio = 0.79; 0·62–0·99; $p = 0{\cdot}045$) [98].

Memantine is another symptomatic treatment option for patients with moderate to severe AD. Beauchet et al. [99] reported a memantine-related decrease in stride time variability among AD outpatients followed in a memory clinic, suggesting that decrease in gait variability may be explained by the combined dopaminergic and glutamatergic effects of memantine.

These preliminary interventional studies provide a basis for testing a variety of approaches in larger clinical trials. If cognitive enhancers can change gait in a meaningful way, it could reduce the risk of falls, and, in turn, have a major impact on individual and societal outcomes. Importantly, a double-blinded placebo-controlled trial found that donepezil improves gait speed during dual-task in individuals with MCI [100]. More clinical trials are necessary to explore the benefits of the combination of pharmacological and non-pharmacological treatments in mobility performance and falls prevention.

Conclusions and Future Directions

Cognitive impairment should be considered as a continuum from normal aging to advanced dementia, and similarly, mobility decline and slowing of gait can be seen as a continuum that co-exists with or even precedes the declines in cognition. Cognitive impairment, gait decline, and falls, singly and together, have a sufficiently high prevalence in older adults to constitute significant population health problems and important causes of disability. Gait variability is an objective measure that reflects cognitive dysfunction and may prove useful prognostically for mobility, cognition, and falls outcomes. Gait assessment under dual-tasking apparently can be used in the clinical encounter as a window into brain function to help detect the impact of cognitive deficits in motor and gait regulations. Dual-task gait seems to predict falls risk, particularly in those with normal gait speed. Disentangling the relationship between early gait and cognitive impairments may help better understand fall risk in aging.

Finally, improving certain aspects of cognition, specifically attention and executive function, in older adults can be a complementary way to treat mobility decline and risk of falls. In the cognitively impaired, this may be critical to reducing fall risk and its attendant disability. Studies have shown that both non-pharmacological and pharmacological interventions targeting cognition may improve gait performance, and consequently, have the potential to reduce fall risk. These interventions may be effective for improving mobility and reducing falls. It remains to be seen whether the pharmacologic and cognitive-training approaches would have a synergistic effect, whether one can substitute for the other or whether one would eclipse the other. While important questions need to be addressed in depth, these initial investigations suggest that a complementary approach to fall prevention can be incorporated into current fall intervention strategies.

Acknowledgments Dr. Montero-Odasso's program in "Gait and Brain Health" is supported by grants from the Canadian Institutes of Health Research (CIHR), the Ontario Ministry of Research and Innovation, the Canadian Consortium on Neurodegeneration in Aging, and the Department of Medicine Program of Experimental Medicine (POEM) Research Award, University of Western Ontario. He is the first recipient of the Schulich Clinician-Scientist Award and holds the Wolf Distinguished Professorship in Aging at Western University, Canada.

References

1. Isaacs B. Are falls a manifestation of brain failure? Age Ageing. 1978;Suppl:97–111.
2. Montero-Odasso M, et al. Mobility and cognition in seniors. Report from the 2008 Institute of Aging (CIHR) Mobility and Cognition Workshop. Can Geriatr J. 2015;18(3):159–67.
3. Montero-Odasso M, et al. Gait and cognition: a complementary approach to understanding brain function and the risk of falling. J Am Geriatr Soc. 2012;60(11):2127–36.
4. van Iersel MB, et al. Systematic review of quantitative clinical gait analysis in patients with dementia. Z Gerontol Geriatr. 2004;37(1):27–32.
5. Tinetti ME, Speechley M, Ginter SF. Risk factors for falls among elderly persons living in the community. N Engl J Med. 1988;319(26):1701–7.
6. Morris JC, et al. Senile dementia of the Alzheimer's type: an important risk factor for serious falls. J Gerontol. 1987;42(4):412–7.
7. Davis JC, et al. International comparison of cost of falls in older adults living in the community: a systematic review. Osteoporos Int. 2010;21(8):1295–306.
8. Woollacott M, Shumway-Cook A. Attention and the control of posture and gait: a review of an emerging area of research. Gait Posture. 2002;16(1):1–14.
9. Yogev-Seligmann G, Hausdorff JM, Giladi N. The role of executive function and attention in gait. Mov Disord. 2008;23(3):329–42; quiz 472.
10. Rosano C, et al. Quantitative measures of gait characteristics indicate prevalence of underlying subclinical structural brain abnormalities in high-functioning older adults. Neuroepidemiology. 2006;26(1):52–60.
11. Herman T, et al. Executive control deficits as a prodrome to falls in healthy older adults: a prospective study linking thinking, walking, and falling. J Gerontol A Biol Sci Med Sci. 2010;65(10):1086–92.
12. Muir SW, Gopaul K, Montero Odasso MM. The role of cognitive impairment in fall risk among older adults: a systematic review and meta-analysis. Age Ageing. 2012;41(3):299–308.
13. Buracchio T, et al. The trajectory of gait speed preceding mild cognitive impairment. Arch Neurol. 2010;67(8):980–6.
14. Petersen RC, et al. Current concepts in mild cognitive impairment. Arch Neurol. 2001;58(12):1985–92.
15. Liu-Ambrose TY, et al. Increased risk of falling in older community-dwelling women with mild cognitive impairment. Phys Ther. 2008;88(12):1482–91.
16. Verghese J, et al. Gait dysfunction in mild cognitive impairment syndromes. J Am Geriatr Soc. 2008;56(7):1244–51.
17. Montero-Odasso M, et al. Dual-tasking and gait in people with mild cognitive impairment. The effect of working memory. BMC Geriatr. 2009;9:41.
18. Pieruccini-Faria F, et al. Mapping associations between gait decline and fall risk in mild cognitive impairment. J Am Geriatr Soc. 2020;68(3):576–84.
19. Hausdorff JM, et al. Walking is more like catching than tapping: gait in the elderly as a complex cognitive task. Exp Brain Res. 2005;164(4):541–8.

20. Pieruccini-Faria F, et al. Association of dual-task gait cost and white matter hyperintensity burden poststroke: results from the ONDRI. Neurorehabil Neural Repair. 2023;37(7):434–43.
21. Robinovitch SN, et al. Video capture of the circumstances of falls in elderly people residing in long-term care: an observational study. Lancet. 2013;381(9860):47–54.
22. Zecevic AA, et al. Utilization of the seniors falls investigation methodology to identify system-wide causes of falls in community-dwelling seniors. Gerontologist. 2009;49(5):685–96.
23. Brown LA, et al. Anxiety-mediated gait adaptations reduce errors of obstacle negotiation among younger and older adults: implications for fall risk. Gait Posture. 2006;24(4):418–23.
24. Brown LA, McKenzie NC, Doan JB. Age-dependent differences in the attentional demands of obstacle negotiation. J Gerontol A Biol Sci Med Sci. 2005;60(7):924–7.
25. Pieruccini-Faria F, Sarquis-Adamson Y, Montero-Odasso M. Mild cognitive impairment affects obstacle negotiation in older adults: results from “Gait and Brain Study”. Gerontology. 2019;65(2):164–73.
26. Sakurai R, et al. Association of age-related cognitive and obstacle avoidance performances. Sci Rep. 2021;11(1):12552.
27. Pieruccini-Faria F, et al. Brain structural correlates of obstacle negotiation in mild cognitive impairment: results from the Gait and Brain Study. Gerontology. 2023;69:1115.
28. Pieruccini-Faria F, Montero-Odasso M. Obstacle negotiation, gait variability, and risk of falling: results from the “Gait and Brain Study”. J Gerontol A Biol Sci Med Sci. 2019;74(9):1422–8.
29. Maki BE, McIlroy WE. Postural control in the older adult. Clin Geriatr Med. 1996;12(4):635–58.
30. Maki BE, McIlroy WE. The role of limb movements in maintaining upright stance: the “change-in-support” strategy. Phys Ther. 1997;77(5):488–507.
31. McIlroy WE, Maki BE. Preferred placement of the feet during quiet stance: development of a standardized foot placement for balance testing. Clin Biomech (Bristol, Avon). 1997;12(1):66–70.
32. McIlroy WE, Maki BE. The control of lateral stability during rapid stepping reactions evoked by antero-posterior perturbation: does anticipatory control play a role? Gait Posture. 1999;9(3):190–8.
33. Montero-Odasso M, and Speechley M. Falls in cognitively impaired older adults: implications for risk assessment and prevention. Journal of the American Geriatrics Society, 2018;66(2):pp.367–75.
34. Fasano A, et al. The neurobiology of falls. Neurol Sci. 2012;33(6):1215–23.
35. Amboni M, Barone P, Hausdorff JM. Cognitive contributions to gait and falls: evidence and implications. Mov Disord. 2013;28(11):1520–33.
36. Montero-Odasso M, Hachinski V. Preludes to brain failure: executive dysfunction and gait disturbances. Neurol Sci. 2014;35(4):601–4.
37. Berner Y, et al. Comorbidity of distal radius (Colles’ type) and hip fractures implies a better outcome in older patients. J Am Geriatr Soc. 2002;50(5):976–7.
38. Alexander NB. Gait disorders in older adults. J Am Geriatr Soc. 1996;44(4):434–51.
39. Montero-Odasso M, et al. Gait velocity in senior people. An easy test for detecting mobility impairment in community elderly. J Nutr Health Aging. 2004;8(5):340–3.
40. Montero-Odasso M, et al. Gait velocity as a single predictor of adverse events in healthy seniors aged 75 years and older. J Gerontol A Biol Sci Med Sci. 2005;60(10):1304–9.
41. Tinetti ME, Speechley M. Prevention of falls among the elderly. N Engl J Med. 1989;320(16):1055–9.
42. Lundin-Olsson L, Nyberg L, Gustafson Y. “Stops walking when talking” as a predictor of falls in elderly people. Lancet. 1997;349(9052):617.
43. Montero-Odasso M, Muir SW, Speechley M. Dual-task complexity affects gait in people with mild cognitive impairment: the interplay between gait variability, dual tasking, and risk of falls. Arch Phys Med Rehabil. 2012;93(2):293–9.

44. Muir SW, et al. Gait assessment in mild cognitive impairment and Alzheimer's disease: the effect of dual-task challenges across the cognitive spectrum. Gait Posture. 2012;35(1):96–100.
45. Leipzig RM, Cumming RG, Tinetti ME. Drugs and falls in older people: a systematic review and meta-analysis: I Psychotropic drugs. J Am Geriatr Soc. 1999;47(1):30–9.
46. Montero-Odasso M, Wells J, Borrie M. Can cognitive enhancers reduce the risk of falls in people with dementia? An open-label study with controls. J Am Geriatr Soc. 2009;57(2):359–60.
47. Montero-Odasso M, et al. Donepezil improves gait performance in older adults with mild Alzheimer's disease: a phase II clinical trial. J Alzheimers Dis. 2015;43(1):193–9.
48. Beurskens R, Bock O. Age-related deficits of dual-task walking: a review. Neural Plast. 2012;2012:131608.
49. Beauchet O, et al. Stops walking when talking: a predictor of falls in older adults? Eur J Neurol. 2009;16(7):786–95.
50. Yamada M, et al. Dual-task walk is a reliable predictor of falls in robust elderly adults. J Am Geriatr Soc. 2011;59(1):163–4.
51. Studenski S, et al. Gait speed and survival in older adults. JAMA. 2011;305(1):50–8.
52. Lord S, et al. Independent domains of gait in older adults and associated motor and nonmotor attributes: validation of a factor analysis approach. J Gerontol A Biol Sci Med Sci. 2013;68(7):820–7.
53. Verghese J, et al. Quantitative gait dysfunction and risk of cognitive decline and dementia. J Neurol Neurosurg Psychiatry. 2007;78(9):929–35.
54. Verghese J, et al. Quantitative gait markers and incident fall risk in older adults. J Gerontol A Biol Sci Med Sci. 2009;64(8):896–901.
55. Hausdorff JM. Gait variability: methods, modeling and meaning. J Neuroeng Rehabil. 2005;2:19.
56. Hausdorff JM. Gait dynamics, fractals and falls: finding meaning in the stride-to-stride fluctuations of human walking. Hum Mov Sci. 2007;26(4):555–89.
57. Montero-Odasso M, et al. Gait variability is associated with frailty in community-dwelling older adults. J Gerontol A Biol Sci Med Sci. 2011;66(5):568–76.
58. Hausdorff JM, et al. Gait variability and basal ganglia disorders: stride-to-stride variations of gait cycle timing in Parkinson's disease and Huntington's disease. Mov Disord. 1998;13(3):428–37.
59. Sheridan PL, et al. Influence of executive function on locomotor function: divided attention increases gait variability in Alzheimer's disease. J Am Geriatr Soc. 2003;51(11):1633–7.
60. Brach JS, et al. Gait variability and the risk of incident mobility disability in community-dwelling older adults. J Gerontol A Biol Sci Med Sci. 2007;62(9):983–8.
61. Herman T, et al. Gait instability and fractal dynamics of older adults with a "cautious" gait: why do certain older adults walk fearfully? Gait Posture. 2005;21(2):178–85.
62. Hausdorff JM, Rios DA, Edelberg HK. Gait variability and fall risk in community-living older adults: a 1-year prospective study. Arch Phys Med Rehabil. 2001;82(8):1050–6.
63. Weerdesteyn V, Hollands KL, Hollands MA. Gait adaptability. Handb Clin Neurol. 2018;159:135–46.
64. Camicioli R, Majumdar SR. Relationship between mild cognitive impairment and falls in older people with and without Parkinson's disease: 1-Year Prospective Cohort Study. Gait Posture. 2010;32(1):87–91.
65. Montero-Odasso M, et al. World guidelines for falls prevention and management for older adults: a global initiative. Age Ageing. 2022;51(9)
66. World Bank. Life expectancy at birth, total (years) | Data (worldbank.org). 2022.
67. Tiedemann A, et al. Older fallers attended to by an ambulance but not transported to hospital: a vulnerable population at high risk of future falls. Aust N Z J Public Health. 2013;37(2):179–85.
68. Mikolaizak AS, et al. A multidisciplinary intervention to prevent subsequent falls and health service use following fall-related paramedic care: a randomised controlled trial. Age Ageing. 2017;46(2):200–7.

69. Nevitt MC, et al. Risk factors for recurrent nonsyncopal falls. A prospective study. JAMA. 1989;261(18):2663–8.
70. Karlsson MK, et al. Prevention of falls in the elderly: a review. Scand J Public Health. 2013;41(5):442–54.
71. Burns ER, et al. Validation and comparison of fall screening tools for predicting future falls among older adults. Arch Gerontol Geriatr. 2022;101:104713.
72. Ganz DA, et al. Will my patient fall? JAMA. 2007;297(1):77–86.
73. Stevens JA. The STEADI Tool Kit: a fall prevention resource for health care providers. IHS Prim Care Provid. 2013;39(9):162–6.
74. Centers for Disease Control and Prevention STEADI. Pocket guide-preventing falls in older patients. Centers for Disease Control and Prevention; 2019.
75. Jepsen B, et al. Predicting falls in older adults: an umbrella review of instruments assessing fait, balance, and functional mobility. BMC Geriatr. 2022;22(615)
76. Ganz DA, Latham NK. Prevention of falls in community-dwelling older adults. N Engl J Med. 2020;382(8):734–43.
77. Fried LP, et al. Frailty in older adults: evidence for a phenotype. J Gerontol A Biol Sci Med Sci. 2001;56(3):M146–56.
78. Rockwood K, et al. A global clinical measure of fitness and frailty in elderly people. CMAJ. 2005;173(5):489–95.
79. Oliver D, et al. Strategies to prevent falls and fractures in hospitals and care homes and effect of cognitive impairment: systematic review and meta-analyses. BMJ. 2007;334(7584):82.
80. Hauer K, et al. Effectiveness of physical training on motor performance and fall prevention in cognitively impaired older persons: a systematic review. Am J Phys Med Rehabil. 2006;85(10):847–57.
81. Verghese J, et al. Effect of cognitive remediation on gait in sedentary seniors. J Gerontol A Biol Sci Med Sci. 2010;65(12):1338–43.
82. Silsupadol P, et al. Effects of single-task versus dual-task training on balance performance in older adults: a double-blind, randomized controlled trial. Arch Phys Med Rehabil. 2009;90(3):381–7.
83. Schwenk M, et al. Dual-task performances can be improved in patients with dementia: a randomized controlled trial. Neurology. 2010;74(24):1961–8.
84. Verghese J, Holtzer R. Walking the walk while talking: cognitive therapy for mobility in dementia? Neurology. 2010;74(24):1938–9.
85. Mirelman A, et al. Virtual reality for gait training: can it induce motor learning to enhance complex walking and reduce fall risk in patients with Parkinson's disease? J Gerontol A Biol Sci Med Sci. 2011;66(2):234–40.
86. van het Reve E, de Bruin ED. Strength-balance supplemented with computerized cognitive training to improve dual task gait and divided attention in older adults: a multicenter randomized-controlled trial. BMC Geriatr. 2014;14:134.
87. Falbo S, et al. Effects of physical-cognitive dual task training on executive function and gait performance in older adults: a randomized controlled trial. Biomed Res Int. 2016;2016:5812092.
88. Smith-Ray RL, Makowski-Woidan B, Hughes SL. A randomized trial to measure the impact of a community-based cognitive training intervention on balance and gait in cognitively intact Black older adults. Health Educ Behav. 2014;41(1 Suppl):62S–9S.
89. van Ooijen MW, et al. The efficacy of treadmill training with and without projected visual context for improving walking ability and reducing fall incidence and fear of falling in older adults with fall-related hip fracture: a randomized controlled trial. BMC Geriatr. 2016;16(1):215.
90. Auriel E, et al. Effects of methylphenidate on cognitive function and gait in patients with Parkinson's disease: a pilot study. Clin Neuropharmacol. 2006;29(1):15–7.
91. Ben-Itzhak R, et al. Can methylphenidate reduce fall risk in community-living older adults? A double-blind, single-dose cross-over study. J Am Geriatr Soc. 2008;56(4):695–700.
92. Bohnen NI, et al. History of falls in Parkinson disease is associated with reduced cholinergic activity. Neurology. 2009;73(20):1670–6.

93. Montero-Odasso M, et al. Can cognitive enhancers reduce the risk of falls in older people with mild cognitive impairment? A protocol for a randomised controlled double blind trial. BMC Neurol. 2009;9:42.
94. Devos D, Defebvre L, Bordet R. Dopaminergic and non-dopaminergic pharmacological hypotheses for gait disorders in Parkinson's disease. Fundam Clin Pharmacol. 2010;24(4):407–21.
95. Drever BD, Riedel G, Platt B. The cholinergic system and hippocampal plasticity. Behav Brain Res. 2011;221(2):505–14.
96. Assal F, et al. Galantamine improves gait performance in patients with Alzheimer's disease. J Am Geriatr Soc. 2008;56(5):946–7.
97. Chung KA, et al. Effects of a central cholinesterase inhibitor on reducing falls in Parkinson disease. Neurology. 2010;75(14):1263–9.
98. Henderson EJ, et al. Rivastigmine for gait stability in patients with Parkinson's disease (ReSPonD): a randomised, double-blind, placebo-controlled, phase 2 trial. Lancet Neurol. 2016;15(3):249–58.
99. Beauchet O, et al. Does memantine improve the gait of individuals with Alzheimer's disease? J Am Geriatr Soc. 2011;59(11):2181–2.
100. Montero-Odasso M, et al. Donepezil for gait and falls in mild cognitive impairment: a randomized controlled trial. Eur J Neurol. 2019;26(4):651–9.
101. You JH, et al. Effects of dual-task cognitive-gait intervention on memory and gait dynamics in older adults with a history of falls: a preliminary investigation. NeuroRehabilitation. 2009;24(2):193–8.
102. Smith-Ray RL, et al. Impact of cognitive training on balance and gait in older adults. J Gerontol B Psychol Sci Soc Sci. 2015;70(3):357–66.
103. Yogev-Seligmann G, et al. Effects of explicit prioritization on dual task walking in patients with Parkinson's disease. Gait Posture. 2012;35(4):641–6.

Gait Initiation in Older People: Concepts, Clinical Implications, and Methodology

10

Paula Hentschel Lobo da Costa and Marcus Fraga Vieira

Abstract

Anticipatory postural adjustments are necessary neuromuscular strategies that help initiate a new gait cycle and take the first step forward safely. For this purpose, postural transients about to occur with imminent forward motion must be controlled. Impairments in this process must be understood in order to reveal pathophysiological mechanisms underlying dynamic balance problems in the older population. The aim of this chapter is twofold: firstly to explain the typical mechanism of gait initiation, some aspects that affect its pattern and the benefits of training interventions for the older population and, secondly, to describe computational methods to assess and quantify this mechanism based on force plate measurements.

Gait Initiation General Aspects

According to Bernstein [1], the execution of each voluntary movement is successfully accomplished by means of two control components: a focal component (related to the segmental motion that performs a goal-directed movement) and a postural component (related to the rest of the body involved in stabilizing reactions). The central nervous system has the task of coordinating these two components, namely movement and posture. In this regard, *gait initiation (GI)* is an interesting process to be studied from the fundamental point of view, because it involves precise coordination between posture and movement, as well as from the clinical one because

P. H. Lobo da Costa (✉)
Department of Physical Education, Federal University of São Carlos, São Carlos, SP, Brazil
e-mail: paulahlc@gmail.com

M. F. Vieira
Bioengineering and Biomechanics Laboratory, Federal University of Goias, Goiania, Brazil

F. A. Barbieri et al. (eds.), *Locomotion and Posture in Older Adults*,
https://doi.org/10.1007/978-3-031-74123-4_10

unbalances during GI have been shown to discriminate between stable and unstable patients [2].

The transition phase from a static to a dynamic condition involves contradictory postural stabilization functions: to prepare for an action and to recover from the perturbation. During this phase, the motor system is in a state of transient disequilibrium, which means that equilibrium will be restored in the next support phase of periodic movements like walking [3]. In this regard, GI is the task used to understand the anticipatory postural adjustments (APAs) needed to make the transition from standing posture to cyclic walking.

GI is a common task performed in daily life that requires a complex muscular synergy to generate the decoupling of the center of mass (COM) and center of pressure (COP) during standing, which results in COM moving forward [4]. It encompasses the period from the preparation for the first step until the reach of a steady-state gait speed.

In the standing position, COP and COM are close to each other. Before GI begins, ankle plantar flexors of both legs are active to maintain COM in a position anterior to the ankle joints. Now the task is to move the body outside the base of support and at the same time prevent falling [5]. GI begins with the posterior and lateral displacement of the COP toward the limb that will oscillate first, namely the swing limb. This increases the anterior–posterior (AP) and medial–lateral (ML) ground reaction forces that, in turn, cause the displacement of the COM in the opposite direction, forward, and toward the supporting foot [6–8]. The result is that COP and COM begin to dissociate.

To better understand the GI function the whole event has been divided into phases (Fig. 10.1). Because COP moves to the swing foot before any detectable foot

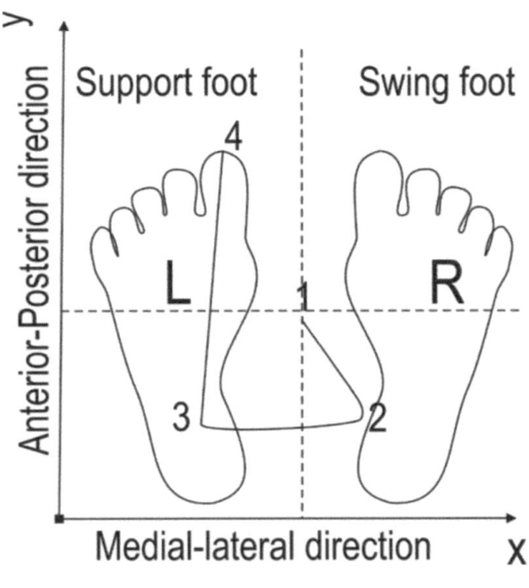

Fig. 10.1 Typical COP path during GI. 1–2: Phase 1—APA phase; 2–3: Phase 2—Swing foot unloading phase; 3–4: Phase 3—Support foot unloading phase. "L" stands for left and "R" for right

movement, the first phase is called the APA phase (1–2 in Fig. 10.1), where the anticipatory adjustments to initiate gait begin.

During the APA phase, the COP backward movement and toward the swing limb are considered an efficient strategy, because it generates the impulse needed to begin walking without requiring the COM to move forward of the base of support [9]. The second phase is called the swing foot unloading phase (2–3 in Fig. 10.1) and it begins with the heel-off of the swing foot and COP movement to the support limb, which is necessary for the subsequent unloading of the swing leg and for shifting body weight from the swing to the support limb, while COM is accelerated forward. By the end of the second phase, the transition from double to single support standing has occurred. The COP now starts to accelerate forward under the support limb [7], and this third phase is called the ***support foot unloading phase*** (3–4 in Fig. 10.1), which encompasses the roll-over of the support foot, while COP moves anteriorly until toe-off of the same foot is completed. COM moves forward through the whole GI process.

The most challenging moment for stability control during gait initiation is considered to be just before the swing foot makes contact with the ground [2]. GI process will be completed when the body reaches a constant walking speed, about the beginning of the third and the end of the eighth step [10]. In steady-state walking or running, the COM is always outside the base of support, except during the double support phase in walking [5]. During walking and running, the swing limb has a trajectory that searches balance conditions during the next support phase, and for this reason, this state of balance has been described as a dynamic balance [5]. Thus, the main goal of GI is to forward propel the body to perform the first step of a new walking cycle while maintaining dynamic balance in order to deal with instabilities during the transition from standing to walking.

The APA in GI is mediated by a central motor program [11]. Muscles of the lower extremities are activated stereotypically and create moments of force around the ankles and hips that rotate the body like an inverted pendulum [5, 12]. During the APA phase, the stereotyped activities of ankle muscles are known to be the inhibition of soleus and gastrocnemius that are followed by activation of tibialis anterior in both legs [11]. Conversely, the ML COP displacements during GI are controlled by the coordinated action of the hip abductor and adductor muscles [13]. While COP moves backward by ankle muscles synergism, swing limb hip abductors move the COP to the swing limb [5] during the anticipatory phase. Next, support foot hip abductors move the COP to the support limb, and the swing limb is unloaded. At the time of swing foot toe-off, the support limb is carrying the total weight of the body. Then, the support limb plantar flexors increase activity and the COP moves forward under this foot [5]. While the stereotyped activity of ankle muscle is well documented, we were not able to find any study that has evidenced stereotyped and invariant characteristics of muscle activities at the hip level in different populations or experimental conditions during GI; therefore, this question needs to be investigated in the future.

Bilateral electromyography of tibialis anterior and gastrocnemius has revealed five pieces of evidence for the existence of this motor program: The invariant relative timing of support (1) and swing limb, (2) tibialis anterior onsets, (3) the fore-aft ground reaction forces, (4) the swing limb toe-off, and (5) the swing limb heel-strike happens at 14, 16, 20, 43, and 87% of the GI process, respectively, regardless of changes in speed [8]. An experiment using two force plates, foot switches, and motion analysis revealed specific limb functions during GI: Since forward impulse increases rapidly after toe-off of the swing limb, the support limb is considered to be responsible for controlling forward impulse, while the swing limb is mainly concerned with weight shift from the swing foot to the support foot because loading of the swing limb in the anticipatory phase occurs simultaneously to the unloading of the support limb and the onset of forward acceleration of the COM [8].

Influencing Factors

Many studies have investigated how the motor pattern of GI is affected by factors related to cognitive demands, foot–floor interface, speed, and initial body posture, among others. Some of these influencing factors will be discussed here.

Fear of falling is a factor that influences GI. Older adults transitioning to frailty are those who do not meet the criteria for either frail or vigorous based on a specific classification scheme [14]. They are highly susceptible to falls and produce smaller and less forceful COP displacements during the APA phase when compared to healthy older adults [15]. The same is known to happen with people with Parkinson's disease (PD) [16, 17], a population that performs even worse in the APA phase of GI than older adults transitioning to frailty [14].

Dual tasking has been shown to affect GI in healthy older adults. Two groups of older adults, one called "fear of falling (Fof)" and another called "no - Fof group" performed GI as a single task while counting backward from 100 to 1. Despite both groups not differing in all clinical measures of functional balance ("Timed Up and Go," "10 m walking," and "Functional Reach" tests), the Fof group produced longer GI phases during dual tasking compared to the single task, whereas for the no-Fof group, no differences were found between both tasks [18]. The prolonged APAs phase for the Fof group is interpreted as an attempt to stabilize the body in order to reduce the risk of falling when attention resources for initiating gait are limited [18].

Footwear type has been shown to influence the number of steps necessary to reach steady-state gait: Using habitual shoes with foot orthoses has helped to reach steady-state walking with fewer steps than when barefoot or wearing habitual shoes without orthoses [19]. When using foot orthoses, ML COM range of motion is reduced during walking and GI, and this advantage has been related to a higher level of stimulation of mechanoreceptors activity and improved dynamic postural stability [19]. Conversely, reduction in the afferent somatosensory information under the foot by means of immersion in iced water results in a reduced ML COP excursion during the anticipatory phase and this loss of sensitivity is not compensated by visual input [20], indicating that plantar cutaneous afferents contribute to the control of GI. Supporting this idea, we have observed that when GI is performed barefoot, ML COP path and velocity during the anticipatory phase are higher than when using footwear, probably because of the enhanced somatosensory perception provided by the barefoot condition [21].

We have also analyzed the relative contribution of each foot to the swing foot loading and unloading processes and evidenced that when GI is performed on a soft surface made of foam, the swing and support foot peak forces in the ML direction are smaller than when the subject is shod or barefoot [21]. Still regarding foam conditions, significant Spearman correlations (Fig. 10.2) between COP integral and force impulse revealed that COP shift is responsible for only about 3.8% of ML impulse production, whereas in barefoot and shod conditions, COP shift is responsible for 26.6% and 37.4% of impulse generation, respectively. Conversely, COP shift is responsible for 89.5%, 84.9%, and 86.7% of impulse production in the AP direction in barefoot, foam, and shod conditions, respectively.

According to our results, we can state that the production of impulse in the AP direction is more dependent on the COP shift than in the ML direction, and thus, the influence of other mechanisms for impulse generation than the COP shift is stronger for the ML direction. Additionally, the foam surface limited the impulse-generating capacity of the COP shift in the anticipation phase of GI and produced smaller force peaks in the ML direction, resulting in limitations to body weight transfer from swing to support foot. Thus, our results suggest that footwear and soft surfaces affect COP patterns and force features during GI, especially in the ML direction of the APA phase [21].

Starting leg, whether freely chosen or predetermined, does not change the muscle activity during GI phases, but when the leading leg is predetermined, the reaction time to start GI is shorter than when using a freely chosen leg for older and younger adults, with the older people needing longer reaction times [22]. Interesting is the fact that tibialis anterior anticipatory activity gradually improves with subsequent trials in a series of ten trials [22], which may suggest a learning effect that could have implications in rehabilitation contexts.

APAs are considered to be under the prospective control [23] and, as such, they are an index for the ability to feedforward control motor actions. Thus limiting factors to properly integrate posture and voluntary locomotion in standing are associated with difficulties in activating the motor program involved in the APAs for GI, especially regarding forward propulsion [24]. Concerning locomotion ability, it is likely that dynamic instabilities during step transitions may be more critical factors in reaching a steady-state walking speed than standing postural control.

GI was investigated when individuals started from inclined surfaces [25]. During the swing phase of GI, an observable pattern emerges wherein the vertical COM velocity is negative, adopting a distinct V-shaped profile. This unequivocally signifies a descending trajectory of the COM; in other words, this indicates that the COM is falling. Nevertheless, a notable reversal of this COM descent becomes evident just prior to the initial contact of the swing foot, manifesting as a discernible reduction in the vertical COM velocity. This particular phenomenon is conventionally characterized as the "braking of the COM fall" (BCOM), as initially described by Chastan et al. [26]. Additionally, the activation of the ankle plantar flexors in the

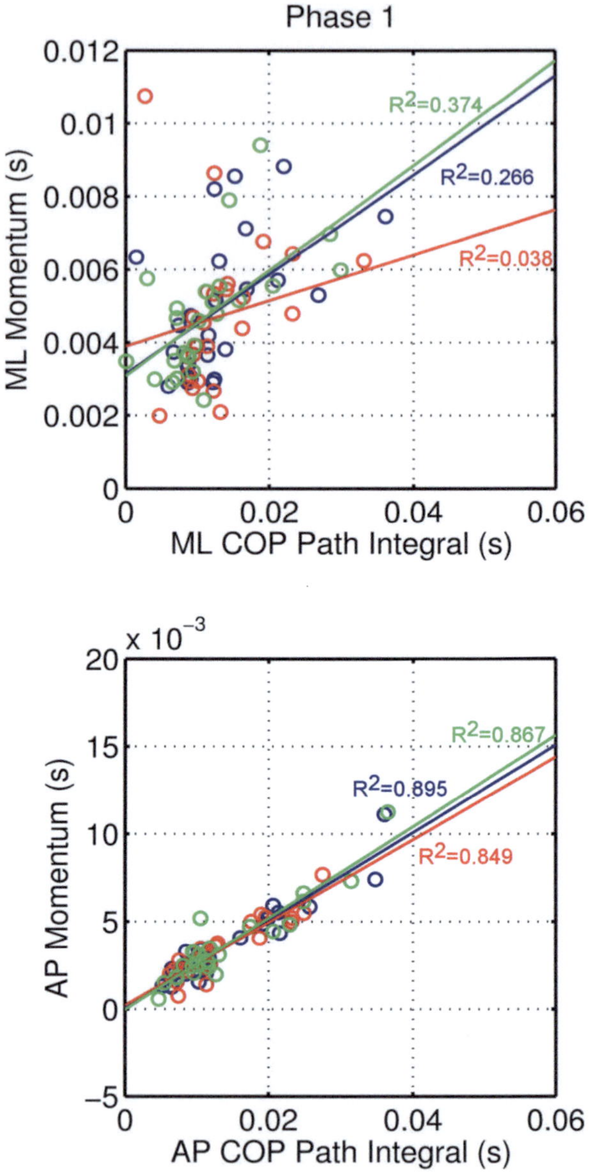

Fig. 10.2 AP impulse x COP path integral graph for phase 1 of GI. See text for explanations. Blue: barefoot condition; Red: foam condition; Green: shod condition

supporting limb counteracts the COM descent before the swing foot's contact with the ground [27].

The reversal of the COM descent during BCOM can be quantified as a ratio between the first COM velocity peak minus the minimum COM velocity (marking the onset of BCOM) over the second COM velocity peak (indicating the end of BCOM) minus the minimum COM velocity, with the resultant value multiplied by 100% [25]. As expected, Vieira et al. [25] established that BCOM was notably diminished when GI was executed on a downward-inclined surface. Thus, the regulatory mechanism of attenuation of the COM fall braking before swing foot contact was detrimentally affected, an effect induced by the slope of the surface. The effective operation of this mechanism was limited by the height difference with respect to gravity between the support foot and the swing foot at the initial contact. Moreover, the eccentric flexion of the knee in the supporting limb and the concurrent activation of the ankle plantar flexors, both observed during GI on a downward-inclined surface, fail to augment the BCOM mechanism as would be anticipated. Consequently, this leads to a diminished damping effect upon the landing of the swing foot on the ground and potentially elevates the biomechanical demands placed upon the musculoskeletal system.

Ankle mobility holds significant importance in facilitating the execution of a functional GI motor pattern, as elucidated by Delafontaine et al. [28]. To explore the short-term effects of stretching the triceps surae in people with PD, a study was conducted. Nineteen PD patients, devoid of freezing or falls, performed ten GI tasks on a force plate both before and after undergoing four 60-second trials of triceps surae stretching, wherein they stood with both feet on a 20-degree inclined wedge positioned in front of a wall. Comparative analysis was carried out by juxtaposing the results of the PD patients with those of a sham group and an age-matched healthy cohort, as conducted by Vialleron et al. [29].

Of particular note, Vialleron et al. [29] introduced a noteworthy aspect to their study by quantifying the frontal plane dynamic stability during the swing foot contact phase of GI. To achieve this, they adapted the concept of the margin of stability [30], which involved calculating the distance between the ML boundary of the base of support and the ML position of the extrapolated center of mass at swing foot contact. Interestingly, enhanced ankle mobility did not exert an influence on ML dynamic stability, thereby indicating that the risk of imbalances in the frontal plane for PD patients remained unchanged after stretching. Conversely, a notable approximately 32% increase in the center of mass forward velocity during the APA phase of GI was observed, suggestive of an acute improvement in the capacity to generate propulsive forces following stretching sessions. Conversely, the same authors did not discern any primary statistical effects, whether related to time or group distinctions nor did they identify any interactions concerning the vertical COM braking. As elucidated previously, the phenomenon involving the reduction of the COM descent prior to the point of the swing foot contact has been well investigated [25, 27]. It requires the engagement of the plantar flexor muscles in the supporting limb's ankle and the eccentric flexion of the knee in the supporting limb. Consequently, it is probable that the implemented stretching sessions did not yield enhancement in the impact attenuation at the initial contact of the swing foot. Additionally, the chronic effects of stretching in the context of GI remain unknown, as does its potential benefit for advanced PD patients [29].

Gait Initiation in Older People

The task of GI challenges the balance control system because the person moves from a relatively stable static balance to a continuously unstable gait [16]. The skills necessary to maintain stability, weight transfer, foot clearance, and propulsion become more critical during transitions like accelerating in GI, decelerating in the gait termination [19], and changing directions [14]. Individuals with postural instabilities and locomotion impairments may experience even more problems reaching equilibrium during GI. Thus, GI represents a risky activity for older people [31], considered a fall-prone population given their well-known problems with static and dynamic balance. It is accepted that the transition from standing to steady-state gait is an ideal paradigm to examine the impact of advancing age on mobility [32], since those changes may not be apparent during quiet support and steady-state walking tests.

GI studies in older people have revealed some important age-related changes in this process. In older people, decreased COP displacements are evidenced during the APA phase [16], and despite the presence of a central motor program for GI, it is less frequently observed in electromyography data than in younger adults [31]. For this reason, COP displacements in the APA phase have been accepted as a sensitive indicator of balance dysfunction [2].

Two measures have revealed that the biomechanical effectiveness of the GI motor program in generating impulse (given as the time integral of GRF in a specific direction) in older people is limited [31]:

1. The relationship of the time integral of backward COP shift and the amount of forward impulse are highly correlated in young as well as in older adults, though older people generate significantly less impulse for each increment in COP displacement (or incremental cop displacement).
2. The relationship between the time integral of the AP COP displacement and walking speed is also highly correlated for both populations, though the correlation coefficients in this case are significantly lower for the older group.

Together these indicators reflect that the older group may generate the impulse needed for the execution of the first step by other strategies than moving the COP backward [31]. Reduced backward COP excursions may be associated with the fact that the soleus and gastrocnemius remain active, while the tibialis anterior becomes active during the anticipatory phase [31].

Although the stereotyped muscle activity of GI remains invariable in healthy older people [16], electromyography studies have demonstrated some alterations in muscle activity durations. The duration of tibial anterior anticipatory activation tends to be shorter for the physically active older than for younger adults [22]. When compared to younger adults, lateral gastrocnemius activity of the support leg starts later and the percentage of delay between tibial anterior and lateral gastrocnemius activations is greater in older people, whereas the mean duration of the simultaneous activation is shorter [22]. Thus, lateral gastrocnemius activation of the support limb does not start before the swing limb has left the ground in the majority of the older individuals studied [22]. This delay may impair not only the propulsion but also the control of the forward movement of the body in preparation for the swing leg to leave the ground [33].

The initial steps of GI are shorter with greater variability for older people, even when step length is normalized to the body height [22]. Step lengths are even shorter in older fallers, as compared to younger adults [34]. Additionally, when investigating the walking cycles of frail older individuals, it is advisable to exclude the initial 2.5 m, as this distance is requisite for achieving steady-state walking in this population [35].

In a study examining GI among both young and older individuals, a multisegment foot model, a three-dimensional motion analysis system, and two adjacent force plates were utilized beneath the same foot to separately measure midfoot and toe joint kinetics [36]. Specialized software was employed to calculate foot kinetics in the sagittal plane. While the results were not explicitly categorized according to the specific phases of the GI task, the older group demonstrated diminished joint moments and powers in the ankle between the metatarsal and hindfoot joints, as well as toe and metatarsal joints. These findings complement the existing knowledge of muscle activation patterns and center of pressure behavior, offering a comprehensive understanding of the mechanisms underpinning the process of gait initiation in the elderly population.

Gait Initiation and Training Effects

Some authors have suggested training strategies that would improve GI in older people, based on results of studies that have compared groups with different characteristics. Pieces of evidence of task memorization [22] indicated that when GI is repeated in a series of successive trials, this task-specific repetitive training could be advised for older people in order to prevent falls. Biofeedback and relaxation exercises [31] have also been suggested to improve the COP shift mechanism and thus probably prevent falls. Other researchers have performed specific interventions and achieved improvements in GI performance.

Tai Chi training [15] as a martial art is considered a potential tool to prevent falls because it emphasizes concentration, awareness of the environment, slow weight shifting, endurance, and strength. When the typical slow transitions from double to single support in Tai Chi techniques are trained by frail older adults for 48 weeks twice weekly, these individuals improved the backward COP shift during the APA phase to values similar to those exhibited by healthy older adults [15]. Furthermore, the movement smoothness values during the swing foot unloading phase were improved in the Tai Chi training group. A comparative group engaged in a wellness education program, including techniques of fall prevention, diet and nutrition advisement, mental health, and other health-related issues, was less efficient in improving backward COP translations and movement smoothness. These results indicate that Tai Chi may help to restore in some aspects the centrally mediated

APAs, soleus inhibition, and tibial anterior activation patterns. Additionally, the smoothness value, as a movement coordination index, is sensitive to this training. Conversely, neither intervention improved ML COP displacements in the anticipatory and swing foot unloading phases.

Training effects should be further investigated to highlight how impairments in GI can be overcome in older adults, especially to prevent falls. Randomized controlled clinical studies are of interest to accomplish this goal.

Additionally, it has already been demonstrated that dividing the GI into its phases provides more information related to specific mechanisms present in the older population than analyzing GI by the overall time [37]. Besides, the median value of multiple measures, instead of the mean, is considered a better summary index in cases where GI is divided into its phases, because of the expected variability of GI behavior and also because the median value better deals with the learning effects expected for successive trials [37]. The time to the first lateral movement may be the best variable to discriminate among different cognitive abilities and attention demands of the task in the elderly population [37].

Forces and Center of Pressure Calculations During Gait Initiation

The GI is frequently studied using force plates. Literature reports some common descriptors and specific variables selected by the authors to identify special aspects of GI. The next section of this chapter will deal with the computational description of the variables we consider relevant that are derived from the dynamometric method using force plates. It is important to mention that electromyography (EMG) and motion analysis provide complementary descriptors of the GI process, but the respective variables are not in the scope of this chapter.

Some authors use the forces recorded by a force plate in the study of GI. These variables can be associated with kinematic variables, obtained through optical systems, or EMG data, and some information can be extracted using multivariate statistics tools like principal component analysis (PCA) and statistical parametric mapping (SPM). However, the COP, a derived variable from the ground reaction forces, is the most used variable to study GI due to its peculiar behavior in this task, especially with respect to APAs. For this reason, we will focus on analyzing the COP in GI, although we will also comment on the ground reaction forces (GRF).

The raw data of the force plate can be sampled at different frequencies (Table 10.1). When kinematic data are acquired by an optic system together with the kinetic data, it is advisable to adopt a sampling frequency that is multiple of the acquisition frequency of the cameras. This will facilitate further operations like synchronization, decimation, and data normalization. However, considering that kinematic and kinetic signals of human movement are low-frequency signals and they primarily occupy the lowest band of the frequency spectrum of the raw data [68], setting the force plate sampling frequency at 100 Hz will be sufficient in most cases.

Table 10.1 Sampling frequency of force plates in GI studies

Sampling frequency (Hz)	Authors
1000	Uemura et al. [18, 42], Lin and Yang [20], Caderby et al. [38], Corbeil and Anaka [39], Gélat et al. [40], Tseng et al. [41]
600	Dibble et al. [43], Martin et al. [44], Tokuno and Eng [45], Tokuno et al. [46]
500	Brunt et al. [6], Chastan et al. [27], Colné et al. [47], Do Nascimento et al. [48], Jian et al. [49], Mouchnino et al. [50], Patchay and Gahéry [51], Ruget et al. [52], Vinti et al. [53], Welter et al. [54], Wicart and Maton [55], Wicart et al. [56], Yiou and Do [57]
250	Delval et al. [58], Yiou and Do [59]
200	Martin et al. ([37], Ledebt et al. [60]
100	Henriksson and Hirschfeld [22], Bruyneel et al. [61], Henriksson et al. [62], Jones et al. [63], Muniz et al. [64], Spencer and Van der Meer [65], Stackhouse et al. [66], Vrieling et al. [67]

It is recommended to filter the raw data to remove noise. The noise can be reduced by adopting a careful protocol to collect data, including an equipment heating period. The force plate manufacturers recommend turning on the equipment for at least 1 h before their use in data collection.

The data should be filtered by a second- or fourth-order low-pass band Butterworth filter. The approximation provided by a Butterworth filter has a flatter frequency response and a phase closer to the linear in relation to other approximations such as Chebyshev or Elliptic. A linear phase is important because it provides an equal delay to all frequencies contained in the original signal. However, the Butterworth filter introduces a delay or phase shift in the filtered signal, and reverse filtering should be performed to eliminate this delay or phase. In other words, the filter must be applied to the raw signal in the forward and reverse direction, canceling the phase introduced by the Butterworth filter. This means that in fact a fourth- or eighth-order filter is applied to the raw data.

The cutoff frequency is a critical point in the filter design and depends on the sampling frequency used in data acquisition and on the maximum relative mean residual allowed [69]. There is no consensus on the cutoff frequency of the filter used in the analysis of the GI (Table 10.2) authors and many of them omit this information.

Considering the low frequency of the signals in the biomechanics [68] and the recommendations for the choice of the cutoff frequency in the filter design [69], we suggest a zero-lag fourth-order low-pass Butterworth filter with a cutoff frequency of 6 Hz and a sampling frequency of at least 100 Hz in GI studies using force plate.

Table 10.2 Filter cutoff frequency to process the force signal

Cutoff frequency	Sampling frequency	Authors
5	Not reported	van Keeken et al. [70]
6	1000	Uemura et al. [18, 42]
10	500 Or 1000	Lin and Yang [20], Corbeil and Anaka [39], Gélat et al. [40]
10.5	500	Do Nascimento et al. [48]
30	500 100	Jian et al. [7], Muniz et al. [64]
50	600 Or 1200	Tokuno and Eng [45], Stackhouse et al. [66]
100	500	Wicart and Maton [55], Wicart et al. [56]

Analyzed Variables

The data collected with one or two force plates are processed to calculate the COP trajectory during the entire task or during each phase of GI or to analyze the behavior of the ground reaction forces. In fact, the COP trajectory is a current index used in basic and clinical research to evaluate balance and locomotion control [51], being an indicator of instability to both healthy and pathological populations [63].

Most studies have considered only discrete parameters from GRF for extraction of information about the GI and other tasks, usually local peaks or minimum values, as reported above. However, different methods of multivariate analysis based on variance estimates, such as PCA and SPM, have been used in the interpretation of GI data. The PCA considers the complete pattern of GRF and can provide additional insight into the GI [64], reducing the dimensionality of the data while keeping their original variability: PCA reduces the number of variables to a subset of orthonormal factors or principal components, which maximize the representation of variance of the original data [71]. Besides, the use of PCA with a pattern recognition tool has been proven to be useful for discriminating different groups [64, 72] or for evaluating how far the gait deviates from a typical pattern [64, 73].

In order to capture features of the entire COP or force time series, a vector analysis using SPM methods should be conducted, as described by Pataky et al. [74]. This statistical approach captures features of the entire time series instead of a few discrete variables and may improve the effectiveness of the GI analysis. Discrete variables fail to capture sufficient portions of the data and covariance among vector components [74]. SPM analysis uses random field theory to identify field regions which co-vary with the experimental protocol [75].

To perform the SPM analysis, each component of the resultant COP or force time series is interpolated with cubic splines to contain 100 points (normalization to 100% of the task). The average over the trials performed by the study participants should be used in the analysis. Next, the components are organized in an array with n rows, one for each participant, 100 columns, and *M* matrices, one for each component X and Y of COP time series (or X, Y, and Z components of GRF time series). One array should be constructed for each condition analyzed in the study.

Taking the COP time series as an example, each column of the ($n \times 100$) COP matrices is regarded as a single-vector field Cop(t) = {$Cop_x(t)$ $Cop_y(t)$}, where t indicates time. Within-subject mean Cop(t) is calculated for each ith subject at each time instant and among the different conditions analyzed, taken two by two:

$$\Delta Cop(t)_i = \left(\text{Cop}(t)_{\text{condition1}}\right)_i - \left(\text{Cop}(t)_{\text{condition2}}\right)_i \tag{10.1}$$

where conditions are before and after an intervention, for example.

The paired Hotelling's T^2 test statistic trajectory is calculated as:

$$T^2(t) = n\left(\Delta\bar{\text{C}}\text{op}(t)\right)W(t)^{-1}\left(\Delta\bar{\text{C}}\text{op}(t)^T\right) \tag{10.2}$$

where n is the number of subjects (number of rows), $\Delta\bar{\text{C}}\text{op}(t)$ is the cross-subject mean, and $W(t)$ is the 2×2 covariance matrix of ΔCop_x and ΔCop_y at time t.

For vector analysis, statistical inference is conducted by calculating the T^2 threshold taking $\alpha = 0.05$. Condition effects are assessed using paired *t-tests* on COPx and COPy, with a Sidák correction threshold, taking $\alpha = 0.05$ producing "p" calculated as follows:

$$p_{\text{critical}} = 1 - (1-\alpha)^{1/N} \tag{10.3}$$

where $N = 2$ is the number of scalars for COP (x and y). Equation (10.3) produces $p = 0.0253$ for $N = 2$.

Additional information and the codes to conduct SPM analysis can be downloaded from www.spm1d.org.

Variables such as COP maximum lateral displacement and COP maximum backward displacement during the APA, as well as the APA duration [18, 37–39, 42, 44, 47, 58, 59, 76–78] are very common in the literature, as well as in studies of child development [24, 60] characterizing the motor behavior during GI of a given population [79].

Some variables can only be calculated using two force plates such as the COP displacement under each foot [62], especially in amputees [46], or the body weight on the swing foot at the beginning and at the end of APA [51, 79], or the force peak on each foot [45]. The trajectory of the COP under the swing foot and the support foot can be analyzed separately, usually normalized by foot length [24]. In the latter case, the use of two force plates is necessary. Specifically, when comparing adults and children, Malouin & Richards [24] proposed an index given by the ratio between the swing foot AP displacement and the support foot AP displacement.

Another variable used is the resultant COP trajectory [14, 66, 80, 81] or the resultant COP displacement in the AP and ML directions [20, 27, 50, 53, 57, 59, 62, 65, 70, 82–84].

The duration of each GI phase and the COP mean velocities in the AP and ML directions, at each phase or during the entire task, are also widely used [14, 15, 33, 40, 56, 65, 85, 86] and can be calculated as suggested in Table 10.3.

Table 10.3 Matlab code suggestions to calculate cop descriptors

Matlab script	Description
path_x = sum (abs (diff (COPx)));	Total COP path in ML direction
path_y = sum (abs (diff (COPy)));	Total COP path in AP direction
duration = length(COPx)/Fs; or duration = length(COPy)/Fs	Duration of corresponding phase
mean_veloc_x = displacement_x / duration;	Mean velocity in ML direction
mean_veloc_y = displacement_y / duration;	Mean velocity in AP direction
smoothness_x trapz((diff(COPx,3)./(1/Fs)^3).^2);	Smoothness in the ML direction
smoothness_y trapz((diff(COPy,3)./(1/Fs)^3).^2);	Smoothness in the AP direction

COPx e COPy—COP trajectory in ML and AP directions, respectively; Fs—sampling frequency

Table 10.4 Matlab code suggestion for filter design

Matlab code	Description
Fs = 100;	Sampling frequency
Fc = 6;	Cutoff frequency
order = 2;	Filter order
Wn = Fc/(Fs/2);	Cutoff frequency in radians relative to the sampling frequency
[b,a]=butter(order,Wn,'low');	Filter coefficients
data=filtfilt(b,a,raw_data);	Zero-lag filtering

raw_data—raw data; data—filtered data

The movement smoothness, a variable used to evaluate the motor performance of healthy and pathological individuals [87–89], has also been used in the study of GI [14, 15]. Maximum smoothness is obtained when the movement oscillations are minimized, indicating that the movement smoothness results from learning processes and better motor coordination [89]. Smoothness is defined as the integral of the square of the third derivative of COP trajectory in the AP and ML directions [15] as presented in Table 10.3.

Another variable used to understand the rocker behavior created by the knee–ankle–foot system is the roll-over, measured by transforming the COP from a laboratory-base coordinate system into the leg-based coordinate system [90], which can be useful in the design of prostheses.

Recommendations for Analytical Studies of Gait Initiation

In order to standardize the analytical procedures to assess GI, some recommendations are suggested to enable future comparisons of different studies.

Table 10.4 presents Matlab code suggestions for filter design.

The *butter* command will design an infinite impulse response (IIR) Butterworth filter. Using, in this case, a second-order filter means assigning a ripple smaller than 3 dB in the pass band and a 60 dB attenuation in the stop band.

The *filtfilt* command will perform an IIR filtering using the filter coefficients calculated by the *butter* command, forward and reverse, canceling the phase

Table 10.5 Matlab code suggestion for COP calculations

Matlab commands	Description
COPx = - ((My + (dz*Fx))./Fz) + dx;	ML COP
COPy = ((Mx - (dz*Fy))./Fz) + dy;	AP COP
COPx = - ((My + ((dz-e)*Fx))./Fz) + dx; COPy = ((Mx - ((dz-e)*Fy))./Fz) + dy;	ML COP with pad on the plate
	AP COP with pad on the plate
COPx_result = ((COPx1.*(Fz1./(Fz1 + Fz2))))+(W_1/2) + ((COPx2.*(Fz2./(Fz1 + Fz2))))-(W_2/2)++	Resultant ML COP between two plates
COPy_result = (COPy1.*(Fz1./(Fz1 + Fz2))) + (COPy2.*(Fz2./(Fz1 + Fz2)))	Resultant AP COP between two plates

Fx = ML GRF component, Fy = AP GRF component, Fz = Vertical GRF component, Mx = ML moment, My = AP moment, dx, dy, dz. = plate true origin coordinates x, y, and z, e = pad thickness on the plate. W_1: force plate 1 width, W_2: force plate 2 width. The indexes 1 and 2 refer to the first and second plates, respectively, when using two force plates. ++ The COP coordinates should be described in relation to the origin of the corresponding force plate. If the COP coordinates are described in relation to the global reference system of the laboratory, $W_1/2$ and $W_2/2$ are not necessary.

introduced by the Butterworth filter. This means using, in fact, a fourth-order filter, as already explained.

The COP instantaneous position is calculated by considering the ground reaction force components, the moments around the AP and ML axes and the data concerning the true origin of the force plate, as reported by the manufacturer. It should be considered that the actual origin of the force plate does not always coincide with the force plate geometrical center due to the limitations in the manufacturing process (Table 10.5).

When the plate has some kind of cover used to hide the plate to prevent the subject to aim at the plate and to modify his step, the pad thickness (e) has to be added to plate true origin z coordinate (Table 10.5).

Analyzing the equations presented in Table 10.5, we can conclude that the COP is sensitive to errors in force and moments values to very small Fz values, commonly acquired at the beginning and the end of foot contact on force plate. Hence, it is important to establish an Fz force threshold, under which the COP will not be calculated. This threshold depends of the analyzed subject. We recommend values around 2% of the average individuals body weight.

While we use the reaction-oriented coordinate system, it is important to observe that some force plate manufactures use action-oriented coordinate system. In this case, a conversion should be done as follows:

Fx → Fx	Mx → Mx	x → -x
Fy → Fy	My → -My	y → y
Fz → Fz	Mz → Mz	z → -z

Calculating the Beginning and the End of Gait Initiation

An important aspect of analyzing GI is the determination of when the task begins. In some studies, the volunteers are instructed to initiate the task after a vocal command, an acoustic stimulus, a cutaneous stimulus, or a visual stimulus. However, even when the laboratory is equipped with devices capable of synchronizing the start command to data acquisition, this does not mean the volunteer will begin the task immediately after the start command. Some procedures have to be done to properly identify the task beginning. Table 10.6 presents different protocols adopted by different authors.

Therefore, for force plate protocols, data should be acquired prior to the start command. The data acquisition has to be triggered at least 2 s before the command to initiate the movement. The individual should be instructed to maintain a quiet posture on the force plate until the start command. If two force plates are being used, the calculations for the beginning of the movement should be made from the ground reaction force of the swing foot force plate and for the end of the movement from the support foot force plate.

The end of the movement is defined by the instant at which the support foot loses contact with the force plate, when the ground reaction force vertical component drops to zero or is smaller than the established threshold. Thus, the data can properly be cut. Table 10.7 gives some examples of Matlab codes for these calculations considering that the data acquisition has begun 2 s before the beginning of the task, with a sampling frequency of 100 Hz and with a threshold of 15 N for the vertical component of ground reaction force.

Table 10.6 Strategies to determine task beginning in GI

Beginning of the task	Authors
When the COP medial–lateral deviation toward the swing foot is greater than three times the standard deviation of the COP average initial position during the first 1.5 s before the stimulus	Uemura et al. [18, 42], Malouin and Richards [24]
When the COP moves beyond 10 mm laterally in relation to its initial position	Jones et al. [63]
When the velocity of the resultant COP is greater than 0.01 m/s	Do Nascimento et al. [48]
By the first medial–lateral COP displacement in frontal plane	Viton et al. [91]
When the first medial–lateral COP deviation toward the swing foot is greater than 4 mm	Melzer et al. [92, 93]
By the first COP trajectory sample toward the swing foot	Martin et al. [17]
At the instant in which occurred a 4 mm displacement in relation to COP baseline with a duration of at least 10 ms	Maki and McIlroy [94]
By an alteration in ground reaction force vertical component immediately before the APA	Muniz et al. [64]
By a detectable increase in swing foot ground reaction force vertical component	Henriksson et al. [62]
At the instant in which the ground reaction force vertical component exceeds its average value plus two times the standard deviation acquired during the first 0.5 s of quiet stance	Hass et al. [9]

Table 10.7 Matlab codes suggestion for calculating the beginning of the task

Matlab script	Description
ind = find(Fz >= (mean(Fz(50:100)) + 2*std(Fz(50:100))); start = ind(1);	Task beginning: Fz>= Fz average during 0.5 s before the movement plus two times the standard deviation. Fz: vertical force of swing foot force plate
ind = find(Fz <= 15.0); end = ind(1);	Fz threshold = 15 N. Fz: vertical force of support foot force plate (around 2% of average body weight)
data = data(start:end,:);	Cutting the data

* We used the protocol suggested by [9, 95]
Fz—vertical ground reaction force component. For data acquired at 100 Hz

Another critical aspect in experimental studies pertains to the acquisition of reliable data for GI metrics. Using inertial measurement units, Seuthe et al. [96] calculated the number of GI trials required to obtain reliable data within a single session for both healthy older adults and PD patients with freezing gait under dopaminergic medication. The study encompassed 38 PD patients and 30 healthy elderly participants, all of whom performed five GI trials followed by walking along a 10-m walkway. The number of trials necessary to achieve reliable metrics varied depending on the specific outcome measure. For the attainment of an estimated intraclass correlation coefficient of 0.75, five trials were deemed sufficient to yield reliable APAs AP and ML peak accelerations, first step range of motion (from toe-off to heel strike), and velocity. In contrast, assessing the latency and duration of APAs required more than ten trials to be reliably measured [96, 8]. Notably, no significant differences were observed between healthy older individuals and PD patients in this regard. This information is of paramount importance, as representative data are indispensable for the comparative analysis and interpretation of GI metrics.

Final Remarks

Considering the importance of the GI process in older people and the studies cited in this chapter, we can point out some final remarks:

- GI studies have improved our understanding of dynamic balance in older people.
- Clinical trials are needed to verify whether GI characteristics are sensitive to interventions.
- Prospective studies are needed to identify whether improvements in GI are related to less frequent falls in the elderly.
- Frontal plane (ML) COP mechanism during GI must be better understood in order to identify invariant characteristics for ankle and hip joint motions during the phases of GI.
- Results of different studies must be compared with caution, considering the respective calculation methods.
- Data processing should consider the characteristics of the process and should focus the search for the underlying mechanism that controls GI.

References

1. Bernstein NA. The co-ordination and regulation of movements. Oxford/New York: Pergamon Press; 1967.
2. Chang H, Krebs PFDE. Dynamic balance control in elders: GI as a screening tool. Arch Phys Med Rehabil. 1999;80(May):490–4.
3. Bouisset S, Do MC. Posture, dynamic stability, and voluntary movement. Neurophysiol Clin. 2008;38:345–62. https://doi.org/10.1016/j.neucli.2008.10.001.
4. Fiolkowski P, Brunt D, Bishop M, Woo R. Does postural instability affect the initiation of human gait? Neurosci Lett. 2002;323:167–70. https://doi.org/10.1016/S0304-3940(02)00158-1.
5. Winter DA. Human balance and posture standing and walking control during, vol. 3; 1995. p. 193.
6. Brunt D, Santos V, Kim HD, Light K, Levy C. Initiation of movement from quiet stance: comparison of gait and stepping in elderly subjects of different levels of functional ability. Gait Posture. 2005;21:297–302. https://doi.org/10.1016/j.gaitpost.2004.03.003.
7. Jian Y, Winter DA, Gilchrist L. Trajectory of the body COG and COP during initiation and termination of gait. Gait Posture. 1993;1(9):9–22.
8. Brunt D, Lafferty MJ, McKeon AB, Goode B, Mulhausen C, Polk P. Invariant characteristics of gait initiation. American Journal of Physical Medicine and Rehabilitation. 1991;70(4):206–212. https://doi.org/10.1097/00002060-199108000-00009.
9. Hass CJ, Buckley TA, Pitsikoulis C, Barthelemy EJ. Progressive resistance training improves GI in individuals with Parkinson' s disease. Gait Posture. 2012;35(4):669–73. https://doi.org/10.1016/j.gaitpost.2011.12.022.
10. Gormley J, Barr D, Bell A, Ravey J, Mollan R. Examination of the duration of GI by use of an electrogoniometer. Gait Posture. 1993;1:85–91. https://doi.org/10.1016/0966-6362(93)90019-W.
11. Crenna BYP, Frigo C. Paolo carlo. J Physiol. 1991;437:635–53.
12. Breniere Y, Do MC. When and how does steady state gait movement induced from upright posture begin? J Biomech. 1986;19(12):1035–40. https://doi.org/10.1016/0021-9290(86)90120-X.
13. Winter DA, Patla AE, Ishac M, Gage WH. Motor mechanisms of balance during quiet standing. J Electromyogr Kinesiol. 2003;13:49–56. https://doi.org/10.1016/S1050-6411(02)00085-8.
14. Hass CJ, Waddell DE, Wolf SL, Juncos JL, Gregor RJ. GI in older adults with postural instability. Clin Biomech. 2008;23:743–53. https://doi.org/10.1016/j.clinbiomech.2008.02.012.
15. Hass CJ, Gregor RJ, Waddell DE, Oliver A, Smith DW, Fleming RP, Wolf SL. The influence of Tai Chi training on the center of pressure trajectory during GI in older adults. Arch Phys Med Rehabil. 2004;85:1593–8. https://doi.org/10.1016/j.apmr.2004.01.020.
16. Halliday SE, Winter DA, Frank JS, Patla AE, Ontario NLG. The initiation of gait in young, elderly, and Parkinson' s disease subjects. Gait Posture. 1998;8:8–14.
17. Martin M, Shinberg M, Kuchibhatla M, Ray L, Carollo JJ, Schenkman ML. GI in community-dwelling adults with Parkinson disease. Phys Ther. 2002;82(6):1264; author reply 1264–5.
18. Uemura K, Yamada M, Nagai K, Tateuchi H, Mori S, Tanaka B, Ichihashi N. Effects of dual-task switch exercise on gait and GI performance in older adults: preliminary results of a randomized controlled trial. Arch Gerontol Geriatr. 2012;54(2):e167–71. https://doi.org/10.1016/j.archger.2012.01.002.
19. Najafi B, Miller D, Jarrett BD, Wrobel JS. Does footwear type impact the number of steps required to reach gait steady state?: An innovative look at the impact of foot orthoses on GI. Gait Posture. 2010;32(1):29–33. https://doi.org/10.1016/j.gaitpost.2010.02.016.
20. Lin SI, Yang WC. Effect of plantar desensitization on postural adjustments prior to step initiation. Gait Posture. 2011;34(4):451–6. https://doi.org/10.1016/j.gaitpost.2011.06.016.
21. Vieira MF, Sacco Ide C, Nora FG, Rosenbaum D, Lobo da Costa PH. Footwear and foam surface alter GI of typical subjects. PLoS ONE. 2015;10(8):e0135821. https://doi.org/10.1371/journal.pone.0135821.

22. Henriksson M, Hirschfeld H. Physically active older adults display alterations in GI. Gait Posture. 2005;21:289–96. https://doi.org/10.1016/j.gaitpost.2004.03.001.
23. Von Hofsten C. An action perspective on motor development. Trends Cogn Sci. 2004;8(6):266–72. https://doi.org/10.1016/j.tics.2004.04.002.
24. Malouin F, Richards CL. Preparatory adjustments during GI in 4–6-year-old children. Gait Posture. 2000;11:239–53.
25. Vieira MF, Brito Junior AA, Lehnen GC, Rodrigues FB. Center of pressure and center of mass behavior during gait initiation on inclined surfaces: a statistical parametric mapping analysis. J Biomech. 2017;3(56):10–8. https://doi.org/10.1016/j.jbiomech.2017.02.018.
26. Chastan N, Do MC, Bonneville F, Torny F, Bloch F, Westby GWM, Dormont D, Agid Y, Welter ML. Gait and balance disorders in Parkinson's disease: impaired active braking of the fall of centre of gravity. Mov Disord. 2009;24:188–95. https://doi.org/10.1002/mds.22269.
27. Chastan, N., Westby, G. W. M., Montcel, S. T. Du, Do, M. C., Chong, R. K., Agid, Y., & Welter, M. L. (2010). Influence of sensory inputs and motor demands on the control of the centre of mass velocity during GI in humans. Neurosci Lett, 469, 400–404. doi:https://doi.org/10.1016/j.neulet.2009.12.038.
28. Delafontaine A, Honeine JL, Do MC, Gagey O, Chong RK. Comparative gait initiation kinematics between simulated unilateral and bilateral ankle hypomobility: does bilateral constraint improve speed performance? Neurosci Lett. 2015;603:55–9.
29. Vialleron T, Delafontaine A, Millerioux I, Memari S, Fourcade P, Yiou E. Acute effects of short-term stretching of the triceps surae on ankle mobility and gait initiation in patients with Parkinson's disease. Clin Biomech. 2021;89:105449. https://doi.org/10.1016/j.clinbiomech.2021.105449.
30. Hof AL, Gazendam MGJ, Sinke WE. The condition for dynamic stability. J Biomech. 2005;38(1):1–8. https://doi.org/10.1016/j.jbiomech.2004.03.025.
31. Polcyn AF, Lipsitz LA, Kerrigan DC, Collins JJ. Age-related changes in the initiation of gait: degradation of central mechanisms for momentum generation. Arch Phys Med Rehabil. 1998;79(December):1582–9. https://doi.org/10.1016/S0003-9993(98)90425-7.
32. Muir BC, Rietdyk S, Haddad JM. GI: the first four steps in adults aged 20–25 years, 65–79 years, and 80–91 years. Gait Posture. 2014;39(1):490–4. https://doi.org/10.1016/j.gaitpost.2013.08.037.
33. Michel V, Do MC. Are stance ankle plantar flexor muscles necessary to generate propulsive force during human GI? Neurosci Lett. 2002;325:139–43. https://doi.org/10.1016/S0304-3940(02)00255-0.
34. Mbourou GA, Lajoie Y, Teasdale N. Step length variability at GI in elderly fallers and non-fallers, and young adults. Gerontology. 2003;49:21–6. https://doi.org/10.1159/000066506.
35. Lindemann U, Najafi B, Zijlstra W, Hauer K, Muche R, Becker C, Aminian K. Distance to achieve steady state walking speed in frail elderly persons. Gait Posture. 2008;27(1):91–6. https://doi.org/10.1016/j.gaitpost.2007.02.005.
36. Satoh Y, Yamada T, Shimamura R, Ohmi T. Comparison of foot kinetics and kinematics during gait initiation between young and elderly participants. J Phys Ther Sci. 2019;31:498–503.
37. Martin K, Blizzard L, Garry M, Thomson R, Mcginley J, Srikanth V. GI in older people—time to first lateral movement may be the measure of choice. Gait Posture. 2011;34(3):374–8. https://doi.org/10.1016/j.gaitpost.2011.06.004.
38. Caderby T, Dalleau G, Leroyer P, Bonazzi B, Chane-Teng D, Do MC. Does an additional load modify the anticipatory postural adjustments in GI? Gait Posture. 2013;37:144–6. https://doi.org/10.1016/j.gaitpost.2012.06.012.
39. Corbeil P, Anaka E. Combined effects of speed and directional change on postural adjustments during GI. J Electromyogr Kinesiol. 2011;21:734–41. https://doi.org/10.1016/j.jelekin.2011.05.005.
40. Gélat T, Coudrat L, Le Pellec A. GI is affected during emotional conflict. Neurosci Lett. 2011;497:64–7. https://doi.org/10.1016/j.neulet.2011.04.030.

41. Tseng SC, Stanhope SJ, Morton SM. Visuomotor adaptation of voluntary step initiation in older adults. Gait Posture. 2010;31:180–4. https://doi.org/10.1016/j.gaitpost.2009.10.001.
42. Uemura K, Yamada M, Nagai K, Tanaka B, Mori S, Ichihashi N. Fear of falling is associated with prolonged anticipatory postural adjustment during GI under dual-task conditions in older adults. Gait Posture. 2012;35(2):282–6. https://doi.org/10.1016/j.gaitpost.2011.09.100.
43. Dibble LE, Nicholson DE, Shultz B, Mac Williams BA, Marcus RL, Moncur C. Sensory cueing effects on maximal speed GI in persons with Parkinson's disease and healthy elders. Gait Posture. 2004;19:215–25. https://doi.org/10.1016/S0966-6362(03)00065-1.
44. Martin M, Shinberg M, Kuchibhatla M, Ray L, Carollo JJ, Schenkman ML. GI in community-dwelling adults with Parkinson disease: comparison with older and younger adults without the disease. Phys Ther. 2002;82:566–77.
45. Tokuno CD, Eng JJ. GI is dependent on the function of the paretic trailing limb in individuals with stroke. Gait Posture. 2006;24:424–8. https://doi.org/10.1016/j.gaitpost.2005.09.012.
46. Tokuno CD, Sanderson DJ, Inglis JT, Chua R. Postural and movement adaptations by individuals with a unilateral below-knee amputation during GI. Gait Posture. 2003;18:158–69. https://doi.org/10.1016/S0966-6362(03)00004-3.
47. Colné P, Frelut ML, Pérès G, Thoumie P. Postural control in obese adolescents assessed by limits of stability and GI. Gait Posture. 2008;28:164–9. https://doi.org/10.1016/j.gaitpost.2007.11.006.
48. Do Nascimento OF, Nielsen KD, Voigt M. Influence of directional orientations during GI and stepping on movement-related cortical potentials. Behav Brain Res. 2005;161:141–54. https://doi.org/10.1016/j.bbr.2005.02.031.
49. Jian Y, Winter D, Ishac M, Gilchrist L. Trajectory of the body COG and COP during initiation and termination of gait. Gait Posture. 1993;1:9–22. https://doi.org/10.1016/0966-6362(93)90038-3.
50. Mouchnino L, Robert G, Ruget H, Blouin J, Simoneau M. Online control of anticipated postural adjustments in step initiation: evidence from behavioral and computational approaches. Gait Posture. 2012;35(4):616–20. https://doi.org/10.1016/j.gaitpost.2011.12.009.
51. Patchay S, Gahéry Y. Effect of asymmetrical limb loading on early postural adjustments associated with GI in young healthy adults. Gait Posture. 2003;18:85–94. https://doi.org/10.1016/S0966-6362(02)00167-4.
52. Ruget H, Blouin J, Teasdale N, Mouchnino L. Can prepared anticipatory postural adjustments be updated by proprioception? Neuroscience. 2008;155:640–8. https://doi.org/10.1016/j.neuroscience.2008.06.021.
53. Vinti M, Couillandre A, Thoumie P. Does somatosensory loss induce adaptation of the GI process? Neurosci Lett. 2010;480(3):178–81. https://doi.org/10.1016/j.neulet.2010.06.017.
54. Welter ML, Do MC, Chastan N, Torny F, Bloch F, Tézenas du Montcel S, Agid Y. Control of vertical components of gait during initiation of walking in normal adults and patients with progressive supranuclear palsy. Gait Posture. 2007;26:393–9. https://doi.org/10.1016/j.gaitpost.2006.10.005.
55. Wicart P, Maton B. Body equilibrium at the end of GI: importance of ankle muscular force as evidenced in clubfoot children. Neurosci Lett. 2003;351:67–70. https://doi.org/10.1016/S0304-3940(03)00619-0.
56. Wicart P, Richardson J, Maton B. Adaptation of GI in children with unilateral idiopathic clubfoot following conservative treatment. J Electromyogr Kinesiol. 2006;16:650–60. https://doi.org/10.1016/j.jelekin.2005.11.005.
57. Yiou E, Do MC. Control of mediolateral stability during rapid step initiation with preferred and non-preferred leg: is it symmetrical? Gait Posture. 2010;32(1):145–7. https://doi.org/10.1016/j.gaitpost.2010.03.018.
58. Delval A, Bleuse S, Simonin C, Delliaux M, Rolland B, Destee A, et al. Are GI parameters early markers of Huntington's disease in pre-manifest mutation carriers? Gait Posture. 2011;34:202–7. https://doi.org/10.1016/j.gaitpost.2011.04.011.

59. Yiou E, Do MC. Effects of medio-lateral postural perturbation induced by voluntary arm raising on the biomechanical organization of rapid step initiation. Mot Control. 2011;15:507–24. https://doi.org/10.1123/mcj.15.4.507.
60. Ledebt A, Bril B, Brenière Y. The build-up of anticipatory behaviour. An analysis of the development of GI in children. Exp Brain Res. 1998;120:9–17. https://doi.org/10.1007/s002210050372.
61. Bruyneel A-V, Chavet P, Bollini G, Mesure S. GI reflects the adaptive biomechanical strategies of adolescents with idiopathic scoliosis. Ann Phys Rehabil Med. 2010;53:372–86. https://doi.org/10.1016/j.rehab.2010.06.005.
62. Henriksson M, Henriksson J, Bergenius J. GI characteristics in elderly patients with unilateral vestibular impairment. Gait Posture. 2011;33(4):661–7. https://doi.org/10.1016/j.gaitpost.2011.02.018.
63. Jones SF, Twigg PC, Scally AJ, Buckley JG. The GI process in unilateral lower-limb amputees when stepping up and stepping down to a new level. Clin Biomech. 2005;20:405–13. https://doi.org/10.1016/j.clinbiomech.2004.11.018.
64. Muniz AMS, Nadal J, Lyons KE, Pahwa R, Liu W. Long-term evaluation of GI in six Parkinson's disease patients with bilateral subthalamic stimulation. Gait Posture. 2012;35(3):452–7. https://doi.org/10.1016/j.gaitpost.2011.11.006.
65. Spencer LM, Van der Meer ALH. Tau G-guidance of dynamic balance control during GI across adulthood. Gait Posture. 2012;36(3):523–6. https://doi.org/10.1016/j.gaitpost.2012.05.017.
66. Stackhouse C, Shewokis PA, Pierce SR, Smith B, McCarthy J, Tucker C. GI in children with cerebral palsy. Gait Posture. 2007;26:301–8. https://doi.org/10.1016/j.gaitpost.2006.09.076.
67. Vrieling AH, van Keeken HG, Schoppen T, Otten E, Halbertsma JPK, Hof AL, Postema K. Gait termination in lower limb amputees. Gait Posture. 2008;27:82–90. https://doi.org/10.1016/j.gaitpost.2007.02.004.
68. Winter, D. (2009). Biomechanics and motor control of human movement. Books.google.com
69. Yu B, Gabriel D, Noble L, An K-N. Estimate of the optimum cutoff frequency for the Butterworth low pass digital filter. J Appl Biomech. 1999;15:318.
70. van Keeken HG, Vrieling AH, Hof AL, Postema K, Otten B. Stabilizing moments of force on a prosthetic knee during stance in the first steps after GI. Med Eng Phys. 2012;34:733–9. https://doi.org/10.1016/j.medengphy.2011.09.017.
71. Chau T. A review of analytical techniques for gait data. Part 1: fuzzy, statistical and fractal methods. Gait Posture. 2001; https://doi.org/10.1016/S0966-6362(00)00094-1.
72. Muniz AMS, Nadal J. Application of principal component analysis in vertical ground reaction force to discriminate normal and abnormal gait. Gait Posture. 2009;29:31–5. https://doi.org/10.1016/j.gaitpost.2008.05.015.
73. Schutte LM, Narayanan U, Stout JL, Selber P, Gage JR, Schwartz MH. An index for quantifying deviations from normal gait. Gait Posture. 2000;11:25–31. https://doi.org/10.1016/S0966-6362(99)00047-8.
74. Pataky TC, Robinson MA, Vanrenterghem J, Savage R, Bates KT, Crompton RH. Vector field statistics for objective center-of-pressure trajectory analysis during gait, with evidence of scalar sensitivity to small coordinate system rotations. Gait Posture. 2014;40(i):255–8. https://doi.org/10.1016/j.gaitpost.2014.01.023.
75. Pataky TC, Robinson MA, Vanrenterghem J. Vector field statistical analysis of kinematic and force trajectories. J Biomech. 2013;46(14):2394–401. https://doi.org/10.1016/j.jbiomech.2013.07.031.
76. Dessery Y, Barbier F, Gillet C, Corbeil P. Does lower limb preference influence GI? Gait Posture. 2011;33(4):550–5. https://doi.org/10.1016/j.gaitpost.2011.01.008.
77. Ito T, Azuma T, Yamashita N. Anticipatory control in the initiation of a single step under biomechanical constraints in humans. Neurosci Lett. 2003;352:207–10. https://doi.org/10.1016/j.neulet.2003.09.002.
78. Roemmich RT, Nocera JR, Vallabhajosula S, Amano S, Naugle KM, Stegemöller EL, Hass CJ. Spatiotemporal variability during GI in Parkinson's disease. Gait Posture. 2012;36:340–3. https://doi.org/10.1016/j.gaitpost.2012.01.018.

79. Halliday SE, Winter DA, Frank JS, Patla AE, Prince F. The initiation of gait in young, elderly, and Parkinson's disease subjects. Gait Posture. 1998;8:8–14. https://doi.org/10.1016/S0966-6362(98)00020-4.
80. Okada Y, Fukumoto T, Takatori K, Nagino K, Hiraoka K. Abnormalities of the first three steps of GI in patients with Parkinson's disease with freezing of gait. Parkinsons Dis. 2011;2011:1. https://doi.org/10.4061/2011/202937.
81. Vrieling AH, van Keeken HG, Schoppen T, Otten E, Halbertsma JPK, Hof AL, Postema K. GI in lower limb amputees. Gait Posture. 2008;27:423–30. https://doi.org/10.1016/j.gaitpost.2007.05.013.
82. Hirschfeld H. Motor control of every day motor tasks: guidance for neurological rehabilitation. Physiol Behav. 2007;92:161–6. https://doi.org/10.1016/j.physbeh.2007.05.018.
83. Laudani L, Casabona A, Perciavalle V, Macaluso A. Control of head stability during GI in young and older women. J Electromyogr Kinesiol. 2006;16:603–10. https://doi.org/10.1016/j.jelekin.2006.08.001.
84. Liu W, McIntire K, Kim SH, Zhang J, Dascalos S, Lyons KE, Pahwa R. Bilateral subthalamic stimulation improves GI in patients with Parkinson's disease. Gait Posture. 2006;23:492–8. https://doi.org/10.1016/j.gaitpost.2005.06.012.
85. Couillandre A, Brenière Y, Maton B. Is human GI program affected by a reduction of the postural basis? Neurosci Lett. 2000;285:150–4. https://doi.org/10.1016/S0304-3940(00)01015-6.
86. Sasaki O, Asawa S, Katsuno S, Usami SI, Taguchi K. Gait initiation in bilateral vestibular loss. Auris Nasus Larynx. 2001;28:295–9. https://doi.org/10.1016/S0385-8146(01)00094-3.
87. Hreljac A. Stride smoothness evaluation of runners and other athletes. Gait Posture. 2000;11(3):199–206.
88. Platz T, Denzler P, Kaden B, Mauritz KH. Motor learning after recovery from hemiparesis. Neuropsychologia. 1994;32(10):1209–23.
89. Rohrer B, Fasoli S, Krebs HI, Hughes R, Volpe B, Frontera WR, et al. Movement smoothness changes during stroke recovery. J Neurosci. 2002;22(18):8297–304.
90. Miff SC, Hansen AH, Childress DS, Gard SA, Meier MR. Roll-over shapes of the able-bodied knee-ankle-foot system during GI, steady-state walking, and gait termination. Gait Posture. 2008;27:316–22. https://doi.org/10.1016/j.gaitpost.2007.04.011.
91. Viton JM, Timsit M, Mesure S, Massion J, Franceschi JP, Delarque A. Asymmetry of GI in patients with unilateral knee arthritis. Arch Phys Med Rehabil. 2000;81(2):194–200.
92. Melzer I, Kurz I, Shahar D, Levi M, Oddsson L. Application of the voluntary step execution test to identify elderly fallers. Age Ageing. 2007;36(June):532–7. https://doi.org/10.1093/ageing/afm068.
93. Melzer I, Shtilman I, Rosenblatt N, Oddsson LIE. Reliability of voluntary step execution behavior under single and dual task conditions. J Neuroeng Rehabil. 2007;4:16. https://doi.org/10.1186/1743-0003-4-16.
94. Maki BE, McIlroy WE. The role of limb movements in maintaining upright stance: the "change-in-support" strategy. Phys Ther. 1997;77(5):488–507.
95. Buckley TA; Pitsikoulis C; Hass CJ. Dynamic postural stability during sit-to-walk transitions in Parkinson disease patients. Movement Disorders. 2008;23(9):1274–80. https://doi.org/10.1002/mds.22079.
96. Seuthe J, D'Cruz N, Ginis P, Blöbaum R, Weisser B, Deuschl G, Nieuwboer A, Schlenstedt C. How many gait initiation trials are necessary to reliably detect anticipatory postural adjustments and first step characteristics in healthy elderly and people with Parkinson's disease? Gait Posture. 2021;88:126–31. https://doi.org/10.1016/j.gaitpost.2021.05.016.

An Overview of the Effects of Experimentally Induced Fatigability on Walking in Aging and Parkinson's Disease

11

Paulo Cezar Rocha dos Santos, Diego Orcioli-Silva, Nicolas Vuillerme, and Fabio Augusto Barbieri

Abstract

One of the most important characteristics of human motor control is the ability to adapt to internal perturbations and cope with environmental situations, task constraints, and internal perturbation. Natural aging and age-related diseases, in particular, Parkinson's disease (PD), may restrict the capacity to cope with perturbation during the performance of motor tasks, such as walking. One way of experimentally examining the ability to adapt walking to internal perturbation is by limiting the availability of internal resources through induced fatigability. Specifically, experimentally induced fatigue state by physical/muscle exercise (muscle fatigability) may reduce the neural and peripheral capacity of controlling and

P. C. R. dos Santos (✉)
IDOR/Pionner Science Initiative, Rio de Janeiro, Rio de Janeiro, Brazil

Center of Advanced Technologies in Rehabilitation, Sheba Medical Center, Ramat Gan, Israel
e-mail: paulo-cezar.rocha-dossantos@weizmann.ac.il

D. Orcioli-Silva
Posture and Gait Studies Laboratory (LEPLO), Institute of Bioscience, São Paulo State University (UNESP), Rio Claro, SP, Brazil

N. Vuillerme
Université Grenoble-Alpes, AGEIS, Grenoble, France

Institut Universitaire de France, Paris, France

LabCom Telecom4Health, Orange Labs & Univ. Grenoble Alpes, CNRS, Inria, Grenoble INP-UGA, Grenoble, France

F. A. Barbieri
Human Movement Research Laboratory (MOVI-LAB), Department of Physical Education, School of Sciences, São Paulo State University (UNESP), Bauru, São Paulo, Brazil
e-mail: fabio.barbieri@unesp.br

F. A. Barbieri et al. (eds.), *Locomotion and Posture in Older Adults*,
https://doi.org/10.1007/978-3-031-74123-4_11

coordinating muscles, while mental exercise-induced fatigue state (mental fatigability) may interfere with the availability of cognitive resources involved in cognitive functions that can consequently interfere with walking performance. In this chapter, we present up-to-date research regarding age- and PD-related walking adaptation to muscle and mental fatigability. We focus on combining such effects from a perspective of fatigability task-specificity as well as different walking conditions. We discuss potential mechanisms of fatigability as an internal perturbation interfering with walking in an age- and PD-specific way and we propose a hypothetical model of those interference and associated factors (e.g., physical activity level). Finally, we discuss potential niches and needs for future studies.

Introduction

One of the most important characteristics of human motor control is the ability to adapt to individual perturbations and cope with environmental situations and task constraints [1–3]. This ability, termed herein as adaptability, may ensure the success of a task as it may indicate the capacity to deal with internal (i.e., a biological reduction in the availability or in the capacity to allocate resources, such as a condition induced by fatigability [4–6]) and external perturbation (e.g., slip, trip, or unexpected induced unbalance situation [2, 7]). Adaptability in motor control is required in several daily tasks, mainly during complex ones, such as job tasks and walking.

Natural aging and related movement disorders (such as Parkinson's disease—PD) reflect a visible decline in walking performance [8–11]. Such declines reflect in 10–20% reductions in gait speed and stride/step length and up to 50% increases in variability and gait instability in older vs. younger individuals [10, 12]. In PD, walking performance is even more impaired. Meta-analyzed data indicated that PD vs. healthy-matched individuals (mainly older people) walked slower, with shorter steps, longer portion of double support, and reduced swing time (moderate to strong effect sizes—0.5–1.0) [9]. Alterations in walking performance in both older and PD populations are associated and/or accompanied by changes in neuromuscular control (e.g., increased antagonistic coactivation [12–14]), decline in muscle functions (e.g., strength [15, 16]), and in cognitive functions (e.g., attention, executive function [17]). Because of the aging and PD typical reductions in neuromuscular, sensorimotor, and cognitive functions, the capacity of those individuals to adapt walking to cope with internal and external perturbations is rather limited.

Experimental designs usually focus on inducing a form of perturbation for examining the limits of gait adaptability in aging and PD. This type of protocol allows researchers to either assess proactive, reactive control to external perturbation [2, 18–20] or analyze the ability to reorganize motor control to cope with limited internal resources, as the state of experimentally induced fatigability [4, 5, 21]. Examining experimentally induced fatigability effects on walking may be relevant as it represents an eminent risk of accidents [21, 22]. Such relevance increases in populations that are more likely to experience fatigue, such as older and people with PD. A clear example is the increased number of trips when adults need to negotiate with obstacles while walking under muscle fatigability accompanied by decreased gait stability [22]. Mental fatigability also leads to an enhanced risk of accidents following a diminished performance in work environments [23–25] or it can even change the physiological state, impairing walking performance in older individuals [26]. Therefore, understanding how fatigability, a form of internal perturbation, affects walking may elucidate and inform the current state-of-the-art and point out future directions for studies in different populations and niches for being explored.

In view of the above, this chapter, thus, aims to integrate the information on the effects of fatigability (mental and physical) on walking in adults across the lifespan and in PD. We aim to extend and update the information from the chapter published in the previous edition [27] by including recent literature, adding information from the literature, and adding evidence related to mental fatigue. The structure of this chapter follows: (i) sections related to the definition of fatigue and fatigability, considering clarifying terms and the use of fatigue as a perturbation model; (ii) explain the physiological mechanism related to experimentally induced muscle and mental fatigability; (iii) present specifically how both mental and muscle fatigability may interfere with gait in aging and neurological population; (iv) discuss about the findings from an integrative perspective front to the literature and raise potential practical applications.

Fatigue and Fatigability as a Perturbation Model

The term fatigue has a diverse set of definitions according to the scope in which fatigue is employed. For example, fatigue may denote a reduction in physical or cognitive performance as an effect of prolonged physical/cognitive tasks but also may represent a feeling of tiredness and reduced energy in old and disease populations [28–30]. Targeting to discern fatigue as symptoms or as a state, Enoka and Duchateau [29] and Kluger et al. [30] discussed a potential taxonomy to accommodate fatigue definitions. Thus, fatigue may be differentiated in a trait (i.e., the amount of fatigue sensations experienced during a period of time—days, weeks, or months) or state (i.e., transient change in specific outcomes and/or increased feelings of exertion due to an exhaustive effort). Differentiating between fatigue as a state and trait is strictly relevant, as it may represent different conditions explained by different mechanisms. For instance, while traits of fatigue may persist for weeks/months, normally due to some neurological condition, the state of fatigue is probably temporary due to over-effort. For example, trait of fatigue may represent a chronic condition of fatigue, defined as a persistent feeling of tiredness associated with diseases and/or treatments [31]. State of fatigue (our focus) may be a result of performance fatigability that represents an exercise-induced reduction in performance (e.g., decrease in force, and/or mental functions), and/or perceived fatigability that indicates an increase of the rate of perceived exertion [29].

Particularly relevant, experimental setups often induce performance fatigability (a fatigue state) to examine the limits of adaptability in motor tasks (e.g., gait) in different populations, such as older adults and people with PD [21, 22, 28, 32–34]. Experimental designs employing induced fatigability are relevant for examining walking adaptability in aging and disease populations because of the fatigability effects on the allocation of internal resources for use during a motor task. Thus, fatigability may be considered as an internal perturbation model [4, 5]. Performance fatigability may lead to a visible alteration in central and peripherical functions [29, 35, 36], although the level of alteration seems to be task-dependent. For instance, the underlying mechanism involved in highly demanding muscle effort differs from a sustained mental task, which may reflect different effects on performance. Prolonged muscle or physical tasks at a high percentage of the available maximal mechanical output can lead to muscle performance fatigability, while prolonged, demanding mental activities interfere with cognitive processes, leading to a state of mental performance fatigability [23, 37, 38].

Muscle Performance Fatigability

Sustaining a demanding muscle effort near maximal available capacity will lead to muscle performance fatigability [29, 38]. This condition will reflect a reduced capacity to produce maximal force, limiting the nervous system's ability to generate a sustained signal and impairing the physiological processes involved in muscle contraction [29, 38]. Because of the complex mechanism related to the development of muscle performance fatigability, this state is also described as an inability to maintain an exercise at a desired level [39]. However, in most cases, the definition is associated with the measured outcome, such as the reduction in the capacity to produce maximal voluntary contraction to characterize the state of muscle fatigability [40, 41]. This definition aligns (to a certain extent) with the one proposed at Ciba Foundation Symposium, held in 1980, in which muscle fatigability was described as "an inability of a physiological process to continue functioning at a particular level and/or the inability of the total organism to maintain predetermined exercise intensity."

It is particularly true that, during the process of developing fatigability during dynamic functional tasks, certain outcomes (e.g., force) cannot always be monitored online, so other complementary/secondary outcomes are attributed to define muscle performance fatigability. For example, some studies inducing fatigability via dynamic muscle contraction characterize muscle fatigability by the inability to sustain a certain movement velocity or frequency [42] and/or by measuring perceived exertion (e.g., increased Borg scale) [22]. Certainly, potential neural mechanisms underlying fatigability effects are task-specific and involve alteration at the peripherical and central levels in a particular manner (see topic 3). As we attempt to attend to most of the behavioral changes, herein, we consider muscle fatigability as a reduction in the capacity to produce maximal voluntary torque or to sustain a motor task at a desired level, accompanying an increase in the rate of perceived exertion.

Mental Performance Fatigability

Similar to muscle performance fatigability, definitions of mental performance fatigability vary according to the key target that the inducing protocols focus on. The overall concept overlaps to some extent with muscle performance fatigability, being a state of exhaustion or tiredness due to prolonged effort [23], but in this specific case, due to a mental effort. This overall concept also fits symptoms of stress and lack of sleep, which are not always the case in experimentally induced mental performance fatigability [43]. Thus, a clear and more specific definition of mental performance fatigability is timely.

Boksem and Tops [44] defined mental fatigability as "a condition characterized by a decrease in mental performance, motivation, and attentional control that results from prolonged periods of cognitive activity and/or inadequate rest or recovery." This definition considers important aspects by relating decreases in mental/cognitive performance (e.g., decrease in attention, executive function, cognitive processing time) with decreases in motivation and with increases in perceived fatigability (i.e., perceived fatigue measured via Visual Analog Scale) [44].

Evidence suggests that specific mental fatigability protocols reflect declines in cognitive functions [45]. For instance, if a mental fatigability protocol requires sustaining a demanding attentional task, the attentional control (i.e., the ability to focus the attention on a specific goal) and the ability to concentrate would be affected [46], while a protocol that requires sustained decision-making task may affect mainly executive functions [45]. Although specific types of mental fatigability protocol would mainly reflect specific declines in cognitive functions, it is unreasonable to ensure an isolated fatigability state in this cognitive domain. Instead, one would expect a more task-specific fatigability impairment in a specific cognitive function (e.g., attention), while lower general fatigability effect overall mental performance [45]. Additionally, because declines in cognitive functions affect the organization of motor inputs (affecting the top-down control of movement—see next topic) [46, 47] and are strictly related to motor performance, including gait [17], mental fatigue affecting cognitive functions may be a reasonable perturbation protocol to examine the limits of gait adaptation in human.

Physiology of Muscle and Mental Fatigability

Either muscle or mental exercise-induced fatigability involves a chain of (neuro) physiological mechanisms that affect the capacity to produce force and/or cognitive functions [29, 35, 38, 44, 48, 49]. In this topic, the approach discusses the potential underlying (neuro)mechanisms related to the impact of muscle and mental fatigability on motor performance.

Muscle Performance Fatigability

Muscle performance fatigability involves complex central and peripherical processes. Centrally, this type of fatigability limits the capacity of the nervous system to generate sustained signals to the muscles. Muscle performance fatigability may affect the organization of motor commands by the central nervous system that are sent via the spinal cord to muscles, affecting motor coordination [4, 29, 35]. Evidence also suggests that (neuro)physiological mechanisms may differ according to the type of task and be mediated by intrinsic motoneuron, spinal and supraspinal factors [35]. For example, Dideriksen and colleagues [50] showed that submaximal maximum voluntary contraction to the failure leads to a decrease in net synaptic input that was attributed to a net decrease in the level of afferent feedback and in the maximal excitation capacity provided by the central nervous system. In addition, Santos and colleagues [5], unlike the literature [51, 52], verified that a multi-joint submaximal dynamic task to failure generated a decrease in muscle activation amplitude instead of an increase, as observed during the last vs. initial repetitions of a repetitive sit-to-stand task. It was argued that characteristics of the task (higher velocity and physical demand) may be a result of a decrease in the number and change in the shape of muscle fiber action potentials and muscle fiber action potentials. On the other hand, some evidence indicates that, during induce-fatigability protocols, it is common to observe a compensatory neural mechanism to fatigability as indicated by either an increase in muscle amplitude [52], synergistic muscle coherence [33, 53] or changes in cortical activity (e.g., increased alpha-2 power at frontal central and parietal brain regions) as measured in postural tasks [54, 55] and increased frontal activity during submaximal voluntary contraction [56]. In summary, centrally, muscle performance fatigability interferes with the cortical organization of motor inputs that reflect in the neural control, organization, and coordination of muscle activation.

Peripherally, the development of muscle fatigability leads to a decrease in oxygen availability in muscles, reducing the nutrients, increasing the accumulation of metabolites into the intracellular milieu, and decreasing the contractile capacity [29, 35, 55, 56]. In terms of neural control, while at the central level, muscle fatigability may result in a failure to generate the output to activate the muscle voluntarily properly, at the peripheral level, it can lead to a chain of change at or distal to the neuromuscular junction [35]. For instance, muscle performance fatigability is associated with changes in membrane and the T-tubular action potential propagations, the coupling mechanism between action potential and calcium release, and calcium regulation at the level of the contractile elements [35, 57]. Thus, an observed functional impact of muscle fatigability in a motor outcome (e.g., force, gait) is mediated by a net of central and peripherical mechanisms.

Mental Performance Fatigability

Physiological aspects underlying mental performance fatigability also involve central and, to a lesser extent, peripheral mechanisms, probably due to the relationship between affected cognitive functions and motor control [58]. Specifically for central mechanisms, mental performance fatigability involves an alteration of cognitive state by inducing neurochemical and functional brain changes. Regarding neurochemical, mental performance fatigability effects on cognitive function may be due to a reduction in the level of acetylcholine and dopamine, affecting the projections of neural commands and functionality of the brain during cognitive processes [44, 59]. Functionally, sustaining demanding mental tasks alters cortical activation, generally causing decreases in activity areas linked to task performance (e.g., sustaining attentional-oriented tasks leads to changes in posterior brain areas [59]), motivation, and evaluation [60]. Cumulative electrophysiological brain data corroborates the idea that mental fatigability may cause a reduction of mental activity by increasing the power of oscillatory activity in the low-frequency band [44, 59]. Fatigability-induced brain changes also involve blood oxygen level-dependent signals, indicating a decrease in response inhibition-associated activity in the corpus callosum, somatosensory association cortex, and anterior cingulate cortex. These changes are linked to a decrease in mental performance [61].

Although the induced alteration in physiological features at central levels is linked to performance, the peripherical physiological mechanisms related to mental fatigability-induced changes in performance are not fully elucidated. For example, decreases in functional physical performance due to mental fatigability are probably more evident during tasks that require a certain level of cognitive involvement. This aligns with previously described findings indicating that mental fatigability did not alter the capacity to produce maximal torque [62] but did affect tasks that require cognitive functions in older adults [26]. In line with the abovementioned information, evidence supports a trend to increase the cortical silent period but not in peripheral neuromuscular function (contractile properties of the muscle, M-wave) under mental fatigability states [49]. This observation suggests that mental fatigability may cause more interference in performance in supraspinal than peripheral mechanisms. In fact, cumulative meta-analyzed evidence suggested that mental fatigability is associated with a visible reduction in the activity of right-lateralized frontal cortical and subcortical areas as well as increased activity in parietal–occipital, posterior cingulate, and primary motor areas [63]. In addition, the activity in frontal brain areas (termed the cognitive control network—CCN) is reduced with mental fatigability [63], which partially explains muscle fatigability affecting performance in tasks in which cognitive resources are required.

Fatigability in Aging

While evidence indicates that traits of fatigue (e.g., the prevalence of general fatigue) are more robust in older adults (up to 98% of older adults report fatigue) [64], in terms of state of fatigue, the age-related presence of fatigue seems to be task dependent. For instance, while inducing a muscle fatigability state via a protocol with sub/maximal local force contraction exercise normalized maximal force (e.g., knee extension), older people may be relatively more resistant to muscle performance fatigability than younger [57, 65]. However, when muscle performance fatigability is induced by functional dynamic contraction or physical protocols (e.g., walking, repetitive sit-to-stand), older are considerably more susceptible to muscle fatigability [5, 28, 41, 42, 66] (discussed below).

The "relatively higher" resistance to muscle fatigability during normalized contractions may be due to a higher percentage of type I fibers in older adults' muscles, showing higher reflex excitability than muscles containing high percentages of type II fibers [57, 67]. Additionally, because such resistance to muscle fatigability is measured relatively to (sub)maximal that is lower in older vs. younger, it may be that the resistance is higher just because the (sub)maximal is substantially lower in older. However, the total natural age-related degeneration of several systems, especially the musculoskeletal system, reflects a higher muscle fatigability state during a functional task. A clear example is the visible decline in repetitive sit-to-stand endurance capacity with aging, accompanied by an increase in self-reported fatigue [5, 29].

Because of the age-related declines in cognitive functions, it is plausible to assume that older adults are more likely to experience mental fatigability. Older vs. younger adults have limited capacity to allocate cognitive functions during a mental task, as indicated by the slowness of a reaction time task [68]. In contrast, there is also evidence indicating age-specific modulation in cortical activation to mental fatigability, so that older and younger adults modulated cortical activation differently (i.e., frontal cortex theta power became larger for older while occipital alpha in younger) by mental fatigability, in a way that differences in mental performance were neutralized [69]. Arnau et al. [69] also point to a possible discussion about the role of task characteristics in the involvement of certain brain areas/functions in mental fatigability. This observation is particularly relevant because age-related neural adaptation and, consequently, changes in performance might be task-dependent (as well as to muscle/physical fatigability). Thus, the appropriate selection of tasks that might be sensible to induce and assess the interference of mental fatigability is highly recommended in experimental setups. For example, if the aim is to target executive functions (i.e., a set of cognitive processes that are responsible for managing and controlling various mental activities, including goal-setting, sequential, planning, organizing, initiating tasks, inhibitory control and monitoring mental tasks), complexes inhibitory tasks may be more appropriate in contrast to simple reaction time task.

Parkinson's Disease and Fatigue

As the most common movement disorder [70], PD is characterized by the death of dopamine-producing cells that leads to a considerable decrease in dopamine levels in the basal ganglia [71, 72]. As this region is involved in the control of movements, PD manifests mainly in the presence of motor symptoms, such as bradykinesia (slowness of movement), tremor, rigidity, hypokinesia (decrease in voluntary movement or muscle activity), and postural instability [71, 72]. Additionally, as the disease progresses, people with PD commonly experience muscle weakness [73], require more energy to walk, and have elevated levels of fatigability [74]. This observation is reinforced by the lower resistance to muscle fatigability by sustaining a repetitive sit-to-stand task in people with PD (94.2 ± 30.4 s; ~47 ± 15 reps) vs.

healthy older adults (265.5 ± 132.8 s; ~133 ± 66 reps), with a similar level of decline in voluntary force (~7%) [32]. In total, the evidence suggests that people with PD, due to specific characteristics of the disease, are more susceptible to muscle performance fatigability.

Mental fatigability may also be constantly experienced by people with PD. Potential reasons involve typical declines that people with PD show in the capacity to sustain an attentionally demanding task due to cognitive function declines [75]. Probable impairments in brain networks involved in attention, such as the alerting, orienting, and executive networks, explain this reduced capacity in PD [76]. As PD affects not only dopaminergic but also noradrenergic, cholinergic, and serotonergic networks and the capacity to integrate somatosensorial information [72, 77], impairments in maintaining the alert state, as well as in the ability to select and integrate appropriate information are observed in people with PD [76]. Additionally, people with PD experience sleep disorders, depression, and anxiety that may also play a role in the impaired capacity to sustain a mental task [78]. This observation is supported by data indicating that individuals with PD, compared to matched control subjects, exhibited worse performance during mental tasks [79]. Thus, while there is no direct evidence of fatigability in mental performance in PD, the cascading decline in cognitive resources may impact the capacity to allocate cognitive resources to sustain demanding mental tasks [80] and reflect in overwhelmed fillings/trait of fatigue [81].

Problems that emerge from fatigability (muscle and mental) and trait of fatigue have overlapping causes. For instance, both mental fatigability and trait of fatigue may occur due to striatal and limbic serotonergic dysfunction [82] that, in turn, is associated with gait abnormalities [83]. However, although an association between mental fatigability (experimentally induced) and functionality in PD may occur, no study on this topic has been found in the literature. Thus, in the next sections, the focus will be on muscle fatigability and walking, and potential hypotheses on how and why mental fatigability would perturb motor control in PD will be further recommended.

Muscle Fatigability and Walking: Remarks and Considerations

Walking is a highly complex motor task that involves interlinked functions (cognitive, psychological, and physical) and high-level organized actions at cortical, subcortical, spinal, and peripherical levels [84]. Thus, any perturbation that interferes with functions may reflect in the control/performance of walking, requiring adaptations to induced perturbations, such as a result of fatigability. Santos [85] illustrated a hypothetical model (adapted version—Fig. 11.1) depicting muscle and mental fatigability effects on human gait. For instance, by interfering with peripheral (e.g., contractile properties) and central (e.g., neuromuscular propagation) characteristics involved in muscular activation [29], muscle fatigability may require adaptation to maintain gait without increasing the risk of accidents/falls. Age and, mainly, PD affect the capacity to adapt gait to a series of perturbations (abovementioned), and,

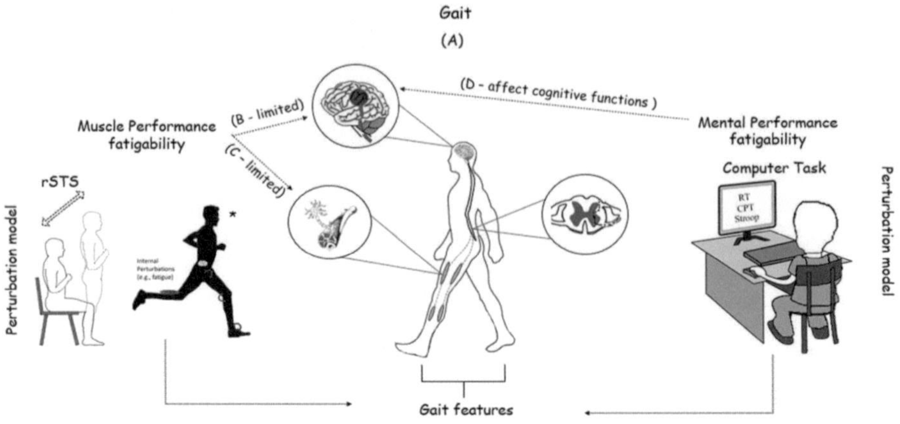

Fig. 11.1 Schematic representation of a hypothetical model of potential reasons for the interference of muscle fatigability on gait. (**a**) Gait is a dynamic and complex task in which the central nervous system sends coordinated commands via the spinal cord to activate muscles that generate gait (measured via, e.g., stride outcomes, dynamic gait features). Muscle performance fatigability perturbs the system by inducing changes at (**b**) the central (e.g., neuromuscular propagation) and (**c**) contraction level (e.g., declines in voluntary force). Mental performance fatigability can interfere with (**d**) cognitive functions (such as intrinsic motivation, executive function, and attention) that are associated with gait performance. (Adapted from Santos [85] and *Van Hooren et al. [86]. rSTS: repetitive sit-to-stand task)

thus, fatigability may be more impactful for gait performance and control in such populations. In this subsection, studies on how muscle fatigability affects gait during lifespan (younger, middle-aged, and healthy older individuals) and in PD will be detailed.

A series of studies have demonstrated that experimentally induced fatigability (mainly muscle performance) leads to adaptation in walking in different populations and walking conditions [22, 28, 32, 34, 87, 88]. The most reported results involve the effects of experimentally induced fatigability on spatial-temporal stride outcomes, including walking speed. Cumulative evidence suggests mixed results, tending to indicate an increase, instead of a decrease, in walking speed after muscle performance fatigability (Fig. 11.2). For a matter of proof here, we meta-analyzed the effects of muscle fatigability on walking speed (Fig. 11.2), considering studies included in previously published systematic reviews [22, 28, 87] and additional studies [32, 34, 88] in PD after a brief search in Pubmed (Terms: “fatigue” and “Parkinson’s” and “walking”). For the meta-analysis, we included population (younger, older, and PD) and walking conditions (overground, obstructed, and dual-task) as subgroup factors. Although not statistically significant (potential reasons below), the meta-analysis indicated a moderate effect size (0.47), suggesting an overall impact of muscle performance fatigability on increasing gait walking speed, regardless of subgroup analyses for populations (younger, older, and PD) and conditions. Despite the moderate effect size, this effect did not reach significance ($p > 0.05$), likely due to high heterogeneity (99.73%). Such high heterogeneity

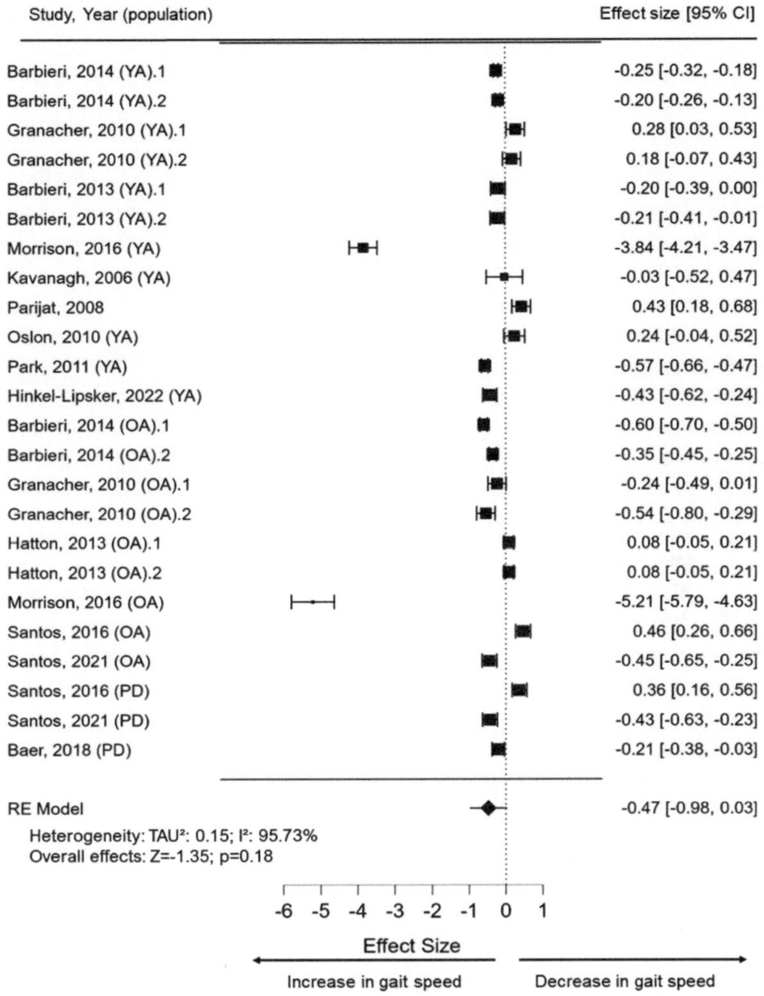

Fig. 11.2 Forest plot of a meta-analysis indicating effects of muscle fatigability on walking speed. The meta-analysis was performed through JASP (v.0.17.3, JASP team, the Netherlands [92]) for this chapter's purpose. We extracted data from studies that clearly reported muscle fatigability effects on gait speed included in three systematic reviews [21, 22, 28, 32, 34, 40, 66, 87, 88, 90, 93–98]. Three additional papers were selected after a search in PubMed by combining "fatigue" and "Parkinson's" and "walking (search performed in 24/08/2023) " Note that for some studies, the numbers in front of the population mean different walking for such conditions (Barbieri, 2014 (population) 1 and 2 = overground and obstructed walking; Barbieri, 2013 (population) 1 and 2 = approach and crossing phase of obstructed walking; Granacher, 2010 (population) 1 and 2 = normal and dual-task overground; Hatton, 2013 (population) 1 and 2, low and high obstacle high for obstructed walking conditions, respectively). For studies that compared different muscle fatigability protocols, those data were averaged. The population of Barbieri et al. [21] and Morrison et al. [66] were polled in age groups—younger (20–49 and 30–49 years old, respectively) and older (>60 years old). Effects sizes ≤0.2, around 0.5 and >0.8 were interpreted as small, moderate, and large effects [99]. Note that some studies from the systematic reviews did not include/or misreported gait speed and, thus, were not included

might be attributed to the diverse characteristics of the included papers (protocols to induce fatigability, walking assessments, experimental design, environment, etc.).

Although such an increase in walking speed might seem unreasonable from the perspective of walking energetics, from a neuromuscular and walking control perspective, fatigability effects may require a compensatory increase in motor units, strength in shared neural drive among synergistic muscle pair [33], and the need to increase the anterior base of the support to increase the stability of enhanced center of mass displacement [89, 90]. The increased anterior base of support was also commonly observed, regardless of the populations—younger, old, PD—in our previous systematic reviews and original studies by calculating step/stride length [21, 22, 28, 32, 87, 91]. The increase in stride length may be a need for counterweights for the increase in anteroposterior trunk acceleration due to muscle fatigability [42].

Muscle fatigability similarly affected stride outcomes of younger, older, and people with PD during level overground walking [22, 28, 87]. Collectively, the literature suggests that the increase in walking speed and stride length is also followed by an increase in gait variability and a decrease in temporal changes in stride outcomes during overground walking [22, 28, 87, 100]. For instance, the consistency of step rhythmicity seems to be affected, as reported by the increase in the trunk acceleration step-by-step variability in older [42] as well as younger individuals [101, 102]. Increasing walking variability due to muscle fatigability may be explained by a combination of different mechanisms, including altered muscle activation patterns and coordination, leading to irregularity in movements; decreased proprioception and reduced joint stability, reflecting in a deviation from the usual gait patterns; and induced compensatory mechanisms, leading to redistribution of joint works and increasing anteroposterior and mediolateral displacement of the center of mass, that leads to inconsistency in the stabilization of the center of mass [42, 91, 103–105].

Particularly from the perspective of compensation due to muscle fatigability, it seems to be the case not only for gait but also for force maintenance and postural control [53, 106]. Sustaining a (sub)maximal voluntary contraction and postural control of muscle fatigability involves a steady increase in muscle activation amplitude [52], accompanying an increase in the coupling in the frequency domain between synergistic muscle pairs [107]. Such increases are discussed as a compensatory augment in the recruitment of motor units to maintain muscle performance. However, this does not always seem to be the case. At a dynamic (relatively) fast task-to-failure, muscle fatigability induces a decrease instead of an increase in the muscle activation amplitude in both old and young populations [5]. Still, it represents a higher metabolic cost (torque or work/ATP per unit muscle) for older vs. younger individuals to perform dynamic movements [108]. This clearly explains the lower performance in dynamic contraction in PD vs. older vs. younger individuals (e.g., the average number of repetitive sit-to-stand movements: 47 vs. 468 vs. 126 reps [5, 21, 32]). Interestingly, overall gait adaptations to such type of fatigability protocol were not aging or PD specific, although slightly more pronounced in some cases for aging and disease, according to the literature [21, 34, 66, 90, 91, 109].

The type of fatigability protocol may lead to specific fatigability effects during walking. For instance, during approaching and crossing phases [91, 109], as well as for recovering walking after an external perturbation [110], ankle muscle fatigability suggests affected the capacity of ankle power generation and biomechanics features of gait. Such effects involving ankle muscle fatigability were even slightly superior to knee muscle fatigability [91, 109]. This observation may be reasonable considering that ankle plantar and dorsiflexors are the main contributors to the work produced to push-off and to body load during level and unlevel walking [111], and is associated with several age-related changes in biomechanical and energetics features of walking [112, 113].

From the perspective of fatigue-type specificity, protocols that target similar characteristics of gait (e.g., treadmill walking or running exercise to fatigability) vs. local muscle fatigue tend to induce more changes in spatial and rhythmic/temporal features of walking. The literature, for example, indicated a substantial increase in velocity (18%, Cohen d >3—strong effect size, Fig. 11.2) after specific gait fatigability protocols, even more evident changes than non-specific gait fatigability protocols (Fig. 11.2). Important to note that even when non-specific muscle fatigability protocol (i.e., repetitive sit-to-stand task) induced slight to moderate changes in spatial and temporal outcomes of gait, these changes remained even after 20 min of rest following the end of the muscle fatigability protocol. Perhaps this inconsistency may be related to the type of walking conditions, treadmill vs. overground walking.

Muscle fatigability, induced by repetitive sit-to-stand, reflected minimal changes in treadmill spatial and temporal walking metrics in young and older adults [62]. Presumably, walking adaptability to fatigability may have been minimized by the reactive and invariant pattern imposed by the treadmill. This idea is partially supported by evidence indicating that treadmill vs. overground constraint biomechanical characteristics of walking [115, 116]. Additionally, treadmill vs. overground walking reflects significantly lower ankle and knee muscle activations in the overall phases of the gait cycle [117]. This observation is particularly relevant mainly in fatigability protocol targeting specific muscles (above discussed). Thus, together with lower muscle activations and invariant biomechanics patterns, walking adaptability to fatigability may have limited effects over protocols assessing walking on the treadmill in young and old populations. It is, however, curious that individuals adapted the neuromuscular control (inferred by intermuscular coherence) in an age-specific way to keep walking on the invariant treadmill walking pattern [33].

While muscle fatigability effects are limited on a treadmill, during more challenging walking conditions (e.g., obstacle avoidance and dual-task walking), such effects are overt and indicate a higher risk of falls. For example, cumulative evidence indicates that muscle fatigability represents a risk of trips while individuals negotiate with obstacles during obstacle crossing walking task [22]. This risk may be higher for older vs. younger adults who had decreased minimum toe clearance during walking due to muscle fatigability [103]. Specifically for dual-task walking, this condition suggests inducing age-specific adjustments, meaning that while older individuals walked with longer and faster strides, younger individuals walked with shorter and slower strides [40]. On the one hand, such previously mentioned age-related differences in speed seem unreasonable since adaptabilities for muscle fatigability are usually observed by increases in length and speed regardless of aging [22, 28, 87]. On the other hand, it may indicate that muscle fatigability added to a challenged condition (i.e., dual-task) may require an extra "compensatory strategy" to increase the anterior center of mass stability to handle the trunk acceleration and variability in older adults [21, 42].

Interestingly, regular practices of physical activity seem to minimize the potential effects of muscle fatigability effects on gait adaptability in people with PD but not younger and older, and only for obstacle avoidance and not for level walking [32, 34, 90]. The results suggested that physically active people with PD, similarly to the control individuals, have less difficulty adapting their gait to negotiate with an obstacle than inactive people with PD. Because the physical activity level interfered with the effects of muscle fatigability on walking only during more complex conditions (e.g., obstacle avoidance vs. overground) in PD, one may argue that in more demanding walking conditions (such as obstacle avoidance) that require more motor control, regular practices of physical activity may help to minimize the system of being perturbed.

Surprisingly, although a wide range of studies elaborated hypotheses based on the muscular effects of sustaining a muscle-demanding task, few focused on examining muscle fatigability effects on neuromuscular control during walking. The few studies indicate consistent results suggesting an increase in relative spectral intensity in the low-frequency band, with enhanced muscle amplitude and muscle fatigability [118–120]. The interpretation is also compatible with the idea of a compensatory increase in motor unit synchronization as an attempt by the central nervous system to ensure control during a motor task [33, 51, 118, 122]. With regard to PD, no study was found in the literature that considered analyzing performance fatigability on muscle activation during walking. Thus, examining fatigability effects on neuromuscular control in PD is a very relevant niche since the disease explicitly affects the muscular tonus, making the participants more susceptible to muscle fatigue state. Such characteristics may hypothetically affect the neuromuscular control during gait in a PD-specific manner. Extending the topic approached here, overall studies involving muscle activation analysis during walking PD are limited to a few, restricting the knowledge on how the disease affects neuromuscular control during walking and the potential underlying mechanism of PD-related effects on walking performance [14].

Mental Fatigability and Walking: Remarks and Considerations

Knowledge of mental performance fatigability effects on gait is limited. To the best of our knowledge, only three studies [26, 62, 100] experimentally induced mental performance fatigability to assess its effects on gait (Table 11.1). These studies focused on the hypothesis that by interfering with cognitive function, mental performance fatigability would perturb the motor system and affect gait. This idea is depicted in Fig. 11.1, where we illustrated that mental performance fatigability potentially interferes with cognitive functions. Because cognitive functions are

Table 11.1 Characteristics of the studies that aimed to verify the effects of mental fatigability on walking

Article	Aim	Sample	Fatigue protocol/ experimental condition	Walking assessment/ condition	Main results
Beherence et al. (2018)	The study aimed to assess single- and dual-task walking performance in young and old participants before and after a randomly assigned mental fatigability and control intervention, respectively	YA: 16 OA: 16	Mental fatigability: Performing a demanding mental stop-signal task for 90 min Control intervention: watching a video for 90 min	Overground—participants walked (6-m walkway) at self-selected gait speed, starting and stopping each trial 2 m before and after the walkway at single- and dual-task walking conditions	Coefficient of variation of the variables increased for OA only for dual-task walking for: Gait speed—Cohen d: 0.66 Length—Cohen d: 0.67 Stance time—Cohen d: 0.59 Swing time—Cohen d: 0.41
Santos et al. (2019)	The study aimed to determine the effects of age, repetitive sit-to-stand, and prolonged mental effort task on the spatial and temporal stride outcomes and gait dynamics during treadmill walking	YA: 12 OA: 12	Mental fatigability: Performing 30-min of demanding mental tasks	Treadmill walking—participants walked at fixed (1.2 m/s) and fast walking conditions (20–30% higher than the comfortable speed)	There was no effect of mental fatigability during treadmill walking
Piche et al. (2023)	The study aimed to evaluate the effect of mental and muscular fatigue on spatiotemporal parameters in dual-task walking in young, non- frail and frail older adults	YA: 20 OA non-frail: 20 OA frail: 19	Metal fatigability: Performing 20 min of Psychomotor vigilance task (PVT)	Overground—participants walked continuously without assistance for 1 min along a 10 m walkway at single- and dual-task	There was no effect of mental fatigability on spatial and temporal stride outcomes and dual-task cost during walking

widely linked with gait [17], mental performance may indirectly induce declines in walking (e.g., gait variability).

It is, however, curious that the current evidence suggests controversial results [26, 62, 100]. While Behrens et al. [26] indicated that older but not younger individuals walked with higher variability in spatiotemporal stride outcomes during dual- but not single-task after mental fatigability (Cohen d range: 0.41–0.67), Piche and colleagues did not reveal any interference of mental performance on dual-task cost during walking [100]. Consistently with the latter, Santos and colleagues did not indicate any effect of mental performance fatigability on treadmill walking [62]. The lack of consistency in the current differences may be attributed to the fatigue and walking assessment/conditions protocols. The mental performance fatigability (induced by 90 min of a demanding mental task) induced changes during dual-task walking, reflecting higher variability [26]. Potentially higher demanding mental tasks (as performed 4.5x more time) may indeed perturb cognitive functions (e.g., attention and arousal) in older adults, reflecting higher gait variability and accentuated risk of falls during walking [17]. Both protocols of the studies that did find effects of mental fatigability on spatiotemporal walking outcomes were relatively shorter (30 and 20 min, respectively) [62, 100] than the abovementioned one [26]. Therefore, it might be that the protocol to induce mental fatigability, although reflected in declines in specific cognitive functions and/or an increase in self-reported fatigue, did not perturb the system enough to induce walking adaptations, even in populations with limited capacity to allocate cognitive resources as older adults. Another potential explanation is that the relatively short mental fatigability protocol did not interfere substantially with the cognitive reserve, allowing the participants to allocate cognitive resources to compensate for mental fatigue effects during walking [121].

Walking conditions also suggest interfering with the potential effects of mental performance fatigability-inducing adaptations. For instance, dual-task cognitive walking requires the allocation of cognitive resources/functions in order for the participants to continue walking and interacting with the secondary task. Thus, considering that mental performance fatigability specifically decreases cognitive functions, dual-task cognitive walking might be an adequate protocol to examine the effects of mental fatigability on walking performance. This argument may explain why Behrens and colleagues did find age-specific mental fatigability effects on walking variability during dual- but not single-task [26]. Such effect only for older individuals is also reasonable considering the age-typical decrease in cognitive functions affecting walking performance [17]. Together, those arguments sign the fact that the appropriate setup to examine gait adaptability to mental fatigability should be composed by inducing fatigability by longer demanding mental task effects on dual-task walking. Hypothetically, such a combination of protocols may perturb even more the system of PD, considering PD-related impairments in cognitive functions and gait.

Limitation, Future Directions, and Final Remarks

In collective, the evidence described in this chapter suggests that induced fatigability protocols can lead to walking adaptations in a task-specific manner. In other words, employing demanding protocols for fatigability that target key elements of walking could serve as a valuable approach to studying gait adaptability in aging and disease.

For example, long-distance walking as muscle/physical fatigability may perturb the system more and induce more adaptations than local muscle fatigue [114]. Additionally, experimentally design protocols targeting the fatigability effects on walking should also focus first on understanding the physiological and/or mechanical aspects behind performing such demanding tasks. This would support advancing setups regarding the arguments of targeting key elements of gait. Still, there is an urgent need for future studies that should not solely focus on stride outcomes but prioritize understanding the neuromuscular mechanisms underlying fatigability effects on gait mechanics. This argument is further supported by the systematic reviews [22, 28, 87] that include just a few studies that focused on neural and muscular control of gait.

Although the use of treadmill has value for investigating age- and PD-related adaptation to perturbation to reduce walking variability and to acquire more gait steps, the effect of the treadmill may have lessened the influence of mental and muscle fatigability on gait. This is because the treadmill represents a more reactive type of walking by providing rhythm and pace information, reflecting in lesser variability than overground walking [115, 123], mitigating potential room for perturbation adaptation, such as mental and muscle fatigability. Therefore, exploring gait adaptability under experimentally induced fatigability conditions in more dynamic gait control scenarios, such as overground walking, as well as more complex conditions, such as obstacle crossing, dual-task walking, and stepping up and down a curb, suggests amplifying the potential impact of fatigability on gait. Given that age- and PD-related gait changes are particularly evident in these complex conditions [22, 124–126], they provide an enriched and more ecological context for studying the interplay between age and fatigability effects on gait.

In the context of mental performance fatigability, investigations exploring its effects on gait should focus on dual-task walking that includes cognitive functions analogous to those predominantly engaged in the mental fatigability protocol. For example, if fatiguing protocols are designed to target attention, the secondary task during dual-task walking should also heavily involve the same cognitive function (in this example, attention). It might be even more comprehensible if such protocols would be accompanied by brain measures/activity to depict the neural mechanisms of the potential interference of mental fatigability on gait adaptation in aging and disease populations. These nuances of the task design are likely pivotal in understanding the effects of mental fatigability on gait adaptability. Additionally, studies involving fatigability effects, mainly mental fatigability, on gait in individuals with PD would be a novel and relevant niche. Since PD affects cognitive functions [17], limits the capacity to allocate cognitive resources [80], and is associated with enhanced fatigability [34, 127], mental fatigability may be associated with walking impairments and represents a high risk of falls during walking in people with PD. Also, a notable research gap lies in the comparative exploration of gait adaptation in individuals with and without self-reported fatigue. These investigations would yield valuable insights into the clinical relevance of gait adaptations occurring in healthy older individuals and people with PD subsequent to the current knowledge in terms of induced mental and muscle fatigability. Additionally, a relevant niche for future studies in the field may be related to the identification of a minimal threshold for fatigability effects on gait.

Based on the insights gleaned from this chapter's findings, muscle fatigability induces walking adaptations across a spectrum of scenarios, including unobstructed, obstructed condition, perturbations, and dual-task, but less evident during habitual treadmill, spanning various age groups such as young adults, older adults, and people with PD. Employing regular physical exercise emerges as a viable strategy to mitigate the emergence of muscle fatigability-related conditions and their subsequent influence on complex walking tasks, mainly in PD. Less consistent evidence supports a potential effect of mental fatigability on walking in aging, while any study was designed in PD, raising a potential gap for future studies. Also, it is important to note that certain gaps persist, necessitating the pursuit of more comprehensive studies in this domain focusing on understanding the neural mechanism of muscle and mental fatigability during walking. Furthermore, it is conceivable that the effects of age and fatigability might manifest more prominently within real-life or intricate walking tasks, such as dual-task or perturbed walking. Consequently, a potentially more efficacious model for investigating gait and age-related adaptability to fatigability should encompass specific gait fatigue types.

Acknowledgment and Fundings Paulo Cezar Rocha dos Santos was supported by the Weizmann-IDOR Pioneer Science Fellowship Program. Diego Orcioli-Silva was supported by the Pró-Reitoria de Pesquisa (PROPe) of São Paulo State University (UNESP). Nicolas Vuillerme was supported by the French National Research Agency (ANR) in the framework of the Investissements d'avenir program (ANR-10-AIRT-05 and ANR-15-IDEX-02), the MIAI @ Grenoble Alpes (ANR-19-P3IA-0003). Fabio Augusto Barbieri was supported by National Council for Scientific and Technological Development—CNPq, and CAPES (Finance Code 001).

References

1. Newell KM, Van Emmerik REA, McDonald PV. Biomechanical constraints and action theory: reaction to G.J. van Ingen Schenau (1989). Hum Mov Sci. 1989;8(4):403–9.
2. McCrum C, Epro G, Meijer K, Zijlstra W, Brüggemann GP, Karamanidis K. Locomotor stability and adaptation during perturbed walking across the adult female lifespan. J Biomech. 2016;49(7):1244–7.
3. Greve C, Zijlstra W, Hortobágyi T, Bongers RM. Not all is lost: old adults retain flexibility in motor behaviour during sit-to-stand. Wenderoth N, editor. PLoS One [Internet]. 2013;8(10):e77760. [cited 2018 Nov 5]. Available from: https://dx.plos.org/10.1371/journal.pone.0077760.
4. Monjo F, Terrier R, Forestier N. Muscle fatigue as an investigative tool in motor control: a review with new insights on internal models and posture-movement coordination. Hum Mov Sci. 2015;44:225–33.
5. dos PCR S, CJC L, LTB G, Zijdewind I, Barbieri FA, Hortobágyi T. Older compared with younger adults performed 467 fewer Sit-to-Stand Trials, accompanied by small changes in muscle activation and voluntary force. Front Aging Neurosci [Internet]. 2021;13:679282. [cited 2021 Jun 22]. Available from: https://www.frontiersin.org/articles/10.3389/fnagi.2021.679282/full.
6. Enoka RM, Duchateau J. Muscle fatigue: what, why and how it influences muscle function. J Physiol [Internet]. 2008;586(1):11–23. [cited 2020 Apr 10]. Available from: http://doi.wiley.com/10.1113/jphysiol.2007.139477.

7. Beretta VS, Carpenter MG, Barbieri FA, Santos PCR, Orcioli-Silva D, Pereira MP, et al. Does the impaired postural control in Parkinson's disease affect the habituation to non-sequential external perturbation trials? Clin Biomech [Internet]. 2021;85:105363. [cited 2021 Apr 28]. Available from: https://linkinghub.elsevier.com/retrieve/pii/S0268003321000930.
8. Aboutorabi A, Arazpour M, Bahramizadeh M, Hutchins SW, Fadayevatan R. The effect of aging on gait parameters in able-bodied older subjects: a literature review. Aging Clin Exp Res [Internet]. 2016;28(3):393–405. [cited 2019 May 28]. Available from: http://link.springer.com/10.1007/s40520-015-0420-6.
9. Zanardi APJ, da Silva ES, Costa RR, Passos-Monteiro E, dos Santos IO, Kruel LFM, et al. Gait parameters of Parkinson's disease compared with healthy controls: a systematic review and meta-analysis. Sci Rep [Internet]. 2021;11(1):752. [cited 2023 Apr 12]. Available from: https://pubmed.ncbi.nlm.nih.gov/33436993/.
10. Menz HB, Lord SR, Fitzpatrick RC. Age-related differences in walking stability. Age Ageing [Internet]. 2003;32(2):137–42. [cited 2023 Apr 12]. Available from: https://academic.oup.com/ageing/article/32/2/137/28914.
11. Orcioli-Silva D, Vitório R, Lirani-Silva E, Santos PCR, Beretta VS, Gobbi LTB. Objective measures of unobstructed walking and obstacle avoidance in Parkinson's disease subtypes. Gait Posture. 2018;62:405.
12. Lee H-J, Chang WH, Choi B-O, Ryu G-H, Kim Y-H. Age-related differences in muscle coactivation during locomotion and their relationship with gait speed: a pilot study. BMC Geriatr [Internet]. 2017;17(1):44. [cited 2019 Oct 7]. Available from: http://www.ncbi.nlm.nih.gov/pubmed/28143609.
13. Hortobágyi T, Solnik S, Gruber A, Rider P, Steinweg K, Helseth J, et al. Interaction between age and gait velocity in the amplitude and timing of antagonist muscle coactivation. Gait Posture. 2009;29(4):558–64.
14. Islam A, Alcock L, Nazarpour K, Rochester L, Pantall A. Effect of Parkinson's disease and two therapeutic interventions on muscle activity during walking: a systematic review. NPJ Park Dis [Internet]. 2020;6(1) [cited 2023 Apr 12]. Available from: /pmc/articles/PMC7481232/.
15. Uematsu A, Hortobágyi T, Tsuchiya K, Kadono N, Kobayashi H, Ogawa T, et al. Lower extremity power training improves healthy old adults' gait biomechanics. Gait Posture. 2018;62:303–10.
16. Allen NE, Sherrington C, Canning CG, Fung VSC. Reduced muscle power is associated with slower walking velocity and falls in people with Parkinson's disease. Park Relat Disord. 2010;16(4):261–4.
17. Morris R, Lord S, Bunce J, Burn D, Rochester L. Gait and cognition: mapping the global and discrete relationships in ageing and neurodegenerative disease. Neurosci Biobehav Rev. 2016;64:326–45.
18. Beretta VS, Santos PCR, Orcioli-Silva D, Jaimes DAR, Pereira MP, Barbieri FA, et al. Cumulative additional information does not improve the neuromuscular control during postural responses to perturbations in postural instability/gait disorders subtype of Parkinson's disease. Exp Gerontol [Internet]. 2022;166:111892. [cited 2022 Jul 16]. Available from: https://linkinghub.elsevier.com/retrieve/pii/S0531556522002005.
19. Hardeman LES, Kal EC, Young WR, van der Kamp J, Ellmers TJ. Visuomotor control of walking in Parkinson's disease: exploring possible links between conscious movement processing and freezing of gait. Behav Brain Res. 2020;395:112837.
20. Hulzinga F, Seuthe J, D'Cruz N, Ginis P, Nieuwboer A, Schlenstedt C. Split-belt treadmill training to improve gait adaptation in Parkinson's disease. Mov Disord [Internet]. 2022; [cited 2022 Oct 19]. Available from: https://onlinelibrary.wiley.com/doi/full/10.1002/mds.29238.
21. Barbieri FA, dos Santos PCR, Simieli L, Orcioli-Silva D, Van Dieën JH, LTB G. Interactions of age and leg muscle fatigue on unobstructed walking and obstacle crossing. Gait Posture [Internet]. 2014;39(3):985–90. [cited 2019 Mar 14]. Available from: https://www.sciencedirect.com/science/article/pii/S0966636213007169.

22. Chardon M, Barbieri FA, Penedo T, Santos PCR, Vuillerme N. The effects of experimentally-induced fatigue on gait parameters during obstacle crossing: a systematic review. Neurosci Biobehav Rev. 2022;142:104854.
23. Van Cutsem J, Marcora S, De Pauw K, Bailey S, Meeusen R, Roelands B. The effects of mental fatigue on physical performance: a systematic review. Sport Med. 2017;47(8):1569–88.
24. Ricci JA, Chee E, Lorandeau AL, Berger J. Fatigue in the U.S. workforce: prevalence and implications for lost productive work time. J Occup Environ Med [Internet]. 2007;49(1):1–10. [cited 2023 Aug 22]. Available from: https://journals.lww.com/joem/fulltext/2007/01000/fatigue_in_the_u_s__workforce__prevalence_and.1.aspx.
25. De Jong M, Bonvanie AM, Jolij J, Lorist MM. Dynamics in typewriting performance reflect mental fatigue during real-life office work. PLoS One [Internet]. 2020;15(10):e0239984. [cited 2023 Aug 22]. Available from: https://journals.plos.org/plosone/article?id=10.1371/journal.pone.0239984.
26. Behrens M, Mau-Moeller A, Lischke A, Katlun F, Gube M, Zschorlich V, et al. Mental fatigue increases gait variability during dual-task walking in old adults. J Gerontol A Biol Sci Med Sci. 2018;73(6):792–7.
27. dos Santos PCR, Orcioli-Silva D, Simieli L, Pereira VIA, Barbieri FA. The influence of muscle fatigue on walking: the role of aging and Parkinson's disease. In: Locomotion and posture in older adults [Internet]. Cham: Springer; 2017. p. 143–59. [cited 2018 Nov 4]. Available from: http://link.springer.com/10.1007/978-3-319-48980-3_10.
28. Santos PCR, Barbieri FA, Zijdewind I, Gobbi LTB, Lamoth C, Hortobágyi T. Effects of experimentally induced fatigue on healthy older adults' gait: a systematic review. PLoS One [Internet]. 2019;14(12):e0226939. [cited 2020 Jan 22]. Available from: https://dx.plos.org/10.1371/journal.pone.0226939.
29. Enoka RM, Duchateau J. Translating fatigue to human performance. Med Sci Sport Exerc. 2016 Nov;48(11):2228–38.
30. Kluger BM, Krupp LB, Enoka RM. Fatigue and fatigability in neurologic illnesses: proposal for a unified taxonomy. Neurology. Wolters Kluwer Health, Inc. on behalf of the American Academy of Neurology. 2013;80:409–16.
31. Millet GY, Bertrand MF, Lapole T, Féasson L, Rozand V, Hupin D. Measuring objective fatigability and autonomic dysfunction in clinical populations: how and why? Front Sport Act Living [Internet]. 2023;5:94. [cited 2023 Apr 13]. Available from: https://www.frontiersin.org/articles/10.3389/fspor.2023.1140833/full.
32. dos Santos PCR, Barbieri FA, Orcioli-Silva D, Beretta VS, Hortobágyi T, Gobbi LTB. Being physically active minimizes the effects of leg muscle fatigue on obstacle negotiation in people with Parkinson's disease. J Biomech [Internet]. 2021;124:110568. [cited 2021 Jun 22]. Available from: https://linkinghub.elsevier.com/retrieve/pii/S0021929021003481.
33. Santos PCR, Lamoth CJC, Barbieri FA, Zijdewind I, Gobbi LTB, Hortobágyi T. Age-specific modulation of intermuscular beta coherence during gait before and after experimentally induced fatigue. Sci Rep [Internet]. 2020;10(1) [cited 2021 Feb 6]. Available from: https://pubmed.ncbi.nlm.nih.gov/32985547/.
34. Santos PCR, Gobbi LTB, Orcioli-Silva D, Simieli L, van Dieën JH, Barbieri FA. Effects of leg muscle fatigue on gait in patients with Parkinson's disease and controls with high and low levels of daily physical activity. Gait Posture [Internet]. 2016;47:86–91. [cited 2018 Sep 20]. Available from: http://www.ncbi.nlm.nih.gov/pubmed/27264409.
35. Gandevia SC. Spinal and supraspinal factors in human muscle fatigue. Physiol Rev. 2001;81(4):1725–89.
36. Kennedy DS, McNeil CJ, Gandevia SC, Taylor JL. Fatigue-related firing of distal muscle nociceptors reduces voluntary activation of proximal muscles of the same limb. J Appl Physiol. 2014;116(4):385–94.
37. Mizuno K, Tanaka M, Yamaguti K, Kajimoto O, Kuratsune H, Watanabe Y. Mental fatigue caused by prolonged cognitive load associated with sympathetic hyperactivity. Behav Brain Func [Internet]. 2011;7:17. [cited 2019 Jan 20]. Available from: http://www.ncbi.nlm.nih.gov/pubmed/21605411.

38. Taylor JL, Amann M, Duchateau J, Meeusen R, Rice CL. Neural contributions to muscle fatigue: from the brain to the muscle and back again. Med Sci Sports Exerc [Internet]. 2016;48(11):2294–306. [cited 2018 Nov 4]. Available from: http://www.ncbi.nlm.nih.gov/pubmed/27003703.
39. Egerton T, Brauer SG, Cresswell AG. Fatigue after physical activity in healthy and balance-impaired elderly. J Aging Phys Act [Internet]. 2009;17(1):89–105. [cited 2019 Aug 2]. Available from: https://journals.humankinetics.com/view/journals/japa/17/1/article-p89.xml.
40. Granacher U, Wolf I, Wehrle A, Bridenbaugh S, Kressig RW. Effects of muscle fatigue on gait characteristics under single and dual-task conditions in young and older adults. J Neuroeng Rehabil. 2010;7(1):56.
41. Bryanton MA, Bilodeau M. The influence of knee extensor fatigue on lower extremity muscle activity during chair rise in young and older adults. Eur J Appl Physiol [Internet]. 2019;119(1):61–71. [cited 2019 Feb 7]. Available from: http://www.ncbi.nlm.nih.gov/pubmed/30317389.
42. Helbostad JL, Leirfall S, Moe-Nilssen R, Sletvold O. Physical fatigue affects gait characteristics in older persons. J Gerontol Ser A Biol Sci Med Sci [Internet]. 2007;62(9):1010–5. [cited 2019 Aug 2]. Available from: https://academic.oup.com/biomedgerontology/article-lookup/doi/10.1093/gerona/62.9.1010.
43. Desmond PA, Hancock PA. Active and passive fatigue states. In: Desmond PA, Hancock PA, editors. Stress, workload, and fatigue. Mahwah: Lawrence Erlbaum Associates Publishers; 2001. p. 455–65.
44. Boksem MAS, Tops M. Mental fatigue: costs and benefits. Brain Res Rev [Internet]. 2008;59(1):125–39. [cited 2019 Feb 17]. Available from: http://www.ncbi.nlm.nih.gov/pubmed/18652844.
45. Chai R, Smith MR, Nguyen TN, Ling SH, Coutts AJ, Nguyen HT. Comparing features extractors in EEG-based cognitive fatigue detection of demanding computer tasks. In 2015 37th Annual International Conference of the IEEE Engineering in Medicine and Biology Society (EMBC). 2015. p. 7594–7.
46. Boksem MAS, Meijman TF, Lorist MM. Effects of mental fatigue on attention: an ERP study. Cogn Brain Res [Internet]. 2005;25(1):107–16. [cited 2019 Mar 20]. Available from: http://www.ncbi.nlm.nih.gov/pubmed/15913965.
47. Lorist MM. Impact of top-down control during mental fatigue. Brain Res [Internet]. 2008;1232:113–23. [cited 2019 Feb 17]. Available from: http://www.ncbi.nlm.nih.gov/pubmed/18687317.
48. Lorist MM, Boksem MAS, Ridderinkhof KR. Impaired cognitive control and reduced cingulate activity during mental fatigue. Cogn Brain Res [Internet]. 2005;24(2):199–205. [cited 2019 Feb 17]. Available from: http://www.ncbi.nlm.nih.gov/pubmed/15993758.
49. Morris AJ, Christie AD. The effect of Mental fatigue on neuromuscular function is similar in young and older women. Brain Sci. 2020;10(4):191.
50. Dideriksen JL, Enoka RM, Farina D. Neuromuscular adjustments that constrain submaximal EMG amplitude at task failure of sustained isometric contractions. J Appl Physiol [Internet]. 2011;111(2):485–94. [cited 2020 Jan 16]. Available from: http://www.ncbi.nlm.nih.gov/pubmed/21596915.
51. Bryanton M, Bilodeau M. The role of thigh muscular efforts in limiting sit-to-stand capacity in healthy young and older adults. Aging Clin Exp Res [Internet]. 2017;29(6):1211–9. [cited 2019 May 21]. Available from: http://link.springer.com/10.1007/s40520-016-0702-7.
52. Bryanton MA, Bilodeau M. The influence of knee extensor fatigue on lower extremity muscle activity during chair rise in young and older adults. Eur J Appl Physiol [Internet]. 2019;119(1):61–71. [cited 2019 Aug 3]. Available from: http://link.springer.com/10.1007/s00421-018-3999-4.
53. Boonstra TW, Daffertshofer A, van Ditshuizen JC, van den Heuvel MRC, Hofman C, Willigenburg NW, et al. Fatigue-related changes in motor-unit synchronization of quadriceps muscles within and across legs. J Electromyogr Kinesiol [Internet]. 2008;18(5):717–31. [cited 2018 Nov 4]. Available from: http://www.ncbi.nlm.nih.gov/pubmed/17462912.

54. Orcioli-Silva D, Beretta VS, Santos PCR, et al (2024) Cerebral and muscle tissue oxygenation during exercise in healthy adults: A systematic review. J Sport Health Sci 13:459–471. https://doi.org/10.1016/J.JSHS.2024.03.003.
55. Gebel A, Busch A, Stelzel C, Hortobágyi T, Granacher U. Effects of physical and mental fatigue on postural sway and cortical activity in healthy young adults. Front Hum Neurosci [Internet]. 2022;16:871930. [cited 2023 Apr 18]. Available from: /pmc/articles/PMC9237223/.
56. Cherouveim ED, Margaritelis NV, Koulouvaris P, Tsolakis C, Malliou VJ, Chatzinikolaou PN, et al. Skeletal muscle and cerebral oxygenation levels during and after submaximal concentric and eccentric isokinetic exercise. J Sports Sci [Internet]. 2021;40(2):195–202. [cited 2023 Apr 18]. Available from: https://www.tandfonline.com/doi/abs/10.1080/02640414.2021.1983248.
57. Allman BL, Rice CL. Neuromuscular fatigue and aging: central and peripheral factors. Muscle Nerve. 2002;25(6):785–96.
58. Smith MR, Chai R, Nguyen HT, Marcora SM, Coutts AJ. Comparing the effects of three cognitive tasks on indicators of mental fatigue. J Psychol Interdiscip Appl [Internet]. 2019;153(8):759–83. [cited 2020 Mar 15]. Available from: http://www.ncbi.nlm.nih.gov/pubmed/31188721.
59. Coull JT. Neural correlates of attention and arousal: insights from electrophysiology, functional neuroimaging and psychopharmacology. Prog Neurobiol. 1998;55(4):343–61.
60. Darnai G, Matuz A, Alhour HA, Perlaki G, Orsi G, Arató Á, et al. The neural correlates of mental fatigue and reward processing: a task-based fMRI study. NeuroImage. 2023;265:119812.
61. Van Cutsem J, Van Schuerbeek P, Pattyn N, Raeymaekers H, De Mey J, Meeusen R, et al. A drop in cognitive performance, whodunit? Subjective mental fatigue, brain deactivation or increased parasympathetic activity? It's complicated! Cortex. 2022;155:30–45.
62. Santos PCR, Hortobágyi T, Zijdewind I, Bucken Gobbi LT, Barbieri FA, Lamoth C. Minimal effects of age and prolonged physical and mental exercise on healthy adults' gait. Gait Posture. 2019;74:205–11.
63. Salihu AT, Hill KD, Jaberzadeh S. Neural mechanisms underlying state mental fatigue: a systematic review and activation likelihood estimation meta-analysis. Rev Neurosci [Internet]. 2022;33(8):889–917. [cited 2023 Jun 12]. Available from: https://pubmed-ncbi-nlm-nih-gov.ezproxy.weizmann.ac.il/35700454/.
64. Liao S, Ferrell BA. Fatigue in an older population. J Am Geriatr Soc [Internet]. 2000;48(4):426–30. [cited 2023 Jun 9]. Available from: https://onlinelibrary.wiley.com/doi/full/10.1111/j.1532-5415.2000.tb04702.x.
65. Stackhouse SK, Stevens JE, Lee SC, Pearce KM, Snyder-Mackler L, Binder-Macleod SA. Maximum voluntary activation in nonfatigued and fatigued muscle of young and elderly individuals. Phys Ther [Internet]. 2001;81(5):1102–9. [cited 2018 Nov 5]. Available from: http://www.ncbi.nlm.nih.gov/pubmed/11319935.
66. Morrison S, Colberg SR, Parson HK, Neumann S, Handel R, Vinik EJ, et al. Walking-induced fatigue leads to increased falls risk in older adults. J Am Med Dir Assoc [Internet]. 2016;17(5):402–9. [cited 2019 Aug 2]. Available from: https://linkinghub.elsevier.com/retrieve/pii/S152586101500763X.
67. Lanza IR, Russ DW, Kent-Braun JA. Age-related enhancement of fatigue resistance is evident in men during both isometric and dynamic tasks. J Appl Physiol [Internet]. 2004;97(3):967–75. [cited 2023 Jun 10]. Available from: https://pubmed.ncbi.nlm.nih.gov/15145914/.
68. Woods DL, Wyma JM, William Yund E, Herron TJ, Reed B. Age-related slowing of response selection and production in a visual choice reaction time task. Front Hum Neurosci. 2015;9(APR):1–12.
69. Arnau S, Möckel T, Rinkenauer G, Wascher E. The interconnection of mental fatigue and aging: An EEG study. Int J Psychophysiol [Internet]. 2017. [cited 2023 Jun 12];117:17–25. https://doi.org/10.1016/j.ijpsycho.2017.04.003.
70. WHO. Parkinson disease [Internet]. 2023. Available from: https://www.who.int/news-room/fact-sheets/detail/parkinson-disease.

71. Samii A, Nutt JG, Ransom BR. Parkinson's disease. Lancet [Internet]. 2004;363(9423):1783–93. [cited 2023 Aug 23]. Available from: http://www.thelancet.com/article/S0140673604163058/fulltext.
72. Kalia LV, Lang AE. Parkinson's disease. Lancet [Internet]. 2015;386(9996):896–912. [cited 2019 Jun 13]. Available from: http://www.ncbi.nlm.nih.gov/pubmed/25904081.
73. Cano-de-la-Cuerda R, Pérez-de-Heredia M, Miangolarra-Page JC, Muñoz-Hellín E, Fernández-de-las-Peñas C. Is there muscular weakness in Parkinson's disease? Am J Phys Med Rehabil [Internet]. 2010;89(1):70–6. [cited 2020 Oct 12]. Available from: http://journals.lww.com/00002060-201001000-00008.
74. Christiansen CL, Schenkman ML, McFann K, Wolfe P, Kohrt WM. Walking economy in people with Parkinson's disease. Mov Disord [Internet]. 2009;24(10):1481. [cited 2023 Jun 12]. Available from: /pmc/articles/PMC2744295/.
75. Burton EJ, McKeith IG, Burn DJ, Williams ED, O'Brien JT. Cerebral atrophy in Parkinson's disease with and without dementia: a comparison with Alzheimer's disease, dementia with Lewy bodies and controls. Brain. 2004;127(4):791–800.
76. Lou JS. Physical and mental fatigue in parkinsons disease: epidemiology, pathophysiology and treatment. Drug Aging [Internet]. 2009;26(3):195–208. [cited 2023 Jun 13]. Available from: https://link.springer.com/article/10.2165/00002512-200926030-00002.
77. Martens KAE, Almeida QJ. Dissociating between sensory and perceptual deficits in PD: more than simply a motor deficit. Mov Disord [Internet]. 2012;27(3):387–92. [cited 2023 Aug 18]. Available from: https://onlinelibrary-wiley-com.ezproxy.weizmann.ac.il/doi/full/10.1002/mds.24042.
78. Reynolds GO, Hanna KK, Neargarder S, Cronin-Golomb A. The relation of anxiety and cognition in Parkinson's disease. Neuropsychology [Internet]. 2017;31(6):596. [cited 2023 Dec 7]. Available from: /pmc/articles/PMC5578881/.
79. Bloxham CA, Dick DJ, Mooret JM. Reaction times and attention in Parkinson's disease. J Neurol Neurosurg Psych [Internet]. 1987;50(9):1178–83. [cited 2023 Aug 23]. Available from: https://jnnp.bmj.com/content/50/9/1178.
80. Orcioli-Silva D, Vitório R, Nóbrega-Sousa P, da Conceição NR, Beretta VS, Lirani-Silva E, et al. Levodopa facilitates prefrontal cortex activation during dual task walking in Parkinson disease. Neurorehabil Neural Repair [Internet]. 2020;34(7):589–99. Available from: http://proxy.kib.ki.se/login?url=http://search.ebscohost.com/login.aspx?direct=true&db=cin20&AN=144336476&site=ehost-live.
81. dos Santos PCR, Barbieri FA, Orcioli-Silva D, Simieli L, Gobbi LTB. Effects of physical activity levels on fatigue perception in patients with Parkinson's disease and neurologically healthy individuals. Health (Irvine Calif). 2014;06(21):2927–33.
82. Pavese N, Metta V, Bose SK, Chaudhuri KR, Brooks DJ. Fatigue in Parkinson's disease is linked to striatal and limbic serotonergic dysfunction. Brain [Internet]. 2010;133(11):3434–43. [cited 2023 Aug 23]. Available from: https://pubmed.ncbi.nlm.nih.gov/20884645/.
83. Rochester L, Jones D, Hetherington V, Nieuwboer A, Willems A-M, Kwakkel G, et al. Gait and gait-related activities and fatigue in Parkinson's disease: what is the relationship? Disabil Rehabil [Internet]. 2006;28(22):1365–71. [cited 2020 Nov 18]. Available from: http://www.tandfonline.com/doi/full/10.1080/09638280600638034.
84. Nielsen JB. How we walk: central control of muscle activity during human walking. Neuroscientist. 2003;9(3):195–204.
85. Santos PCR. Effects of age and fatigue on human gait [Internet]. University of Groningen; 2020. Available from: https://research.rug.nl/en/publications/effects-of-age-and-fatigue-on-human-gait.
86. Van Hooren B, Meijer K, McCrum C. Attractive gait training: applying dynamical systems theory to the improvement of locomotor performance across the lifespan. Front Physiol. 2019;10(JAN):416836.
87. Barbieri FA, dos Santos PCR, Lirani-Silva E, Vitório R, LTB G, van Diëen JH. Systematic review of the effects of fatigue on spatiotemporal gait parameters. J Back Musculoskelet

Rehabil [Internet]. 2013;26(2):125–31. [cited 2019 Aug 2]. Available from: http://www.medra.org/servlet/aliasResolver?alias=iospress&doi=10.3233/BMR-130371.

88. Baer M, Klemetson B, Scott D, Murtishaw AS, Navalta JW, Kinney JW, et al. Effects of fatigue on balance in individuals with Parkinson disease: influence of medication and brain-derived neurotrophic factor genotype. J Neurol Phys Ther [Internet]. 2018;42(2):61–71. [cited 2023 Jul 30]. Available from: https://journals-lww-com.ezproxy.weizmann.ac.il/jnpt/Fulltext/2018/04000/Effects_of_Fatigue_on_Balance_in_Individuals_With.2.aspx.
89. Santos PCR, Lamoth C, Vuillerme N, Barbieri FA. Faster walking under muscle fatigability: a strategy to improve stability or a warm-up effect? Brazilian J Mot Behav [Internet]. 2021;15(3):149–52. [cited 2023 Jul 31]. Available from: https://socibracom.com/bjmb/index.php/bjmb/article/view/241/214.
90. Barbieri FA, Santos PCR, Vitório R, van Dieën JH, Gobbi LTB. Effect of muscle fatigue and physical activity level in motor control of the gait of young adults. Gait Posture [Internet]. 2013;38(4):702–7. [cited 2021 Feb 11]. Available from: https://pubmed.ncbi.nlm.nih.gov/23557595/.
91. Barbieri FA, Lee Y-J, Gobbi LTB, Pijnappels M, Van Dieën JH. The effect of muscle fatigue on the last stride before stepping down a curb. Gait Posture [Internet]. 2013;37(4):542–6. [cited 2019 Aug 2]. Available from: https://linkinghub.elsevier.com/retrieve/pii/S096663621200361X.
92. Team JASP. JASP. 2023.
93. Kavanagh JJ, Morrison S, Barrett RS. Lumbar and cervical erector spinae fatigue elicit compensatory postural responses to assist in maintaining head stability during walking. J Appl Physiol [Internet]. 2006;101(4):1118–26. [cited 2018 Jul 4]. Available from: http://www.ncbi.nlm.nih.gov/pubmed/16763109.
94. Parijat P, Lockhart TE. Effects of quadriceps fatigue on the biomechanics of gait and slip propensity. Gait Posture [Internet]. 2008;28(4):568–73. [cited 2019 Aug 2]. Available from: https://linkinghub.elsevier.com/retrieve/pii/S0966636208000969.
95. Park K, Rosengren KS, Horn GP, Smith DL, Hsiao-Wecksler ET. Assessing gait changes in firefighters due to fatigue and protective clothing. Saf Sci [Internet]. 2011;49(5):719–26. [cited 2019 Aug 2]. Available from: https://linkinghub.elsevier.com/retrieve/pii/S0925753511000208.
96. Hinkel-Lipsker JW, Stoehr NM, Lachica IJ, Rogers SM. Gait adaptations to physical fatigue during the negotiation of variable and unexpected obstacles. Hum Factors [Internet]. 2021;64(8):1317–30. [cited 2021 Jun 13]. Available from: http://www.ncbi.nlm.nih.gov/pubmed/33851893.
97. Olson MW. Trunk extensor fatigue influences trunk muscle activities during walking gait. J Electromyogr Kinesiol [Internet]. 2010;20(1):17–24. [cited 2023 Aug 23]. Available from: https://pubmed.ncbi.nlm.nih.gov/19435670/.
98. Hatton AL, Menant JC, Lord SR, Lo JCM, Sturnieks DL. The effect of lower limb muscle fatigue on obstacle negotiation during walking in older adults. Gait Posture [Internet]. 2013;37(4):506–10. [cited 2019 Aug 2]. Available from: https://linkinghub.elsevier.com/retrieve/pii/S0966636212003311.
99. Cohen J. Statistical power analysis for the behavioral sciences. 2nd ed. Hillsdale: Lawrence Erlbaum Associates; 1988. 567 p
100. Piche E, Gerus P, Zory R, Jaafar A, Guerin O, Chorin F. Effects of muscular and mental fatigue on spatiotemporal gait parameters in dual task walking in young, non-frail and frail older adults. Aging Clin Exp Res [Internet]. 2023; [cited 2023 Aug 4]; Available from: https://pubmed.ncbi.nlm.nih.gov/37535312/.
101. Yoshino K, Motoshige T, Araki T, Matsuoka K. Effect of prolonged free-walking fatigue on gait and physiological rhythm. J Biomech [Internet]. 2004;37(8):1271–80. [cited 2023 Aug 3]. Available from: https://pubmed.ncbi.nlm.nih.gov/15212933/.
102. Qu X. Uncontrolled manifold analysis of gait variability: effects of load carriage and fatigue. Gait Posture [Internet]. 2012;36(2):325–9. [cited 2019 Aug 3]. Available from: https://linkinghub.elsevier.com/retrieve/pii/S096663621200080X.

103. Nagano H, James L, Sparrow WA, Begg RK. Effects of walking-induced fatigue on gait function and tripping risks in older adults. J Neuroeng Rehabil [Internet]. 2014;11(1):155. [cited 2019 Aug 2]. Available from: http://jneuroengrehab.biomedcentral.com/articles/10.1186/1743-0003-11-155.
104. Toebes MJP, Hoozemans MJM, Dekker J, van Dieën JH. Effects of unilateral leg muscle fatigue on balance control in perturbed and unperturbed gait in healthy elderly. Gait Posture [Internet]. 2014;40(1):215–9. [cited 2019 Aug 2]. Available from: https://linkinghub.elsevier.com/retrieve/pii/S096663621400294X.
105. Kao P-C, Pierro MA, Booras K. Effects of motor fatigue on walking stability and variability during concurrent cognitive challenges. Jan Y-K, editor. PLoS One. 2018;13(7):e0201433.
106. Vuillerme N, Boisgontier M. Changes in the relative contribution of each leg to the control of quiet two-legged stance following unilateral plantar-flexor muscles fatigue. Eur J Appl Physiol. 2010;110(1):207–13.
107. Danna-Dos Santos A, Poston B, Jesunathadas M, Bobich LR, Hamm TM, Santello M. Influence of fatigue on hand muscle coordination and EMG-EMG coherence during three-digit grasping. J Neurophysiol [Internet]. 2010;104(6):3576–87. [cited 2019 Nov 7]. Available from: http://www.ncbi.nlm.nih.gov/pubmed/20926609.
108. Fitzgerald LF, Bartlett MF, Nagarajan R, Francisco EJ, Sup FC, Kent JA. Effects of old age and contraction mode on knee extensor muscle ATP flux and metabolic economy in vivo. J Physiol [Internet]. 2021;599(12):3063–80. [cited 2023 Aug 4]. Available from: https://pubmed-ncbi-nlm-nih-gov.ezproxy.weizmann.ac.il/33876434/.
109. Barbieri FA, Gobbi LTB, Lee YJ, Pijnappels M, van Dieën JH. Effect of triceps surae and quadriceps muscle fatigue on the mechanics of landing in stepping down in ongoing gait. Ergonomics. 2014;57(6):934–42.
110. Granacher U, Gruber M, Förderer D, Strass D, Gollhofer A. Effects of ankle fatigue on functional reflex activity during gait perturbations in young and elderly men. Gait Posture [Internet]. 2010;32(1):107–12. [cited 2018 Jul 4]. Available from: http://linkinghub.elsevier.com/retrieve/pii/S0966636210001001.
111. Waanders JB, Hortobágyi T, Murgia A, DeVita P, Franz JR. Advanced age redistributes positive but not negative leg joint work during walking. Med Sci Sport Exerc [Internet]. 2019;51(4):615–23. [cited 2019 Nov 6]. Available from: http://www.ncbi.nlm.nih.gov/pubmed/30395049.
112. Boyer KA, Johnson RT, Banks JJ, Jewell C, Hafer JF. Systematic review and meta-analysis of gait mechanics in young and older adults. Exp Gerontol [Internet]. 2017;95:63–70. [cited 2022 Sep 25]. Available from: https://pubmed-ncbi-nlm-nih-gov.ezproxy.weizmann.ac.il/28499954/.
113. Boyer KA, Hayes KL, Umberger BR, Adamczyk PG, Bean JF, Brach JS, et al. Age-related changes in gait biomechanics and their impact on the metabolic cost of walking: report from a National Institute on Aging workshop. Exp Gerontol [Internet]. 2023;173. [cited 2023 Aug 4]. Available from: https://pubmed.ncbi.nlm.nih.gov/36693530/.
114. Wai-Chi Wong D, Lam W-K, Chiu-Chun Lee W. Gait asymmetry and variability in older adults during long-distance walking: implications for gait instability. 2019. [cited 2020 Apr 6]. Available from: www.elsevier.com/locate/clinbiomech.
115. Hollman JH, Watkins MK, Imhoff AC, Braun CE, Akervik KA, Ness DK. A comparison of variability in spatiotemporal gait parameters between treadmill and overground walking conditions. Gait Posture. 2016;43:204–9.
116. Hagoort I, Vuillerme N, Hortobágyi T, CJC L. Age and walking conditions differently affect domains of gait. Hum Mov Sci [Internet]. 2023;89:103075. [cited 2023 Mar 26]. Available from: http://creativecommons.org/licenses/by/4.0/.
117. Lee SJ, Hidler J. Biomechanics of overground vs. treadmill walking in healthy individuals. J Appl Physiol. 2008;104:747–55.
118. Fidalgo-Herrera A, Miangolarra-Page JC, Carratalá-Tejada M. Electromyographic traces of motor unit synchronization of fatigued lower limb muscles during gait. Hum Mov Sci. 2021;75:102750.

119. Barbieri FA, Beretta SS, Pereira VAI, Simieli L, Orcioli-Silva D, dos Santos PCR, et al. Recovery of gait after quadriceps muscle fatigue. Gait Posture [Internet]. 2016;43:270–4. [cited 2019 Aug 3]. Available from: https://linkinghub.elsevier.com/retrieve/pii/S0966636215009236.
120. Antonopoulos C, Patikas D, Koutlianos N, Papadopoulou SD, Chatzopoulos D, Hatzikotoulas K, et al. The effect of fatigue on electromyographic characteristics during obstacle crossing of different heights in young adults. J Sports Sci Med [Internet]. 2014;13(4):724. [cited 2023 Aug 15]. Available from: /pmc/articles/PMC4234939/.
121. Santos PCR, Barbieri FA, Lamoth C, Hortobágyi T Wavelet-based time-frequency intermuscular beta-band coherence decreases with age but increases after mental fatigue in ankle muscles during gait independent of age. Journal of Electromyography and Kinesiology. In Press.
122. McManus L, Hu X, Rymer WZ, Suresh NL, Lowery MM. Muscle fatigue increases beta-band coherence between the firing times of simultaneously active motor units in the first dorsal interosseous muscle. J Neurophysiol [Internet]. 2016;115(6):2830–9. [cited 2019 Nov 7]. Available from: http://www.ncbi.nlm.nih.gov/pubmed/26984420.
123. Dingwell JB, Cusumano JP, Cavanagh PR, Sternad D. Local dynamic stability versus kinematic variability of continuous overground and treadmill walking. J Biomech Eng. 2001;123(1):27–32.
124. Galna B, Peters A, Murphy AT, Morris ME. Obstacle crossing deficits in older adults: a systematic review. Gait Posture [Internet]. 2009;30(3):270–5. [cited 2019 May 14]. Available from: https://www.sciencedirect.com/science/article/pii/S0966636209001568?via%3Dihub.
125. Hortobágyi T, Mizelle C, Beam S, DeVita P. Old adults perform activities of daily living near their maximal capabilities. J Gerontol A Biol Sci Med Sci [Internet] 2003 May [cited 2018 Jul 18];58(5):M453–M460. Available from: http://www.ncbi.nlm.nih.gov/pubmed/12730256.
126. Orcioli-Silva D, Barbieri FA, dos Santos PCR, Beretta VS, Simieli L, Vitorio R, et al. Double obstacles increase gait asymmetry during obstacle crossing in people with Parkinson's disease and healthy older adults: a pilot study. Sci Rep. 2020;10(1):1–8.
127. Pereira VAI, Barbieri FA, Zagatto AM, Dos Santos PCR, Simieli L, Barbieri RA, et al. Muscle fatigue does not change the effects on lower limbs strength caused by aging and Parkinson's disease. Aging Dis [Internet]. 2018;9(6):988–98. [cited 2023 Aug 21]. Available from: https://pubmed.ncbi.nlm.nih.gov/30574412/.

Parkinson's Disease and Gait Asymmetry 12

Fabio Augusto Barbieri, Aline Prieto Silveira-Ciola,
Tiago Penedo, and Murilo Henrique Faria

Abstract

The aim of this chapter was to deepen into the topic of gait asymmetry (GA) among individuals with Parkinson's disease (PD). This chapter commenced by furnishing a comprehensive definition of GA, accompanied by an exploration of its manifestation and the theoretical constructs that elucidate the origins of motor asymmetry within the context of PD. The subsequent section spotlighted the principal findings concerning GA in the PD population, focusing on three pivotal domains: gait initiation, overground walking, and challenging walking (obstacle avoidance and dual-tasking). Intriguingly, although individuals with PD do not exhibit motor asymmetry during gait initiation, they do manifest cortical activity asymmetry. On the other hand, asymmetry is observed in multiple gait parameters during overground walking and challenging walking tasks. Notably, challenging walking accentuates GA, barring instances of obstacle circumvention coupled with dual-tasking, where GA appears to diminish. The simultaneous effort of consciously controlling walking while skillfully avoiding obstacles may, in fact, outweigh the available resources, consequently leading to changes in GA. Subsequently, potential mechanisms that could elucidate the genesis of GA within the PD population were presented. While the correlation between asymmetrical brain degeneration and GA appears logical, the precise neural mechanisms remain largely uncharted. This chapter was concluded with several recommendations pertinent to the realm of rehabilitation strategies were proffered. These recommendations are poised to augment our comprehension of GA in PD and, in turn, potentially steer interventions tailored to alleviate this condition.

F. A. Barbieri (✉) · A. P. Silveira-Ciola · T. Penedo · M. H. Faria
Human Movement Research Laboratory (MOVI-LAB), Department of Physical Education, School of Sciences, São Paulo State University (UNESP), Bauru, São Paulo, Brazil
e-mail: fabio.barbieri@unesp.br

F. A. Barbieri et al. (eds.), *Locomotion and Posture in Older Adults*,
https://doi.org/10.1007/978-3-031-74123-4_12

Introduction

It is conventionally accepted that walking is a symmetrical task for children and young adults [1]. However, gait asymmetry (GA) is often an indicator of underlying pathology, such as Parkinson's disease (PD) and represents as a significant clinical concern within the domain of movement disorders rehabilitation [1]. PD is characterized by a prevalence of unilateral motor symptoms, including tremor, rigidity, and bradykinesia [2], which are the result of asymmetrical degeneration in the brain, particularly affecting the basal ganglia [3, 4].

The impact of PD on gait is notable due to this unilateral degeneration, leading to asymmetry in gait patterns within the PD population [5–8]. This accentuated asymmetry play a pivotal role as an independent gait impairment among individuals with PD. Furthermore, together to gait variability, GA has been demonstrated to have a direct correlation with more severe gait deficits, including freezing of gait (FoG) and instances of falls [7]. A comprehensive understanding of how PD affects gait symmetry/asymmetry could potentially reduce the incidence of fall-related hospitalizations and associated costs. Furthermore, an appreciation of the alterations in GA might serve as a valuable tool for early PD diagnosis and offer insights into the efficacy of interventions, ultimately enhancing gait rehabilitation training.

The aim of this chapter is to delve into the topic of GA among individuals with PD. In order to achieve this, the following structure has been adopted. Firstly, a comprehensive definition of asymmetry is provided. Subsequently, a detailed overview is offered, encompassing unilateral motor impairments and the manifestation of asymmetry in individuals with PD. This includes an exploration of the theories that elucidate the underlying mechanisms of motor asymmetry in the context of PD. The following section highlights the primary findings regarding GA in PD populations. The findings are classified into three key aspects: gait initiation, overground walking, and challenging walking (obstacle avoidance and dual-tasking). Subsequently, the discussion turns to a detailed analysis of the potential mechanisms that may contribute to the emergence of GA in individuals with PD. A comprehensive debate is conducted in order to determine the relative merits of these candidate mechanisms. In conclusion, this chapter offers recommendations relevant to rehabilitation strategies. These suggestions have the potential to enhance our understanding of GA in PD and potentially guide interventions aimed to improve this condition.

Asymmetry Definition

As defined by the dictionary, symmetry is defined as "the quality of being made up of exactly similar parts facing each other or around an axis; a correct or pleasing proportion of the parts of a thing" (https://www.lexico.com). In the context of the human body, mirror symmetry along the coronal axis, which essentially divides the body into left and right halves, is typically considered. As results, asymmetry is defined as the "lack of equality or equivalence between parts or aspects of something; lack of symmetry; deviation from mirror symmetry across the coronal axis is termed bilateral asymmetry" (https://www.lexico.com). The term, asymmetry, encompasses both structural and functional dissimilarities between the left and right sides of the body [9].

In context of motor control, the term 'asymmetry' is used to describe differences in performance and control between the two sides of the body [10]. These differences results in individuals exhibiting a preference for using one side of their body during motor tasks, a phenomenon referred to as laterality [10]. For instance, approximately 90% of individuals exhibit a preference for using their right hand for manipulative tasks, whereas only 25–45% demonstrate a preference for the right lower limb during actions [11]. Therefore, asymmetry is an adverse factor affecting performance, despite some research findings that do not wholly support the association between preference and asymmetry [12].

As this chapter primarily concerned with GA, it is essential to provide a clear definition of this term too. In parallel with the concept of asymmetry, the literature first defines the term gait symmetry. This is described as a state of perfect alignment between the actions of the lower limbs or when no statistically significant differences are observed in bilaterally measured parameters [1]. A common thread across diverse definitions is that the term "gait symmetry" is applicable when both limbs exhibit identical behavior [1]. Therefore, GA can be defined as the (significant) differences in control and performance of the right and left limbs during walking, as evidenced by parameters measured bilaterally [13].

The emergence of motor asymmetry in humans is the result of a complex interplay between genetic and environmental factors, the precise nature of which remains unclear [14]. This phenomenon becomes apparent even during the gestational period, as fetuses display a predilection for movements on one side of the body, a preference that seems to impact subsequent performance asymmetries [15]. However, the evidence suggests that lateralization is only 10–20% genetically determined, with the remaining 80–90% being influenced by postnatal environmental factors [14]. There is an ongoing debate in the literature regarding the most suitable approach for explaining motor asymmetry. A multitude of intertwined factors contribute to the development of handedness and footedness, including parental education, cultural influences, genetics, and imitation behaviors, among others [14, 16].

Asymmetry can be categorized into three distinct types (Fig. 12.1) [12]: (a) directional asymmetry—a consistent attribute that develops towards a specific side (e.g., the position of internal organs in the human body); (b) antisymmetry—an attribute that evolves towards a particular side, but with variable sides of occurrence (e.g., footedness and handedness); (c) fluctuating asymmetry—an attribute that would normally evolve symmetrically but deviates due to environmental stress, disease, and the evolutionary "health" of an organism (e.g., unilateral PD symptoms). Directional asymmetries and antisymmetries are commonly controlled and adapted. However, fluctuating asymmetry is frequently linked to adverse implications, such as those seen in PD.

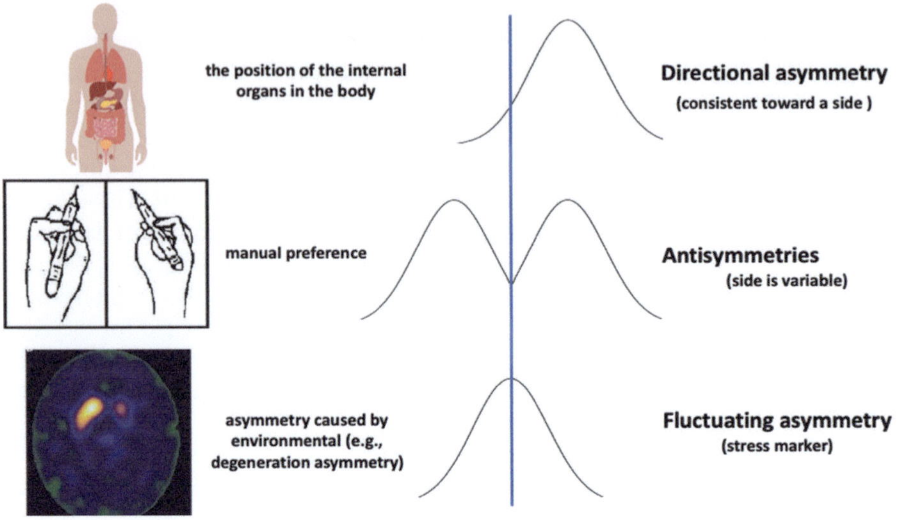

Fig. 12.1 The distribution curves represent the directional asymmetry, antisymmetry, and fluctuating asymmetry. In addition to the curves, there are illustrative examples of each type of asymmetry. These includes directional asymmetry—the position of the internal organs in the body; antisymmetry—manual preference; fluctuating asymmetry—asymmetry caused by environmental factors such as degeneration asymmetry in the basal ganglia of individuals with PD

The determination of lower limb preference is typically achieved through the observation of the preferred leg for kicking or the utilization of inventories. The quantification of asymmetries usually involves the calculation of the asymmetry index [17], left-to-right ratios [13], or the utilisation of statistical procedures [18]. Of the aforementioned techniques, the asymmetry index is the most commonly employed in studies focusing on asymmetry.

Numerous available asymmetry indexes are available for quantification of motor asymmetries, including the Symmetry Index [17], Gait Asymmetry [19], Ratio Index [20], Symmetry Angle [18], or the Normalized Symmetry Index [21], are used to quantify motor asymmetries. However, there is no consensus on a standardised approach to the calculation method of motor asymmetry or the parameters used for its assessment. For example there is no agreement on the most effective method of measuring GA, particularly given the use of multiple variables, including forces, distances, angles, and moments, are often employed. Moreover, these asymmetry indexes exhibit several shortcomings, including an artificial inflation [22], normalization to a reference value [22] and lack of sensitivity [23, 24]. These limitations preclude the comparison of irregular signals frequently observed in pathological gait [25]. As a result, the applicability of existing methods for assessing motor asymmetry, including GA, across varying injury severities and disease conditions remains considerably constrained in its scope.

Parkinson's Disease and Asymmetry

The asymmetric onset of motor symptoms represents a significant "red flag" favoring the diagnosis of PD, as outlined by the criteria set forth by the Movement Disorder Society [26]. Indeed, the London Brain Bank criteria include marked asymmetry as a supportive characteristic for the diagnosis of PD [2]. It has traditionally been observed that while both sides of the nervous system are affected by the pathological and clinical progression of the disease, the initial motor symptoms on the affected side tend to remain more pronounced throughout the course of the disease. Nevertheless, these asymmetries may become less pronounced in the advanced stages of PD [4].

It is estimated that approximately 87.5%, 69.7%, and 66.4% of individuals with PD present with unilateral initial symptoms of tremor, rigidity, and bradykinesia, respectively [4]. The magnitude of these asymmetries may be influenced by factors such as age, duration of PD, and daily habits [27]. In addition, the symmetric distribution of motor signs is associated with an accelerated disease progression [28], an elevated risk of balance disorder [29], an increased limitations in daily activities [30], a heightened higher susceptibility to restless legs syndrome [31], a poor mental state [30] and an elevated risk of cognitive impairment [32] and dementia [33]. Also, van der Hoorn and collaborators [34] put forth a hypothesis suggesting a correlation between laterality and the dominance of symptoms in PD, with symptoms exhibiting a proclivity to manifest more frequently on the side corresponding to the preferred hand.

The most evident rationale for motor asymmetry in PD is the unequal degeneration of dopaminergic neurons, particularly within the basal ganglia region of the substantia nigra. This hypothesis is based on the premise that motor symptoms manifest when approximately 50–70% of dopaminergic neurons have undergone degeneration, exhibiting an unilateral predominance [4]. Literature has shown significant differences between the hemisphere that is most affected (contralateral to the side of the body most affected by PD) and the least affected by PD. The predominant effects were observed in the basal ganglia, including the putamen, globus pallidus, and substantia nigra, which lends support to the hypothesis of asymmetric neurodegeneration in the nigrostriatal pathways [35]. Furthermore, evidence suggests that asymmetry in brain activity and connectivity between brain regions also occurs. There is evidence of asymmetry in the connectivity between brain regions. Functional magnetic resonance imaging studies have identified functional asymmetry within the basal ganglia and asymmetric connectivity between the ipsilateral inferior orbitofrontal and contralateral inferior parietal regions [36], which is linked to the severity and lateralization of motor symptoms in PD. Also, diagnosed with PD exhibit heightened asymmetry in cortical activity relative to those without neurological impairments [37]. Moreover, the extent of impairment in the lower and upper limbs of individuals with PD corresponds to the degree of brain damage to regions containing dopamine in each hemisphere [38]. Individuals with unilateral PD demonstrate notable discrepancies in striatal uptake between sides, manifesting in both the caudate and putamen nuclei [39]. In addition, the dominant hemisphere exhibits a more widespread distribution in the thalamic circuitry [40].

Two theories have emerged in attempts to elucidate the unilateral nature of motor symptoms in PD and the resulting motor asymmetry. The theory proposed by Djaldetti and colleagues [41] suggest that the unilateral manifestation of motor symptoms may be attributed to two main factors. Firstly, it is possible that normal inborn variations in the numbers of nigral dopaminergic neurons may result in a discrepancy in the count of these neurons on one side compared to the other from birth. Given that the degenerative process of the disease affects both sides equally, the side with the initially reduced number of neurons may reach a critical point of vulnerability sooner. Secondly, the theory postulates that the substantia nigra on one side of the brain may be more susceptible due to structural or environmental influences, such as greater use of one side. Consequently, once the degenerative process has commenced, there is a possibility of accelerated cell death occurring initially on the side where the degeneration was initiated. This theory considers both neural and structural factors, as well as environmental and motor factors, in order to explain the observed motor asymmetry in PD.

A more recent theory presented by Borghammer [42] in (Fig. 12.2) highlights the role of the initial site of α-synuclein accumulation and Lewy body formation within the central nervous system, as well as symmetry/asymmetry aspects, in influencing the clinical phenotype of individuals with PD. This theory posits two distinct patterns of distinguishes between two types of PD progression: body-first PD and brain-first PD. In the case of body-first PD, the origin of α-synuclein pathology is in

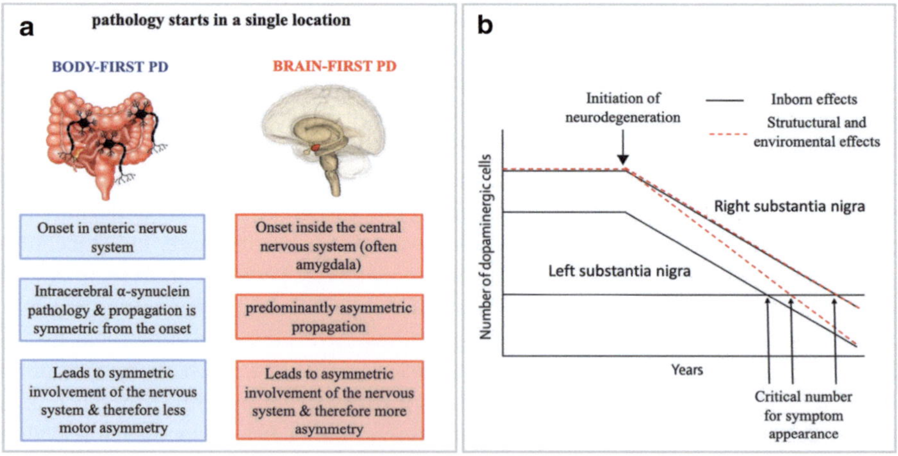

Fig. 12.2 (**a**) An exemplification of Borghammer's theory, which highlights that symmetry/asymmetry aspects are influenced by two types of PD progression patterns: body-first and brain-first α-synuclein pathology. (**b**) Exemplification of Djaldetti's theory, which attributes the unilateral manifestation of motor symptoms to two main factors: normal inborn variations in the numbers of nigral dopaminergic neurons, and the susceptibility of one side of the brain (i.e., substantia nigra) to degeneration

the enteric nervous system, with subsequent bilateral spread to the brain via the parasympathetic and sympathetic connectome. This mode of progression is associated with a more symmetrical pattern of central nervous system degeneration. Conversely, in brain-first PD, the onset of symptoms is more heterogeneous, with propagation occuring in multiple directions. In instances where symptoms commence unilaterally in the amygdala or locus coeruleus, the ipsilateral central nervous system is observed to degenerate at an earlier stage than the contralateral counterpart. Nevertheless, these theories remain untested and await further validation. Importantly, the prodromal phase of PD, which can extend for over 20 years, suggests a slow neuron-to-neuron propagation of the α-synuclein pathology [43]. Despite the consistent understanding of the lateralization of motor symptoms in PD, evidence of GA requires further clarification and depth. Additionally, no theory has been specifically designed to explain GA to date.

Gait Asymmetry in Individuals with Parkinson's Disease

GA has consistently been observed in individuals with PD, manifesting as an accentuated asymmetry in various gait parameters. Robust data underscores that individuals with PD exhibit pronounced asymmetry in the step length [7, 44] and duration [7] as well as in the swing phase [13, 19, 45] when compared to their neurologically healthy peers. It is noteworthy that the extent of GA may be influenced by environmental challenges encountered during the act of walking and the specific phase of the gait cycle in individuals with PD. The following sections delineate the behaviour of GA during specific gait phases, including gait initiation, overground walking, and challenging walking, such as obstacle avoidance (crossing and circumventing) and dual-tasking.

Gait Initiation

Gait initiation, as a functional daily living task, represents a valuable investigative tool for elucidating postural control changes and mobility alterations associated with disability [46]. It is particularly pertinent to individuals with PD that gait initiation can prove problematic and even trigger instances of FoG [47]. Individuals with PD exhibit distinctive characteristics in gait initiation, including reduced velocity and magnitude of center of pressure displacements, as well as a slower first step [48]. This indicates a less pronounced anticipatory postural adjustment [47, 49]. These alterations are associated with reduced or absent tibial anterior muscle activation and a shortened first step in comparison to individuals without neurological impairment [47]. Therefore, the quantification of gait initiation behavior not only provides insights into postural control deficiencies in PD [50] but also offers a potential explanation for GA in this population.

In light of the pervasive motor asymmetry observed in individuals with PD, it is reasonable to expect that those with PD would demonstrate an increase in asymmetry during gait initiation. However, intriguingly, individuals with PD do not exhibit motor asymmetry (in terms of anticipatory postural adjustments and stepping parameters) during gait initiation (Fig. 12.3). Instead, they display higher cortical activity asymmetry in comparison to their healthy peers [37], which indicates an adaptive change to enhance gait initiation. One may argue that cortical activity asymmetry represets an adaptive change, given that damaged areas of the most affected hemisphere are substituted by residual networks within both hemispheres [51, 52]. The reorganization of degenerated areas in the less affected hemisphere resulted in heightened activity within its motor cortex, The remapping of functional representation from degenerated areas onto homologous areas within the least-degenerated hemisphere causes an increased activity in the least affected motor cortex [51], thereby leading to increased cortical activity asymmetry. Therefore, the observation that individuals with PD who manifest lower motor asymmetry during gait initiation also exhibit higher cortical activity asymmetry provides further evidence in support of the hypothesis that an adaptive mechanism is in place with the aim of enhancing motor behaviour during gait initiation.

The diminished asymmetry in anticipatory postural adjustments observed in individuals with PD during gait initiation suggests that they employ a similar postural adjustment strategy regardless of which limb is initiating the gait. This is in contrast to the findings observed in other populations, including hemiparetic patients [53], individuals with severe unilateral knee arthritis [54] and hemiplegic patients [55], who exhibited asymmetry during gait initiation. This inconsistency extends to previous studies that have analyzed level walking, which have reported higher asymmetry in individuals with PD compared to their neurologically healthy peers [7, 13]. This inconsistency in the findings can be understood through two perspectives.

Firstly, a consistent finding in the literature is that individuals with PD tend to employ a more rigid strategy, maintaining uniform motor behavior across trials, particularly when the task is not particularly challenging. This behavior is driven by

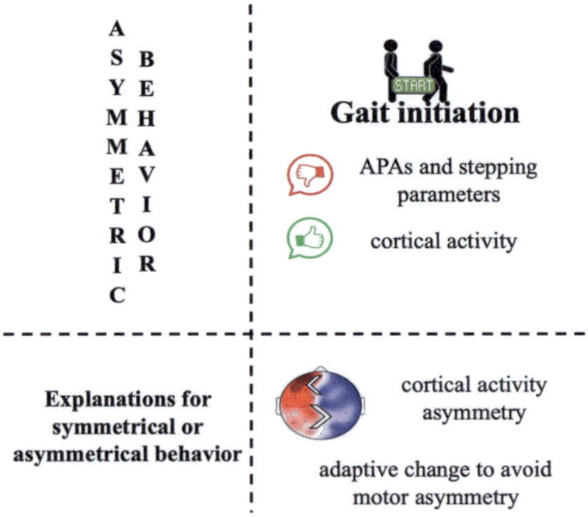

Fig. 12.3 The main findings of GA during gait initiation and a potential rationale for motor symmetric behavior. indicates symmetric behavior; indicates asymmetric behavior

a desire to avoid instability, additional mechanical effort, and to prioritize safety [56]. It may be posited that the utilization of analogous anticipatory postural adjustments regardless of the initiating limb could be interpreted as a cautious strategy, particularly since none of the individuals in the study experienced falls or FoG episodes during gait initiation. However, it is important to note that this symmetric behavior may not necessarily be advantageous for gait initiation. This is because individuals with PD tend to exhibit slower movements and smaller center of pressure displacements during gait initiation, which results in impaired initiation of gait [47].

A second potential explanation for the inconsistent change in asymmetry across populations may be related to impairments in the dopaminergic system. The neurodegeneration of dopaminergic neurons, particularly in the substantia nigra pars compacta, disrupts the thalamocortical and brainstem motor systems [57], resulting in impaired motor adjustments during gait initiation [47]. Additionally, neural neurodegeneration is asymmetric in the PD [3, 4], resulting in functional asymmetry between hemispheres, with a relative reduction of neural excitability on the most affected hemisphere and a supposed increase in the least affected one. Also, individuals with PD present reduced transcallosal sensorimotor structural connectivity [7], which plays a role in balancing mutual inhibitory control in the motor cortex [58]. The unequal balance of transcallosal inhibitory circuits between motor areas in both hemispheres in PD may contribute to asymmetries in the cortical activity [7]. The higher asymmetry in cortical activity parameters, particularly in the frontal region [59], may lead to bradykinesia and akinesia symptoms during movement. These symptoms may potentially inhibit effective postural adjustments during gait initiation, thereby explaining the lack of change in anticipatory postural adjustments observed in individuals with PD.

Overground Walking

The existing body of evidence strongly suggests that individuals with PD demonstrate a marked asymmetry in spatial-temporal parameters during overground walking (Table 12.1). Specifically, parameters such as the swing time [71, 73, 75], step duration [6, 7, 67, 73], and step length [7, 73, 68, 72] are consistently reported as the main asymmetric parameters during overground walking in individuals with PD. On the other hand, other spatial-temporal parameters, such as step speed, are not tipically found to be asymmetric in individuals with PD. In addition, a significant number of studies have reported the absence of GA in individuals with PD [63, 69, 74].

Dopaminergic medication appears to play an important role in the regulation of asymmetry in kinematic parameters during overground walking [73]. Individuals with PD exhibit a reduction in step duration asymmetry when under the effects of dopaminergic medication (vs. OFF state). However, even when the medication is in a state of efficacy, individuals with PD continuos to demonstrate a greater GA compared to their peers, particularly in step duration, step length, and swing time [73]. Interestingly, the presence of GA is evident even in the early stages of PD [76] as

Table 12.1 Main findings of the studies that investigated GA during overground walking in individuals with PD

Study	Groups (n)	Main findings
Miller et al. [60]	PD = 19 CG = 18	PD—lower symmetry in the MG and TA muscles VL symmetry—PD = CG PD—greater asymmetry in TA after a gait training program
Plotnik et al. [19]	PD + FoG = 24 PD-FoG = 12	PD + FoG—greater asymmetry in swing time vs. PD-FoG No correlation between GA and UPDRS score - GA is not a direct reflection of asymmetry in PD symptoms
Baltadjieva et al. [61]	PD = 35 CG = 22	PD—greater asymmetry in gait temporal parameters but not in the ground reaction forces
Galna et al. [62]	PD = 121 CG = 184	PD—greater asymmetry in step duration, swing time and stance time vs. CG
Grajić et al. [63]	PD = 40 CG = 43	No difference in GA between PD and CG
Su et al. [64]	PD = 89 CG = 72	PD—greater GA vs. CG
Griet Vervoort et al. [65]	PIGD = 43 TD = 22 CG = 20	No differences in GA between PIGD and TD
Del Din et al. [66]	PD = 47 CG = 50	PD and CG—greater GA in free-living environment vs laboratory environment for step time, swing time, stance time and step length PD—greater GA (step length) in free-living environment vs. CG
Djurić-Jovičić et al. [67]	PD = 40 CG = 40	Asymmetry of step duration—an indicator to classify the disease in early stages
Morris et al. [68, 69]	PD = 67 CG = 103	Free-living—greater asymmetry in stride length vs. laboratory in both groups
Ren et al. [70]	PD = 93 CG = 72	PD—GA is more evident in earlier stages of the disease
Fling et al. [7]	PD = 39 CG = 20	PD—greater asymmetry in step duration and length vs. CG PD—lower transcallosal fiber tract integrity of the pre-SMA and S1 associated with greater asymmetry in step length asymmetry
Barbieri, Simieli, et al. [6]	PD = 13 CG = 13	ON—lower GA vs. OFF
Martínez et al. [71]	PD = 11 CG = 12 YC = 16	PD—greater GA vs. CG and YC GA—predicted by the affected side related to clinical onset, cognitive status and motor scale
Son et al. [72]	PD + FoG = 10 PD-FoG = 16	PD + FoG—greater asymmetry in step length during backward vs. PD-FoG
Gilmore et al. [73]	PD = 62 CG = 11	Forward walking: (a) ON—lower step duration asymmetry vs OFF, (b) PD—greater asymmetry in step length and swing time vs. CG (both in ON and OFF) Backwards walking: PD—greater asymmetry in step duration and swing time vs. CG (both in ON and OFF)
Koh et al. [74]	PD = 41 CG = 23	PD - shoulder and elbow asymmetries affect arm swing asymmetry Asymmetries in spatial-temporal parameters—no predicted arm swing asymmetry

Note: *CG* control group of healthy individuals, *+FoG* presence of FoG, *–FoG* absence of FoG, *MG* medial gastrocnemius, *PD* Parkinson's disease group, *PIGD* postural instability and gait disorder, *TA* tibialis anterior, *TD* tremor dominant, *VL* vastus lateralis, *SMA* supplementary motor areas, *S1* primary somatosensory cortices, *YC* young control group well as in de novo patients, who already exhibit increased swing time asymmetry [61] despite the findings are inconclusive yet [63]. On the other hand, when comparing individuals with PD who have undergone long-term dopaminergic treatment with their healthy peers, the pronounced GA in PD becomes more pronounced. These individuals consistently demonstrate greater degree of asymmetry in both temporal [7, 71, 73] and spatial parameters [7, 73] during overground walking.

Although there is a substantial body of evidence supporting the confirmation of GA in PD through the analysis of spatial-temporal gait parameters, joint angular, kinetic, and muscle activity parameters have often been overlooked in this context. Only two studies have investigated asymmetry in angular parameters (range of motion) during walking: one involving upper limbs [74] and another involving lower limbs [72].

Koh et al. [74] reported that asymmetries in the shoulder and elbow joints influence arm swing asymmetry in early-stage of PD. The authors posit that asymmetry in arm swing may precede gait dysfunctions related to the lower limb, highlighting the importance of analyzing upper limb asymmetry during gait assessments for individuals with PD. In addition, Son et al. [72] found greater ankle range of motion asymmetry during stepping with the most affected limb compared to the least affected limb in individuals experiencing FoG (freezers). These findings, in conjunction with the observation of heightened spatial-temporal asymmetries in stepping (swing time, step time, and step length) in individuals experiencing FoG [77], suggest a potential relationship between GA and FoG in PD.

Regarding kinetics parameters, Baltadjieva et al. [61] investigated patients with PD *de novo* and found greater degree of asymmetry in temporal stepping parameters, but not in the kinetic parameters (i.e., ground reaction forces). Similarly, Martínez and collaborators [71] found no significant asymmetry in the kinetics parameter among individuals with PD. However, Su and collaborators [64] reported greater asymmetry in ground reaction forces in individuals with PD. The discrepancy in findings may be attributed to variations in data analysis methodologies. Su et al. [64] employed a novel method involving the decomposition of ground reaction forces into components of different frequency sub-bands using the wavelet transform, whereas Baltadjieva et al. [61] and Martínez et al. [71] analyzed the magnitude of ground reaction forces.

Only one study has evaluated muscular asymmetry during overground walking in patients with PD [60]. The authors assessed bilateral asymmetry in the medial gastrocnemius, tibial anterior, and vastus lateralis muscles using a latency-corrected ensemble average method. The findings revealed that individuals with PD exhibited significantly lower shape symmetry (greater asymmetry) in the medial gastrocnemius and tibial anterior muscles when compared to neurologically healthy individuals. However, no asymmetry was identified in the vastus lateralis muscle.

Challenging Walking

GA increases during obstacle avoidance in individuals with PD, as demonstrated in various comparative studies: overground walking vs. single obstacle avoidance [6], overground walking vs. obstacle circumvention [5] and single vs. double obstacle avoidance [8] (Fig. 12.4). While stepping over a single obstacle primarily impacts the asymmetry of temporal parameters (i.e., step duration), stepping over of double obstacles and obstacle circumvention primarily influence the asymmetry of spatial parameters, particularly safe parameters such as toe clearance and body clearance, respectively. This finding indicates that more challenging tasks tend to affect spatial parameter asymmetry while leaving temporal parameter asymmetry unchanged [8]. In addition, the effect of obstacle avoidance on GA is influenced by the distance between the obstacles (shorter vs. longer distances), particularly when the most affected limb is involved in stepping over or circumventing the obstacle [8]. Furthermore, obstacle circumvention to the most affected side is risky for individuals with PD [5]. The motor adjustments required during obstacle avoidance are complex adaptations for individuals with PD, which result in an exacerbation of GA and an increased likelihood of detecting gait disability better.

The demands of obstacle avoidance can exceed the available motor resources, leading to gait adjustments and heightened asymmetry. Negotiating obstacles while walking requires that individuals implement specific adaptations. For example, stepping over an obstacle requires a more conservative and cautious strategy

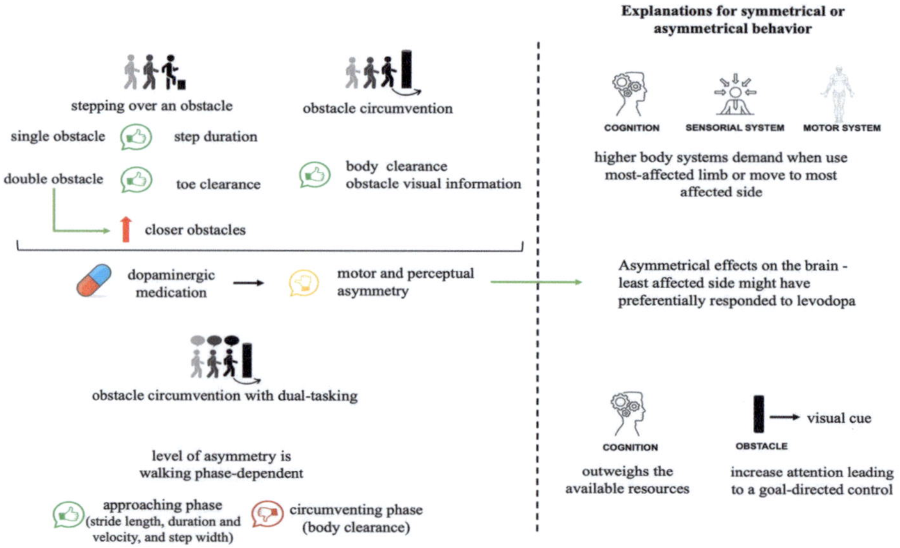

Fig. 12.4 The main findings of GA during obstacle avoidance and a possible explanation for motor symmetric behavior. [red icon] indicates symmetric behavior; [green icon] indicates asymmetric behavior; [yellow icon] indicates possible asymmetric behavior

approach characterized by reduced velocity, shorter step length, and wider step width [78, 79]. This task requires the rapid planning and execution of adaptive movements, which intensifies the motor demands and engages complex brain circuitry within both the central and peripheral nervous systems [80]. The combination of conscious control of walking and deliberate avoidance of obstacles may indeed outweigh the available resources, resulting in gait adjustments that exacerbate GA [6, 8].

The altered neural underpinnings observed in PD underscore the increased GA observed during obstacle avoidance [41]. For example, Fling et al. [7] showed that a reduction in the microstructural integrity of callosal white matter tracts connecting the pre-supplementary motor area and supplementary motor areas is crucial factor in the development of GA. Also, the degeneration of nigral dopaminergic neurons in the basal ganglia is associated with motor (e.g., balance and sequential and rhythmic movements) and sensory (e.g., visuospatial processing) deficits [81] that could contribute to GA in PD. In neurologically healthy individuals, GA was observed to be heightened when faced with more challenging locomotion tasks. This pattern was also observed in older individuals [82], suggesting that GA is not exclusively associated to PD-related impairments but may also be influenced by the aging process.

Individuals with PD exhibit greater degree of asymmetry in leading and trailing toe clearance when stepping over double obstacles compared to their peers [8], indicating that the role of each limb during obstacle crossing is of considerable importance. Notably, the most affected limb tends to cross the obstacle at a shorter vertical distance than the least affected limb. Careful management of toe clearance is crucial, as reduced clearance increases the risk of stumbling over obstacles [79]. It is consistent in the literature that individuals with PD display decreased toe clearance parameters in comparison to neurologically healthy individuals [83–85]. Negotiating environments with obstacles increases the cognitive (processing and action planning), sensory (information from the environment), and motor (adaptive movements) demands to perform the task [86]. As a consequence of age-related impairments in motor, cognitive, and sensory systems [86], the act of locomotion in environments with obstacles becomes a challenging task, which can heighten GA.

Obstacle circumvention has been also demonstrated to increase GA in PD. Individuals with PD adopt a risky strategy when circumventing an obstacle towards their most affected side [5]. They begin the obstacle circumvention closer to the obstacle, resulting in shorter horizontal body clearance and smaller medial-lateral body clearance compared to circumventing the obstacle towards the least affected side. In addition, they increase the number and time of fixations on the ground and decrease these gaze parameters on the obstacle during the circumvention process towards the most affected side. This approach appears to accentuate the necessity for precise foot placement and trajectory to successfully circumvent the obstacle. In order to cope with this strategy, individuals with PD reduce their walking speed during both the approach and circumvention phases when circumventing the obstacle towards their most affected side [5]. This reduction of speed allows more time for planning foot placement accurately and executing precise foot movements [87].

The presence of proprioceptive deficits [88] and working memory impairments [89] is a common observation in individuals with PD. This renders them more reliant on real-time visual information to precisely adjust foot placement accuracy [79]. Speculatively, degeneration in the most affected brain hemisphere could also extend to perceptual brain regions. Previous studies have suggested that veering is side affected-dependent in individuals with PD [76]. Perceptual/sensorial asymmetry is a characteristic that manifest in the earliest stages of the disease [90], with its manifestation depending on the basal ganglia-cortical loops activated by the visual and motor demands of a given task [90].

Obstacle circumvention with dual-tasking increases GA during the approaching phase while reduces GA during the circumventing phase in individuals with PD [91]. Also, symmetry in stride duration, velocity, and double support time increases during the obstacle-avoidance phase under dual-tasking conditions. These findings highlight that the influence of dual-tasking on GA in individuals with PD is walking phase-dependent: GA increases during the late planning phase of obstacle circumvention and diminishes when the obstacle guides the movement. As the obstacle serves as a visual cue during obstacle circumvention, prompting goal-directed control of gait, these findings provides a basis for proposing that goal-directed movement control may regulate GA in individuals with PD. In light of the capacity sharing theory [92], one may argue that walking with dual-tasking in a challenging context may shift attention towards gait, thereby reducing GA. This finding contrasts with scenarios where individuals with PD engage in dual-tasking during overground walking, where the influence of dual-tasking heightens due to attention demands [93]. This insight holds practical implications. Healthcare professionals should incorporate goal-directed control activities into interventions for individuals with PD, enhancing ecologically-based training programs with the potential to diminish GA and better prepare individuals for challenging walking situations throughout the day [91].

Candidate Mechanisms to Explain Gait Asymmetry in Parkinson's Disease

Given that GA is exacerbated in individuals with PD, it is imperative to delve into potential mechanisms that may underlie this phenomenon. Figure 12.5 depicts the principal candidates to explain GA in PD. It is important to emphasize that our current understanding of the pathophysiology and mechanisms underlying GA in PD is still limited. While the connection between brain degeneration asymmetry and GA seems plausible, the neural mechanisms involved have yet to be extensively explored. Here, we outline six potential mechanisms that could account for GA in individuals with PD.

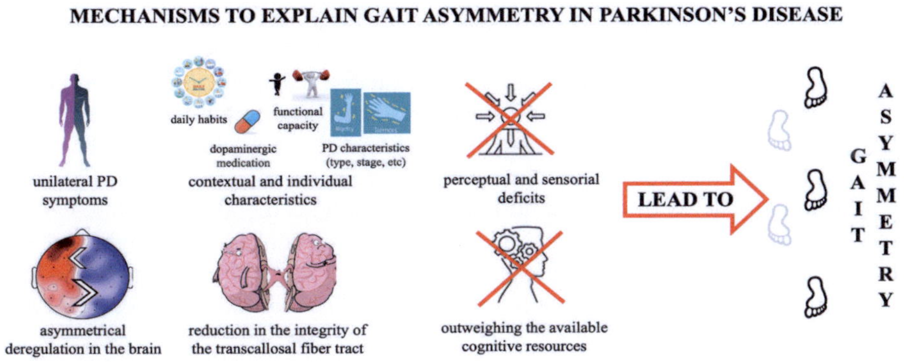

Fig. 12.5 Potential mechanisms to explain GA in individuals with PD

Unilateral PD Symptoms

It can be reasonably deduced that GA is primarily attributable to unilateral motor degradation. While GA is already observable in neurologically healthy individuals, largely due to the effects of aging, the exacerbation of this asymmetry in individuals with PD can be attributed to the unilateral motor degradation [5–8]. This can be understood within the context of the "state of asymmetry" [94], which reflects the unilateral progression of motor symptoms in PD resulting from asymmetric degeneration of nigral dopaminergic neurons. Additionally, the asymmetry in the distribution of these cells across the cortical-basal ganglia-thalamic circuitry also contributes [39]. Therefore, the observed increase in GA in PD suggests that the issue is more closely related to motor control rather than to mechanical factors.

Asymmetrical Deregulation/Degeneration in the Brain

GA observed in PD can be attributed to an asymmetrical depletion of dopamine in the substantia nigra [95], which results in an imbalanced in the regulation of the striatum and subsequent dysfunction in various circuits involving the basal ganglia and cortical regions [96]. The basal ganglia play a role in the generation and control of automatic and well-learned motor movements [97]. Firstly, the basal ganglia generate internal cues or triggers to facilitate the initiation of movement sequences without (or with minimal) attention. Secondly, they contribute to the cortical "motor set", thereby enabling the appropriate execution of motor functions. Consequently, dysfunction within the basal ganglia directly impacts gait control.

The gait deficits observed in PD are closely basal ganglia dysfunction and alterations in the size of key components, including the striatum, caudate, putamen, and globus pallidus [98]. Asymmetrical degeneration of the basal ganglia leads to uncoordinated limb movements in PD, resulting in GA [93]. This theory is consistent with the well-documented correlation between asymmetric motor symptoms and contralateral basal ganglia dopaminergic deficits [99]. Moreover, beyond the basal ganglia, other structural and functional aspects of the brain, such as the cerebral cortex, also ontribute to the elucidation of the precise mechanisms of GA in PD.

The malfunction of the cerebral cortex, particularly the motor, sensory, and frontal regions, is also directly related to gait issues in individuals with PD [98]. Furthemore, the literature also indicates that changes in cortical activity in PD occur with distinct patterns of cortical atrophy between the cerebral hemispheres as the disease progresses [3]. The impaired neuroanatomy connecting the right and left higher-order motor planning regions of the sensorimotor cortical hemispheres and the primary somatosensory cortices reduces the ability to spatially coordinate and control leg movements during gait in PD [7].

The progression of the disease appears to result in atrophy in specific cortical areas, with frontal brain regions being primarily affected in the early stages and the posterior regions being affected as the disease progresses [100]. Notably, a left hemisphere-predominant appendicular symptom increases the risk of developing FoG in the PD [101]. Given the close relationship between FoG and GA [19], it is suggested that the heightened involvement of the right hemisphere in PD is associated with an earlier and more frequent disturbances in the gait control [102], potentially contributing to GA in PD. A reduction in the activation of the right posterior parietal cortex is strongly correlated with the severity of gait disturbances [103]. These findings, when considered alongside other studies that have identified alterations in the right hemisphere of the brain in individuals with PD [104], suggest that abnormalities in the right hemisphere circuits associated with locomotion may contribute to the development of GA in PD.

Reduction in the Integrity of the Transcallosal Fiber Tract of the Pre-supplementary and Supplementary Motor Areas

Transcallosal communication via the corpus callosum plays a key role in the production of integrated motor behavior to generate appropriate and coordinated motor responses on both sides of the body [105, 106]. The primary motor cortices are linked to the contralateral muscles responsible for movement control and are extensively interconnected via the corpus callosum, thereby facilitating the transfer of information between the hemispheres. The precise bilateral coordination of movements in terms of timing and spatial aspects, such as walking, is dependent on interhemispheric communication. This process involves where the activation of one limb, which has an inhibitory effect on the ipsilateral motor cortex [107].

Fling and collaborators [105, 106] observed a robust associations between the integrity of callosal fiber tracts connecting the pre-supplementary and primary somatosensory cortical regions and step length asymmetries in individuals with PD. These findings suggest that reduced transcallosal sensorimotor structural connectivity may represent a pivotal mechanism underlying GA in individuals with PD. In addition, individuals with PD exhibit diminished microstructural integrity of white matter fibers connecting the pre-supplementary and supplementary regions responsible for higher-order motor control in both hemispheres. Specifically, the study points to trans-callosal connections between the pre-supplementary and primary somatosensory cortices as crucial fiber tracts associated with the diminished symmetrical control of gait in PD. Impaired connectivity between bilateral pre-supplementary areas results in a decreased ability to generate consistent steps in the spatial domain for individuals with PD [105, 106]. This mechanism provides the most substantial scientific evidence for explaining GA in PD to date.

Contextual and Individual Characteristics Trigger Gait Asymmetry in PD

Contextual factors play a significant role in the explanation of GA in individuals with PD. Studies have demonstrated differences in cerebral activity between the most and least affected sides, with levodopa exhibiting a preferential impact on brain activations in task-relevant regions [108]. The least affected side has demonstrated a preferential response to levodopa, which may be atributted to the lesser degeneration of the nigrostriatal dopaminergic terminals on that side [109]. Therefore, the medication state represents a crucial contextual factor in the explanation of GA in PD.

Asymmetries in functional capacity components, including postural control, strength, and coordination are also been linked to GA [94, 110]. Particularly, step temporal parameter asymmetry is strongly associated with the functional outcomes [111]. Swing time asymmetry may result from challenges in propelling the leading limb forward during the swing phase or maintaining balance during the stance phase [111]. Besides, general characteristics, such as age and daily habits, as well as clinical features like disease type and stage, can also exert an influence on the level of GA [4].

Motor asymmetry tends to decrease as PD progresses [4, 112]. A similar trend may occur in GA. In addition, the postural instability and gait disturbances PD subtype is associated with a greater degree degeneration of the left hemisphere [113], which is involved in movement planning and control [114]. Therefore, the side of PD onset may be associated with motor asymmetry (GA), indicating disparate neural degeneration patterns between patients whose initial symptoms manifested on the right and left sides of the body [115]. These contextual factors collectively contribute to the complex and multifaceted picture of GA in PD.

Outweighing the Available Cognitive Resources During Walking

The motor cortical regions, which encompass the primary motor cortex, supplementary motor area, and premotor area, are intricately connected with the basal ganglia and cerebellum, forming a motor loop that is crucial for the execution of gait and the programming of motor actions [98]. As the basal ganglia increase inhibitory output to thalamocortical projections and cognitive information processing diminishes in individuals with PD, the capacity to generate motor programs in response to changing contexts becomes compromised [98]. Consequently, individuals not only demonstrated a reduction in automatism during walking but also encounter difficulties in generating the appropriate postural adjustments that are essential for maintenace of a safe and efficient gait. This suggests that individuals with PD face heightened cognitive demands in gait control due to reduced excitability in motor cortical areas [98].

Given the cognitive deficits often present in individuals with PD, their limited cognitive capacity makes even basic motor programming tasks, such as walking, require an additional cognitive load. Consequently, individuals with PD experience difficulties in augmenting the cognitive demands required for efficient gait programming, resulting in an imbalance between the necessary and available cognitive resources, which ultimately contributes to GA. In addition, higher cognitive demand placed on individuals with PD may be considered a maladaptive change due to the increased neural and/or hemodynamic activity required for the same computation task, ultimately leading to neural inefficiency [51, 52]. This complex interaction between cognitive demand, motor programming, and neural efficiency is a significant key factor in understanding the phenomenon of GA in PD.

Perceptual and Sensorial Deficits in PD

Individuals with PD demonstrate an increased reliance on perceptual and sensorial information, particularly visual cues, during walking, particularly in situations involving obstacle avoidance and dual-tasking. Possibly, the greater dependency on perceptual and sensorial information is attributed to damage in the basal ganglia [39], as well as damage to the right hemisphere, which is responsible for visuospatial processing [116]. Evidence suggests that the basal ganglia play a pivotal role in sensorimotor integration [97]. It has been demonstrated that striatal cells demonstrate robust activation is response to the presentation of sensory cues that trigger movements. However, the loss of dopamine in the striatum, which is common in PD, can impede the effective transfer of essential information to the basal ganglia, resulting in a reduced ability to detect crucial internal sensory and movement cues [116]. Such disruption in the relay of information to the basal ganglia can exacerbate difficulties in movement selection and sequencing within the dopamine-depleted striatum, leading to gait abnormalities [117], including GA.

The pattern of motor deficits observed in individuals with PD is consistent with a disruption of sensorimotor integration mechanisms. Individuals with PD may be compelled to increasingly rely on external stimuli to initiate and shape their motor actions due to the lack of critical proprioceptive information [118]. Importantly, it should be noted that the damage to the basal ganglia is asymmetric in PD. Therefore, it can be surmised that the asymmetrical control of the basal ganglia suggests that deficits in utilizing the most affected limb or circumventing obstacles on the most affected side extend beyond the motor system impairment to encompass the sensorial and perceptual domains. It is reasonable to suggest that the degeneration observed in the more affected hemisphere of the brain also extends to the areas responsible for sensory and perceptual processing, further contributing to the explanation of GA in PD.

Recommendations for Gait Asymmetry Rehabilitation in Parkinson's Disease

Motor and non-motor interventions have potential to mitigate GA in individuals with PD. It is widely acknowledged that dopaminergic medication serves as the primary treatment for PD. Notwithstanding its efficacy in ameliorating motor symptoms and reducing GA, the impact of dopaminergic medication diminishes gradually over time, accompanied by the emergence of side effects, such as dyskinesias, which impede gait [57]. Furthermore pharmacological therapy has been demonstrated to be ineffective in addressing certain aspects of motor control, including cadence and postural adjustments [119]. As a result, complementary interventions have become an indispensable component of PD treatment. Motor training represents as an intriguing strategy for addressing GA in individuals with PD. However, to date, there is a limited knowledge regarding interventions that can mitigate GA in this population, necessitating validation through future studies. Despite that, certain strategies for GA rehabilitation can be recommended:

1. *Balance Training for Postural Control Asymmetry:* A reduction in the degree of asymmetry in postural control may represent an initial step towards the alleviation of GA in individuals with PD. As postural control asymmetry correlates with falls and plays a pivotal role in stability [120], it is advisable to integrate balance exercises that target each leg specifically in order to rectify postural control asymmetry. Improved balance can facilitate greater stability and improved compensatory mechanisms between the legs, consequently leading to reduced GA.
2. *Incorporation of Visual Cues:* The utilisation of visual cues, such as obstacles, has been demonstrated to enhance gait control, particularly in the more affected limb. This approach has the potential to reduce the impact of GA. The utilization of visual cues, such as obstacles, has been demonstrated to trigger a shift in gait control towards goal-directed mechanisms [91, 121], thereby facilitating the implementation of more deliberate motor control strategies. This approach circumvents portions of the basal ganglia that are implicated in automated motor control, relying on regions (such as the rostromedial striatum) less impacted by dopaminergic loss [121], which regulates GA. Furthermore, visual cues also have the potential to reduce cortical activity asymmetry [37, 122]. A higher level of cortical activity asymmetry may be regarded as a maladaptive change [51, 52], thus resulting in a greater degree of asymmetry.
3. *Goal-Directed Control Activities:* The incorporation of goal-directed control activities within ecologically-based training programes can enhance gait efficiency and reduce asymmetry. Such activities prepare individuals with PD with the capacity to adapt to challenging walking scenarios encountered in daily life.

Considering the diminished automaticity of gait in individuals with PD and their dificculties with automatic walking [123], coordination activities that require goal-directed control may prove an effective strategy for enhancing gait control.

4. *Minimization of Most Affected Limb Usage:* Advising individuals with PD to minimize using the most affected limb when stepping over or navigating obstacles, particularly during periods of medication depletion, can help to prevent unsafe gait adaptations and attenuate GA. Nevertheless, implementing this recommendation is challenging due to the complexities of daily locomotion and the limited time available for individuals to choose the least affected limb. Alternatively, a more viable approach may train the most affected limb to perform locomotor activities with greater efficacy, which could result in a reduction in GA.
5. *Training Targeted at the Most Affected Limb:* The potential benefits of targeted training for the most affected limb in terms of enhancing mobility, stability, and gait coordination holds promise. Asymmetric training exercises have the potential to enhance the function of the weaker limb, which may subsequently lead to a reduction in GA. Previous studies have demonstrated that extra doses of exercise, particularly in the most affected limb, facilitate enhanced mobility and gait stability, thereby mitigating GA [124].

Final Remarks

Accentuated GA is a distinctive trait among individuals with PD. An understanding of the underlying dynamics of this phenomenon is of significance in the context of managing gait-related interventions for individuals with PD. Intriguingly, despite the absence of motor asymmetry during gait initiation in individuals with PD, cortical activity asymmetry is evident. On the other hand, asymmetry emerges in multiple gait parameters during overground walking and challenging walking tasks, such as obstacle avoidance and dual-tasking. Notably, challenging walking accentuates GA,with the exception of instances of obstacle circumvention coupled with dual-tasking, where GA appears to diminish. The simultaneous effort of consciously controlling walking while skillfully avoiding obstacles may, in fact, outweigh the available resources, consequently leading to a change in GA.

In order to elucidate the intricate mechanisms underpinning GA, it is imperative to unravel the underlying causative factors. This comprehension is pivotal not only in explaining this behavior but also in formulating efficacious strategies for rehabilitation. Regrettably, our understanding of the pathophysiological underpinnings and the driving mechanisms behind GA in PD remains limited. Although the link between asymmetrical brain degeneration and GA appears plausible, the precise neural mechanisms remain largely uncharted. Consequently, while recommendations aimed at addressing GA can be proposed, their effectiveness still necessitates robust validation.

Acknowledgments This study was financially supported by São Paulo Research Foundation (FAPESP, #2016/14950-6; #2018/21870-7; #2019/24752-8; #2022/09235-0; #2022/02971-2) and partly supported by the Coordenação de Aperfeiçoamento de Pessoal de Nível Superior-Brasil (CAPES)-Finance Code 001, and the National Council for Scientific and Technological Development—CNPq.

References

1. Sadeghi H, Allard P, Prince F, Labelle H. Symmetry and limb dominance in able-bodied gait: a review. Gait Posture. 2000;12(1):34–45. https://doi.org/10.1016/S0966-6362(00)00070-9.
2. Hughes AJ, Daniel SE, Kilford L, Lees AJ. Accuracy of clinical diagnosis of idiopathic Parkinson's disease: a clinico-pathological study of 100 cases. J Neurol Neurosurg Psychiatry. 1992;55(3):181–4. https://doi.org/10.1136/jnnp.55.3.181.
3. Claassen DO, McDonell KE, Donahue M, Rawal S, Wylie SA, Neimat JS, Kang H, Hedera P, Zald D, Landman B, Dawant B, Rane S. Cortical asymmetry in Parkinson's disease: early susceptibility of the left hemisphere. Brain Behav. 2016;6(12):e00573.
4. Riederer P, Sian-Hülsmann J. The significance of neuronal lateralisation in Parkinson's disease. J Neural Transm. 2012;119(8):953–62. https://doi.org/10.1007/s00702-012-0775-1.
5. Barbieri FA, Polastri PF, Gobbi LTB, Simieli L, Pereira VIA, Baptista AM, Moretto GF, Fiorelli CM, Imaizumi LFI, Rodrigues ST. Obstacle circumvention and eye coordination during walking to least and most affected side in people with Parkinson's disease. Behav Brain Res. 2018;346:105–14. https://doi.org/10.1016/j.bbr.2017.11.032.
6. Barbieri FA, Simieli L, Orcioli-Silva D, Baptista AM, Borkowske Pestana M, Spiandor Beretta V, dos Santos PCR, Bucken Gobbi LT. Obstacle avoidance increases asymmetry of crossing step in individuals with Parkinson's disease and neurologically healthy individuals. J Mot Behav. 2018;50(1):17–25. https://doi.org/10.1080/00222895.2016.1271303.
7. Fling BW, Curtze C, Horak FB. Gait asymmetry in people with Parkinson's disease is linked to reduced integrity of callosal sensorimotor regions. Front Neurol. 2018;9 https://doi.org/10.3389/fneur.2018.00215.
8. Orcioli-Silva D, Barbieri FA, dos Santos PCR, Beretta VS, Simieli L, Vitorio R, Lirani-Silva E, Gobbi LTB. Double obstacles increase gait asymmetry during obstacle crossing in people with Parkinson's disease and healthy older adults: a pilot study. Sci Rep. 2020;10(1):2272. https://doi.org/10.1038/s41598-020-59266-y.
9. Hugdahl K. Symmetry and asymmetry in the human brain. Eur Rev. 2005;13(S2):119–33. https://doi.org/10.1017/S1062798705000700.
10. Anne Shumway-Cook MHW. Motor control: translating research into clinical practiceno title. Baltimore: Lippincott Williams & Wilkins; 2016. p. 680.
11. Tommasi L. Mechanisms and functions of brain and behavioural asymmetries. Philos Trans R Soc Lond Ser B Biol Sci. 2009;364(1519):855–9. https://doi.org/10.1098/RSTB.2008.0293.
12. Maloney SJ. The relationship between asymmetry and athletic performance: a critical review. J Strength Cond Res. 2019;33(9):2579–93. https://doi.org/10.1519/JSC.0000000000002608.
13. Plotnik M, Hausdorff JM. The role of gait rhythmicity and bilateral coordination of stepping in the pathophysiology of freezing of gait in Parkinson's disease. Mov Disord. 2008;23(S2):S444–50. https://doi.org/10.1002/mds.21984.
14. Güntürkün O, Ocklenburg S. Ontogenesis of lateralization. Neuron. 2017;94(2):249–63. https://doi.org/10.1016/J.NEURON.2017.02.045.
15. Carpes FP, Mota CB, Faria IE. On the bilateral asymmetry during running and cycling—a review considering leg preference. Phys Ther Sport. 2010;11(4):136–42. https://doi.org/10.1016/j.ptsp.2010.06.005.
16. Marcori AJ, Okazaki VHA. A historical, systematic review of handedness origins. Laterality. 2020;25(1):87–108. https://doi.org/10.1080/1357650X.2019.1614597.

17. Robinson RO, Herzog W, Nigg BM. Use of force platform variables to quantify the effects of chiropractic manipulation on gait symmetry. J Manip Physiol Ther. 1987;10(4):172–6. http://www.ncbi.nlm.nih.gov/pubmed/2958572
18. Zifchock RA, Davis I, Higginson J, Royer T. The symmetry angle: a novel, robust method of quantifying asymmetry. Gait Posture. 2008;27(4):622–7. https://doi.org/10.1016/J.GAITPOST.2007.08.006.
19. Plotnik M, Giladi N, Balash Y, Peretz C, Hausdorff JM. Is freezing of gait in Parkinson's disease related to asymmetric motor function? Ann Neurol. 2005;57(5):656–63. https://doi.org/10.1002/ana.20452.
20. Ganguli S, Mukherji P, Bose KS. Gait evaluation of unilateral below-knee amputees fitted with patellar-tendon-bearing prostheses. J Indian Med Assoc. 1974;63(8):256–9. http://www.ncbi.nlm.nih.gov/pubmed/4443595
21. Queen R, Dickerson L, Ranganathan S, Schmitt D. A novel method for measuring asymmetry in kinematic and kinetic variables: the Normalized Symmetry Index. J Biomech. 2020;99:109531. https://doi.org/10.1016/J.JBIOMECH.2019.109531.
22. Błażkiewicz M, Wiszomirska I, Wit A. Comparison of four methods of calculating the symmetry of spatial-temporal parameters of gait. Acta Bioeng Biomech. 2014;16(1):29–35. http://www.ncbi.nlm.nih.gov/pubmed/24708092
23. Cabral S, Resende RA, Clansey AC, Deluzio KJ, Selbie WS, Veloso AP. A global gait asymmetry index. J Appl Biomech. 2016;32(2):171–7. https://doi.org/10.1123/jab.2015-0114.
24. Hill A, Nantel J. Sensitivity of discrete symmetry metrics: implications for metric choice. PLoS One. 2022;17(5):e0268581. https://doi.org/10.1371/journal.pone.0268581.
25. Alves SA, Ehrig RM, Raffalt PC, Bender A, Duda GN, Agres AN. Quantifying asymmetry in gait: the weighted universal symmetry index to evaluate 3D ground reaction forces. Front Bioeng Biotechnol. 2020;8(October) https://doi.org/10.3389/fbioe.2020.579511.
26. Postuma RB, Berg D, Stern M, Poewe W, Olanow CW, Oertel W, Obeso J, Marek K, Litvan I, Lang AE, Halliday G, Goetz CG, Gasser T, Dubois B, Chan P, Bloem BR, Adler CH, Deuschl G. MDS clinical diagnostic criteria for Parkinson's disease. Mov Disord. 2015;30(12):1591–601. https://doi.org/10.1002/mds.26424.
27. Uitti RJ, Baba Y, Whaley NR, Wszolek ZK, Putzke JD. Parkinson disease: handedness predicts asymmetry. Neurology. 2005;64(11):1925–30. https://doi.org/10.1212/01.WNL.0000163993.82388.C8.
28. Gasparoli E, Delibori D, Polesello G, Santeli L, Ermani M, Battistin L, Bracco F. Clinical predictors in Parkinson's disease. Neurolog Sci. 2002;23(SUPPL. 2):s77. https://doi.org/10.1007/S100720200078.
29. Hely MA, Morris JGL, Reid WGJ, O'Sullivan DJ, Williamson PM, Broe GA, Adena MA. Age at onset: the major determinant of outcome in Parkinson's disease. Acta Neurol Scand. 1995;92(6):455–63. https://doi.org/10.1111/J.1600-0404.1995.TB00480.X.
30. Gómez-Esteban JC, Tijero B, Ciordia R, Berganzo K, Somme J, Lezcano E, Zarranz JJ. Factors influencing the symmetry of Parkinson's disease symptoms. Clin Neurol Neurosurg. 2010;112(4):302–5. https://doi.org/10.1016/J.CLINEURO.2009.12.017.
31. Munhoz RP, Teive HA, Eleftherohorinou H, Coin LJ, Lees AJ, Silveira-Moriyama L. Demographic and motor features associated with the occurrence of neuropsychiatric and sleep complications of Parkinson's disease. J Neurol Neurosurg Psychiatry. 2013;84(8):883–7. https://doi.org/10.1136/JNNP-2012-304440.
32. Uc EY, McDermott MP, Marder KS, Anderson SW, Litvan I, Como PG, Auinger P, Chou KL, Growdon JC. Incidence of and risk factors for cognitive impairment in an early Parkinson disease clinical trial cohort. Neurology. 2009;73(18):1469–77. https://doi.org/10.1212/WNL.0B013E3181BF992F.
33. Aarsland D, Andersen K, Larsen JP, Lolk A, Kragh-Sørensen P. Prevalence and characteristics of dementia in Parkinson disease: an 8-year prospective study. Arch Neurol. 2003;60(3):387–92. https://doi.org/10.1001/ARCHNEUR.60.3.387.

34. van der Hoorn A, Bartels AL, Leenders KL, de Jong BM. Handedness and dominant side of symptoms in Parkinson's disease. Parkinsonism Relat Disord. 2011;17(1):58–60. https://doi.org/10.1016/j.parkreldis.2010.10.002.
35. Huang P, Tan YY, Liu DQ, Herzallah MM, Lapidow E, Wang Y, Zang YF, Gluck MA, Chen SD. Motor-symptom laterality affects acquisition in Parkinson's disease: a cognitive and functional magnetic resonance imaging study. Mov Disord. 2017;32(7):1047–55. https://doi.org/10.1002/MDS.27000.
36. Yoo K, Chung SJ, Kim HS, Choung OH, Lee YB, Kim MJ, You S, Jeong Y. Neural substrates of motor and non-motor symptoms in Parkinson's disease: a resting fMRI study. PLoS One. 2015;10(4):e0125455. https://doi.org/10.1371/JOURNAL.PONE.0125455.
37. Faria MH, Simieli L, Rietdyk S, Penedo T, Santinelli FB, Barbieri FA. (A) Symmetry during gait initiation in people with Parkinson's disease: a motor and cortical activity exploratory study. Front Aging Neurosci. 2023;15:1142540.
38. Lewis SJG, Barker RA. A pathophysiological model of freezing of gait in Parkinson's disease. Parkinsonism Relat Disord. 2009;15(5):333–8. https://doi.org/10.1016/j.parkreldis.2008.08.006.
39. Tatsch K, Schwarz J, Mozley PD, Linke R, Pogarell O, Oertel WH, Fieber RS, Hahn K, Kung HF. Relationship between clinical features of Parkinson's disease and presynaptic dopamine transporter binding assessed with [123I]IPT and single-photon emission tomography. Eur J Nucl Med. 1997;24(4):415–21. https://doi.org/10.1007/BF00881814.
40. Potgieser ARE, De Jong BM. Different distal-proximal movement balances in right- and left-hand writing may hint at differential premotor cortex involvement. Hum Mov Sci. 2011;30(6):1072–8. https://doi.org/10.1016/j.humov.2011.02.005.
41. Djaldetti R, Ziv I, Melamed E. The mystery of motor asymmetry in Parkinson's disease. Lancet Neurol. 2006;5(9):796–802. https://doi.org/10.1016/S1474-4422(06)70549-X.
42. Borghammer P. The α-Synuclein Origin and Connectome model (SOC model) of Parkinson's disease: explaining motor asymmetry, non-motor phenotypes, and cognitive decline. J Parkinsons Dis. 2021;11(2):455–74. https://doi.org/10.3233/JPD-202481.
43. Savica R, Bradley BF, Mielke MM. When do α-synucleinopathies start? An epidemiological timeline: a review. JAMA Neurol. 2018;75(4):503–9. https://doi.org/10.1001/JAMANEUROL.2017.4243.
44. Roemmich RT, Nocera JR, Stegemöller EL, Hassan A, Okun MS, Hass CJ. Locomotor adaptation and locomotor adaptive learning in Parkinson's disease and normal aging. Clin Neurophysiol. 2014;125(2):313–9. https://doi.org/10.1016/j.clinph.2013.07.003.
45. Yogev G, Plotnik M, Peretz C, Giladi N, Hausdorff JM. Gait asymmetry in patients with Parkinson's disease and elderly fallers: when does the bilateral coordination of gait require attention? Exp Brain Res. 2007;177(3):336–46. https://doi.org/10.1007/s00221-006-0676-3.
46. Nocera JR, Roemmich R, Elrod J, Altmann LJP, Hass CJ. Effects of cognitive task on gait initiation in Parkinson disease: evidence of motor prioritization? J Rehabil Res Dev. 2013;50(5):699. https://doi.org/10.1682/JRRD.2012.06.0114.
47. Delval A, Tard C, Defebvre L. Why we should study gait initiation in Parkinson's disease. Neurophysiologie Clinique/Clin Neurophysiol. 2014;44(1):69–76.
48. Simieli, L.. Effect of Parkinson's disease on gait initiation: a sytematic review. J Parkinsonism Rel Disord. 2021.
49. Boonstra TA, van Kordelaar J, Engelhart D, van Vugt JP, van der Kooij H. Asymmetries in reactive and anticipatory balance control are of similar magnitude in Parkinson's disease patients. Gait Posture. 2016;43:108–13. https://doi.org/10.1016/j.gaitpost.2015.08.014. Epub 2015 Sep 26. PMID: 26475760
50. Hass CJ, Waddell DE, Fleming RP, Juncos JL, Gregor RJ. Gait initiation and dynamic balance control in Parkinson's disease. Arch Phys Med Rehabil. 2005;86(11):2172–6.
51. Berenguer-Rocha M, Baltar A, Rocha S, Shirahige L, Brito R, Monte-Silva K. Interhemispheric asymmetry of the motor cortex excitability in stroke: relationship with sensory-motor impairment and injury chronicity. Neurol Sci. 2020;41(9):2591–8. https://doi.org/10.1007/s10072-020-04350-4.

52. Knights E, Morcom AM, Henson RN. Does hemispheric asymmetry reduction in older adults in motor cortex reflect compensation? J Neurosci. 2021;41(45):9361–73. https://doi.org/10.1523/JNEUROSCI.1111-21.2021.
53. Hesse S, Reiter F, Jahnke M, Dawson M, Sarkodie-Gyan T, Mauritz KH. Asymmetry of gait initiation in hemiparetic stroke subjects. Arch Phys Med Rehabil. 1997;78(7):719–24. https://doi.org/10.1016/S0003-9993(97)90079-4.
54. Viton JM, Timsit M, Mesure S, Massion J, Franceschi JP, Delarque A. Asymmetry of gait initiation in patients with unilateral knee arthritis. Arch Phys Med Rehabil. 2000;81(2):194–200. https://doi.org/10.1053/apmr.2000.0810194.
55. Bensoussan L, Mesure S, Viton JM, Delarque A. Kinematic and kinetic asymmetries in hemiplegic patients' gait initiation patterns. J Rehabil Med. 2006;38(5):287–94. https://doi.org/10.1080/16501970600694859.
56. Yogev-Seligmann G, Hausdorff JM, Giladi N. Do we always prioritize balance when walking? Towards an integrated model of task prioritization. Mov Disord. 2012;27(6):765–70. https://doi.org/10.1002/mds.24963.
57. Obeso JA, Rodríguez-Oroz MC, Benitez-Temino B, Blesa FJ, Guridi J, Marin C, Rodriguez M. Functional organization of the basal ganglia: therapeutic implications for Parkinson's disease. Mov Disord. 2008;23(S3):S548–59. https://doi.org/10.1002/mds.22062.
58. Fling BW, Peltier SJ, Bo J, Welsh RC, Seidler RD. Age differences in interhemispheric interactions: callosal structure, physiological function, and behavior. Front Neurosci. 2011;5(MAR) https://doi.org/10.3389/FNINS.2011.00038.
59. Mostile G, Nicoletti A, Dibilio V, Luca A, Pappalardo I, Giuliano L, Cicero CE, Sciacca G, Raciti L, Contrafatto D, Bruno E, Sofia V, Zappia M. Electroencephalographic lateralization, clinical correlates and pharmacological response in untreated Parkinson's disease. Parkinsonism Relat Disord. 2015;21(8):948–53. https://doi.org/10.1016/j.parkreldis.2015.06.006.
60. Miller RA, Thaut MH, McIntosh GC, Rice RR. Components of EMG symmetry and variability in parkinsonian and healthy elderly gait. Electroencephalogr Clin Neurophysiol. 1996;101(1):1–7. https://doi.org/10.1016/0013-4694(95)00209-X.
61. Baltadjieva R, Giladi N, Gruendlinger L, Peretz C, Hausdorff JM. Marked alterations in the gait timing and rhythmicity of patients with de novo Parkinson's disease. Eur J Neurosci. 2006;24(6):1815–20. https://doi.org/10.1111/J.1460-9568.2006.05033.X.
62. Galna B, Lord S, Burn DJ, Rochester L. Progression of gait dysfunction in incident Parkinson's disease: impact of medication and phenotype. Mov Disord. 2015;30(3):359–67. https://doi.org/10.1002/mds.26110.
63. Grajić M, Stanković I, Radovanović S, Kostić V. Gait in drug naïve patients with de novo Parkinson's disease—altered but symmetric. Neurol Res. 2015;37(8):712–6. https://doi.org/10.1179/1743132815Y.0000000043.
64. Su BL, Song R, Guo LY, Yen CW. Characterizing gait asymmetry via frequency sub-band components of the ground reaction force. Biomed Signal Process Control. 2015;18:56–60. https://doi.org/10.1016/J.BSPC.2014.11.008.
65. Vervoort G, Bengevoord A, Nackaerts E, Heremans E, Vandenberghe W, Nieuwboer A. Distal motor deficit contributions to postural instability and gait disorder in Parkinson's disease. Behav Brain Res. 2015;287:1–7. https://doi.org/10.1016/j.bbr.2015.03.026.
66. Del Din S, Godfrey A, Galna B, Lord S, Rochester L. Free-living gait characteristics in ageing and Parkinson's disease: impact of environment and ambulatory bout length. J Neuroeng Rehabil. 2016;13(1):46. https://doi.org/10.1186/S12984-016-0154-5.
67. Djurić-Jovičić M, Belić M, Stanković I, Radovanović S, Kostić VS. Selection of gait parameters for differential diagnostics of patients with de novo Parkinson's disease. Neurol Res. 2017;39(10):853–61. https://doi.org/10.1080/01616412.2017.1348690.
68. Morris R, Hickey A, Del Din S, Godfrey A, Lord S, Rochester L. A model of free-living gait: a factor analysis in Parkinson's disease. Gait Posture. 2017;52:68–71. https://doi.org/10.1016/j.gaitpost.2016.11.024.

69. Morris R, Lord S, Lawson RA, Coleman S, Galna B, Duncan GW, Khoo TK, Yarnall AJ, Burn DJ, Rochester L. Gait rather than cognition predicts decline in specific cognitive domains in early Parkinson's disease. J Gerontol A Biol Sci Med Sci. 2017;72(12):1656–62. https://doi.org/10.1093/GERONA/GLX071.
70. Ren P, Karahan E, Chen C, Luo R, Geng Y, Bosch Bayard JF, Bringas ML, Yao D, Kendrick KM, Valdes-Sosa PA. Gait influence diagrams in Parkinson's disease. IEEE Trans Neural Syst Rehabil Eng. 2017;25(8):1257–67. https://doi.org/10.1109/TNSRE.2016.2622285.
71. Martínez M, Villagra F, Castellote JM, Pastor MA. Kinematic and kinetic patterns related to free-walking in Parkinson's disease. Sensors (Basel, Switzerland). 2018;18(12) https://doi.org/10.3390/S18124224.
72. Son M, Cheon SM, Youm C, Kim Y, Kim JW. Impacts of freezing of gait on forward and backward gait in Parkinson's disease. Gait Posture. 2018;61:320–4. https://doi.org/10.1016/j.gaitpost.2018.01.034.
73. Gilmore G, Gouelle A, Adamson MB, Pieterman M, Jog M. Forward and backward walking in Parkinson disease: a factor analysis. Gait Posture. 2019;74:14–9. https://doi.org/10.1016/j.gaitpost.2019.08.005.
74. Koh S-B, Park Y-M, Kim M-J, Kim W-S. Influences of elbow, shoulder, trunk motion and temporospatial parameters on arm swing asymmetry of Parkinson's disease during walking. Hum Mov Sci. 2019;68(May):102527. https://doi.org/10.1016/j.humov.2019.102527.
75. Del Din S, Godfrey A, Coleman S, Galna B, Lord S, Rochester L. Time-dependent changes in postural control in early Parkinson's disease: what are we missing? Med Biol Eng Comput. 2016;54(2–3):401–10. https://doi.org/10.1007/s11517-015-1324-5.
76. Ren X, Salazar R, Neargarder S, Roy S, Ellis TD, Saltzman E, Cronin-Golomb A. Veering in hemi-Parkinson's disease: primacy of visual over motor contributions. Vis Res. 2015;115(Pt A):119–27. https://doi.org/10.1016/J.VISRES.2015.08.011.
77. Lord S, Galna B, Yarnall AJ, Coleman S, Burn D, Rochester L. Predicting first fall in newly diagnosed Parkinson's disease: insights from a fall-naïve cohort. J Mov Disord. 2016;31(12):1829–36. https://doi.org/10.1002/MDS.26742.
78. Alcock L, Galna B, Hausdorff JM, Lord S, Rochester L. Gait & Posture special issue: gait adaptations in response to obstacle type in fallers with Parkinson's disease. Gait Posture. 2018;61(January):368–74. https://doi.org/10.1016/j.gaitpost.2018.01.030.
79. Vitório R, Lirani-Silva E, Baptista AM, Barbieri FA, dos Santos PCR, Teixeira-Arroyo C, Gobbi LTB. Disease severity affects obstacle crossing in people with Parkinson's disease. Gait Posture. 2014;40(1):266–9. https://doi.org/10.1016/j.gaitpost.2014.03.003.
80. Snijders AH, Weerdesteyn V, Hagen YJ, Duysens J, Giladi N, Bloem BR. Obstacle avoidance to elicit freezing of gait during treadmill walking. Mov Disord. 2010;25(1):57–63. https://doi.org/10.1002/MDS.22894.
81. Magrinelli F, Picelli A, Tocco P, Federico A, Roncari L, Smania N, Zanette G, Tamburin S. Pathophysiology of motor dysfunction in Parkinson's disease as the rationale for drug treatment and rehabilitation. J Parkinson's Dis. 2016;2016:1–18. https://doi.org/10.1155/2016/9832839.
82. Wong DW-C, Lam W-K, Lee WC-C. Gait asymmetry and variability in older adults during long-distance walking: implications for gait instability. Clin Biomech. 2020;72:37–43. https://doi.org/10.1016/j.clinbiomech.2019.11.023.
83. Orcioli-Silva D, Barbieri FA, Simieli L, Vitorio R, dos Santos PCR, Beretta VS, Gobbi LTB, Rocha PC, Santos D, Spiandor Beretta V, Teresa L, Gobbi B. Walking behavior over multiple obstacles in people with Parkinson's disease. Gait Posture. 2017;58:510–5. https://doi.org/10.1016/j.gaitpost.2017.09.021.
84. Orcioli-Silva D, Vitório R, Lirani-Silva E, Santos PCR, Beretta VS, Gobbi LTB. Objective measures of unobstructed walking and obstacle avoidance in Parkinson's disease subtypes. Gait Posture. 2018;62:405–8. https://doi.org/10.1016/J.GAITPOST.2018.03.046.
85. Simieli L, Barbieri FA, Orcioli-Silva D, Lirani-Silva E, Beretta VS, dos Santos PCR, Gobbi LTB. Variability of crossing phase in older people with Parkinson's disease is dependent of obstacle height. Sci Rep. 2018;8(1):14852. https://doi.org/10.1038/s41598-018-33312-2.

86. Kovacs CR. Age-related changes in gait and obstacle avoidance capabilities in older adults: a review. J Appl Gerontol. 2016;24(1):21–34. https://doi.org/10.1177/0733464804271279.
87. Barbieri FA, dos Santos PCR, Simieli L, Orcioli-Silva D, van Dieën JH, Gobbi LTB. Interactions of age and leg muscle fatigue on unobstructed walking and obstacle crossing. Gait Posture. 2014;39(3):985–90. https://doi.org/10.1016/j.gaitpost.2013.12.021.
88. Konczak J, Corcos DM, Horak F, Poizner H, Shapiro M, Tuite P, Volkmann J, Maschke M. Proprioception and motor control in Parkinson's disease. J Mot Behav. 2009;41(6):543–52. https://doi.org/10.3200/35-09-002.
89. Lee AC, Harris JP, Atkinson EA, Fowler MS. Disruption of estimation of body-scaled aperture width in Hemiparkinson's disease. Neuropsychologia. 2001;39(10):1097–104. https://doi.org/10.1016/S0028-3932(01)00032-X.
90. Harris JP, Atkinson EA, Lee AC, Nithi K, Fowler MS. Hemispace differences in the visual perception of size in left hemiParkinson's disease. Neuropsychologia. 2003;41(7):795–807. https://doi.org/10.1016/S0028-3932(02)00285-3.
91. Corradini JR, Silveira-Ciola AP, Pereira VAI, Kuroda MH, Faria MH, Simieli L, Tavares JMRS, Barbieri FA. Dual tasking reduces gait asymmetry of trajectory deviation during obstacle circumvention in people with Parkinson's disease. Hum Mov Sci. 2022;83:102938. https://doi.org/10.1016/j.humov.2022.102938.
92. Tombu M, Jolicœur P. A central capacity sharing model of dual-task performance. J Exp Psychol Hum Percept Perform. 2003;29(1):3–18. https://doi.org/10.1037/0096-1523.29.1.3.
93. Plotnik M, Giladi N, Hausdorff JM. Bilateral coordination of gait and Parkinson's disease: the effects of dual tasking. J Neurol Neurosurg Psychiatry. 2009;80(3):347–50. https://doi.org/10.1136/jnnp.2008.157362.
94. Beretta VS, Gobbi LTB, Lirani-Silva E, Simieli L, Orcioli-Silva D, Barbieri FA. Challenging postural tasks increase asymmetry in patients with Parkinson's disease. PLoS One. 2015;10(9):1–11. https://doi.org/10.1371/journal.pone.0137722.
95. Kaasinen V, Nurmi E, Bergman J, Eskola O, Solin O, Sonninen P, Rinne J. Personality traits and brain dopaminergic function in Parkinson's disease. Proc Natl Acad Sci. 2001;98(23):13272–7.
96. Clower DM, Dum RP, Strick PL. Basal ganglia and cerebellar inputs to "AIP". Cerebral Cortex (New York, NY: 1991). 2005;15(7):913–20. https://doi.org/10.1093/CERCOR/BHH190.
97. Muthukrishnan N, Abbas JJ, Shill HA, Krishnamurthi N. Cueing paradigms to improve gait and posture in Parkinson's disease: a narrative review. Sensors (Basel, Switzerland). 2019;19(24) https://doi.org/10.3390/S19245468.
98. Takakusaki K. Functional neuroanatomy for posture and gait control. J Mov Disord. 2017;10(1):1–17. https://doi.org/10.14802/jmd.16062.
99. Prasad S, Saini J, Yadav R, Pal PK. Motor asymmetry and neuromelanin imaging: concordance in Parkinson's disease. Parkinsonism Relat Disord. 2018;53:28–32.
100. Wang J, Yang QX, Sun X, Vesek J, Mosher Z, Vasavada M, Chu J, Kanekar S, Shivkumar V, Venkiteswaran K, Subramanian T. MRI evaluation of asymmetry of nigrostriatal damage in the early stage of early-onset Parkinson's disease. Parkinsonism Relat Disord. 2015;21(6):590–6. https://doi.org/10.1016/j.parkreldis.2015.03.012.
101. Giladi N, McDermott MP, Fahn S, Przedborski S, Jankovic J, Stern M, Tanner C. Freezing of gait in PD: prospective assessment in the DATATOP cohort. Neurology. 2001;56(12):1712–21. https://doi.org/10.1212/WNL.56.12.1712.
102. Lizarraga KJ, Luca CC, De Salles A, Gorgulho A, Lang AE, Fasano A. Asymmetric neuromodulation of motor circuits in Parkinson's disease: the role of subthalamic deep brain stimulation. Surg Neurol Int. 2017;8(1):261. https://doi.org/10.4103/SNI.SNI_292_17.
103. Crémers J, D'Ostilio K, Stamatakis J, Delvaux V, Garraux G. Brain activation pattern related to gait disturbances in Parkinson's disease. Mov Disord. 2012;27(12):1498–505.
104. Tessitore A, Amboni M, Esposito F, Russo A, Picillo M, Marcuccio L, Pellecchia MT, Vitale C, Cirillo M, Tedeschi G, Barone P. Resting-state brain connectivity in patients with Parkinson's disease and freezing of gait. Parkinsonism Relat Disord. 2012;18(6):781–7. https://doi.org/10.1016/J.PARKRELDIS.2012.03.018.

105. Fling BW, Seidler RD. Fundamental differences in callosal structure, neurophysiologic function, and bimanual control in young and older adults. Cereb Cortex. 2012;22(11):2643–52. https://doi.org/10.1093/CERCOR/BHR349.
106. Fling BW, Seidler RD. Task-dependent effects of interhemispheric inhibition on motor control. Behav Brain Res. 2012;226(1):211–7. https://doi.org/10.1016/j.bbr.2011.09.018.
107. Sohn YH, Jung HY, Kaelin-Lang A, Hallett M. Excitability of the ipsilateral motor cortex during phasic voluntary hand movement. Exper Brain Res. 2003;148(2):176–85. https://doi.org/10.1007/S00221-002-1292-5.
108. Behrens TEJ, Woolrich MW, Jenkinson M, Johansen-Berg H, Nunes RG, Clare S, Matthews PM, Brady JM, Smith SM. Characterization and propagation of uncertainty in diffusion-weighted MR imaging. Magn Reson Med. 2003;50(5):1077–88. https://doi.org/10.1002/MRM.10609.
109. Feigin A, Fukuda M, Dhawan V, Przedborski S, Jackson–Lewis V, Mentis MJ, Moeller JR, Eidelberg D. Metabolic correlates of levodopa response in Parkinson's disease. Neurology. 2001;57(11):2083–8.
110. Boonstra TA, Schouten AC, Van Vugt JPP, Bloem BR, Van Der Kooij H. Parkinson's disease patients compensate for balance control asymmetry. J Neurophysiol. 2014;112:3227–39. https://doi.org/10.1152/jn.00813.2013.-In.
111. Guadagnin EC, Barbieri FA, Simieli L, Carpes FP. Is muscular and functional performance related to gait asymmetry in older adults? A systematic review. Arch Gerontol Geriatr. 2019;84:103899. https://doi.org/10.1016/j.archger.2019.103899.
112. Miller-Patterson C, Buesa R, McLaughlin N, Jones R, Akbar U, Friedman JH. Motor asymmetry over time in Parkinson's disease. J Neurol Sci. 2018;393:14–7. https://doi.org/10.1016/j.jns.2018.08.001.
113. Steinbach MJ, Campbell RW, DeVore BB, Harrison DW. Laterality in Parkinson's disease: a neuropsychological review. Appl Neuropsychol Adult. 2023;30(1):126–40.
114. Haaland KY, Harrington DL. Limb-sequencing deficits after left but not right hemisphere damage. Brain Cogn. 1994;24(1):104–22. https://doi.org/10.1006/BRCG.1994.1006.
115. Li K, Su W, Chen M, Li C-M, Ma X-X, Wang R, Lou B-H, Zhao H, Chen H-B, Yan C-Z. Abnormal spontaneous brain activity in left-onset Parkinson disease: a resting-state functional MRI study. Front Neurol. 2020;11(July):1–8. https://doi.org/10.3389/fneur.2020.00727.
116. Benninger F, Khlebtovsky A, Roditi Y, Keret O, Steiner I, Melamed E, Djaldetti R. Beneficial effect of levodopa therapy on stooped posture in Parkinson's disease. Gait Posture. 2015;42(3):263–8.
117. Weiss D, Schoellmann A, Fox MD, Bohnen NI, Factor SA, Nieuwboer A, Hallett M, Lewis SJG. Freezing of gait: understanding the complexity of an enigmatic phenomenon. Brain: J Neurol. 2020;143(1):14–30. https://doi.org/10.1093/BRAIN/AWZ314.
118. Abbruzzese G, Berardelli A. Sensorimotor integration in movement disorders. Mov Disord. 2003;18(3):231–40. https://doi.org/10.1002/MDS.10327.
119. Curtze C, Nutt JG, Carlson-Kuhta P, Mancini M, Horak FB. Levodopa is a double-edged sword for balance and gait in people with Parkinson's disease. Mov Disord. 2015;30(10):1361–70. https://doi.org/10.1002/mds.26269.
120. Beretta VS, Barbieri FA, Orcioli-Silva D, dos Santos PCR, Simieli L, Vitório R, Gobbi LTB. Can postural control asymmetry predict falls in people with Parkinson's disease? Mot Control. 2018;22(4):449–61. https://doi.org/10.1123/mc.2017-0033.
121. Redgrave P, Rodriguez M, Smith Y, Rodriguez-Oroz MC, Lehericy S, Bergman H, Agid Y, DeLong MR, Obeso JA. Goal-directed and habitual control in the basal ganglia: implications for Parkinson's disease. Nat Rev Neurosci. 2010;11(11):760–72.
122. Drucker JH, Sathian K, Crosson B, Krishnamurthy V, McGregor KM, Bozzorg A, Gopinath K, Krishnamurthy LC, Wolf SL, Hart AR, Evatt M, Corcos DM, Hackney ME. Internally guided lower limb movement recruits compensatory cerebellar activity in people with Parkinson's disease. Front Neurol. 2019;10 https://doi.org/10.3389/fneur.2019.00537.

123. Nonnekes J, Růžička E, Nieuwboer A, Hallett M, Fasano A, Bloem BR. Compensation strategies for gait impairments in Parkinson disease: a review. JAMA Neurol. 2019;76(6):718–25.
124. Ricciardi L, Ricciardi D, Lena F, Plotnik M, Petracca M, Barricella S, Bentivoglio AR, Modugno N, Bernabei R, Fasano A. Working on asymmetry in Parkinson's disease: randomized, controlled pilot study. Neurol Sci. 2015;36(8):1337–43. https://doi.org/10.1007/s10072-015-2082-8.

Freezing of Gait in Parkinson's Disease: Balance, Gait, and Neurophysiological Aspects

13

Claudia Eunice Neves de Oliveira, Layla Cupertino, Vanessa Milanese, and Daniel Boari Coelho

Abstract

Freezing of gait (FoG) is quite prevalent in individuals with Parkinson's disease (PD). It can be classified according to its behavioral manifestation associated with the movement of the legs with short and fast steps, alternating leg tremors, and akinetic. FoG is characterized by an abrupt and unforeseen cessation of movement, leading to an impaired capacity to regain balance and subsequently increasing the risk of falling. The occurrence of FoG is a prevalent cause of falls among individuals with PD. Finding disparities in postural control between people with PD who have FOG and those who do not freeze can help us understand why people are more likely to fall in freezers and how training programs could be tailored to address these impairments. We aimed to assess further the biomechanical aspects of balance, gait, and the neurophysiological mechanisms of FoG.

C. E. N. de Oliveira · L. Cupertino
Center for Mathematics, Computation, and Cognition, Federal University of ABC, São Bernardo do Campo, Brazil

V. Milanese
Department of Neurosurgery, Mayo Clinic Florida, Jacksonville, FL, USA

Department of Neurosurgery, Center of Neurology and Neurosurgery Associates (NeuroCENNA), Beneficencia Portuguesa of São Paulo Hospital, São Paulo, Brazil

R. Capitão-mor Roque Barreto, São Paulo, SP, Brazil

D. B. Coelho (✉)
Center for Mathematics, Computation, and Cognition, Federal University of ABC, São Bernardo do Campo, Brazil

Biomedical Engineering, Federal University of ABC, São Paulo, Brazil
e-mail: daniel.boari@ufabc.edu.br

F. A. Barbieri et al. (eds.), *Locomotion and Posture in Older Adults*,
https://doi.org/10.1007/978-3-031-74123-4_13

Introduction

Freezing of gait (FoG) is quite prevalent in individuals with Parkinson's disease (PD) and becomes more so the longer the disease has been present. FoG can also occur mildly in untreated patients and relatively early stages of PD. This distinct and incapacitating clinical syndrome is defined by brief episodes of being unable to walk or taking very few steps [1]. Freezing episodes are often described as "the feet are glued to the floor" while the body's center of mass continues to move forward, sometimes resulting in a forward fall. FoG is usually a transient and short-lived episode. It can be triggered in different situations, such as at the gait initiation, during a turn, or when passing through narrow places or obstacles. Still, it can also occur for no apparent reason during any moment of gait. FoG can be classified according to its behavioral manifestation associated with the movement of the legs in FoG with short and fast steps; FoG with alternating leg tremor; and akinetic FoG when there is no movement in the legs [2, 3]. FoG can also be classified as responsive, resistant, or induced by dopaminergic medication, suggesting the existence of subtypes [4].

Individuals with FoG usually have more severe motor and cognitive symptoms, longer disease duration, and use higher doses of antiparkinsonian medication [5]. When analyzing prospective studies that followed individuals with PD from the early stages, a meta-analysis by Gao et al. [6] showed that gait disturbances could predict the development of FoG, with the postural instability and gait disturbance (PIGD) subtype of PD being one of the risk factors for the development of this symptom. Furthermore, this same study showed that nonmotor factors, such as depression and anxiety, cognitive impairment, and lower educational level, can also be considered risk factors for the development of FoG, but with limited evidence in the literature.

The physiological triggering mechanisms of FoG have not yet been fully elucidated, and there are several hypotheses in the literature based on different FoG phenotypes [6, 7]. Two models deserve mention: (a) threshold model [8] and (b) interference model [9]. The first model is based on the gait disturbances exhibited by individuals with FoG (i.e., decreased stride length, impaired gait coordination, and increased step timing variability) and assumes that when these gait disturbances accumulate to a certain threshold, there is a point of motor collapse that triggers FoG. Therefore, according to the authors of the model, by improving gait of individuals with PD, it is possible to reduce the propensity to FoG [8]. The second model is based on the competitive and complementary relationship between the motor, cognitive, and limbic circuits through the basal ganglia, which integrates information from different sensory inputs and coordinates an efficient functional response [9]. The authors of this model suggest that the simultaneous processing of cognitive and/or limbic information during motor tasks would overload a system already affected by the dopaminergic deficit. Vitorio et al. [10] showed that freezers had greater prefrontal cortical activation during both single and dual-task walking than nonfreezers. This finding highlights the overload of the executive locomotor network (i.e., executive/attentional resources) in those who freeze even in the absence of an actual freezing episode (as the analyzed data did not include freezing episodes). This overload would result in the inactivation of the pedunculopontine nucleus (PPN), responsible for regulating the functional motor response, thus serving as a trigger-to-trigger FoG episodes. In addition, the authors add that this overload can be reversed by inducing the focus of attention of the individual with PD to a single external sensory cue (i.e., a line on the floor or an obstacle to be crossed), thus reducing the number of sensory inputs and stimulating the NPP again. It is noteworthy that the models proposed in the literature are not mutually exclusive and understanding the possible physiological mechanisms that trigger FoG can help in treatment strategies, whether pharmacological or not.

In this chapter, we review the biomechanical aspects of balance and gait (Fig. 13.1) and the neurophysiological mechanisms of FoG. These losses in the postural and gait control domains, associated with FoG, lead to falls. FoG is one of the most frequent causes of falls in people with PD because it can cause an imbalance with a diminished capacity to take a step to restore equilibrium [11]. FoG is also one of the leading predictors of falls [12].

Hypotheses for Pathogenesis

Nutt et al. [1] review five hypotheses, not necessarily exclusive, on the pathogenesis of FoG:

1. Abnormal Gait Pattern Generation: Distinctive gait characteristics linked to FoG result from atypical control outputs originating from the central pattern generators. FoG events could be attributed to interrupting the supraspinal control signals regulating the central pattern generator. These control signals are vital for turning, pausing, navigating obstacles, and adjusting locomotion objectives. The absence of effective coordination among dopaminergic modulation networks gives rise to inhibitions within the globus pallidus internus/substantia nigra pars reticulate (GPi/SNr) pathway, ultimately leading to impaired regulation of rhythmic gait [13].
2. A problem with central drive and automaticity of movement: Individuals with PD may experience impairments in implicit learning and automatic task execution [14]. These deficits may be particularly pronounced in patients with FoG. FoG may be attributed to the impaired ability of the basal ganglia to automatically update motor programs, resulting in a deficit in multitasking capabilities. FoG could be initiated by interacting with complementary but conflicting basal ganglia signals from motor, cognitive, and limbic cortical regions. The occurrence of FoG can be attributed to the heightened inhibition in brainstem locomotor areas, which results from synchronized firing in the output nuclei of

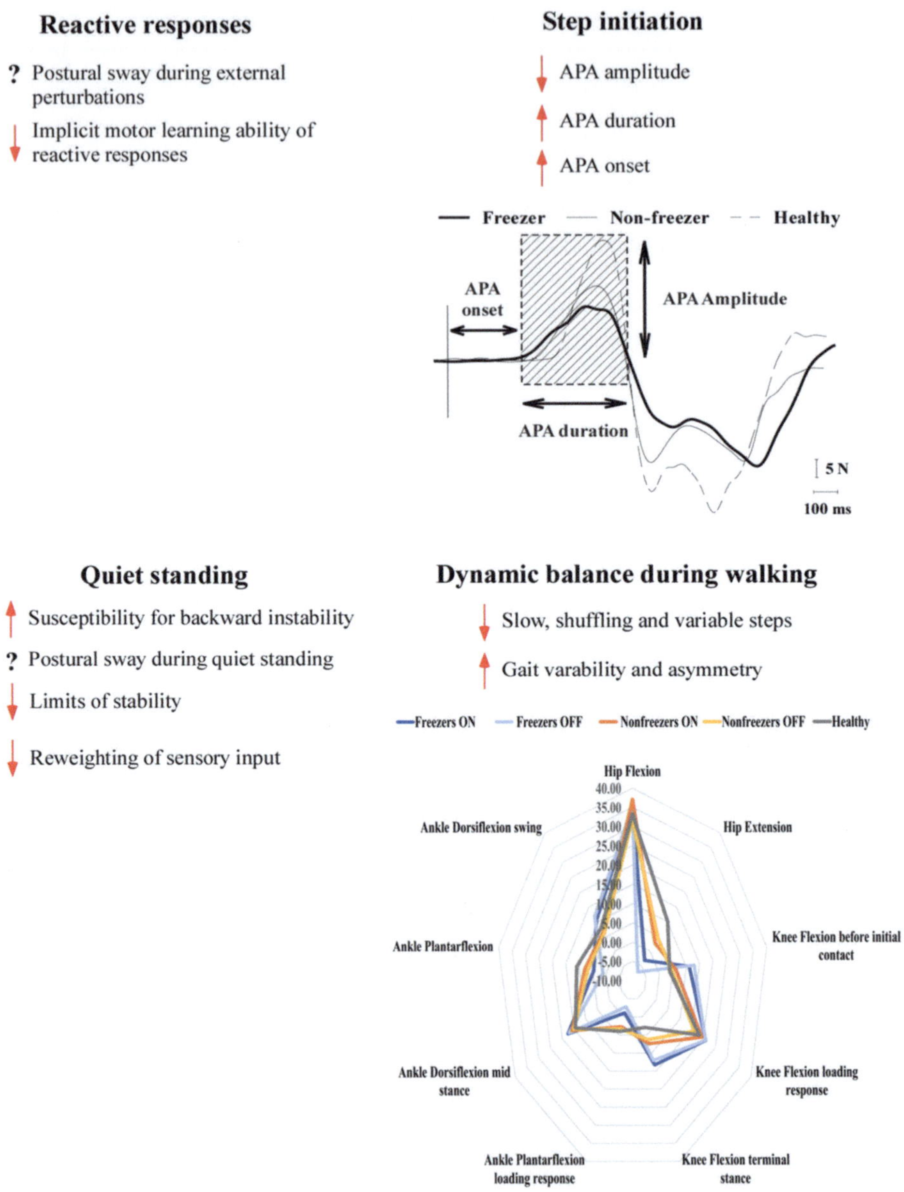

Fig. 13.1. Balance dysfunction in freezers. The red color indicates worse indices for the freezers. The up arrow indicates an increase, while the down arrow indicates a decrease in specified aspects of movement. The question mark indicates that the studies are controversial. APA: Anticipatory postural adjustments

the basal ganglia under the proposed model. The associative striatum and frontal-parietal cortices exhibit a very limited impact during the disease's initial stages, enabling freezers to employ goal-directed methods in gait regulation. Nevertheless, consequently, the process of walking becomes less automatic and more susceptible to disruption from concurrent tasks that can interfere with the regulation of walking.
3. Abnormal Coupling of Posture with Gait: Breakdown in the coupling between posture preparation by the SMA and step initiation by the motor cortex leads to multiple anticipatory postural adjustments (APA) preceding FoG events [15].
4. A Perceptual Malfunction: The phenomenon commonly observed in patients experiencing a temporary inability to initiate movement while traversing a doorway indicates a potential issue related to the perceptual processing of environmental cues for navigation [16]. Indeed, the perception-based processing of environmental restrictions leads to a deceleration in walking speed directly proportional to the width of the doorway in healthy participants.
5. A Frontal Executive Dysfunction: FoG sometimes arises when there is a need to transition between motor programs due to turns or to avoid obstacles. The capacity to rapidly modify motor programs is believed to be facilitated by the basal ganglia's processing of information derived from divergent motor, cognitive, and limbic complementary and competitive inputs. FoG seems to occur more frequently when individuals engage in demanding walking tasks that necessitate heightened attention, problem-solving abilities, and the suppression of improper reactions [17]. Additionally, FoG is associated with difficulties in set-shifting, further supporting the notion that executive dysfunction plays a role in the manifestation of FoG.

Balance

Postural control refers to the ability to maintain balance and stability during various activities, such as standing, walking, and turning. Parkinson's disease can lead to postural instability, increasing the fall risk. Specifically, freezers perform worse on clinical balance tests, such as the Mini-BEST and Berg Balance Scale, than non-freezers (for a review, see [18]).

The relationship between FoG and postural control in PD is complex and multifactorial [19]. Effective management of these symptoms may require a multifaceted approach that addresses sensory/perceptual, motor, and cognitive aspects of PD. While the precise mechanisms underlying this relationship are not fully understood, several possible explanations have been proposed [1, 20]:

(a) Impaired Postural Control May Contribute to FoG: PD can cause postural instability, increasing the risk of falls. Impaired postural control can also affect gait initiation, as maintaining balance is essential for initiating and maintaining gait. People with PD with more severe postural instability are more likely to experience FoG.

(b) FoG May Contribute to Postural Instability: FoG can lead to sudden stopping or freezing during movement, disrupting the body's sense of balance and leading to falls. In addition, FOG episodes can be unpredictable and difficult to anticipate, increasing anxiety and further destabilizing posture.
(c) Common Underlying Neural Circuitry: FoG and postural control may share a common neural circuitry involving the basal ganglia and other brain regions involved in motor planning and execution. Dysfunction in this circuitry due to the loss of dopamine-producing cells in PD can result in both FoG and postural instability.
(d) Attentional Control: People with PD may have difficulty with attentional control [21], leading to FoG and postural instability. Attentional control is important for maintaining posture and adjusting gait in response to environmental cues, and disruptions in this process can contribute to FoG and postural instability.

Five out of eight studies on postural sway indicated no differences between quiet standing with eyes open in individuals with FoG (freezers) versus those without FoG (nonfreezers) (for a review, see [20]). However, the studies report abnormalities in the anterior–posterior direction both in the ON in OFF medication with a backward shift of the body center of pressure (CoP) [22]. Nevertheless, in both freezers and nonfreezers, sway increased in velocity and area with eyes closed compared to eyes open, similarly to controls, and there were no group differences [23]. Therefore, we can conclude that there is no difference between the groups of freezers and nonfreezers for quiet standing. Still, the susceptibility for backward postural instability in people with FoG is increased. It is unclear if sensory weighting to control postural sway in quiet standing differs between freezers and nonfreezers [22, 24–27]. Few small studies show contradictory results, probably because these studies did not account for disease severity, the challenge of recognizing freezers, and the effects of medication on testing patients.

Freezers demonstrated a deficit in voluntary tilting in the forward and backward directions compared to nonfreezers, as measured by limits of stability [22]. This could reflect decreased proprioception or kinesthesia, increased fall fear, less flexed postural alignment, or decreased strength. Schlenstedt et al. [22] showed that limits of stability are correlated with FoG severity. Deficits in this domain may not reflect a primary pathway to explain FoG and postural instability.

Except for those evoked by startle, reactive postural control measures are slower and smaller but otherwise substantially intact in freezers compared to nonfreezers. Comparing freezers and nonfreezers, it was found that freezers had smaller and slower corrective stepping reactions [28]. Still, other studies reported that reactive postural control was similar between freezers and nonfreezers [29, 30], or even better in freezers [24]. Therefore, we conclude that reactive postural instability appears less affected in freezers than in nonfreezers. Additionally, freezers with repeated practice in responding to surface translations showed no progress in protective postural responses or could maintain it [30].

Anticipatory postural adjustments (APAs) are pre-programmed muscle movements that occur in preparation for a voluntary movement, such as reaching or stepping. These adjustments help maintain balance and stability during the movement. Specifically, freezers may exhibit abnormal APAs, such as reduced amplitude, duration, and timing of APAs [31–34] compared to nonfreezers. This can lead to unstable posture and difficulty maintaining balance during voluntary movements. Due to their inability to swiftly stop an active motor program or activate a pre-existing motor program, freezers produce anomalous APAs when faced with time restrictions. Inappropriate APAs prior to step initiation, as shown by more asymmetric and dysrhythmic [35, 36], also indicate problems in weight-shifting caused by FoG. The behavioral pattern seen prior to a FoG episode, in which freezes exhibit smaller step sizes, rhythmicity, and symmetry of the gait cycles, is mimicked by the variations observed in parameters of stepping in place by freezers compared to nonfreezers. This resemblance would suggest that FoG and dynamic postural control share a small portion of a single neural circuit.

Turning in freezers is characterized by (1) a closer coupling between the head and pelvis and a delay in head rotation, indicating reduced trunk movement during turning [37]; (2) reduced step width [38]; (3) at the end of the turn, when FoG episodes were most frequent, segmental rigidity and reduced step widths were most noticeable [38]; (4) wider and sharper turns, which are correlated with higher step time variability and more freezing [39]; and (5) longer turn duration, slower peak turn velocity, more steps, and faster cadence than nonfreezers [40]. It is unknown why turning induces FoG, but it may involve the close coupling between APAs and top-down modification of the stepping pattern to maintain stability and change direction.

Gait

The gait differences observed in freezers are likely related to the difficulty initiating movement associated with FoG. Patients may hesitate before taking a step, take several smaller steps to get started, or take longer to plan and execute each step. The reduced stride length and slower gait speed can also contribute to a shuffling gait pattern, increasing the risk of falls, and other mobility-related problems. Additionally, the pauses and hesitation associated with FOG can disrupt the normal gait rhythm, making it more difficult for patients to navigate their environment. Gait of freezers differs from nonfreezers in several ways. Some of the differences are:

(a) Reduced Stride Length: Freezers tend to take shorter steps, which can make their gait appear shuffling. This is likely due to the difficulty initiating movement associated with FOG. Patients may hesitate to take a step or take several smaller steps to get started.
(b) Slower Gait Speed: Freezers tend to move slower than those without FoG. This may be related to the reduced stride length and difficulty initiating movement. Patients may need more time to plan and execute each step.

(c) More Variability in Step Length and Duration: Freezers tend to have more variable step length and duration, meaning their gait is less consistent. Higher variability is also associated with attentional/executive control of movement (relative to automatic control). This is likely related to the hesitation and difficulty initiating movement associated with FOG. Patients may take smaller or larger steps depending on how they feel now.
(d) Increased Number of Steps: Freezers may take more steps to cover the same distance as those without FoG due to hesitation and difficulty initiating movement. This can make their gait appear less efficient.
(e) Reduced Arm Swing: Freezers may have reduced arm swing on the side affected by FoG, making their gait asymmetric. This is likely related to the dysfunction in the basal ganglia-thalamocortical circuits that control movement in PD.
(f) The kinematic differences presented between the freezers and nonfreezers groups are mainly in distal joints, with freezers having greater knee flexion at initial contact, greater minimal knee flexion in terminal stance, lower ankle plantar flexion peak in load response, and higher ankle dorsiflexion during the swing phase compared to the nonfreezers [41].
(g) When compensatory executive control mechanisms are ineffective, freezers may use visuospatial strategies to control gait under challenging circumstances [42].
(h) Additionally, there is a greater dual-task cost on gait in freezers than in nonfreezers. Even after adjusting for disease severity, serial subtraction had a greater impact on stride length and first-step time in freezers than in nonfreezers [23].

These differences in gait are thought to be related to the underlying pathophysiology of FOG in PD, which involves dysfunction in the basal ganglia-thalamocortical circuits that control movement. This would lead to a loss of gait automaticity in freezers. Freezers employ executive functions to alleviate the loss of movement automaticity, as evidenced by increased recruitment of the prefrontal cortex during gait (for a review, see [43]).

How to Measure FoG Episodes?

Although there is evidence that FoG can be detected at home [44], the diversity of triggers and heterogeneity of the presentation of this symptom makes its prediction difficult. A distinct and objective definition based on observable motor behaviors of what constitutes an episode of FoG and its relationship to other motor and nonmotor symptoms would facilitate the development of methods to detect and predict such episodes. Further, it may be advantageous to identify markers that can predict which patients will exhibit FoG. Nonetheless, therapy and prevention are likely suboptimal without objective measures and comprehension of the issue.

The presence of FOG can be quantified subjectively or objectively. Although validated and reliable [45], the New Freezing of Gait Questionnaire (nFoG-q) for assessing FoG is subjective. Consequently, it might not represent the real severity of the freezing. Future studies should implement biomechanical measurements and an adequate environment to provoke and assess the severity of FoG. However, the subjective record from the patient and family is important and should be used with objective methods, given the challenge of provoking FoG in a clinical setup.

Objective measures quantifying the severity of FoG should be validated using standardized procedures to facilitate comparability and reproducibility of research and clinical protocols.

Several freezing-provoking tasks have been described, such as rapid 360-degree turns [46], dual-tasking, and walking with short rapid steps [47]. Asking the patient to attempt a 360-degree turn in place to the right and then the left is one of the most reliable methods of observing FoG in the clinic [46].

In the past decade, wearable inertial sensors, which typically incorporate a triaxial accelerometer, gyroscope, and magnetometer, have been increasingly utilized to measure FoG objectively. Methods for FoG detection differ in complexity, and numerous algorithms have been implemented in wearable sensors. The thigh and ankle were the most popular device location, and the combination of accelerometer and gyroscope was the most frequently used wearable inertial sensor. Several features are used, such as Fourier transform [46, 48, 49], wavelet transforms [50], and multiple machine-learning techniques, such as neural networks [51], nearest neighbor [52], support vector machines [53], random forests [54], and deep residual network [55].

One of the measurements derived from inertial sensors is the FoG ratio. The FoG ratio is calculated from the power spectrum as the area under the curve for trembling, freezing frequencies (3.5–8 Hz) divided by the area under the curve for the stepping frequencies (0.5–3 Hz). The FoG ratio also correlates with the nFoG-q and video rating performed by expert neurologists. Nonetheless, the subtypes of FoG are based on the type of leg movements: Start hesitation characterized by alternating trembling of the legs with a frequency of 3–8 Hz; akinetic FOG when no movements of the legs; patients make very small shuffling steps. Using inertial sensors and a frequency analysis that identifies the locomotor and a freezing band, FoG ratio does not measure all FoG subtypes [46].

In a systematic review, Cupertino et al. [56] analyzed the biomechanical characteristics that precede FoG episodes. The most consistent results indicate a dramatic reduction of movement excursions with (1) decrease in stride length; (2) decreased gait speed; (3) postural instability with the increased double support phase; (4) incoordination of anterior tibial and gastrocnemius; (5) increased range of motion of biceps femoris; (6) decreased range of motion in the sagittal plane at the ankle and hip joints; and (7) anterior pelvic tilt.

Brain Circuitry Abnormalities

Unfortunately, FoG has a complex pathophysiology that remains poorly understood. FoG has been linked to alterations in several brain networks, encompassing both motor and nonmotor domains, including frontal and frontostriatal networks, parietal-occipital cortices, basal ganglia, thalamus, brainstem, cerebellum, and limbic system, resulting in both structural and functional modifications [57, 58]. Below, we summarize the main non-exclusive results comparing freezers versus nonfreezers:

1. Recent theoretical frameworks propose that the manifestation of FoG may be attributed to transient over-activation in the inhibitory striatal output nuclei that project to the motor thalamus and brainstem locomotor regions, such as the pedunculopontine nucleus [59]. Additionally, dysfunctional cortical and cerebellar projections to these subcortical and brainstem regions are believed to play a role in the development of FoG [60]. This concept suggests that the presence of FoG may be associated with neural circuitry that enhances the firing rate of the striatal output nuclei, such as through modified processing in the cortico-basal ganglia system, or disrupts the connections between the cortex and brainstem, as well as the cerebellum and brainstem, potentially caused by additional pathology in the substantia nigra [61].
2. Freezers exhibit a disrupted connection between the sensorimotor [62] and frontoparietal and visual networks [63] and subcortical regions.
3. Several other studies point to impaired integration of the cognitive control network, including the executive and attentive domains [63–65]. These neuroimaging findings would support the loss of automaticity hypothesis found in FOG.
4. Freezers exhibit functional changes in the subcortical changes regions, especially in the mesencephalic locomotor region (MLR) [66, 67] and cerebellum [68].
5. Freezers have atypical emotional brain circuitry [69], potentially elucidating the frequent co-occurrence of anxiety and panic attacks during freezing episodes.
6. Freezers show an attenuated mid-frontal theta (4–8 Hz) power associated with cognitive control impairments [70].
7. During lower limb pedaling in freezers, it was shown that the beta band exhibited an increase in the frontal region (for a review, see [71]). This increase suggests the involvement of anticipatory modifications and the execution of motor plans through top-down signaling.
8. Freezers show an increased high-beta (21–35 Hz) power observed in the STN during the OFF state.

Conclusion

Freezing is a transient and intermittent condition characterized by the inability to initiate movement, accompanied by the sensation that one's feet are firmly affixed to the ground. The phenomenon known as freezing of gait is prevalent in a significant proportion of individuals with PD and is frequently linked to instances of falling as the condition advances.

Freezers exhibit a higher prevalence of balance abnormalities compared to nonfreezers. This is notably evident in the context of step initiation and gait. Freezers exhibit notable deviations in the structure and function of brain circuitry compared to individuals without freezing symptoms. However, it is challenging to account for the varying degrees of disease severity, as FoG tends to become more prevalent as the disease advances.

Conflict of Interest Statement None.

References

1. Nutt JG, Bloem BR, Giladi N, Hallett M, Horak FB, Nieuwboer A. Freezing of gait: moving forward on a mysterious clinical phenomenon. Lancet Neurol. 2011;10(8):734–44.
2. Thompson PD, Marsden CD. Walking disorders. In: Bradley WG, Daroff RB, Fenichel GM, Marsden CD, editors. Neurology in clinical practice: principles of diagnosis and management. Boston, MA: Butterworth-Heinemann; 1995. p. 321–34.
3. Schaafsma JD, Balash Y, Gurevich T, Bartels AL, Hausdorff JM, Giladi N. Characterization of freezing of gait subtypes and the response of each to levodopa in Parkinson's disease. Eur J Neurol. 2003;10(4):391–8.
4. Ehgoetz Martens KA, Hall JM, Georgiades MJ, Gilat M, Walton CC, Matar E, Lewis SJG, Shine JM. The functional network signature of heterogeneity in freezing of gait. Brain. 2018;141(4):1145–60.
5. Lord SR, Bindels H, Ketheeswaran M, Brodie MA, Lawrence AD, Close JCT, Whone AL, Ben-Shlomo Y, Henderson EJ. Freezing of gait in people with Parkinson's disease: nature, occurrence, and risk factors. J Parkinsons Dis. 2020;10(2):631–40.
6. Gao C, Liu J, Tan Y, Chen S. Freezing of gait in Parkinson's disease: pathophysiology, risk factors and treatments. Transl Neurodegener. 2020;9:12.
7. Nieuwboer A, Giladi N. Characterizing freezing of gait in Parkinson's disease: models of an episodic phenomenon. Mov Disord. 2013;28(11):1509–19.
8. Plotnik M, Giladi N, Hausdorff JM. Is freezing of gait in Parkinson's disease a result of multiple gait impairments? Implications for treatment. Parkinsons Dis. 2012;2012:459321.
9. Lewis SJ, Barker RA. A pathophysiological model of freezing of gait in Parkinson's disease. Parkinsonism Relat Disord. 2009;15(5):333–8.
10. Vitorio R, Stuart S, Mancini M. Executive control of walking in people with Parkinson's disease with freezing of gait. Neurorehabil Neural Repair. 2020;34(12):1138–49.
11. Paul SS, Canning CG, Sherrington C, Lord SR, Close JC, Fung VS. Three simple clinical tests to accurately predict falls in people with Parkinson's disease. Mov Disord. 2013;28(5):655–62.
12. Kerr GK, Worringham CJ, Cole MH, Lacherez PF, Wood JM, Silburn PA. Predictors of future falls in Parkinson disease. Neurology. 2010;75(2):116–24.
13. Lewis SJ, Shine JM. The next step: a common neural mechanism for freezing of gait. Neuroscientist. 2016;22(1):72–82.
14. Peterson DS, Dijkstra BW, Horak FB. Postural motor learning in people with Parkinson's disease. J Neurol. 2016;263(8):1518–29.
15. Jacobs JV, Lou JS, Kraakevik JA, Horak FB. The supplementary motor area contributes to the timing of the anticipatory postural adjustment during step initiation in participants with and without Parkinson's disease. Neuroscience. 2009;164(2):877–85.
16. Higuchi T, Cinelli ME, Greig MA, Patla AE. Locomotion through apertures when wider space for locomotion is necessary: adaptation to artificially altered bodily states. Exp Brain Res. 2006;175(1):50–9.
17. Snijders AH, Leunissen I, Bakker M, Overeem S, Helmich RC, Bloem BR, Toni I. Gait-related cerebral alterations in patients with Parkinson's disease with freezing of gait. Brain. 2011;134(Pt 1):59–72.

18. Bekkers EMJ, Dijkstra BW, Dockx K, Heremans E, Verschueren SMP, Nieuwboer A. Clinical balance scales indicate worse postural control in people with Parkinson's disease who exhibit freezing of gait compared to those who do not: a meta-analysis. Gait Posture. 2017;56:134–40.
19. Coelho DB, Ribeiro de Souza C, de Lima-Pardini AC, Treza RC, Shida TKF, Silva-Batista C, Teixeira LA. Is freezing of gait correlated with postural control in patients with moderate-to-severe Parkinson's disease? Eur J Neurosci. 2021;53(4):1189–96.
20. Bekkers EMJ, Dijkstra BW, Heremans E, Verschueren SMP, Bloem BR, Nieuwboer A. Balancing between the two: are freezing of gait and postural instability in Parkinson's disease connected? Neurosci Biobehav Rev. 2018;94:113–25.
21. Monaghan AS, Gordon E, Graham L, Hughes E, Peterson DS, Morris R. Cognition and freezing of gait in Parkinson's disease: a systematic review and meta-analysis. Neurosci Biobehav Rev. 2023;147:105068.
22. Schlenstedt C, Muthuraman M, Witt K, Weisser B, Fasano A, Deuschl G. Postural control and freezing of gait in Parkinson's disease. Parkinsonism Relat Disord. 2016;24:107–12.
23. de Souza Fortaleza AC, Mancini M, Carlson-Kuhta P, King LA, Nutt JG, Chagas EF, Freitas IFJ, Horak FB. Dual task interference on postural sway, postural transitions and gait in people with Parkinson's disease and freezing of gait. Gait Posture. 2017;56:76–81.
24. Vervoort G, Nackaerts E, Mohammadi F, Heremans E, Verschueren S, Nieuwboer A, Vercruysse S. Which aspects of postural control differentiate between patients with Parkinson's disease with and without freezing of gait? Parkinsons Dis. 2013;2013:971480.
25. Pelykh O, Klein AM, Botzel K, Kosutzka Z, Ilmberger J. Dynamics of postural control in Parkinson patients with and without symptoms of freezing of gait. Gait Posture. 2015;42(3):246–50.
26. Huh YE, Hwang S, Kim K, Chung WH, Youn J, Cho JW. Postural sensory correlates of freezing of gait in Parkinson's disease. Parkinsonism Relat Disord. 2016;25:72–7.
27. Feller KJ, Peterka RJ, Horak FB. Sensory re-weighting for postural control in Parkinson's disease. Front Hum Neurosci. 2019;13:126.
28. Sutter EN, Seidler KJ, Duncan RP, Earhart GM, McNeely ME. Low to moderate relationships between gait and postural responses in Parkinson disease. J Rehabil Med. 2017;49(6):505–11.
29. Nonnekes J, de Kam D, Oude Nijhuis LB, van Geel K, Bloem BR, Geurts A, Weerdesteyn V. StartReact effects support different pathophysiological mechanisms underlying freezing of gait and postural instability in Parkinson's disease. PLoS One. 2015;10(3):e0122064.
30. Peterson DS, Horak FB. Effects of freezing of gait on postural motor learning in people with Parkinson's disease. Neuroscience. 2016;334:283–9.
31. Cohen RG, Nutt JG, Horak FB. Recovery from multiple APAs delays gait initiation in Parkinson's disease. Front Hum Neurosci. 2017;11:60.
32. Lira JLO, Ugrinowitsch C, Coelho DB, Teixeira LA, de Lima-Pardini AC, Magalhaes FH, Barbosa ER, Horak FB, Silva-Batista C. Loss of presynaptic inhibition for step initiation in Parkinsonian individuals with freezing of gait. J Physiol. 2020;598(8):1611–24.
33. Delval A, Moreau C, Bleuse S, Tard C, Ryckewaert G, Devos D, Defebvre L. Auditory cueing of gait initiation in Parkinson's disease patients with freezing of gait. Clin Neurophysiol. 2014;125(8):1675–81.
34. Tard C, Dujardin K, Bourriez JL, Destee A, Derambure P, Defebvre L, Delval A. Attention modulates step initiation postural adjustments in Parkinson freezers. Parkinsonism Relat Disord. 2014;20(3):284–9.
35. Nantel J, de Solages C, Bronte-Stewart H. Repetitive stepping in place identifies and measures freezing episodes in subjects with Parkinson's disease. Gait Posture. 2011;34(3):329–33.
36. Nantel J, Bronte-Stewart H. The effect of medication and the role of postural instability in different components of freezing of gait (FOG). Parkinsonism Relat Disord. 2014;20(4):447–51.
37. Spildooren J, Vercruysse S, Heremans E, Galna B, Vandenbossche J, Desloovere K, Vandenberghe W, Nieuwboer A. Head-pelvis coupling is increased during turning in patients with Parkinson's disease and freezing of gait. Mov Dis. 2013;28(5):619–25.

38. Bengevoord A, Vervoort G, Spildooren J, Heremans E, Vandenberghe W, Bloem BR, Nieuwboer A. Center of mass trajectories during turning in patients with Parkinson's disease with and without freezing of gait. Gait Posture. 2016;43:54–9.
39. Spildooren J, Vinken C, Van Baekel L, Nieuwboer A. Turning problems and freezing of gait in Parkinson's disease: a systematic review and meta-analysis. Disabil Rehabil. 2019;41(25):2994–3004.
40. Mancini M, Weiss A, Herman T, Hausdorff JM. Turn around freezing: community-living turning behavior in people with Parkinson's disease. Front Neurol. 2018;9:18.
41. Shida TKF, de Oliveira CEN, da Silva Fragoso de Campos D, Los Angeles E, Bernardo C, Dos Santos de Oliveira L, ESLC S, Novaes TM, Shokur S, Bouri M, et al. Effect of freezing of gait and dopaminergic medication in the biomechanics of lower limbs in the gait of patients with Parkinson's disease compared to neurologically healthy. Neurosci Lett. 2023;806:137250.
42. Piramide N, Agosta F, Sarasso E, Canu E, Volonte MA, Filippi M. Brain activity during lower limb movements in Parkinson's disease patients with and without freezing of gait. J Neurol. 2020;267(4):1116–26.
43. Bardakan MM, Fink GR, Zapparoli L, Bottini G, Paulesu E, Weiss PH. Imaging the neural underpinnings of freezing of gait in Parkinson's disease. Neuroimage Clin. 2022;35:103123.
44. Mancini M, Shah VV, Stuart S, Curtze C, Horak FB, Safarpour D, Nutt JG. Measuring freezing of gait during daily-life: an open-source, wearable sensors approach. J Neuroeng Rehabil. 2021;18(1):1.
45. Nieuwboer A, Rochester L, Herman T, Vandenberghe W, Emil GE, Thomaes T, Giladi N. Reliability of the new freezing of gait questionnaire: agreement between patients with Parkinson's disease and their carers. Gait Posture. 2009;30(4):459–63.
46. Mancini M, Smulders K, Cohen RG, Horak FB, Giladi N, Nutt JG. The clinical significance of freezing while turning in Parkinson's disease. Neuroscience. 2017;343:222–8.
47. Nonnekes J, Janssen AM, Mensink SH, Oude Nijhuis LB, Bloem BR, Snijders AH. Short rapid steps to provoke freezing of gait in Parkinson's disease. J Neurol. 2014;261(9):1763–7.
48. Moore ST, MacDougall HG, Ondo WG. Ambulatory monitoring of freezing of gait in Parkinson's disease. J Neurosci Methods. 2008;167(2):340–8.
49. Moore ST, Yungher DA, Morris TR, Dilda V, MacDougall HG, Shine JM, Naismith SL, Lewis SJ. Autonomous identification of freezing of gait in Parkinson's disease from lower-body segmental accelerometry. J Neuroeng Rehabil. 2013;10:19.
50. Punin C, Barzallo B, Clotet R, Bermeo A, Bravo M, Bermeo JP, Llumiguano C. A non-invasive medical device for Parkinson's patients with episodes of freezing of gait. Sensors. 2019;19(3):737. https://doi.org/10.3390/s19030737.
51. Ahn D, Chung H, Lee HW, Kang K, Ko PW, Kim NS, Park T. Smart gait-aid glasses for Parkinson's disease patients. IEEE Trans Biomed Eng. 2017;64(10):2394–402.
52. Mazilu S, Calatroni A, Gazit E, Mirelman A, Hausdorff JM, Troster G. Prediction of freezing of gait in Parkinson's from physiological wearables: an exploratory study. IEEE J Biomed Health Inform. 2015;19(6):1843–54.
53. Rodriguez-Martin D, Sama A, Perez-Lopez C, Catala A, Moreno Arostegui JM, Cabestany J, Bayes A, Alcaine S, Mestre B, Prats A, et al. Home detection of freezing of gait using support vector machines through a single waist-worn triaxial accelerometer. PLoS One. 2017;12(2):e0171764.
54. Tripoliti EE, Tzallas AT, Tsipouras MG, Rigas G, Bougia P, Leontiou M, Konitsiotis S, Chondrogiorgi M, Tsouli S, Fotiadis DI. Automatic detection of freezing of gait events in patients with Parkinson's disease. Comput Methods Prog Biomed. 2013;110(1):12–26.
55. Miao R, Shokur S, de Lima-Pardini AC, Coelho DB, Bouri M. Detecting freezing of gait in Parkinson's disease patient via deep residual network. In: IEEE, editor. 2021 20th IEEE international conference on machine learning and applications (ICMLA). Pasadena, CA: IEEE; 2021. p. 320–5. https://doi.org/10.1109/ICMLA52953.2021.00056.
56. Cupertino L, Dos Reis TG, Los Angeles E, Costa TM, Shokur S, Bouri M, de Lima-Pardini AC, Coelho DB. Biomechanical aspects that precede freezing episode during gait in individuals with Parkinson's disease: a systematic review. Gait Posture. 2022;91:149–54.

57. Song W, Raza HK, Lu L, Zhang Z, Zu J, Zhang W, Dong L, Xu C, Gong X, Lv B, et al. Functional MRI in Parkinson's disease with freezing of gait: a systematic review of the literature. Neurol Sci. 2021;42(5):1759–71.
58. Fonoff ET, de Lima-Pardini AC, Coelho DB, Monaco BA, Machado B, Pinto de Souza C, Dos Santos Ghilardi MG, Hamani C. Spinal cord stimulation for freezing of gait: from bench to bedside. Front Neurol. 2019;10:905.
59. Holanda VM, Okun MS, Middlebrooks EH, Gungor A, Barry ME, Forder J, Foote KD. Postmortem dissections of common targets for lesion and deep brain stimulation surgeries. Neurosurgery. 2020;86(6):860–72.
60. Snijders AH, Takakusaki K, Debu B, Lozano AM, Krishna V, Fasano A, Aziz TZ, Papa SM, Factor SA, Hallett M. Physiology of freezing of gait. Ann Neurol. 2016;80(5):644–59.
61. Gilat M, Silva L, de Lima A, Bloem BR, Shine JM, Nonnekes J, Lewis SJG. Freezing of gait: promising avenues for future treatment. Parkinsonism Relat Disord. 2018;52:7–16.
62. Wang M, Jiang S, Yuan Y, Zhang L, Ding J, Wang J, Zhang J, Zhang K, Wang J. Alterations of functional and structural connectivity of freezing of gait in Parkinson's disease. J Neurol. 2016;263(8):1583–92.
63. Canu E, Agosta F, Sarasso E, Volonte MA, Basaia S, Stojkovic T, Stefanova E, Comi G, Falini A, Kostic VS, et al. Brain structural and functional connectivity in Parkinson's disease with freezing of gait. Hum Brain Mapp. 2015;36(12):5064–78.
64. Shine JM, Matar E, Ward PB, Frank MJ, Moustafa AA, Pearson M, Naismith SL, Lewis SJ. Freezing of gait in Parkinson's disease is associated with functional decoupling between the cognitive control network and the basal ganglia. Brain. 2013;136(Pt 12):3671–81.
65. Shine JM, Matar E, Ward PB, Bolitho SJ, Gilat M, Pearson M, Naismith SL, Lewis SJ. Exploring the cortical and subcortical functional magnetic resonance imaging changes associated with freezing in Parkinson's disease. Brain. 2013;136(Pt 4):1204–15.
66. Fling BW, Cohen RG, Mancini M, Carpenter SD, Fair DA, Nutt JG, Horak FB. Functional reorganization of the locomotor network in Parkinson patients with freezing of gait. PLoS One. 2014;9(6):e100291.
67. Lench DH, Embry A, Hydar A, Hanlon CA, Revuelta G. Increased on-state cortico-mesencephalic functional connectivity in Parkinson disease with freezing of gait. Parkinsonism Relat Disord. 2020;72:31–6.
68. Bharti K, Suppa A, Pietracupa S, Upadhyay N, Gianni C, Leodori G, Di Biasio F, Modugno N, Petsas N, Grillea G, et al. Abnormal cerebellar connectivity patterns in patients with Parkinson's disease and freezing of gait. Cerebellum. 2019;18(3):298–308.
69. de Lima-Pardini AC, Coelho DB, Nucci MP, Boffino CC, Batista AX, de Azevedo Neto RM, Silva-Batista C, Barbosa ER, Cohen RG, Horak FB, et al. Brain networks associated with anticipatory postural adjustments in Parkinson's disease patients with freezing of gait. Neuroimage Clin. 2020;28:102461.
70. Singh A, Cole RC, Espinoza AI, Brown D, Cavanagh JF, Narayanan NS. Frontal theta and beta oscillations during lower-limb movement in Parkinson's disease. Clin Neurophysiol. 2020;131(3):694–702.
71. Marquez JS, Hasan SMS, Siddiquee MR, Luca CC, Mishra VR, Mari Z, Bai O. Neural correlates of freezing of gait in Parkinson's disease: an electrophysiology mini-review. Front Neurol. 2020;11:571086.

Part III

Posture

14 Motor and Sensory Changes in Postural Control of Older Adults

Caio Ferraz Cruz and José Angelo Barela

Abstract

Postural control involves a complex relationship between sensory information and muscular activity, with the purpose of postural orientation and postural equilibrium. The aging process leads to several changes in the sensory and motor systems, with consequent deterioration of the postural control functioning. In this chapter, we start from the definition of aging by Spirduso WW, Francis KL, MacRae PG. Physical dimensions of aging. 2nd ed. Champaign: Human Kinetics; 2005, which makes reference to the lack of adaptability, to develop a line of discussion on postural control and aging, analyzing the effects of sensory and motor changes typical of aging on the mechanisms and strategies for controlling the standing posture in older people. Special attention is given to the role of physical activity as a factor in preventing losses in obtaining sensory information and, consequently, deterioration of postural control. Finally, we present sensory reweighting as an adaptation strategy for older people to maintain the functionality of the postural control system and ensure safety in their motor actions. We conclude that the aging process, with regard to postural control, does not necessarily cause a loss of adaptability, but it is a matter of readaptation in older people to their new sensory and motor conditions, which require changes in the sensorimotor relationship to perform with lesser risk to the demands of their daily life tasks.

C. F. Cruz
Center for Studies and Practices of Physical Activities, Graduate Program in Gerontology, School of Arts, Sciences and Humanities, University of São Paulo (USP), São Paulo, SP, Brazil
e-mail: caiofcruz@usp.br

J. A. Barela (✉)
Laboratory for Movement Studies, Department of Physical Education, Institute of Biosciences, São Paulo State University (UNESP), Rio Claro, SP, Brazil
e-mail: jose.barela@unesp.br

F. A. Barbieri et al. (eds.), *Locomotion and Posture in Older Adults*,
https://doi.org/10.1007/978-3-031-74123-4_14

Introduction

Nowadays, the maintenance of quality of life during aging is an important issue. With the increase in longevity worldwide, the aging population has also grown considerably, making it crucial to maintain a good quality of life during this phase. However, this is not a simple matter, as various factors can impact life quality. Thus, studies and scientific knowledge regarding aging and well-being are even more important and needed.

In general, the aging process is defined as natural changes in the organism that occur throughout life leading to a lack of *adaptability* [1]. Moreover, the lack of adaptability leads to functional deficits, implying that the relationship between the person and the environment is altered impacting daily life activity performance.

Despite the frequent and pertinent use of this definition and concept, there are several issues and questions that arise. First, lack of adaptability of what? What are the implications of somebody being less adaptable? Finally, can such a lack or loss of adaptability be minimized and/or reverted by any specific activity, such as exercises or practice of physical activity? Certainly these questions are intriguing, but they are quite large and, necessarily, any discussion about them needs to be based upon a specific context and major.

To further understand adaptability changes in older adults, the purpose of this chapter will focus on motor behavior, specifically the postural control of older adults. Such an approach seems to be pertinent and appropriate because postural control involves both motor activity and the use of sensory information and many issues of these aspects can be manipulated. Therefore, the purpose of this chapter is to discuss changes that occur in postural control due to the aging process, aiming to understand the differences and the underlying processes that might be related to the lack of adaptability in older adults.

Postural Control and Aging

According to Horak and Macpherson [2], postural control has two main behavioral goals: postural orientation and postural equilibrium. Postural orientation refers to the relative position of body segments to each other and to the environment in a certain posture. Postural equilibrium refers to balancing all the forces acting on the body. In this case, we can group those forces as internal, the forces produced by muscle contractions, and external, the forces coming from objects of the environment in contact with the body.

For these two behavioral goals to be achieved, an intricate relationship between sensory information and muscle activity is required and necessary [2, 3]. Sensory stimuli from several channels provide sensory cues to the central nervous system (CNS) that can identify position of segments in relation to other segments and in relation to the environment and the forces acting on the body. Considering that in any assumed posture, there is a need for muscle activity to achieve and assume it, the CNS needs to constantly use sensory information to organize and to specify appropriate muscle activity. When that occurs repeatedly, posture maintenance results from a perception–action cycle [4].

One of the alterations observed with advancing age is the deterioration in the performance of postural control. Several studies have shown that after a certain age, usually around 60 years old, while maintaining a quiet upright posture, a larger amplitude or higher velocity of body sway is observed [5–7]. This higher body sway is understood as an indication of deterioration in postural control functioning. That deterioration, over the years, would be related to a more serious problem such as a greater predisposition to falls [8].

Certainly, deterioration of body sway control, such as larger sway magnitude and higher sway velocity, and the increase in incidence of falls in older people represent a *loss of adaptability*, as has been used in the definition of aging. Older adults are not able to maintain the same relationship with the environment, compared to younger adults, during the maintenance of quiet upright posture and in situations of dynamic postural orientation. This finding leads us to the first question raised in the introduction: Loss of "adaptability" of what? A possible answer that we would like to suggest, at this moment, is a loss of adaptability regarding the relationship with the environment: Older people are not able to maintain the same efficiency in performing the actions as previously occurred and, as a consequence, the performance of achieved actions is lower than previously observed.

Based on the understanding that postural control requires an intricate relationship between sensory information and motor action, we initially suggested that changes in postural control would be due to changes in this relationship and, in a first attempt, we further examined more deeply and carefully the relationship between sensory information and motor action in older adults [9]. For instance, we examined this relationship employing the moving room paradigm, when older adults maintained upright stance inside a special room (2.1 × 2.1 × 2.1 m) in which the walls could be moved forward and backward by a servomechanism while the floor would stay stationary. The movement of the walls promotes optic flow changes and induces corresponding body sway of the standing participant.[1] Figure 14.1 depicts time series of an older adult in the room moving continuously, back and forward, for 60 s, at frequencies of 0.1, 0.17, and 0.5 Hz.

As can be seen from Fig. 14.1, older people were influenced by the room movement, presenting coherent and corresponding body sway with the visual manipulation. The initial hypothesis was that older people, because they had worse performance in the postural control system, would be less influenced by the visual manipulation information. Our hypothesis was refuted as older adults were not only influenced by the room movement but also presented a better relationship between visual information and body sway than young adults [9]. Figure 14.2 depicts the mean coherence values, which indicate the relationship between the movement of the room (visual information) and body sway, for the older and young adults, and it

[1] The moving room sway inducing somehow reproduces, in a controlled manner, the effect that we eventually experience when we are in a car and the car next to us moves creating the illusion that we are moving.

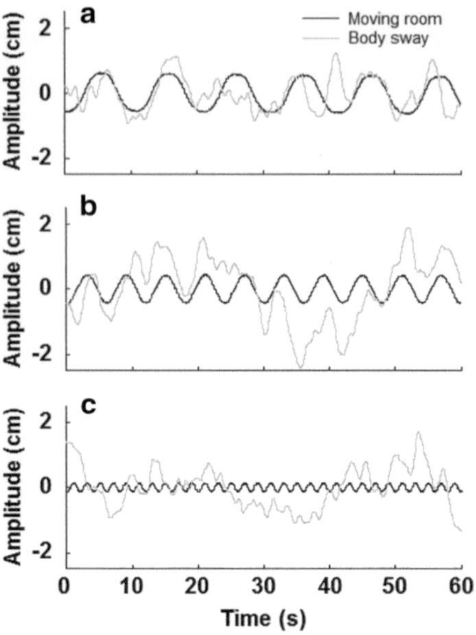

Fig. 14.1 Example of three trials of an older individual. Panels (**a**), (**b**), and (**c**) show the position of the moving room sway and body sway, over one trial, at the frequencies of 0.1 Hz, 0.17 Hz, and 0.5 Hz, respectively

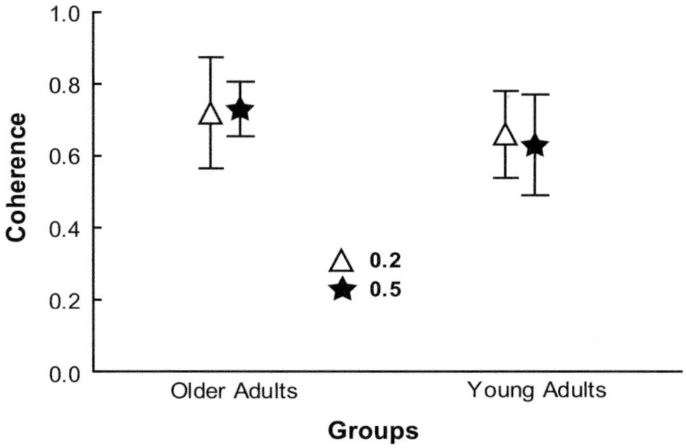

Fig. 14.2 Mean and standard deviation of coherence between the room movement and body sway of the older and younger adults, at the frequencies of 0.2 and 0.5 Hz

is shown that older adults show higher coherence values than those observed for the young adults.

How to reconcile worse performance in postural control, for example, larger amplitude of body sway during upright stance and higher incidence of falls, with a better relationship between sensory information and motor action? It is worth mentioning that in this initial study [9], we qualitatively observed a very interesting fact: While young adults were able to discriminate that the room was moved, no older participant was able to do so as none of them discriminated that the room had been moved.

A quick review of a few studies on the subject led us to the study by Wade and colleagues [10], in which it was observed that older adults were more influenced than younger adults by the movement of a room that was moved toward or away from the participants. Despite the discrete movement of the room, it also induced corresponding body sway in older adults.

In addition to triggering corresponding body sway, the magnitude of sway induced by the room was larger in older than in young adults [10]. These results are consistent with what we observed [9], making the investigation of the relationship between sensory information and motor action in older people even more intriguing. It is noteworthy that the higher influence of the manipulation of visual information, in a discrete way, on the body sway in older adults was replicated in a posterior study conducted by our group [11].

Physical Activity and Postural Control of Older Adults

Despite the numerous questions we had about the functioning of postural control in older people, we decided to add another and important aspect: the practice of physical activity. In this case, we decided to compare the relationship between visual information and body sway, in continuous and discrete moving room conditions, between young adults, sedentary older adults, and older adults who were engaged in a physical activity program [11]. Figure 14.3 presents the coherence values and Fig. 14.4 presents the body displacement values, indicating how much the room movement induced the body movement in the continuous and discrete conditions,

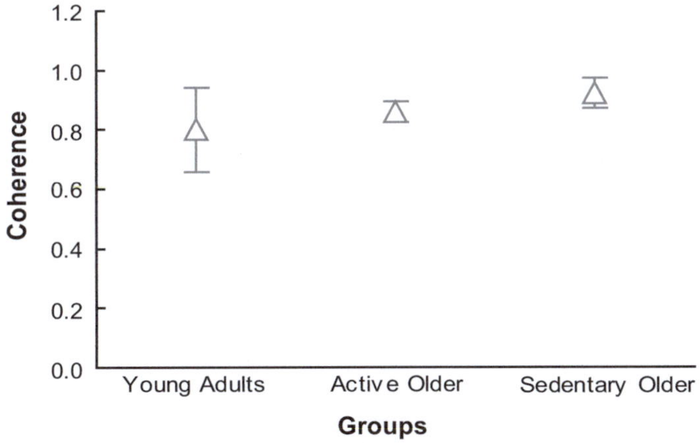

Fig. 14.3 Mean and standard deviation of coherence between room movement and body sway in young adults, active older adults, and sedentary older adults in the condition of continuous movement of the moving room, at the frequency of 0.2 Hz

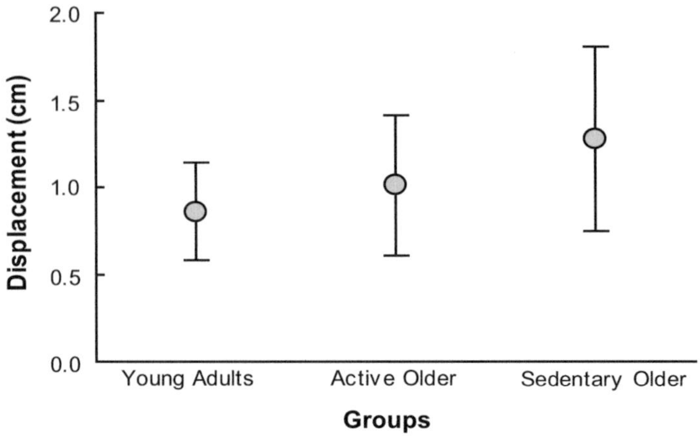

Fig. 14.4 Mean and standard deviation of body displacement triggered by discrete movement of the room backward in young adults, active older adults, and sedentary older adults

respectively. As can be seen, while older adults were more influenced by the room movement than young adults in the continuous condition, with no difference between active and sedentary older adults, in the discrete condition, active older and young adults were less influenced than sedentary older adults by the room movement.

It is important to note that the results do not provide an explanation for the differences between young and older adults in terms of their use of sensory information. However, they do suggest that physical activity can generally enhance the functioning of the postural control system, at least in the specific condition of room movement. However, these results also raise another (one more!) intriguing question: What is the reason for the difference between older and young adults in the continuous and discrete conditions of the room movement?

Based on these results and the many emerging questions, we began to wonder and look for some answers and explanations for these intriguing findings. The first explanation that we forwarded was that despite the sensory alterations and specifically the reduction in visual capacity, older people still kept the relationship between sensory information and motor action intact, performing body sway corresponding to the manipulation, as observed in results from the reported studies. Therefore, although several aspects of the visual system undergo changes due to the aging process, these changes do not prevent or severely deteriorate the relationship between visual information and body sway.

The second finding was that older adults also and still maintain the capability of producing coherent responses and actions based on sensory cues, in this case, visual information. Older adults responded with coherent movement and even higher intensity to the visual manipulation than younger adults. Again, despite the changes that occur in the muscular system with aging, these changes do not prevent the production of motor responses coherent with the visual information being provided.

Despite these two findings, we still question the reason for the more coherent responses [9] and larger magnitude [10, 11] in older adults compared to younger adults when visual information is manipulated. What physical activity could provide in terms of benefits to resolve or minimize these differences between older and younger adults?

To answer these questions, we began to analyze the movement of the moving room in a conflicting sensory situation. Older adults are more influenced by the discrete movement of the moving room, because in this condition there is a sensory conflict that older people need to solve with precision and in a short period of time. The approaching of the moving room frontal wall in relation to the person standing inside of the room erroneously indicates to the person that he/she swayed forward and induces the person to produce backward body sway. With the onset of backward sway, the visual change no longer occurs, but the person begins to change the pressure on the soles of the feet and the position of the ankle joint and also obtains vestibular cues both informing that the body and head are changing. Therefore, there is a sensory conflict between visual information and somatosensory and vestibular information. If the person continues to sway backward with the moving room, using visual information and disregarding somatosensory and vestibular information, he/she may even lose balance and fall. In this situation, older adults need a larger displacement to reverse the displacement initially triggered by the room movement, at least those who are sedentary, as the active ones presented body displacement similar to younger adults.

In the continuous condition of the movement of the room, there is also sensory conflict, but this conflict does not need to be resolved with time pressure, as the movement of the room is smaller and does not compromise the maintenance of upright posture to the point of leading to a fall. Not compromising the upright posture, visual cues provide mean for the CNS of older adults to produce even larger and more coherent postural sway than that observed for young adults. Moreover, despite inducing continuous body sway, the body sway has a much lower magnitude than that triggered by discrete movement of the room and, therefore, it is more difficult for participants to discriminate the conflict between visual and other sensory cues. We remember that in our first study [9], young adults discriminated that the room had been moved, whereas no older adult was able to discriminate against such manipulation.

Wade and colleagues [10] suggested that older people were more influenced by the discrete movement of the room, as they did not have proprioceptive information so refined as to avoid the influence of visual information. This argument can be used to explain results observed in both conditions of continuous and discrete movement of the moving room. With lower resolution or accuracy of the cues coming from the lower limbs and feet, the older adults needed larger amplitude of body sway and, consequently, larger changes in the ankle joint and changes in plantar pressure to discriminate the erroneous movement of swaying based on visual information. Furthermore, with regular physical activity, the older adults could better discriminate the cues coming from the lower limbs allowing the CNS to furnish a piece of much precise information and, thus, not be so influenced by visual manipulation, at least in the discrete condition of the room movement.

Although coherent, an alternative explanation could be suggested: muscle strength. With aging, numerous studies have shown that older adults have reduced muscle torque production capacity and, therefore, this could be the reason for higher body sway resulting from visual manipulation. With a lower capacity to produce muscle torque, older people would produce larger body sway magnitude, as they would take longer to brake and reverse the body sway that had started. Physical activity, however, would cause an increase in the production of joint torque, and thus, active older adults would not differ from young adults. This explanation is plausible for the discrete condition of the moving room but would not help to explain the differences in the continuous condition and, thus, the muscle strength explanation is not sufficient for the changes observed in the older adults.

Sensory or Motor Changes on Postural Control in Older Adults?

It is clear that older adults use sensory information and produce corresponding body sway in the same fashion as young adults, despite the decline of both systems with aging. However, some aspect differs between older and young adults, because the older adults sway with larger magnitude and respond with larger displacement than young adults in the situation of visual manipulation.

Therefore, the next step would be to try to discriminate what could be different in the sensory and motor aspects and what would be the contribution of these possible differences in the postural control of older adults [12, 13]. Toledo [12] initially compared the performance of older and young adults in sensory and motor tests. Sensory tests involved acuity and visual contrast testing (vision), cutaneous sensitivity of the sole of the foot and passive motion detection sensitivity of the ankle and knee (somatosensory), and motor tests involved muscle torque production around the knee and ankle and muscle activation latency after standing posture disturbance. In addition to these tests, the magnitude of postural sway was examined in the semi-tandem standing position.

The results indicated lower performance in older adults compared to younger adults on sensory and motor tests and larger sway magnitude. These results were expected, as the older adults show deterioration and lower performance in the functioning of the sensory systems and reduced capacity to produce muscular torque [13].

In addition to this comparison, we also had the objective of using all these tests to account for body sway performance in this case, larger sway magnitude in the older than in young adults. Using the performance of sensory and motor tests in a multiple regression analysis to explain postural control sway magnitude, the only variable that was associated with older adults' larger body sway was the detection of passive movement in the lower limb joints [13]. Moreover, the passive motion detection contribution to explain larger sway is even more important when the postural task is more challenging [12].

Therefore, although older adults show deterioration of the sensory and motor systems, in order to maintain a standing posture, the difficulty in detecting movement around the ankle joint was the aspect that contributed to larger body sway in older adults. Thus, the answer to the question about which alterations contribute to the decline in the functioning of the postural control system, at least for the conditions that we studied regarding the maintenance of standing posture, are sensory changes and not motor ones. In the case of a person inside the moving room, the deterioration in detecting small changes around the ankle joint leads this person to respond to visual manipulation without any conflict with the somatosensory cues and as a consequence with a larger sway to the visual scenario.

Effect of Physical Activity on Sensory Changes and Postural Control of Older Adults

Prioli and colleagues [11] showed that active older adults responded similarly to younger adults and less than sedentary older people to the manipulation of visual information, in the discrete condition of the room movement. Could such a difference also be due to sensory changes caused by the practice of physical activity? The answer seems to be yes.

Recently, Razuk, Lopes, and Barela [14] showed that older diabetic patients present higher body sway and need higher displacement to detect passive movement of the ankle than active older people. Interestingly, active diabetic patients behaved similarly to active older adults, reducing body sway and displacement to detect passive movement in lower limb joints. Figure 14.5 presents the angular displacement

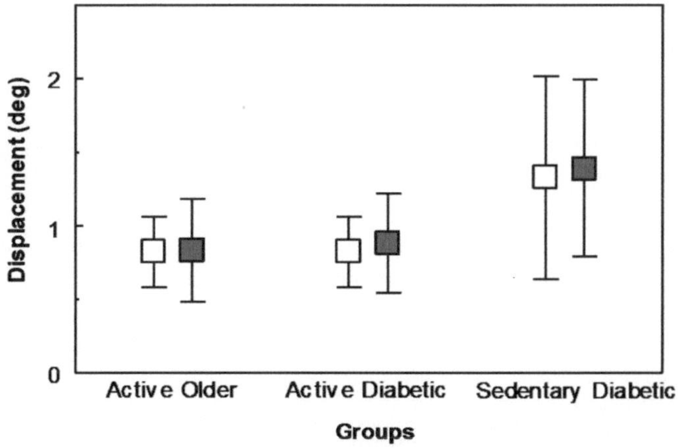

Fig. 14.5 Mean and standard deviation of ankle joint angular displacement in dorsiflexion (open square) and plantar flexion (solid square) to detect passive motion in active older adults, active diabetic patients, and sedentary diabetic patients

values that the participants needed to detect passive movement around the ankle for dorsiflexion and plantar flexion.

As one can observe, both active groups, older and diabetic adults, showed much smaller displacement magnitude compared to the sedentary diabetics adults. Such observation is much important as physical activity seems to preserve and maintain functional performance in discriminating movement around the joint, leading to a much improved performance. It is important and still needed to examine if this improvement due to physical activity is peripheral or central, but despite this doubt, such results are much important and impressive.

Postural Control in Older Adults: Sensory and Motor Changes

Based on the results observed in active and sedentary older people, it can be suggested that the larger body sway observed in several studies involving older participants is due to the deterioration in obtaining accurate sensory cues. With less accurate sensory cues, larger magnitude of body occurs so that the sensors can provide the CNS with information about the sway that is occurring and, thus, muscular activity is triggered to reverse the body sway. Such suggestion was even further examined by providing an additional source of somatosensory cues to older adults when participants used a light touch during upright standing [15]. The higher threshold in detecting passive ankle joint contributed to increased body sway but sway improvement in older adults was observed when enhanced cues were provided by lightly contacting the fingertip with a rigid surface. Specifically, the use of light touch may override peripheral sensory loss of the lower limbs improving postural control performance [15].

Although our recent studies [13, 14] have shown that changes in the detection of passive movement are related to higher body sway in older people maintaining an upright posture and that enhanced cues improve postural control performance [15], it is important to highlight that it would not only be the deterioration of the somatosensory system responsible for changes in postural control in older adults. With aging, older people undergo changes in the visual and somatosensory systems and in the production of muscle torque. However, to maintain an upright posture, the need for muscle torque production is low and, therefore, the reduction observed in older adults does not seem to be crucial. This finding would not be the same if it were observed in a situation of disturbed standing posture, with drastic alteration of postural balance, when the ability to produce muscle torque was perhaps more important and crucial.

Concerning the sensory systems, the decline observed in the various channels causes the need for greater alteration of segments or the whole body, so that such alteration is obtained by the central nervous system and used to obtain information about postural orientation. Thus, for any body adjustment to occur, there is a need for higher displacement to be detected, producing higher sway. Such a situation has been demonstrated involving the somatosensory system responsible for detecting movement around the ankle and knee joints.

Physical activity, however, helps to at least minimize the deterioration or "wear and tear" of sensory stimuli [14]. In this case, it was observed that physical activity maintains the level of detection of passive movement around the joints of the lower limbs similar to that observed in young adults and much lower than that observed for non-active older people. Likewise, physical activity also promotes improvement in several motor skills, for example, joint torque production capacity around the ankle and knee joints. However, these motor changes are not crucial and are not associated with maintaining a more stable upright posture [13].

Postural Control in Older Adults: Lack of Adaptability

Based on what was exposed in this chapter, we can suggest that the lack of adaptability, used in the definition of aging [1], in the case of postural control, permeates the difficulty of older people in using sensory information to obtain accurate information and use it to trigger appropriate muscle activation to keep or achieve a given posture. With the obtaining of less accurate information, older adults have a lower functioning of postural control than that observed in young adults and in many cases are unable to adapt to the demands of maintaining postural orientation and balance, reaching the drastic situation of incurring falls. Even in less drastic situations, the lack of adaptability can also reflect a higher magnitude of body sway.

Finally, changes in the functioning of postural control and deterioration in the use of sensory information to keep the desired body position can at least be minimized by the practice of physical activity. Physical exercises and formal and structured physical activity promote improvement in obtaining sensory information, making the information more accurate and that used by the postural control system can minimize the deterioration of performance of postural control.

Sensory Reweighting and Postural Control in Older Adults

If, on the one hand, physical activity plays an important role in enhancing sensory cue acquisition and muscular responses and, therefore, minimizing the deterioration of postural control observed with aging, on the other hand, the postural control system of older people can use a strategy to modify the use of information from each sensory channel. Considering that the crucial sensory information for the nervous system to control postural orientation and postural equilibrium comes from the somatosensory, vestibular, and visual systems, in many cases, cues from one of these systems generally prevail over cues from the others, depending on the environmental conditions and demands of the motor task. Furthermore, situations of changes in the environment—which modify the availability of sensory information—and the motor task may occur and, moreover, situations in which the different sensory channels provide divergent or conflicting information. In these cases, the CNS needs to manage and select the cues that provide the most relevant information to perform the intended task, thus attributing more importance—or weight—to a certain sensory channel while minimizing the influence (weight) of other channels. This process of adjustment—or adaptation—of the relative contributions of each sensory system to postural control has been named sensory reweighting [16, 17].

Sensory reweighting can occur intentionally, a condition in which the person consciously and voluntarily alters the use of sensory information, or automatically, when the CNS alters the selection and use of sensory information without the person discriminating or having conscious knowledge of such change. Intentional sensory reweighting to control upright posture requires cognitive resources. In studies using the moving room paradigm, visuomotor coupling decreased when participants were informed about the manipulation of visual information, which they had not previously discriminated [18, 19] or when they were asked to resist to the influence of visual information on their postural sway [19, 20]. This means that such people intentionally attributed less weight to visual information, seeking other sources of sensory information, e.g., somatosensory, for their postural control. Similarly, older people and even those with some neurological changes, for instance, Parkinson's disease, can make use of this adaptive mechanism. When older and middle-aged people, with and without Parkinson's disease, were exposed to visual manipulation in the moving room and asked to resist its influence on their body sway, they similarly decreased the magnitude of the sway and the relationship between visual information and body sway, showing that they were also able to intentionally reweight the use of visual information for postural control [21].

Conversely, the ability to automatically reweight the use of sensory information implies the minimum involvement of cognition to control posture, allowing the person to make available a greater reserve of her/his attentional resources to capture environmental and body information relevant to a certain motor task. Furthermore, they can direct their attention to greater use of their executive functions and the planning of motor actions that require a greater degree of intentionality. Thereby, automatic sensory reweighting can contribute to better performance and safety of a voluntary task. Considering that the aging process can lead to a decrease in cognitive capabilities, these adaptive adjustments become especially important for older people to prevent falls and increase their independence in daily life tasks.

The experimental designs of studies examining sensory reweighing in postural control typically add or remove cues from one or more distinct sensory channels, such as vision, proprioception, or touch [22–24] or modify the stimulus variables (e.g., amplitude and frequency) of the same sensory modality [25, 26]. In the case of older people, considering that the aging process causes sensory deterioration and, consequently, a deterioration in the postural control functioning [5–7], the manipulation of sensory information can be used to study sensory reweighting as an adaptive strategy that older people can use to adjust their postural control. The ability to reweigh sensory information, and more importantly, the ability to quickly switch between sensory modalities, is crucial for older people to deal with sudden or unpredictable environmental changes, such as when walking on uneven floors or with variations in lighting, thus minimizing the risk of falls. Indeed, it has been observed that sensory reweighing processes degrade with increasing age and are particularly deficient in fall-prone adults compared to healthy adults [22, 24, 27]. However,

Allison, Kiemel, and Jeka [28] demonstrated that multisensory reweighing was intact in older fallers and non-fallers as well as in young adults. One explanation is that they used much longer trials than previous studies, thus managing to demonstrate that older people may be able to reweight visual and somatosensory information, but perhaps not as quickly as young adults. In a later study, Jeka, Allison, and Kiemel [25] exposed young and older adults to a sudden change in the amplitude of the sinusoidal visual stimulus and examined the postural response, noting that visual reweighting was slower in the older adults, which makes them more vulnerable to disturbances that can compromise their standing posture. Because they observed no differences between groups in the initial response to the sudden change in visual stimulus, they suggested that vision may not play a large role in recovery from perturbations, but more in the ongoing stability of postural control. However, Barela, Genoves, Alleoni, and Barela [29] observed that, with an abrupt change in the amplitude and velocity of the visual stimulus, older participants increased the magnitude of body sway and decreased the relationship between visual information and body sway, but not in the same magnitude than young adults. This suggests that older people are less adaptable to changes in environmental stimuli, probably due to less accurate sensory cues captured by sensory systems.

Final Remarks

Based upon the initial definition of Spirduso et al. [1], which considers the aging process as natural changes in the organism that occur throughout life, leading to a lack of adaptability, we initially questioned what this adaptability referred to and what the implications would be for someone being less adaptable. Presenting studies on postural control, which examined both the performance of postural control and the relationship between sensory information and body sway, we showed that the deterioration in postural control functioning that occurs with aging is due to sensory and motor changes, especially the decreased ability to detect sensory cues, in our case somatosensory, in the lower limbs. However, these difficulties can be minimized through the practice of physical activity, which maintains the level of detection of passive movement around the joints of the lower limbs similar to that observed in young adults. In addition to the important role of physical activity, sensory reweighing is a crucial strategy for older people to adapt their postural control system, with the aim of maintaining a functional and safe performance of their motor actions. Thus, it can be inferred that the aging process, specifically with regard to postural control, does not necessarily lead to a lack of adaptability but is a matter of an adaptation that older people have to deal with their new sensory and motor conditions, which require changes in the sensorimotor relationship to perform the demands of their daily life tasks with less risk.

References

1. Spirduso WW, Francis KL, MacRae PG. Physical dimensions of aging. 2nd ed. Champaign, IL: Human Kinetics; 2005.
2. Horak FB, Macpherson JM. Postural orientation and equilibrium. In: Rowell L, Shepherd J, editors. Handbook of physiology. New York, NY: Oxford University Press; 1996. p. 255–92.
3. Barela JA. Aquisição de habilidades motoras: do inexperiente ao habilidoso. Mot Rev Educ Física. 1999;5(1):53–7.
4. Barela JA. Estratégias de controle em movimentos complexos: ciclo percepção-ação no controle postural. Rev Paul Educ Física. 2000;2000(supl.3):79–88.
5. Berger L, Chuzel M, Buisson G, Rougier P. Undisturbed upright stance control in the elderly: part 1. Age-related changes in undisturbed upright stance control. J Mot Behav [Internet]. 2005;37(5):348–58. Available from: http://www.tandfonline.com/doi/abs/10.3200/JMBR.37.5.348-358.
6. Freitas Júnior P, Barela JA. Alterações no funcionamento do sistema de controle postural de idosos. Uso da informação visual. Rev Port Ciências do Desporto. 2006;2006(1):94–105.
7. Prioli AC, Cardozo AS, de Freitas Júnior PB, Barela JA. Task demand effects on postural control in older adults. Hum Mov Sci [Internet]. 2006;25(3):435–46. Available from: https://linkinghub.elsevier.com/retrieve/pii/S0167945706000297.
8. Perracini MR, Ramos LR. Fatores associados a quedas em uma coorte de idosos residentes na comunidade. Rev Saude Publica [Internet]. 2002;36(6):709–16. Available from: http://www.scielo.br/scielo.php?script=sci_arttext&pid=S0034-89102002000700008&lng=pt&tlng=pt.
9. Polastri PF, Barela AMF, Barela JA. Controle postural em idosos: relacionamento entre informação visual e oscilação corporal. In: Anais do IX Congresso Brasileiro de Biomecânica. Gramado, RS; 2001. p. 133–7.
10. Wade MG, Lindquist R, Taylor JR, Treat-Jacobson D. Optical flow, spatial orientation, and the control of posture in the elderly. J Gerontol Ser B Psychol Sci Soc Sci [Internet]. 1995;50B(1):P51–4. Available from: https://academic.oup.com/psychsocgerontology/article-lookup/doi/10.1093/geronb/50B.1.P51.
11. Prioli AC, Freitas Júnior PB, Barela JA. Physical activity and postural control in the elderly: coupling between visual information and body sway. Gerontology [Internet]. 2005;51(3):145–8. Available from: https://www.karger.com/Article/FullText/83984.
12. Toledo DR. Alterações sensoriais e motoras associadas ao envelhecimento e controle postural de idosos. São Paulo: Universidade Estadual Paulista; 2008.
13. Toledo DR, Barela JA. Sensory and motor differences between young and older adults: somatosensory contribution to postural control. Rev Bras Fisioter [Internet]. 2010;14(3):267–75. Available from: http://www.ncbi.nlm.nih.gov/pubmed/20730372.
14. Razuk M, Lopes AG, Barela JA. Controle postural e informação somatosensorial em idosos diabéticos praticantes e não praticantes de atividade física. Rev Bras Ciência [Internet]. 2010;18(1):26–34. Available from: http://portalrevistas.ucb.br/index.php/RBCM/article/viewArticle/1278.
15. Barela AMF, Caporicci S, de Freitas PB, Jeka JJ, Barela JA. Light touch compensates peripheral somatosensory degradation in postural control of older adults. Hum Mov Sci [Internet]. 2018;60(June):122–30. Available from: https://linkinghub.elsevier.com/retrieve/pii/S0167945717302543.
16. Assländer L, Peterka RJ. Sensory reweighting dynamics in human postural control. J Neurophysiol [Internet]. 2014;111(9):1852–64. Available from: https://www.physiology.org/doi/10.1152/jn.00669.2013.
17. Nashner L, Berthoz A. Visual contribution to rapid motor responses during postural control. Brain Res [Internet]. 1978;150(2):403–7. Available from: https://linkinghub.elsevier.com/retrieve/pii/0006899378902913.

18. Freitas Júnior PB, Barela JA. Postural control as a function of self- and object-motion perception. Neurosci Lett [Internet]. 2004;369(1):64–8. Available from: http://linkinghub.elsevier.com/retrieve/pii/S0304394004009590.
19. Aguiar SA, Gramani-Say K, Lopes AG, Barela JA. Dual task interferes with sensorimotor coupling in postural control. Psychol Neurosci [Internet]. 2014;7(4):593–9. Available from: http://doi.apa.org/getdoi.cfm?doi=10.3922/j.psns.2014.4.19.
20. Barela AMF, Barela JA, Rinaldi NM, Toledo DR. Influence of imposed optic flow characteristics and intention on postural responses. Mot Control. 2009;13:119–29.
21. Cruz CF, Genoves GG, Doná F, Ferraz HB, Barela JA. People in early stages of Parkinson's disease are able to intentionally reweight the use of visual information for postural control. PeerJ [Internet]. 2020;8:e8552. Available from: https://peerj.com/articles/8552.
22. Hay L, Bard C, Fleury M, Teasdale N. Availability of visual and proprioceptive afferent messages and postural control in elderly adults. Exp Brain Res [Internet]. 1996;108(1):129–39. Available from: http://link.springer.com/10.1007/BF00242910.
23. Sozzi S, Do M-C, Monti A, Schieppati M. Sensorimotor integration during stance: processing time of active or passive addition or withdrawal of visual or haptic information. Neuroscience [Internet]. 2012;212:59–76. Available from: https://linkinghub.elsevier.com/retrieve/pii/S0306452212003132.
24. Teasdale N, Stelmach GE, Breunig A, Meeuwsen HJ. Age differences in visual sensory integration. Exp Brain Res [Internet]. 1991;85(3):691–6. Available from: http://link.springer.com/10.1007/BF00231755.
25. Jeka JJ, Allison LK, Kiemel T. The dynamics of visual reweighting in healthy and fall-prone older adults. J Mot Behav [Internet]. 2010;42(4):197–208. Available from: https://www.tandfonline.com/doi/full/10.1080/00222895.2010.481693.
26. Polastri PF, Barela JA, Kiemel T, Jeka JJ. Dynamics of inter-modality re-weighting during human postural control. Exp Brain Res [Internet]. 2012;223(1):99–108. Available from: http://link.springer.com/10.1007/s00221-012-3244-z.
27. Woollacott MH. Editorial: systems contributing to balance disorders in older adults. J Gerontol Ser A Biol Sci Med Sci [Internet]. 2000;55(8):M424–8. Available from: https://academic.oup.com/biomedgerontology/article-lookup/doi/10.1093/gerona/55.8.M424.
28. Allison LK, Kiemel T, Jeka JJ. Multisensory reweighting of vision and touch is intact in healthy and fall-prone older adults. Exp Brain Res [Internet]. 2006;175(2):342–52. Available from: http://link.springer.com/10.1007/s00221-006-0559-7.
29. Barela JA, Genoves GG, Alleoni B, Barela AMF. Visual reweighting in postural control is less adaptative in older adults. Health (Irvine Calif). 2013;5:74–9.

Effects of Vision on Postural Control in Neurologically Healthy Individuals

15

Sérgio Tosi Rodrigues, Gisele Chiozi Gotardi, and Stefane Aline Aguiar

Abstract

The purpose of this chapter is to characterize how the postural system of healthy individuals is capable of adaption when facing distinct levels of challenge, all planned to vary the visual context involved. A series of postural studies showed a variety of circumstances in which the postural control system faced both stronger, mechanical and subtle, sensorial perturbations. Effects of vision were tested in tasks such as moving line-of-gaze in space (during saccadic and smooth pursuit eye movements), grasping an object (under different optic flow conditions), three-ball juggling (under narrow and wide stances), performing a ballet skill (with eyes opened and blindfolded), and driving a car (under simulated conditions); additionally, effects of aging on posture are discussed. In summary, the authors suggest that studies on posture and vision must consider both multiple levels of the visual system functioning (eyes, head, trunk, and whole-body movements) and lifespan postural changes in order to advance our knowledge of the process of acquisition and use of visual information to stabilize posture.

Introduction

The maintenance of balance and body orientation in static and dynamic situations is a core element for the performance of daily life, work, exercise, and sport activities [1]. Postural control requires maintaining position of body segments with respect to both other segments and environment (orientation) and controlling internal forces to compensate external forces acting on the body (balance) [2]. To achieve these behavioral goals, the postural control system needs sensory information regarding

S. T. Rodrigues (✉) · G. C. Gotardi · S. A. Aguiar
Department of Physical Education, Universidade Estadual Paulista, Bauru, SP, Brazil
e-mail: sergio.tosi@unesp.br; gisele.gotardi@unesp.br

F. A. Barbieri et al. (eds.), *Locomotion and Posture in Older Adults*,
https://doi.org/10.1007/978-3-031-74123-4_15

relative position of body parts and forces acting on it to, then, trigger appropriate muscular contractions in order to maintain or change a given postural position. The sensory bases of this perception-action linkage are complex as information arriving from visual, vestibular, and somatosensory channels must be integrated by the superior levels of central nervous system [3]. Conversely, any motor action related to the maintenance or achievement of a given body position requires that the effector system works with a multi-segment body, applying specific strategies and muscle activities to constrain many organism degrees of freedom and have them acting as a functional unit [2].

Analyzing the so-called quiet stance, when individuals standing upright are looking straight ahead, is a standard method in posturography that offers the opportunity of better understanding the perceptuomotor complexity of posture [4]. However, exploring situations in which the postural system is challenged by subtle stimuli or dynamical actions may reveal a more comprehensive perspective on postural adaptability and allow novel manipulations of visual information. Thus, the purpose of this chapter is to characterize how the postural system of healthy individuals is capable of adaption when facing distinct levels of challenge, all planned to vary the visual context involved. A series of postural studies is summarized where the effects of vision were tested in tasks such as moving their line-of-gaze in space (during saccadic and smooth pursuit eye movements), grasping an object (under different optic flow conditions), three-ball juggling (under narrow and wide stances), performing a ballet skill (with eyes opened and blindfolded), and driving a car (under simulated conditions), as shown in the following sections. In addition, a section on a particular type of postural adaptation due to the aging process is presented to describe the effects of progressive perceptual, motor, and cognitive challenges faced by older adults, which is followed by final considerations.

Static Posture and Eye Movements

Specific characteristics define different gaze behaviors such as fixation, saccades, and smooth pursuit eye movements. In fixation, the eyes remain stationary focusing at a given point in the environment so as to stabilize the visual image on the fovea region allowing the extraction and processing of visual information in detail. Saccades are fast eye movements used to bring a new part of the visual field to the fovea region [5]. Due to this high velocity, the processing of visual information during the saccade is extremely poor, a phenomenon known as saccadic suppression [6]. Smooth pursuit is the visual tracking of a moving target in which a continuous movement rotates the eyes to compensate for the motion of the visual object, minimizing blur and therefore occurring within a non-stationary frame of reference [7].

The influence of each one of these behaviors on the control of static posture has been the object of innumerous investigations [8, 9]. Besides their great importance on daily life activities, the fact that eye movements do not generate great biomechanical constraints on posture and large center of mass displacements has made the study of their effects on balance even more attractive. In this section, we explore these effects as well as their interaction with the complexity of the postural and visual tasks.

Effects of Distance to Fixed Object

Lee and Lishman [10] argued that the magnitude of the optic flow resulting from movements of the head is a function of the linear distance between visual object and observer. Consequently, bigger changes in optic flow will be produced while fixating an object nearby compared to a distant one when the observer produces a head movement of the same amplitude. Evidence for this interpretation has been provided by the authors by showing that body sway decreases when subjects are fixating nearby targets (0.4 m) compared to distant ones (3 m). Since greater changes in optic flow will be produced for head displacements when the observer is fixating nearby targets, body sway becomes more "detectable" and would be minimized more precisely to stabilize the fixed object in the visual field. Conversely, for distant targets greater magnitude of body oscillation can be allowed without having a large effect on the stabilization of the visual image [10].

Stoffregen et al. [11] extended this finding demonstrating that, when the subject is fixating a distant object but the object nearby is still present in the visual field, body sway is still greater than when the nearby object is being fixated. The authors argue that even though visual information on the nearby object is still available in the optic array, body sway occurred as a function of the task at hand. This means that oscillation was still greater because the subject was fixating a distant target, regardless on the available visual information that might be "automatically" detected by the postural control system but was not part of the suprapostural task [11].

This study has been replicated in further investigations, which moved on to show how these effects interact with more complex postures [12]. Rodrigues et al. [12] explored the effects of object distance on body sway during the maintenance of the kiba-dachi posture, a karate stance which challenges balance specially in the anterior–posterior direction since it requires the person to maintain their legs very distant from each other (larger than shoulder width) with knees flexed and trunk aligned with the feet. Results revealed decreased body sway while fixating a nearby object as compared to a distant one, showing that the effect of distance is also present during the control of such complex posture [12].

Effects of Saccades on Posture

Although a few studies suggested that eye movements might actually increase body sway, this finding was only present in very specific contexts, such as adding cognitive tasks while performing eye movements [13] and exploring these effects in patients with spontaneous nystagmus as opposed to planned voluntary saccades [8, 14]. Overall, the literature provides solid evidence that saccades decrease body sway in neurologically healthy individuals [15]. This is exemplified by experiments showing reduced body oscillation during saccades performed both horizontally and vertically [16] and at near and far distances between observer and visual object [17]. Several studies confirm this pattern of results [18, 19]. Interestingly, eye movements performed with eyes closed do not reduce body sway [19].

Stoffregen et al. [9] argue that the reason why body oscillation is reduced during eye movements is to achieve the goal of stabilizing the visual scene, allowing eye movements to be performed more accurately. Two mechanisms are thought to be responsible for visually detecting body sway and stabilizing posture, which are referred to as afferent and efferent motion perception or ocular and extraocular mechanisms, respectively [20]. The first, afferent motion perception, is a feedback-based mechanism which uses information contained in the optic flow to minimize retinal slip and therefore stabilize the distance between the eye and the visual environment. The second, efferent motion perception, is based on either the copy of the motor command, named efference copy—which is a feedforward mechanism that predicts the sensory consequences of the movement produced—or the extraocular muscle afferents, named reafferences, that are consecutive to eye movements [20].

Rodrigues et al. [18] investigated not only the effects of saccades on postural stabilization but also their interaction with the complexity of the postural and eye movement tasks. While performing horizontal saccades at different frequencies (0.5 and 1.1 Hz), young adults controlled their balance by standing either with feet apart at shoulder width or pressed together reducing stability especially in medial-lateral axis. Results indicated in general reduced body sway during saccades compared to fixation and in narrow compared to wide stance, as expected. Also, specifically in the anterior–posterior axis, body sway was greater for narrow compared to wide stance only in the condition of high frequency (1.1 Hz) saccades. This shows that the reduction in body sway that took place during eye movements was actually stronger with the combination of the most complex postural (narrow stance) and eye movements (1.1 Hz saccades) tasks. Therefore, the reduced time for the planning of the next saccade which occurs for the high frequency saccades compared to the low frequency ones might have required greater stabilization of posture in the non-stable narrow stance condition in order to accurately fulfill the demands of the eye movement task being performed. The authors argue that the fact that the frequency of saccades could affect posture differently according to the stance condition is in line with an adaptive resource-sharing model, proposed by Mitra and Fraizer [21–23], which postulates that postural and suprapostural tasks compete for the same limited resources which will be dedicated to either one of these tasks according to the demands of each one [18].

Brito et al. [24] further investigated the relationship between gaze and posture, analyzing an even more dynamical context; effects of predictable and unpredictable saccadic eye movements in stationary and moving visual scenarios on posture were compared. They found that while mean amplitude of center of pressure displacements was lower in the saccadic tasks compared to the gaze fixation, in predictable and unpredictable conditions, they were higher in the moving scenario than in the stationary condition. Variability of center of pressure displacements was lower in the unpredictable saccades than gaze fixation task; saccadic reaction time was longer in the unpredictable as compared to the predictable task. The authors concluded that postural displacements were reduced to facilitate the saccadic tasks regardless of predictability conditions and task complexity, with lower variability used by participants to deal with increased attentional demands of unpredictable saccades [24].

Effects of Smooth Pursuit on Posture

Although saccades clearly stabilize posture, contradictory results have been presented on whether performing smooth pursuit eye movements decreases or increases body oscillation. Visual tracking of a moving target has been shown to cause larger body sway, especially when the target appeared in a dark background [8, 25]. The lack of spatial reference of a dark background together with additional manipulations on stance conditions in these studies—using complex tasks such as heel-to-toe position and standing on a foam cushion—makes these results able to be interpreted only in very specific contexts.

Recent evidence has been provided, however, indicating that smooth pursuit eye movements performed in a regular spatial frame of reference—i.e., not in darkness—which is the most common situation observed in daily life activities, actually decrease body sway, stabilizing posture similarly to saccades [26]. In this investigation, Rodrigues et al. [26] varied the velocity of saccades and smooth pursuit eye movements and demonstrated that both types of eye movements decreased body oscillation compared to fixation, regardless of their velocities.

There are relevant differences between saccades and smooth pursuit eye movements. First difference is related to saccadic suppression, which drastically reduces the capacity for processing of visual information during saccades but does not exist for smooth pursuit. Second difference is the non-stationary spatial frame of reference that occurs during smooth pursuit but not during saccades. Third difference, and perhaps the most important one, is the fact that while smooth pursuit are movements entirely based on feedback to keep the target at the fovea region continuously, saccades need to be planned beforehand due to their high velocity, leaving no space for corrections during their execution. Nevertheless, even with these different aspects, both eye movement tasks seem to reduce body sway, leaving authors to conclude that the mechanisms involved in the execution of saccades and smooth pursuit eye movements share similarities in postural control [26], possibly due to the fact that greater postural stabilization is required to perform both tasks accurately [9].

Posture, Optic Flow, and Arm Movements

Effects of Grasping Movements Under Different Optic Flow Conditions

Many environmental aspects such as the optical flow and one's own movement can affect posture stabilization. However, little is known about how these two features can be combined as participants maintain upright stance during grasping actions. Rodrigues et al. [26] examined the effects of discrete movements of a moving room (approaching to or moving back from participants) combined with grasping an object on postural control stability. Twelve participants stood upright inside a moving room, which moved discretely approaching or moving away from the participants, as they had to remain still or grasp a stationary or an approaching ball, totalizing nine experimental conditions (Table 15.1).

A pulley system was connected to a servo-mechanism in order to move simultaneously the room and a shaft, which had a ball (6 cm of diameter) fixed in its end. Forward and backward movements of the room were associated with clockwise and anti-clockwise rotations of the pulley system, moving the shaft in speed and amplitude proportional to the movement of the room in the same or opposite directions. Participants were instructed to stay in the starting position as stable as possible and keep it through the end of the experimental trials with no grasping (conditions 1, 4, and 5), grasping the ball after the light being turned on with no movement of the room and of the ball (condition 2), and grasping the ball after the light being turned on simultaneously to the room and shaft movements initiation (conditions 3, 6, 7, 8, and 9). The discrete movement of the room had approximate duration of 2 s, with peak velocity of 2.6 cm/s and amplitude of 2.5 cm [27]; the shaft approached the participant, being moved approximately during 2 s, with peak velocity of 74.8 cm/s and amplitude of 53 cm. During all conditions, participants were required to stand upright for 18 s, maintaining fixation with their eyes on the ball. Each trial was divided into four-time windows: prior to room movement initiation (4 s), during room movement (2 s), after room movement—first and second periods (4 s each), totalizing 14 s; the remaining time was excluded from analysis. The variables body displacement and correlation coefficient were obtained during the room movement;

Table 15.1 Rodrigues et al.'s [26] experimental conditions combining manipulations of moving room, ball, and catching action

Condition	Room	Ball	Grasping
1	Stationary	Stationary	Absent
2	Stationary	Stationary	Present
3	Stationary	Approaching	Present
4	Approaching	Stationary	Absent
5	Moving back	Stationary	Absent
6	Approaching	Stationary	Present
7	Moving back	Stationary	Present
8	Approaching	Approaching	Present
9	Moving back	Approaching	Present

the variable mean sway amplitude was used to infer stability prior to and after movement of the room.

Rodrigues et al. [26] found that grasping leads to increased effect of moving room on induced body sway, as body displacement is larger during grasping. However, body sway is more related to room movement when the room is moved back compared to the approaching movement. Despite inducing larger body sway during the movement of the moving room, grasping disruption of postural equilibrium is even larger when there is no moving room visual flow. These results also showed that grasping a stationary ball in a moving scenario is worse, leading to larger body sway induced by the moving room and such effect is even larger in the moving back movement of the room. Such postural equilibrium disruption is still observed after the grasping has ended (following 4 s).

It was surprising that grasping during room discrete movement leads to a larger sway; literature had pointed out only correspondent body sway in children [28], adults [27], and even in older adults [29]. This new finding can be explained by the fact that when adults have to gather information about the ball position, they are more influenced by the peripheral flow. In the context of a moving room with no arm movement involved, it is known that flow with large lamellar (peripheral) structure generates stronger sway response than more radially (centrally) structured flow [30]. In line with this reasoning is that, although vision of the hand in Rodrigues et al.'s [26] experiment is peripherally available during its initial movement, the use of central vision during the later stages of grasping is advantageous for controlling movement amplitude as the limb decelerates [31].

The correlation coefficient in the moving back condition, which indicates the relationship between moving room and body sway, was dependent on direction, being stronger in the condition of backward optical flow, with the room moving away from the participant. It is well-known that infant rhesus monkeys [32] and infant humans [33] show defensive reactions to approaching (looming) patterns of optic flow; these responses were in clear contrast to those related to objects approaching on a non-collision path or a shrinking (as opposed to a looming) pattern [34]. In the moving room paradigm, the room approaches the observers who respond to the optical flow (looming) as if it arose from their own postural sway [35], attempting to keep a constant relation with the room's walls. As in Rodrigues et al.'s [26] experiment, a grasping action was required, the postural adjustment in response to the approaching movement of the room would result in increase of hand-ball distance; instead, a sway stabilization took place to allow a proper grasping movement. Differently, the room moving back from participants seemed to have facilitated grasping as they both were in the same direction.

In short, Rodrigues et al. [26] showed that grasping leads to increased effect of moving room on induced body sway. In this context, posture was more affected when the room was moved back compared to the approaching movement. Based upon these results, the authors suggest that postural control takes advantage of the structured optical flow available due to room movement, even when posture might be destabilized due to one's own movement, to maintain postural equilibrium.

Effects of Juggling Movements Under Different Bases of Support Conditions

Cascade ball juggling is a complex perceptual-motor skill, which requires an efficient postural stabilization. Experience in the juggling task may play a role in the linkage between manual and postural tasks. To clarify how the postural system works in this context, Rodrigues et al. [36] investigated effects of experience (expert and intermediate groups) and feet distance (wide and narrow stances) on body sway of jugglers during three-ball cascade juggling. Participants stood barefoot on the force plate (some participants wore a gaze tracking system), with feet maintained in wide and narrow conditions and performed three 40 s trials of the three-ball juggling task.

The main finding of Rodrigues et al. [36] was that only intermediate jugglers showed smaller oscillation in the narrow as compared to wide stance. Expert jugglers showed a superior postural stabilization in both stances, with more consistent patterns of center of pressure displacements characterized by measures of mean velocity and amplitude in both anteroposterior and mediolateral axes, corroborating the notion according to which juggling skill level is associated with decreased body sway. Previous studies have shown that expertise similarly affects other motor skills, such as rifle shooting, manual rhythmic movements, circus activities, and gymnastics [37–41]. In a study with jugglers, Leroy et al. [42] found that, although experts and intermediate participants showed similar body sway amplitude (measured through sacrum lateral displacement), the skilled group was able to perform anticipatory postural adjustments differently from novice jugglers.

Interestingly, gaze behavior seems to participate in controlling more complex postural tasks. The increased body sway of intermediate jugglers could be explained by the larger area of gaze displacement observed throughout each trial. A more stable, spatially reduced gaze pattern, named gaze-through strategy [43], may improve movement planning via the attentional system [44, 45]. During a gaze fixation, balls move in the retinal periphery, which most likely involves a stage operating in gaze-centered coordinates that is more accurate [43, 46]. With a more stable gaze, movement planning is improved because the entire visual background is stable since allocentric and gaze-centered representations become aligned [43, 47]. Although visual information acquisition through fixation patterns (number of fixations, mean duration of fixations and its variability) was not affected by group or condition in Rodrigues et al.'s study [36], the significant base of support by group interaction found for the area of gaze displacement seems to corroborate the experts' gaze-through strategy, suggesting an attentional linkage between postural (center of pressure) and visual (gaze) stability, as shown in typical examples of the time series of center of pressure and line-of-gaze displacement (Fig. 15.1). Although acknowledging the small sample size of gaze data, the authors interpreted these results as a confirmation that experts were less dependent of foveal vision and more capable of decoupling the control of posture and bimanual rhythmic arm movements [37, 47].

Rodrigues et al. [36] found a surprising significant effect of base of support; greater postural instability was expected during more challenging tasks, but the

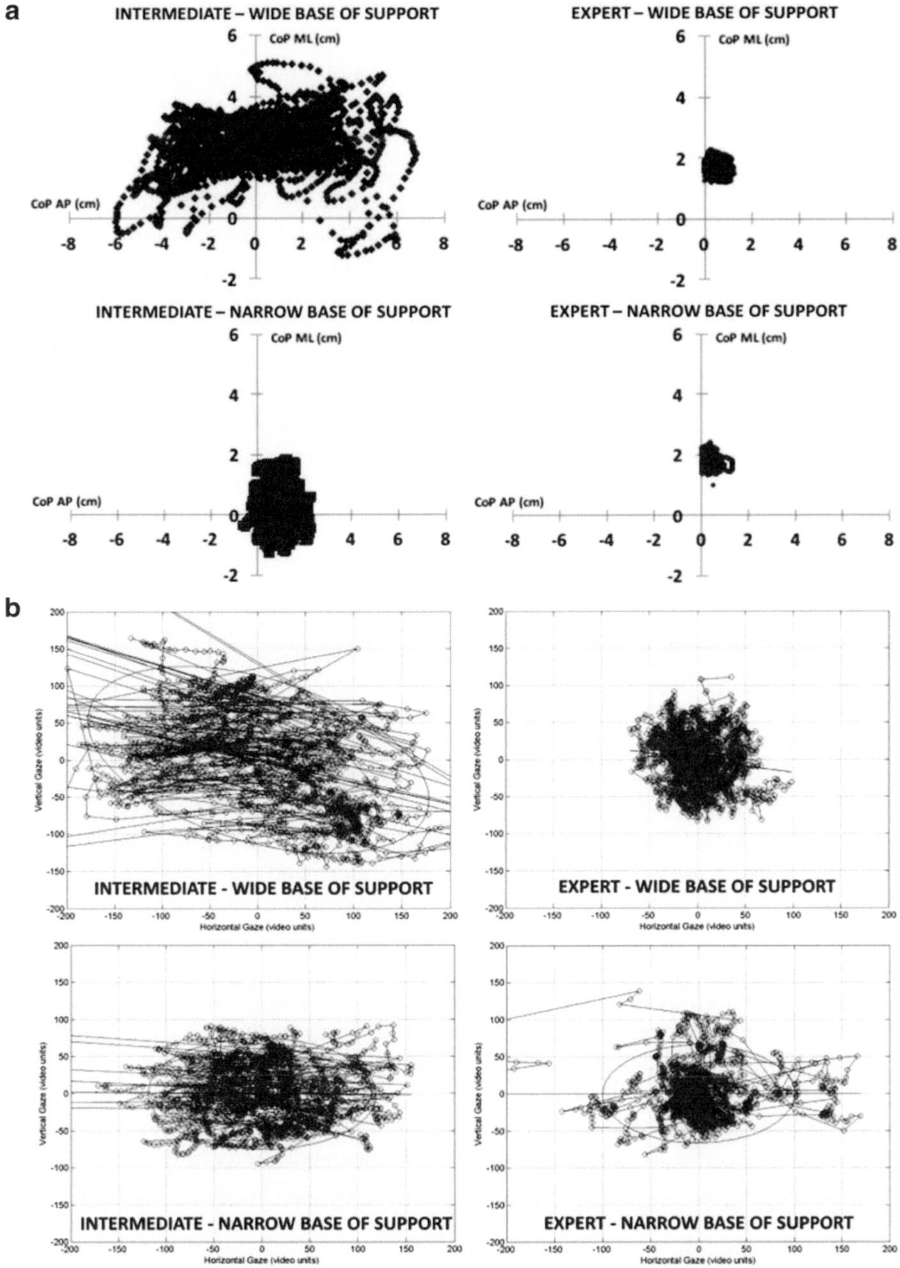

Fig. 15.1 Rodrigues et al.'s [36] typical examples of the time series of center of pressure (**a**) and line-of-gaze displacement (**b**) during cascade juggling on wide and narrow bases of support in intermediate (left panels) and expert (right panels) jugglers. Ellipses represent area containing 85% of gaze data

opposite was observed. Particularly, intermediate jugglers increased the sway laterally more than experts to facilitate their arms movement pattern, as shown by the significant main effect of group on the ML sway amplitude. Additionally, intermediate jugglers showed significantly smaller oscillation in the narrow stance, indicating that experts were less affected by the basis of support reduction than intermediate jugglers. Expert jugglers showed differences in body oscillation between narrow and wide stances, which were not significant while the intermediate group was clearly affected by the smaller basis of support and had to reduce more drastically their body sway to keep balance and the juggling task ongoing. The authors interpreted their results as corroborating previous studies which showed effects of the experience and motor specialization on the improvement of postural control [42, 48–50].

In sum, Rodrigues et al. [36] concluded that experts' body sway was characterized by lower velocity and smaller amplitude as compared to intermediate group. Interestingly, the authors found that the more challenging (narrow) basis of support caused significant attenuation in body sway only for the intermediate group, suggesting that expertise in cascade juggling was associated with refined postural control.

Eye–Head Stabilization in Complex Contexts

The role of visual information on the control of movement has been investigated in a variety of complex contexts such as everyday life and sport activities [51–54]. The eyes move around the environment to align fovea region to a specific portion of visual scene for processing of visual information in detail [52]. Acquisition of useful visual information in dynamical postures involves controlled coordination between body, head, and eye movements. Eye and head stabilization during the execution of motor actions is an important mechanism to keep stationary the image on the retina in order to ensure a clearer visual processing during the execution of motor actions [53, 54].

Two kinds of compensatory mechanisms participate in the stabilization of eyes and head during dynamical postures, making the eyes to move in line with head rotations. In the vestibulo-ocular reflex, head rotation velocity is detected by semicircular channels (vestibular system), which provide sensory signals to the oculomotor system to move the eyes in the opposite direction. The second mechanism, the optokinetic reflex, is engaged in adjusting the actual velocity of the retinal image with the velocity of eyes rotation in the same direction [52]. In this section, it will be discussed the role of eye and head stabilization in several everyday life and sport activities that directly affect visual information acquisition and the maintenance of dynamical stability.

Stabilizing Posture During Dynamical Skills: Ballet and Table Tennis

Visual information during the execution of a ballet pirouette is the crucial sensory input used to maintain postural stability. However, visual processing is impaired during the rotation of the trunk, head, and eyes that can affect dynamical posture. Denardi et al. [54] investigated the role of visual information on postural control of expert ballet dancers with analyses of trunk, head, and eyes movements during the execution of a pirouette with (opened eyes) and without (blindfolded eyes) vision available. Gaze stability for as long as possible during performance is an important strategy to minimize rotational flow on the retina generated by the movement of whole body [53–55]. In Denardi et al.'s [54] experiment, gaze stability strategy was checked with analyses of the quiet eye period. The concept of quiet eye proposed by Vickers [55, 56] suggested that a longer final fixation before the initiation of movement is used to extract the maximum of the critical information from environment to define details of motor performance. Denardi et al. [54] observed a longer quiet eye period in the beginning of the pirouette turns; however, there was absence of correlation between quiet eye duration and postural stability. In contrast with previous studies [53, 55, 57], a longer period of quiet eye did not cause changes on pirouette performance. However, the authors assumed that visual information acquired during gaze stability period was sufficient for expert ballet dancers to achieve dynamical postural requirements of the task [54]. In addition, a clear sequence of trunk, head, and eyes rotations in the execution of the pirouette with opened eyes was observed. In the initiation of movement, trunk rotation starts to turn following with the rotation of the head and finishing with the delayed eyes rotation. At the end, eyes rotation starts following to the head and trunk rotations sequentially. Interestingly, in the experimental conditions without visual information (blindfolded eyes), the rotations of the head and trunk were coupled [54]. These findings showed evidence that when visual information was available, head movements were delayed to maintain the gaze stability as long as possible in order to ensure a useful extraction of information during quiet eye period. Eye and head stabilization during quiet eye period facilitated visual information acquisition to perform the task [54].

Rodrigues, Vickers, and Williams [53] investigated the coordination of head, eye, and arm movements of skilled and less skilled table tennis players; although they did not focus directly on postural control, head contribution to visual stability may help in understanding the role played by vision in posture. Their experimental task consisted of a forehand drive shot to one of the two cued target areas, which was illuminated in order to generate distinct temporal conditions: pre-cue, before serve; early-cue, during the initial portion of ball flight; late-cue, during the final portion of ball flight. The duration of quiet eye was reduced according to the increase in complexity of the task (from pre- to early-cue and from early- to late-cue conditions). Eye–head stabilization was defined as the period in which head and eye were aligned. During the most difficult condition (late-cue), eye–head stabilization was less frequent suggesting that task complexity disrupted optimal conditions for information acquisition via eye–head stability, which occurred along with a reduction in the quiet eye duration. These changes in eye–head stabilization and quiet eye period during more complex task induced a lower accuracy performance for all players [52, 53].

Eye and Head Stabilization During Driving

Driving a car is a particularly complex type of locomotion supported by visual information available in the surrounding environment. Eye and head movements have been studied during driving situations to determine drivers' visual search strategies [51, 52, 58–61]. Land and Lee [62] investigated the steering control on a road with steeper bends, recording steering wheel angle and drivers' gaze direction. The authors found that, before the car entering on the bend, drivers spent much of time fixating the tangent point—defined as the most salient point inside of the bend—and also observed a clear correlation between gaze and steering wheel angle, with gaze movements preceding the rotation of the steering wheel by about 0.8 s. The authors suggested that gaze angle directed at the tangent point can provide the signal needed for the arms to control of the steering wheel [62]. In another study, Land and Tatler [58] examined the eye and head movements of a Formula 3 racing driver in a winding road. The racing driver fixated most of the time close to, but not exactly at, the tangent point before starting to turn the steering wheel [58]. Interestingly, head movements from central line of the lane to the tangent point begun 1.5 s before starting cornering, and the correlation between driver's head direction and the rotation of the vehicle was stronger ($r = 0.96$) than correlation between gaze and head direction ($r = 0.3$). The authors suggested that, even though the racing driver did not displace his gaze exactly to the tangent point location, driver's head direction provided sufficient information for the steering wheel control [57].

Carizio [51] investigated the effects of cognitive workload (use of cell phone) on gaze and head stability during simulated driving. The use of a cell phone in speakerphone mode or holding the device in the driver's hand can interfere in the attentional mechanism of drivers and tend to disrupt perceptual and motor performance. Drivers had eyes and head movements recorded while driving in a driver simulator under three experimental conditions: control (no talking, no cell phone), speakerphone mode (talking, with cell phone in speakerphone mode), and holding in hand (talking, with cell phone held in the hand). Results revealed that drivers performed a higher number of fixations per time unit and a higher spread of fixation locations in the horizontal and vertical axes during both cell phone conditions as compared to the control condition. Similarly to gaze behavior, variance of head position and orientation also increased during both speakerphone mode and holding in hand conditions of mobile phone use. These findings suggest that increased cognitive workload/task complexity provoked a decrease in eye and head stabilization [51], corroborating previous studies on eye–head stabilization in sports [53]. Carizio et al. [63], based on data from the same experiment [51], measured cognitive workload through pupil dilation. Interestingly, greater pupil dilation during talking on the cell phone (handheld and hands-free conditions) while driving occurred only for the novice group. Experience level of the two groups modulated cognitive workload imposed by the dual task of talking on a cell phone, altering acquisition of visual information and impairing postural responses and driving behavior [51, 63].

Another interest in investigating gaze behavior in driving is due to the relationship between the adoption of risky visual strategies (e.g., more fixations toward irrelevant areas in the visual scene) and a greater likelihood of accident involvement. Gotardi and colleagues [59] induced state-anxiety on experienced- and inexperienced-drivers while driving in a car simulator. In the high-anxiety condition, both groups were involved in more collisions and reduced the number of fixations toward the lane ahead (main source of relevant information) compared to the low-anxiety condition. Interestingly, the anxiety-induced shift in attention differed across experience: inexperienced drivers under pressure spent more time looking at other cars on the road, while experienced drivers increased the number of fixations on the speedometer. The authors argued that high levels of state-anxiety disturb drivers' visual attention differently: inexperienced drivers tended to shift attention to threatening stimuli, while experienced drivers were more likely to engage in conscious motor processing behavior. However, both attentional shifts were accompanied by a higher rate of collisions [59]. In addition to the complexity of sensory stimuli and motor actions involved in natural situations, the aging process represents a progressive challenge and requires important adaptation of older adults. Gotardi and colleagues [61] investigated the potential effects of aging process and/or age-related neurological diseases, such as Parkinson's disease (PD), on gaze behavior and performance of drivers. Neurologically healthy older drivers, older drivers with PD, and neurologically healthy young drivers were asked to drive in a car simulator for 3 min while keeping the speed at 100–120 km/h. Both PD and aging process caused a drop in driving performance. Drivers with PD made fewer fixations on task-relevant information and showed higher visual entropy than young adults, whereas older drivers restricted their visual search to the lane than other areas of interest [61]. In natural contexts as those referred above [51, 53, 54, 58, 59], eye and head movements seem to work together to extract useful visual information from a relevant location at a proper time. Particularly, head control plays a critical role in maintaining gaze stability in such complex contexts, which is in line with previous evidence of linkage between eye movements and postural control discussed above [51, 53, 54]. The coordinated activity of eyes, head, trunk, and whole body emphasizes the organism's collective effort toward an optimal acquisition of useful visual information; the observed coupling between gaze and motor behavior is evidence that visual information is essential for planning motor actions and maintaining dynamical posture in complex contexts [51–55].

Effects of Aging on Eye Movements and Postural Control

Aging is known to affect both the motor and sensory systems which are intimately related in the control of static posture [64]. Older adults show poorer performance compared to young adults in both postural control [64–66] and eye movement tasks

[67–69]. Specifically, postural control has been shown to be affected by aging in both simple [70] and complex postural tasks [71]. For this reason, the risk of falls in older adults has received great attention from researchers and authorities representing an important public health issue [72]. Mechanisms contributing to poorer postural control in older adults include motor deficits such as muscle weakness [73], sensory deficits in visual [74], vestibular [75], and somatosensory systems [76] and limitations in attentional capabilities [77]. Importantly, besides causing specific deficits in both motor and sensory systems contributing to postural control, aging has been shown to affect also sensorimotor integration in the control of posture [71, 78].

Deficits caused by aging specifically in the visual system such as a reduced visual acuity [79] and a poorer contrast sensibility [80] provoke an impaired visual perception to older adults. Furthermore, the effect of aging on performance of eye movement tasks has also been well documented. Older adults perform saccades less accurately [68], with slower reaction times [81] and with reduced amplitude, velocity, and frequency [82] compared to young adults. The gain [83] and accuracy [69] of smooth pursuit eye movements are also affected by aging. A comparison between the performance of eye movements in real world and laboratory situations has shown that in real world performance of saccades is greatly deteriorated by aging, while performance on tracking movements can remain unaffected by aging probably due to the use of additional sensory cues compensating for aging deficits [82]. Interestingly, the effects of aging on eye movements performance have been shown also for common tasks such as reading [84] and have been even proposed as an indicator on driver's ability in older adult drivers [85] and as a tool for detecting mild cognitive impairments [86].

Similar to results shown previously from young adults [18], Aguiar et al. [64] also explored the effects of saccades at different frequencies and different stance conditions in postural control but in a population of older adults. Discussions around the adaptive resource-sharing model would be enriched with this investigation since the sensory and motor deficits presented by older adults would potentially alter these limited resources available for postural and suprapostural tasks and therefore how the postural control system would give priority to one task over another. Results showed decrease in body sway during saccades compared to fixation, which is the same result encountered in young adults. Interestingly, no difference was found between narrow and wide stance conditions according to the frequency of saccades, which was present for young adults. The authors concluded that older adults present a more rigid postural control strategy, which does not allow larger body sway during a more complex postural task [64]. However, Laufer et al. [65] investigated postural stability in young and older adults during upright stance on restricted basis of support, 85 cm above ground level, with both opened and closed eyes. Postural threat did not affect young adults; however, older adults showed a greater mean power frequency of displacement of center of pressure [65]. The authors concluded that older adults adopted an inadequate postural response during postural threat that increased body sway. The increasing of complexity of the postural task may be a challenge to older adults since the postural control system is affected by aging. In

Aguiar et al.'s experiment [64], even with a more complex postural task (restricted basis of support), older adults maintained their body sway unaltered with different frequencies of horizontal saccadic eye movements. According to the authors, older adults performed a more rigid postural strategy to prioritize the postural performance during a threatening situation, which did not allow the influence of saccadic eye movements on body sway. Interestingly, Paquette and Fung [67] found that older adults performed more corrective saccadic movements and with greater latency between stimulus onset and saccadic eye movement onset with a moving surface compared to young adults. The authors suggested that older adults have visual and postural performance impaired during threatening stability situations. In general, saccadic eye movements reduce body sway of young and older adults; however, during more challenging postural tasks, the relationship between eye movements and postural control seems to be altered with aging.

Final Considerations

Understanding the effects of vision on postural control in healthy individuals requires an extended notion of visual system which includes postural elements. For instance, the notion that "eyes-in-the-head-on-the-body-resting-on-the-ground" [87] are continuously searching for relevant information in the optic flow favors the simultaneous consideration of gaze and postural data to discuss balance control. Postural adjustments seem to support optimal gaze behavior during simple and complex actions. Although optic flow results from translational components of head movement in space and eye movements add rotational components to the flow on the retina [88, 89], a process of minimization of rotational consequences to the flow, called gaze stabilization [90], seems advantageous to optimize translational information acquisition with respect to the perceiver. As human visual input depends on the dynamics of all body parts, studies on posture should explore this collective postural effort (resulting from movements of eyes, head, trunk, and whole body) to acquire the relevant information available in the optic flow, needed to successful action.

Following this suggestion, the series of studies presented in this chapter showed a variety of circumstances in which the postural control system faced both stronger, mechanical perturbations and subtle, sensory challenges. During quiet stance, posture is more stabilized when the fixed object is nearby as compared to a distant one, a principle which holds for complex stances, such as karate kiba-dachi; besides distinct control mechanisms, saccadic and smooth pursuit eye movements directed to predictable and continuous stimulus also tend to reduce body sway.

In contexts with more complex postural requirements, adaptations in the perception-action linkage are multivariate. Grasping action leads to increased effect of optic flow (moving room) on induced body sway; posture was more affected when the room was moved back compared to the approaching movement, suggesting that postural control takes advantage of the structured optical flow available, even when posture might be destabilized due to one's own movement, to maintain postural balance. In cascade juggling, expertise reduces body sway of participants; the more challenging (narrow) basis of support caused significant attenuation in body sway only for the intermediate group, suggesting that experts have a refined postural control. During a pirouette in ballet or a forehand drive in table tennis, eye and head stabilization was strategically adopted in order to facilitate the extraction of useful information to control the motor behavior; increasing of task complexity (removing visual information in ballet or delaying the visual cue in table tennis) caused impairment on eye–head stabilization which disrupted performance. In simulated driving, an increase in cognitive load generated by the use of cell phone resulted in higher relative number of fixations and spatial spread of fixation locations, as well as increased variance of head position and orientation, suggesting a worsening of postural stability and visual information acquisition.

Particularly, characterizing the effects of vision on postural control in healthy older adults adds even more complexity to the debate. The natural perceptual, motor, and cognitive deficits due to the aging process push the limits of adaptation. In general, the older adults show a more rigid postural control strategy, with increased probabilities of instability and risk of falls. In summary, the authors suggest that studies on posture and vision must consider both multiple levels of the visual system functioning (eyes, head, trunk, and whole-body movements) and lifespan postural changes in order to advance our knowledge of the process of acquisition and use of visual information to stabilize posture.

References

1. Zatsiorsky VM. Kinematics of human motion. Champaign, IL: Human Kinetics; 1998.
2. Horak FB, MacPherson JM. Postural orientation and equilibrium. In: Rowell LB, Sherpherd JT, editors. Handbook of physiology. Exercise: Regulation and integration of multiple systems. New York: Oxford University Press; 1996.
3. Nashner LM. Analysis of stance posture in humans. In: Towe AL, Luschei ES, editors. Motor coordination. Handbook of behavioral physiology. New York: Plenum Press; 1981. p. 527–65.
4. Duarte M, Freitas SMSF. Revision of posturography based on force plate for balance evaluation. Rev Bras Fisioter. 2010;14:183–92.
5. Carpenter RHS. Movements of the eyes. London: Pion Limited; 1988.
6. Volkmann FC, Schick AM, Riggs LA. Time course of visual inhibition during voluntary saccades. J Opt Soc Am. 1968;58:562–9.
7. Krauzlis R. Recasting the smooth pursuit eye movement system. J Neurophysiol. 2004;91:591–603.
8. Glasauer S, Schneider E, Jahn K, Strupp M, Brandt T. How the eyes move the body. Neurology. 2005;65:1291–3.
9. Stoffregen T, Bardy B, Bonnet C, Hove P, Oullier O. Postural sway and the frequency of horizontal eye movements. Mot Control. 2007;11:86–102.
10. Lee DN, Lishman JR. Visual proprioceptive control of stance. J Hum Mov Stud. 1975;1:87–95.
11. Stoffregen TA, Pagulayan RJ, Bardy BG, Hettinger LJ. Modulating postural control to facilitate visual performance. Hum Mov Sci. 2000;19:203–20.
12. Rodrigues ST, Jardim JG, Siqueira NS, Paula F, Aguiar SA, et al. Estabilização postural do olhar : Efeitos da distância do objeto [Postural stabilization of looking: effects of distance to target]. Brazilian J Motor Behav. 2011;6:7–15.

13. Hunter MC, Hoffman MA. Postural control: visual and cognitive manipulations. Gait Posture. 2001;13:41–8.
14. Jahn K, Strupp M, Krafczyc S, Schüler O, Glasauer S, Brandt T. Suppression of eye movements improves balance. Brain. 2002;125:2005–11.
15. Bonnet CT, Baudry S. Active vision task and postural control in healthy, young adults: synergy and probably not duality. Gait Posture. 2016;48:57–63.
16. Rougier P, Garin M. Performing saccadic eye movements or blinking improves postural control. Mot Control. 2007;11:213–23.
17. Rey F, Lê T, Bertin R, Kapoula Z. Saccades horizontal or vertical at near or at far do not deteriorate postural control. Auris Nasus Larynx. 2008;35:185–91.
18. Rodrigues S, Aguiar S, Polastri P, Godoi D, Moraes R, Barela J. Effects of saccadic eye movements on postural control stabilization. Motriz. 2013;19:614–9.
19. Stoffregen T, Bardy B, Bonnet C, Pagulayan R. Postural stabilization of visually guided eye movements. Ecol Psychol. 2006;18:191–222.
20. Guerraz M, Bronstein AM. Ocular versus extraocular control of posture and equilibrium. Neurophysiol Clin. 2008;38(6):391–8. https://doi.org/10.1016/j.neucli.2008.09.007.
21. Mitra S. Adaptive utilization of optical variables during postural and suprapostural dual-task performance: comment on Stoffregen, smart, Bardy, and Pagulayan. J Exp Psychol Hum Percept Perform. 2004;30:28–38.
22. Mitra S, Fraizer E. Effects of explicit sway minimization postural-suprapostural dual-task performance. Hum Mov Sci. 2004;23:1–20.
23. Mitra S. Postural costs of suprapostural task load. Hum Mov Sci. 2003;22:253–70.
24. Brito MB, Gotardi GC, Rodrigues ST, Cavalieri BC, Lima DN, Moraes LR, et al. Variability of visually-induced center of pressure displacements is reduced while young adults perform unpredictable saccadic eye movements inside a moving room. Neurosci Lett. 2021;764:136276.
25. Laurens J, Awai L, Bockish C, Hegemann S, van Hedel H, Dietz V, et al. Visual contribution to postural stability: interaction between target fixation or tracking and static or dynamic large-field stimulus. Gait Posture. 2010;31:37–41.
26. Rodrigues S, Bertoloni G, Moraes R, Barela A, Savelsbergh G, Barela J. Controlling posture during grasping with different optical flow conditions. In: Advances in Visual Perception Research. Hauppauge, NY: Nova Science Publishers; 2015. p. 1–18. http://hdl.handle.net/11449/220551.
27. Prioli A, Freitas Júnior P, Barela J. Physical activity and postural control in the elderly: coupling between visual information and body sway. Gerontology. 2005;51:145–8.
28. Perotti Júnior A, Barela J, Polastri P, Tani G. Influência de diferentes informações comportamentais na dinâmica intrínseca entre informação visual e oscilação corporal [Influence of different behavioral informations in intrinsic dynamics between visual information and body sway]. Brazilian J Mot Behav. 2007;2:40–50.
29. Wade M, Lindquist R, Taylor J, Treat-Jacobson D. Optical flow, spatial orientation, and the control of posture in the elderly. J Gerontol Ser B Psychol Sci Soc Sci. 1995;50:51–4.
30. Stoffregen T. Flow structure versus retinal location in the optical control of stance. J Exp Psychol Hum Percept Perform. 1985;11:554–65.
31. Lawrence G, Khan M, Buckolz E, Oldham A. The contribution of peripheral and central vision in the control of movement amplitude. Hum Mov Sci. 2006;25:326–38.
32. Schiff W, Caviness J, Gibson J. Persistent fear responses in rhesus to the optical stimulus of "looming". Science (80-). 1962;136:982–3.
33. Bower T, Broughton J, Moore M. Infant responses to approaching objects: an indicator of response to distal variables. Percept Psychophys. 1971;9:193–6.
34. Bruce V, Green P. Visual perception: physiology, psychology and ecology. 2nd ed. Hove: Lawrence Erlbaum Associates Ltd; 1990.
35. Stoffregen T, Riccio G. Responses to optical looming in the retinal center and periphery. Ecol Psychol. 1990;2:251–74.

36. Rodrigues ST, Polastri PF, Gotardi GC, Aguiar SA, Mesaros MR, Pestana MB, et al. Postural control during cascade ball juggling: effects of expertise and base of support. Percept Mot Skills. 2016;123(1):279–94. https://doi.org/10.1177/0031512516660718.
37. Amado AC, Palmer CJ, Hamill J, van Emmerik REA. Coupling of postural and manual tasks in expert performers. Hum Mov Sci. 2016;46:251–60.
38. Era P, Konttinen N, Mehto P, Saarela P, Lyytinen H. Postural stability and skilled performance—a study on toplevel and naive rifle shooters. J Biomech. 1996;29:301–6.
39. Garcia RS, Hayes SJ, Williams AM, Bennett SJ. Multisensory perception and action in 3-ball cascade juggling. J Mot Behav. 2013;45:29–36.
40. Sahli S, Ghroubia S, Rebaic H, Chaâbaned M, Yahiaa A, Pérennoue D, et al. The effect of circus activity training on postural control of 5-6-year-old children. Sci Sports. 2013;28:11–6.
41. Gautier G, Thouvarecq R, Larue J. Influence of experience on postural control: effect of expertise in gymnastics. J Mot Behav. 2008;40:400–8.
42. Leroy D, Thouvarecq R, Gautier G. Postural organization during cascade juggling: influence of expertise. Gait Posture. 2008;28:265–70.
43. Dessing JC, Rey FP, Beek PJ. Gaze fixation improves the stability of expert juggling. Exp Brain Res. 2012;216:635–44.
44. Williams AM, Davids K. Visual search strategy, selective attention, and expertise in soccer. Res Q Exerc Sport. 1998;69:111–28.
45. Shulman GL, Remington RW, Mclean JP. Moving attention through visual space. J Exp Psychol Hum Percept Perform. 1979;5:522–6.
46. Dessing JC, Crawford JD, Medendorp WP. Spatial updating across saccades during manual interception. J Vis. 2011;11:1–18.
47. Huys R, Beek PJ. The coupling between point-of-gaze and ball movements in three-ball cascade juggling: the effects of expertise, pattern and tempo. J Sports Sci. 2002;20:171–86.
48. Marin L, Bardy BG, Bootsma RJ. Level of gymnastic skill as an intrinsic constraint on postural coordination. J Sports Sci. 1999;17:615–26.
49. Perrin P, Deviterne D, Hugel F, Perrot C. Judo, better than dance, develops sensorimotor adaptabilities involved in balance control. Gait Posture. 2002;15:187–94.
50. Yoshitomi SK, Tanaka C, Duarte M, Lima F, Morya E, Hazime F. Respostas posturais à perturbação externa inesperada em judocas de diferentes níveis de habilidade [Postural responses to unexpected external perturbations in judo athletes of different skill levels]. Rev Bras Med do Esporte. 2006;12:159–63.
51. Carizio BG. Efeito distrator do telefone celular sobre a condução simulada de automóveis: situações de uso manual e viva-voz (Dissertação) [Distractor effect of cell phone on the simulated car driving: In hand and speakerphone mode situations (Dissertation)]. Bauru: Faculdade de Arquitetura, Artes e Comunicação [Faculty of Architecture, Arts and Comunication], Universidade Estadual Paulista [São Paulo State University]; 2016.
52. Land MF. Eye movements and the control of actions in everyday life. Prog Retin Eye Res. 2006;25:296–324.
53. Rodrigues ST, Vickers JN, Williams M. Head, eye and arm coordination in table tennis. J Sports Sci. 2002;20:187–200.
54. Denardi R, Ferracioli M, Rodrigues S. Informação visual e controle postural durante a execução da pirouette no ballet [Visual information and postural control during a pirouette in ballet]. Rev Port Ciências do Desporto. 2008;8:241–50.
55. Vickers JN. Visual control when aiming at a far target. J Exp Psychol Hum Percept Perform. 1996;22:342–54.
56. Vickers JN. Origins and current issues in quiet eye research. Curr Issues Sport Sci. 2016;1:101.
57. Vickers JN, Adolphe RM. Gaze behaviour during a ball tracking and aiming skill. Int J Sport Vis. 1997;4:18–27.
58. Land MF, Tatler BW. Steering with the head: the visual strategy of a racing driver. Curr Biol. 2001;11:1215–20.
59. Gotardi GC, Polastri PF, Schor P, Navarro M, Oudejans RRD, van der Kamp J, Savelsbergh GJP, Rodrigues ST. Adverse effects of anxiety on attentional control differ as a function of

experience: a simulated driving study. Appl Ergon. 2019;74:41–7. https://doi.org/10.1016/j.apergo.2018.08.009.
60. Gotardi GC, Kuga GK, Simão RO, Brito MB, Paschoalino GP, Silva GA, Barbieri FA, Polastri PF, Schor P, Navarro M, Rodrigues ST. Combining experiences of race gaming and natural driving affects gaze location strategy in simulated context. Ergonomics. 2019;62(11):1392–9. https://doi.org/10.1080/00140139.2019.1652770.
61. Gotardi GC, Barbieri FA, Simão RO, Pereira VA, Baptista AM, Imaizumi LF, Moretto G, Navarro M, Polastri PF, Rodrigues ST. Parkinson's disease affects gaze behaviour and performance of drivers. Ergonomics. 2022;65(9):1302–11. https://doi.org/10.1080/00140139.2022.2028901.
62. Land MF, Lee DN. Where we look when we steer. Nature. 1994;369:742–4.
63. Carizio BG, Silva GA, Paschoalino GP, Angelo J, Gotardi GC, Zago PFP, et al. Pupil dilation as indicative of cognitive workload while driving a car: effects of cell phone use and driver experience in young adults. Brazilian J Motor Behav. 2021;15:391–402.
64. Aguiar SA, Polastri PF, Godoi D, Moraes R, Barela JA, Rodrigues ST. Effects of saccadic eye movements on postural control in older adults. Psychol Neurosci. 2015;8:19–27.
65. Laufer Y, Barak Y, Chemel I. Age-related differences in the effect of a perceived threat to stability on postural control. J Gerontol A Biol Sci Med Sci. 2006;61:500–4.
66. Prioli AC, Freitas Junior PB, Barela JA. Physical activity and postural control in the elderly: coupling between visual information and body sway. Gerontology [Internet]. 2005;51:145–8. https://doi.org/10.1159/000083984.
67. Paquette C, Fung J. Old age affects gaze and postural coordination. Gait Posture [Internet]. 2011;33:227–32. https://doi.org/10.1016/j.gaitpost.2010.11.010.
68. Warren DE, Thurtell MJ, Carroll JN, Wall M. Perimetric evaluation of saccadic latency, saccadic accuracy, and visual threshold for peripheral visual stimuli in young compared with older adults. Invest Ophthalmol Vis Sci. 2013;54:5778–87.
69. Bozhkova VP, Surovicheva NS, Nikolaev DP, Nikolaev IP, Bolshakov AS. Smooth pursuit in elderly adults studied with apparent motion. Perception. 2015;44:1040–53.
70. Cattagni T, Scaglioni G, Laroche D, Gremeaux V, Martin A. The involvement of ankle muscles in maintaining balance in the upright posture is higher in elderly fallers. Exp Gerontol. 2016;77:38–45.
71. Prioli AC, Cardozo AS, de Freitas Junior PB, Barela JA. Task demand effects on postural control in older adults. Hum Mov Sci. 2006;25:435–46.
72. Ambrose AF, Cruz L, Paul G. Falls and fractures: a systematic approach to screening and prevention. Maturitas. 2015;82:85–93.
73. Orr R. Contribution of muscle weakness to postural instability in the elderly. A systematic review. Eur J Phys Rehabil Med. 2010;46:183–220.
74. Bennett PJ, Sekuler R, Sekuler AB. The effects of aging on motion detection and direction identification. Vis Res. 2007;47:799–809.
75. Fife TD, Baloh RW. Disequilibrium of unknown cause in older people. Ann Neurol. 1993;34:694–702.
76. Toledo DR, Barela JA. Sensory and motor differences between young and older adults: somatosensory contribution to postural control. Rev Bras Fisioter. 2010;14:267–75.
77. Shumway-Cook A, Woollacott M, Kerns KA, Baldwin M. The effects of two types of cognitive tasks on postural stability in older adults with and without a history of falls. J Gerontol A Biol Sci Med Sci. 1997;52:232–40.
78. Prioli AC, Freitas Junior PB, Barela JA. Physical activity and postural control in the elderly: coupling between visual information and body sway. Gerontology. 2005;51:145–8.
79. Owsley C. Aging and vision. Vis Res. 2011;51:1610–22.
80. West SK, Munoz B, Rubin GS, Schein OD, Bandeen-Roche K, Zeger S, et al. Function and visual impairment in a population-based study of older adults the SEE project. Invest Ophthalmol Vis Sci [Internet]. 1997;38:72–82. Recuperado de: http://www.ncbi.nlm.nih.gov/pubmed/9008632.
81. Moschner C, Baloh RW. Age-related changes in visual tracking. J Gerontol. 1994;49:235–8.

82. Dowiasch S, Marx S, Einhauser W, Bremmer F. Effects of aging on eye movements in the real world. Front Hum Neurosci. 2015;9:46. https://doi.org/10.3389/fnhum.2015.00046.
83. Ross RG, Olincy A, Harris JG, Radant A, Adler LE, Compagnon N, et al. The effects of age on a smooth pursuit tracking task in adults with schizophrenia and normal subjects. Biol Psychiatry. 1999;46:383–91.
84. Wang J, Li L, Li S, Xie F, Chang M, Paterson KB, et al. Adult age differences in eye movements during reading: the evidence from Chinese. J Gerontol B Psychol Sci Soc Sci. 2018;73(4):584–93. https://doi.org/10.1093/geronb/gbw036.
85. Schmitt KU, Seeger R, Fischer H, Lanz C, Muser M, Walz F, et al. Saccadic eye movement performance as an indicator of driving ability in elderly drivers. Swiss Med Wkly. 2015;145:w14098. https://doi.org/10.4414/smw.2015.14098.
86. Seligman SC, Giovannetti T. The potential utility of eye movements in the detection and characterization of everyday functional difficulties in mild cognitive impairment. Neuropsychol Rev. 2015;25:199–215.
87. Gibson J. The ecological approach to visual perception. Boston, MA: Houghton-Mifflin Company; 1979.
88. Cutting JE. Wayfinding from multiple sources of local information in retinal flow. J Exp Psychol Hum Percept Perform. 1996;22:1299–313.
89. Kim N, Turvey MT, Growney R. Wayfinding and the sampling of optical flow by eye movements. J Exp Psychol Hum Percept Perform. 1996;22:1314–9.
90. Daniel BM, Lee DN. Development of looking with head and eyes. J Exp Child Psychol. 1990;50:200–16.

Falls and Postural Control in Older Adults: Effects of the Physical Exercise and the Implications for Activities of Daily Living

16

Paula Fávaro Polastri, Daniela Godoi-Jacomassi, and Karina Gramani-Say

Abstract

The risk of falling is associated with aging-related motor and sensory declines. A higher incidence of falls has been observed in individuals over 60 years who are known to have balance problems. The current knowledge regarding the mechanisms involved in the recovery of postural orientation and body equilibrium shows that the main changes occur as individuals become older and in those who are sedentary or are affected by some diseases. Extensive research and preventive measures have been extensively undertaken to gain a comprehensive understanding of the causes and consequences of falling. Fortunately, older individuals who engage in regular physical activity lead a healthy lifestyle and have a reduced risk and occurrence of falls. This may be attributed to the proper functioning of their postural control system. Recently, public health policies have been adopted by many countries to improve the quality of life of older individuals and reduce the high number of fallers among the adult population.

P. F. Polastri (✉)
Laboratory of Information, Vision, and Action, Department of Physical Education, São Paulo State University – UNESP, Bauru, Brazil
e-mail: paula.polastri@unesp.br

D. Godoi-Jacomassi
Dinâmica—Motor Behavior Laboratory, Department of Physical Education, Federal University of Sao Carlos—UFSCar, São Carlos, Brazil
e-mail: danielagodoij@ufscar.br

K. Gramani-Say
LADORFE—Laboratory for the Study of Pain and Functionality in Aging, Department of Gerontology, Federal University of Sao Carlos—UFSCar, São Carlos, Brazil
e-mail: gramanisay@ufscar.br

F. A. Barbieri et al. (eds.), *Locomotion and Posture in Older Adults*,
https://doi.org/10.1007/978-3-031-74123-4_16

Introduction

As we age, our bodies undergo various constraints that affect us both physically and mentally. These can include organic, physiological, and psychosocial factors, which may make even simple tasks more challenging to complete. Brazil has one of the largest populations of people aged 60 years and above in the world, currently comprising 32% of the population and will increase from 33.679.986 (15.1% of the population) to 73 million people by 2060 [1]. Health professionals who work with this population are still concerned about the high incidence and risk of falls in older individuals and seek strategies to prevent the causes of this phenomenon [2].

A fall can be defined as an "unintentional event that causes the body to move downward from its starting position, with no time to correct the disability, caused by multifactorial circumstances that compromise stability" [3]. Intrinsic and extrinsic characteristics of older adults may lead to a risk of falling. The intrinsic factors are related to physiological alterations during aging, such as decreased visual acuity; the abusive use of drugs/medication; chronic diseases such as hypertension, diabetes, arthritis, osteoarthritis, and osteoporosis, causing deficits in muscle strength, balance, and gait; and the psychological status, such as fear of falling, which affects, for instance, gait performance [4]. The extrinsic factors are environmental and social circumstances in which the older people are included, such as inadequate lighting, slippery surfaces, carpets without anti-slip coatings or with folds, obstacles when walking, no handrail support, high or narrow steps, and public pathways with holes or irregularities, among others [5]. As falls are a multifactorial event, current interventions aim to identify non-modifiable (chronic diseases) and modifiable risk factors to act with physical and cognitive interventions to reduce or control modifiable risk factors (medications, vitamin D deficiency, visual acuity, heart rate and rhythm, postural hypotension, pain, gait, balance, mobility, and muscle strength, evaluation of feet and shoes, and safety at home).

According to the Brazilian Health Ministry, the Public Health System has significant annual expenses related to fracture treatments in older individuals, mainly associated with hip fractures [6], which are the leading cause of morbidity and mortality in this population. The occurrence of falls in Brazil was 1798 in 2019, with an increase of 23% in 2021 (2211 cases) [6]. Accidental falls significantly impair the functional capacity of older individuals. A recent study [7] found that falls are among the most common causes of years lived with disability, ranking 16th for individuals up to 74 years old and eighth for those above 75.

The literature suggests that falls are often associated with the frailty syndrome, particularly in elderly individuals over the age of 80. For both the aging process and frailty syndrome, prevention programs, education, and case management can be used to treat older individuals. Developing programs and services for older individuals is fundamental [8]. Fear or concern about recurrent falls is also associated with reduced mobility, loss of balance confidence, and activity restriction in older adults [8, 9]. The process of evaluation can be challenging as it may encompass various aspects such as physical, behavioral, and functional limitations [9]. For these reasons, it is necessary to identify possible causes and risk factors and propose several interventions to prevent falls in older adults.

Studies have shown that peripheral structure impairments, such as muscle weakness, loss of bone mineral density, sensorial constraints, nerve transmission delays, and a slower reaction time are characteristics associated with older fallers [10, 11]. For instance, older adults with impaired neurotransmission and sensory constraints show delays in initiating the postural response after an environmental disturbance. These delays may lead to a higher center of mass excursion and torque production at the ankle and hip joints. As older adults appear to present age-related muscle weakness, balance recovery may not occur.

In addition to these peripheral constraints, studies have indicated that balance disorders in older adults may also occur due to altered central mechanisms. In particular, older adults demonstrate a loss of central neurons and synaptic connections, which reduces processing speed and the ability to perform multiple activities simultaneously, predominantly those involving postural control [12, 13]. Some differences in brain structure (loss of global brain mass, a decline in volume of gray and white matter), biochemistry (dopaminergic degeneration), and function (limited recruitment in prefrontal resources) were found [14] when comparing older adults with younger ones. Overall results have demonstrated that brain activation alters as age increases [15–19], mainly in areas such as the cerebellum, precuneus, occipital cortex, and basal ganglia, which seem to be associated with ankle muscle activation. Older adults, but not younger ones, have the brain areas related to ankle dorsiflexion movements increasingly activated [15]. A recent study [18] has revealed that bidirectional connectivity between the premotor cortex (PMC) and primary motor area (M1) is associated with ankle force precision. Neurons activation patterns and magnitude are different in older adults compared to young adults. Specifically, young adults demonstrate backward M1-PMC and forward PMC-M1 coupling strongly associated with worse ankle force precision. Older adults also show stronger coupling between M1 and PMC associated with poorer ankle task performance, but it is lower than young adults. Moreover, contrarily, older adults exhibit stronger coupling between PMC and M1, which is associated with better ankle force precision. Since these cortico-cerebellar areas contribute to higher-order cognitive processes [20] and postural and balance control [17, 21], these neural changes have been interpreted as compensatory responses to age-related deficits in sensorimotor control of the distal lower limbs [15, 18].

Therefore, functional constraints in the central and peripheral nervous systems seem to lead to inappropriate age-related postural responses to a constantly changing sensory environment, which could be associated with an increased risk of falling among this population. For instance, many fall events occur while performing activities of daily living (ADLs) that simultaneously associate two or more tasks [20]. A dual-task is defined as the simultaneous performance of a primary task, e.g., postural, in association with another task, denominated secondary, which could be a cognitive task (speaking, counting down, or speaking different names), a simple motor task (holding a glass of water or carrying a tray), a complex motor task (changing pocket coins), or cognitive/motor task (using a telephone while walking)

[15, 20]. Typically, adequate dual-task performance involves dividing attention and making more effort to process postural control and sensory input [12, 13]. Older adults, when performing a dual task, present changes in the maintenance of postural control due to competition between the secondary task performance and the effectiveness of the relationship between motor responses and sensory input, increasing the body sway to maintain balance [13]. One reason for these results might be the fact that both postural control and cognitive/motor tasks occur at the cortical level, so to perform these activities simultaneously implies competition for cortical processing, causing a reduction in the automatism of the older people to perform simultaneous activities [12, 16, 17].

There are a variety of physical exercises and activities that are recommended to help maintain optimal performance across multiple operating systems. These benefits can also improve postural control. In recent years, there has been a growing understanding of the neural mechanisms involved in anticipatory and reactive balance control. It has provided new insights into the ability of older adults to adapt their postural responses to varying environmental conditions. This chapter aims to demonstrate changes in postural control over the years and the recent advances in understanding the neural mechanisms underlying the recovery of body stability of older adults. We will first discuss the factors that affect the postural control system and then explore a multifactorial approach to prevent falls and related injuries.

Aging and Postural Control

Historically, postural control was considered a summation of parallel and hierarchical reflex pathways [10, 22, 23]. Currently, it is understood as the complex interaction between multiple neural systems underlying two functional goals: postural orientation refers to the positioning of body segments about the environment, whereas postural equilibrium denotes a state where the body is balanced, with all forces acting on it in harmony [22].

Postural control involves balance and the ability to assume and maintain a desired orientation; thus, every movement involves postural control [22]. Therefore, the accurate functioning of the postural control system allows us to efficiently interact and adapt to constant changes in the environment [24]. However, a decline in postural control performance is well documented in the older population [25, 26]. Furthermore, these changes in the postural control system due to aging have been associated with individuals who experience falls [27–30]. Piirtola and Era [28] suggested that parameters of mean speed and the root mean square of center of pressure (CoP) may be a predictor of the number of falls in older adults during upright stance. Studies have indicated differences between older adults with and without a history of falls for global CoP descriptors [27, 29, 30], structural, and spectral CoP descriptors [29]. Therefore, it is crucial to comprehend the mechanisms that cause changes in the postural control system to prevent falls [29].

The postural control system involves different control mechanisms and behavioral strategies, such as: compensatory or reactive (feedback) and anticipatory (feedforward) postural adjustments. Compensatory postural adjustments operate as a closed-loop control [31]; thus, afferent feedback controls the body position when the initial setting is disturbed [32]. On the other hand, anticipatory postural control relies on predictive control [31]; higher-order processing anticipates muscle activation before the occurrence of the disturbance. Usually, the central nervous system (CNS) uses feedback control to respond to an external and unpredictable perturbation and feedforward control to deal with disturbances due to the movements themselves (self-motion) [33].

In older adults, the feedforward postural control mechanism is not used effectively [34–37], and, for this reason, it seems that older adults rely more on feedback control [34]. For Dault and coworkers [34], the inability of older individuals to use feedforward control could be related to motor and sensory modifications associated with aging. That is a problem for the postural control system because feedback and feedforward mechanisms must work together to achieve optimal motor control functioning [38]. If muscle activation begins before the disturbance, it minimizes the perturbation to vertical posture and, consequently, requires less feedback postural control. On the other hand, if anticipatory muscle activation is not as effective, body position will be severely disturbed, and compensatory postural adjustments may not be enough to balance recovery.

Behavioral strategies are required to recover balance after disturbances, and they have been widely described [10, 22, 39]. The ankle strategy is the most common postural adjustment triggered during slow and small perturbations [22]. In this strategy, the ankle muscles alone act to recover the balance by producing torque at the ankle joint when the vertical alignment alters due to perturbation [40]. The CNS uses the hip strategy when the ankle muscles are not as efficient to restore body balance [40]. The hip strategy occurs during rapid or large amplitude disturbances [22]. It consists of flexing the hip, moving the center of mass posteriorly, or extending the hip to move the center of mass anteriorly [40]. Additionally, there is the stepping strategy, which is triggered when the ankle and hip strategies are inadequate to maintain the center of mass within the limits of stability during large and fast perturbations [10, 22]. Some studies have shown that older individuals switch from ankle to hip strategies to recover postural stability even after a small (feedback control) but unpredictable perturbation [11, 41, 42]. As individuals age, their postural control functioning may begin to deteriorate [10, 25, 26]. Therefore, they tend to rely more on the hip strategy or a combination of ankle and hip strategies [43] to improve their postural stability.

Recent studies have revealed that although these strategies may seem fast and completely automatic (i.e., control at a subcortical level, for instance, via neural circuits at the spinal level), the cortex plays a role in reactive balance control (e.g., [44, 45]., with evidence of activity in a balance control network while standing, and a rearrangement in brain topology temporally associated with postural instability [46]. However, it is still unclear whether and how the brain activity linked with moments of losing balance is affected in older adults and those who are prone to falling ([47] for details). Investigating the causes and consequences of high fall risk is crucial for individuals affected by this issue.

Integration of sensory inputs is crucial to provide accurate information for postural control system functioning. For instance, the CNS uses sensory inputs to adjust self-initiated balance disturbances (feedforward) and also to detect externally triggered disturbances (feedback) [31, 48]. As the body oscillates, a wide variety of receptors are activated and provide different information to the central nervous system (CNS) to generate appropriate muscular contractions, depending on the goals of the desired task in a specific environmental condition [48].

Generally, information from three sensory systems is available to the postural control system: visual, vestibular, and somatosensory [49, 50]. The visual system provides information about the position and movement of an object in space and the body segments in the environment. The aging process reduces acuity, contrast sensitivity, depth perception, and rapid adaptation to changing depth [26, 48], which could make older adults more susceptible to falling. The somatosensory system provides information on the body's position in space relative to the supporting surface and the position information and relative speed between body segments. The sensors of this system include muscle proprioceptors (Golgi tendon organ and muscle spindles) and joint and skin mechanoreceptors. The reduction in density and sensitivity of dermal mechanoreceptors, the stiffness of tissue, and the degeneration of peripheral nerves may be related to decreased skin sensitivity over the years [26, 48]. The vestibular system provides information about the orientation and movement of the head, and the speed of information processing may reduce with age, also resulting in an increased risk of falls.

Falls in older adults are associated with multiple underlying causes, such as the sensory reweighting process [10]. Under normal conditions, the sensory systems provide redundant information to the CNS about the position and orientation of the body segments [50]. However, in constantly changing environments, some sensory cues may become more reliable than others to achieve the movement task. When this happens, visual, vestibular, and somatosensory inputs must be dynamically reweighted to optimize the control of postural stability [22]. Upweights and downweights of different sensory modalities suggest a nonlinear process [24, 51]. Some evidence points out that older individuals are not able to reweight sensory information appropriately [13, 26, 52]; however, it is still unclear whether such differences are due to central [52, 53] or peripheral mechanisms [54].

Toledo and Barela [54] found evidence that sensory reweighting in older adults might involve peripheral deterioration. In this study, the authors evaluated the central and peripheral mechanisms of the postural control of older adults. Sensory (visual acuity, visual contrast sensitivity, tactile foot sensitivity, and detection of passive ankle motion) and motor assessments (isometric ankle torque, muscular activity latency after stance perturbation) evaluated the integrity of peripheral mechanisms; postural control assessment (body sway during upright stance and induced by movement of a visual scene) evaluated the integrity of central mechanisms. The results revealed that less accurate sensitivity to passive ankle joint motion was related to large body sway in sensory conflicting situations (induced by movement of a visual scene). Thus, peripheral sensation appears to be sufficiently intact; there is no difference in the sensory reweighting process between young and older adults (fallers and non-fallers) [55], suggesting that age-related changes in the reweighting process seem more likely to be due to peripheral mechanisms.

Studies have shown that physical exercise may improve the underlying mechanisms responsible for sensory reweighting in older adults' postural control. Allison, Kiemel, and Jeka [56], for example, observed that 8 weeks of a sensory-challenge balance exercise program led to improvement in sensory reweighting in older adults with a history of falls. Furthermore, other studies (e.g., [57, 58]) have shown that older adults who engage in different physical exercise programs demonstrate more effective performance of the postural control system in many daily activities. Besides the functional fitness improvements from regular physical exercise practice (strength, flexibility, coordination, balance, and cardiovascular endurance), active older adults are constantly encouraged to interact with changing environments during exercise practice, and it requires integration between useful sensory information and appropriate muscle contractions which could benefit the postural control functioning. Based on these results, many professionals have considered the multifactorial aspects to develop exercise programs and prevent falls.

Physical Exercise and Postural Control of Older Adults

The participation of older adults in specific or multimodal exercise programs is crucial to prevent and rehabilitate multiple aspects associated with falls, such as muscle weakness, deterioration in postural control, balance recovery, and committed instability during locomotion (e.g., [59–61]). Although prevention of falls has been the goal of several exercise programs, with different contributions to the health style of older people (e.g., [62–65]), understanding the aspects that might change one or more factors associated with the risk of falling is still being investigated. Meta-analyses and reviews [63, 66, 67] about this issue have pointed out, in many cases, incomplete methodologies without strict definitions of the groups or training methods (frequency, intensity, duration) applied in physical activity programs for older adults. It compromises the knowledge of consistent results on the effects of exercise in reducing falls in this population.

Despite this lack of information, overall results have shown that the practice of different types of physical exercise has beneficial effects on the health and quality of life of older individuals, mainly due to the maintenance of their functional and neural capacity, independent mobility, and ability to carry out ADLs, which is associated with lower risk and fear of falling [14, 68–70]. Table 16.1 summarizes the main findings regarding the effects of exercise/physical activity training on the postural and functional parameters, which likely is associated with the risk of falling in older individuals.

Strength/resistance, balance, and aerobic training are the most popular activities practiced by older adults and the most commonly prescribed among health professionals to prevent the risk of falling [56, 57, 66]. The American Geriatrics Society (https://www.americangeriatrics.org/) and British Geriatrics Society Clinical Practice Guidelines (https://www.bgs.org.uk/resources/resource-series/clinical-

Table 16.1 Summarized exercise/physical activities training effects on postural and functional parameters

Author	Main objectives	Mean age	Intervention/Evaluation	Main assessments	Main results
Perrin et al. [84]	Examine the influence of continuous PSA practice on postural control in the elderly	AA: 73.9 years; IA: 71.9 years; AI:67.9 years; II: 73.7 years.	The period during which the subjects were Engaged in PSA	- Posturographic tests (static, dynamic with a single and fast upward tilt, and dynamic with slow sinusoidal oscillations or electromyography responses;	The postural control performance decreased in the order AA>IA > AI>II;
Hess and Woollacott [82]	Evaluate the effect of 10-week, high-intensity strength-training program	EG: 80.9 years; CG: 82.5 years;	EG: 10-week (3 days/week); I: High-intensity strength-training program (quadriceps, hamstrings, tibialis anterior, gastrocnemius muscles);	Pre and post-training evaluation: - Berg balance scale; - TUG; - Balance confidence scale;	EG: Improvements on Berg balance scale ($p = 0.030$); TUG ($p = 0.045$); balance confidence scale ($p = 0.038$);
Colcombe et al. [70]	Examined whether aerobic fitness training of older adults can increase brain volume in regions associated with age-related declines	EG: 65.5 years; CG:66.9 years; YA: 18–30 years.	EG: 6 months (3 days/week); I: Aerobic exercises (cardiorespiratory fitness prescribed by HR); CG: 6 months (3 days/week); I: Aerobic exercises (whole-body stretching and toning);	EG and CG: VO2 and MRI images; YA: MRI images;	EG: Increases in brain volume (gray and white matter regions);
Bruin and Murer [64]	Evaluate the additional effect of functional exercises on balance and lower extremity function in strength training of older adults	EG: 86.3 years; CG: 86.5 years;	EG: 12-week (2 days/week); I: Strength and functional exercises (45 min + 30 min); CG: 12-weeks (2 days/week); I: Strength exercises (45 min);	- Tinetti Scal; - physical performance tests (timed walking measure, chair stand test, tandem stand); - balance test; - maximal isometric knee extensor muscle force;	EG: Improvement on Tinetti test ($p = 0.026$); chair stand test ($p = 0.012$); balance test ($p = 0.009$);
Martínez-Amat et al. [74]	Evaluate the effect of a 12-week specific proprioceptive training program on postural stability, gait, balance, and fall prevention	EG: 79.35 years; CG: 77.0 years;	EG 12-week (2 days/week); CG: Maintain activity levels and medication during the 12-week intervention period;	Pre and post-training evaluation: - Tinetti scale (postural stability, gait, balance, and risk of falling); - Berg balance test;	EG: Improvements on ML body sway with EO ($p < 0.05$) and AP body sway with EC ($p < 0.01$); Romberg quotient about Surface ($p < 0.05$) and speed ($p < 0.01$); Gait (Tinetti test): Improved 14.66%; Balance (Berg test scores): 11.47%;

Lee et al. [62]	Evaluate effects of a multifactorial fall prevention program on fall incidence and physical function in community-dwelling older adults	EG: 75.4 years; CG: 76.0 years;	EG: 3-month multifactorial intervention program (8-week, 1 day/week + daily home exercise); I: Health education, home hazards evaluation/modification, exercise training (strengthening, balance, Cardiorespiratory endurance, and flexibility); CG: 3-month multifactorial intervention program; I: Health education brochures, referrals, and recommendations without direct exercise intervention;	Pre and post-training evaluation: - fall incidence (1 fall during the 12-month follow-up); - PPA risk index (vision, muscular Strength, reaction time, postural sway, and proprioception); - TUG test; - GDS; - FES; - IPAQ;	Cumulative 1-year fall incidence: EG: 25.2% and CG: 27.6%; EG: PPA improvements on fall risk index, reaction time, postural sway with EO, TUG test, and GDS, especially for marked fall risk older individuals;
Pau et al. [72]	Assess the effects of vigorous and light physical activity on static balance, gait, and sit-to-stand (STS) tasks in a cohort of healthy older adults	VPA: 69.8 years; LPA: 70.3 years;	VPA: 12-week (3 days/week); I: 45 min with %HRR in the range 60–84% (aerobic and anaerobic exercises); LPA: 12-week (3 days/week); I: %HRR below 40% (static and dynamic exercises for posture and balance, joint and spine mobility);	Pre and post-training evaluation: - bipedal stances (EO and EC); - Unipedal stance (left and right); - gait: SpatiotemporalFparameters; - sit-to-stand test;	VPA: Improvements on gait parameters ($p < 0.001$) and STS time ($p < 0.001$); reduced body sway with EC ($p < 0.01$); LPA: Decreased swing phase duration ($p = 0.042$); and reduced body sway with EC ($p < 0.05$);
Gianoudis et al. [57]	Evaluate the effectiveness and feasibility of a multimodal exercise program in older adults.	EG: 67.7 years; CG: 67.2 years;	EG: 12 months (3 days/ week)—Osteo-cise exercise program; I: HV-PRT, weight-bearing impact, and challenging balance/ mobility activities; CG: To continue usual care and to take charge of own musculoskeletal health;	- femoral neck and lumbar spine BMD; - muscle strength; - functional muscle power (timed stair climb test); - dynamic balance (four square step and sit-to-stand tests); - TUG; - falls rate;	EG: Gains in femoral neck and lumbar spine BMD ($p < 0.05$); muscle strength ($p < 0.05$); functional muscle power ($p < 0.05$), and dynamic balance ($p < 0.01$);

(continued)

Table 16.1 (continued)

Author	Main objectives	Mean age	Intervention/Evaluation	Main assessments	Main results
Allison et al. [56]	Measure whether sensory challenge exercises influenced MSR Determine whether MSR changes were associated with Clinical measures of balance and fall risk	78 years-old adults with a history of falls in the prior year	8-weeks baseline (control) period; 8-week intervention (2 days/week—45 min) with computerized sensory-challenge balance exercises;	Pre and post-intervention: - MSR variables (center of mass gain and phase, position, and velocity variability); - clinical tests (activities-specific Balance confidence scale, Berg balance scale, SOT, limits of stability test, and lower extremity strength and range of motion);	Post-intervention: Decrease in the coupling (touch gain, $p < 0.006$) and temporal relationship (phase, $p < 0.05$) between somatosensory information and postural sway; Better results for the Berg balance scale ($p < 0.002$), SOT ($p < 0.002$); limits of stability ($p < 0.001$), and lower extremity strength score ($p < 0.005$);
Osti et al. [79]	Evaluate the stand-up paddling training for the promotion of body balance stability gains in older adults.	OA: 61.7 years	EG: 2 months (3 days/week), SUP training (50 min); CG: 2 months (3 days/week), general cardiovascular endurance training (50 min);	Pre-, training, and post-training evaluation: -body balance: Tandem Romberg (EO, EC) and tiptoes posture (30 sec); -body sway: Markers;	Pre- vs. post-training: -Romberg test: EG reduced trunk sway in post-training evaluation ($p < 0.02$); CG: No difference; - tiptoes posture: EG reduced ML trunk sway compared to EC in post-training evaluation ($p < 0.03$);

Rogge et al. [85]	Examine structural changes induced by balance training	HA: 19–65 years	Participants were randomly assigned to: Balance training (BT): 12-week (2 days/week), 50 min; -circuit training (8 stations/5 min each) -difficulty: Static vs. dynamic stability, eyes open vs. eyes closed, narrowed base of support, stable and unstable undergrounds; Relaxation training (RT): 12-week (2 days/week), 50 min; -progressive muscle relaxation (6 weeks): Tension (5–7 sec) and relaxation (45 sec) of single muscles (2 rep/per session); -autogenic training: Concentration on the breathing rhythm and heartbeat and imagination of body parts (3–4 rep/session);	Pre- and post-training evaluation: -balance performance; - MRI processing for: - cortical thickness; - subcortical gray matter Volume (hippocampus and Basal ganglia);	Balance performance: BT > RT ($p = 0.008$); Cortical thickness: BT > RT ($p < 0.05$); Hippocampus volume: BT = RT; Basal ganglia: BT decreased gray matter volume of putamen bilaterally (left -$p = 0.019$; right - $p < 0.028$);
Bubela et al. [75]	Compare performance on measures related to the risk of falling in older tai chi practitioners and non-tai chi practitioners	EG: 80.4 years; EC: 71.2 years;	EG: 16 weeks (2–3 days/ week—60 min) -tai chi exercises; EC: 16 weeks (2–3 days/ week—60 min) -daily routine;	Pre- and post-training evaluation: Outcomes: -strength (knee extensor strength and 5-time sit-to-stand); -balance (functional reach and BBS); -functional mobility (TUG e FFWT); -fear of falling (ABC scale);	EG older than EC ($p < 0.0001$); Greater lower extremity strength for EC (knee extensor strength) (left: $p < 0.02$; right: $p < 0.001$); Greater confidence in standing in a chair and reaching for an object in CG than EC ($p < 0.001$); EG: Higher TUG score after training ($p < 0.001$); EG improved confidence on the ABC scale ($p < 0.05$); No significant changes in balance and functional mobility between EG and EC;

(continued)

Table 16.1 (continued)

Author	Main objectives	Mean age	Intervention/Evaluation	Main assessments	Main results
Phu et al. [78]	Compare individualized virtual reality training using BRU to community-based OEP intervention	BRU: 79 years; OEP: 76 years; CG: 79 years;	BRU: 6 weeks (2 days/week—30 min): -individual virtual-reality balance training (limits of stability exercises); OEP: 6 weeks (2 days/week—60 min): -individually progressed home-based exercises (strength and balance training); CG: Non-intervention group;	Pre- and post-training evaluation: -physical performance (5-times sit-to-stand, TUG, FSST, handgrip, gait speed); -Posturography assessment (COP) on the BRU platform (EO, EC, firm and foam surface, saccadic task); FES-I score;	Pre-test: -better results in TUG ($p < 0.005$) and gait speed ($p < 0.002$) for the OEP group than BRU and CG; Post-test: -limits of stability and performance in EC, foam surface condition improves for BRU and OEP compared to EC ($p < 0.001$); -better results for BRU in EC, firm surface condition; TUG, gait speed, FES-I score, and handgrip strength changed in the BRU and OEP groups;
Sipila et al. [77]	Examine the effectiveness of combining physical and cognitive training with physical training alone	EG: 74.4 years; EC: 74.5 years;	PT: 2 days/week + home exercises: -walking and dynamic balance training (45 min); -resistance and balance training (60 min) - moderate aerobic activity (total of 150 min per week); - strengthening and balance home exercises (20–30 min, 2–3 days/week); PTCT: 2 days/week + cognitive training: -physical training + home exercises (similar PT group); - *i*PASS program: 2–3 days/week, 15–25 min - inhibition, set-shifting, and updating of working memory;	Baseline, 6- and 12 months: Outcomes: –10-meter maximal gait Speed; –6-min walking distance; -dual-task cost in gait speed; -executive functions (Stroop color-word test and trail making test B-A);	-gait speed and 6-min walking distance: Increase in both PT and PTCT groups; - dual-task cost in gait speed: Improvements for both groups; - Stroop color-word test: Declined effect in PTCT more than PT after 6 months; - trail making test B-A: Increase in the PTCT group, but was similar to the PT group during baseline;

guidelines) for the prevention of falls in older persons recommend additional training for gait and coordination that should be performed 1–3 times a week, with different exercise intensities, and at least 12 months to achieve the necessary preventive benefits to reduce falls. In the last year, as part of a global initiative (https://worldfallsguidelines.com/), a team of 96 multidisciplinary experts from 39 countries (World Falls Task Force) produced a guideline with recommendations for fall prevention and management for older adults. Older adults at low risk of falling must engage in 150–300 minutes of moderate-intensity physical activity per week or 75–150 minutes of high-intensity physical activity per week [71]. Pau and collaborators [72] investigated the effects of exercise intensity (light or vigorous) on sitting and standing, static balance, and gait tasks in older adults. The results indicated that vigorous-intensity physical activity may reduce body sway in static and dynamic situations and improve gait parameters in older adults during the performance of ADLs. Similarly, the results showed that light physical activity may benefit older adults, but only in static balance tasks. These findings can aid in the design and implementation of more specific fall prevention programs for older people.

In particular, the decline in postural control and increase in the incidence and risk of falling due to the aging process [27, 28] have led older adults to practice exercises to improve or maintain adequate levels of functioning of this system [57, 58]. For instance, community-dwelling older adults at intermediate and high fall risk must engage in multimodal interventions with supervised and individualized exercises three or more times a week, with progression in intensity for at least 12 weeks or more [71]. The program should include challenging exercises targeting balance and strength training that support the performance of daily tasks [71], and it can reduce fall risk by almost 40% [73]. These exercises are based on generating situations involving balance and postural orientation, increased mobility through the environment, volitional and reactive stepping, shifts of movement direction, postural disturbances through known and sudden events (reactive and anticipatory training), and sensory system manipulation [63, 72, 73]. These situations lead the postural control system to produce effective and adaptable motor responses due to the disturbances suffered in these contexts and can reduce falls by about 50% [73]. Prioli and collaborators [52] showed that sedentary older individuals presented great body sway compared to active older and young adults in response to changing visual stimuli. In addition, active older adults responded more quickly and accurately to situations of sensory conflict than their sedentary peers. These results suggest that exercise practice might improve the perceptual motor skills of older adults, decreasing the risk of falls associated with the deterioration of the postural control system.

Many studies have examined and compared the effectiveness of different types of exercise on the postural control performance of healthy older people. Stretching and multisensory training [74]; strength and flexibility exercises [66]; functional exercises [64]; Tai Chi, Pilates, and Yoga [58, 75]; physical and cognitive training and training with virtual reality [69, 76–78]; on-water balance training [79]; resistance exercises [80] and, recently, ecological training [81] are some of these exercises. For instance, Hess and collaborators [82] showed that high-intensity strength training improved the postural stability levels and balance confidence of

80-year-old individuals after 10 weeks of training. More recently, a systematic review and network meta-analysis pointed out that balance exercise programs composed of one or more mechanical postural perturbations that induce balance recovery similar to real-life situations are more effective in improving reactive balance than other programs [83]. Overall, all these studies show that practicing more than one type of exercise may reduce postural instability and improve functional tasks and ADL performance, preventing the risk of falling.

Therefore, participating in physical exercise programs can be critical in maintaining and enhancing postural control performance over time. It is worth mentioning that the period during which this practice occurred affects postural control. As an example [84], older people who have been active in physical and sporting activities throughout their lifetime generally show better postural control performance as they get older. This is followed by older individuals who have recently started engaging in these activities, and those who only participated in physical or sports activities in their earlier years but are not currently practicing. Older individuals who have never practiced regular physical/sports activity present the worst performance of this system, demonstrating greater postural instability compared to the other groups [84].

Recent studies have shown that the benefits of this practice extend beyond the neuromuscular and sensory alterations observed in the peripheral nervous system [14]. Colcombe and collaborators [70] observed an increase in the brain volume of healthy subjects aged 60–79 years after only 6 months of regular aerobic training. In addition, Rogge and colleagues [85] found neuroplasticity of brain regions associated with visual and vestibular self-motion perception after 12 weeks of balance training. There is evidence that exercise may increase the performance of prefrontal brain regions, enabling better control of movement and compensation in the functioning of brain areas directly affected by the aging process, which causes balance disorders, lower coordination, and slower movement, mainly during gait [14, 69, 70, 85].

Unfortunately, there is no agreement among the literature as to which exercise is superior for maintaining or enhancing postural control and thus preventing falls. It is most likely because there are no specific exercises to prevent falls. More importantly, regardless of the type, regular physical exercises enable older people to act on the environment and receive sensory information to produce adequate muscular activation. In this sense, active older adults might better calibrate their postural responses to environmental contexts.

The main program for the prevention of falls recommended by the World Health Organization [86] comprises educational health, exercise practice, dual-task training, and identification of the risks of falling (individual, environmental, and social). There are many successful programs to prevent falls around the world [87, 88], according to Table 16.2. According to studies, intervention programs should last for at least 12 weeks to effectively prevent falls. These programs should involve physical exercises performed at least twice a week, either in groups or individually, with 50-minute sessions that include personalized load and difficulty progressions. Additionally, it is important to evaluate the older adult's home environment, footwear, and individual risk factors.

Table 16.2 Preventive multimodal programs of falls

Multimodal program	Main topics of the organization	Overview
Prevention of Falls in Older People: American Geriatrics Society and British Geriatrics Society	– 12 weeks – 1–3 times per week – Individualized or in a group	– Gait, balance, and muscle strength training – Flexibility and aerobic endurance training but not isolated – Individualized progression
Exercise to prevent falls in older adults	– 3 h per week – Individualized or in a group – Complete with home exercises – Identify other factors related to falls	– Balance training (base of support, mobility training without using the arms for support or trying to reduce dependence on the upper limbs) – Gait training (vigorous gait programs should not be prescribed in individuals at high risk of falls) – Strength training can be performed along with balance
Multisensory exercise program	– 16 weeks – 3 times per week – 50 min per session – Progression every 4 weeks – Not individualized	– Multisensory exercise program – Improvement in cognition, balance, mobility, and functional performance – Improvement in muscle strength in the lower limb – Improvement in postural balance and mobility
Balance exercise circuit	– 12 weeks – Twice a week – 50 min per session – Progression every 3 weeks – Not individualized	– Improvement in muscle strength in the lower limb – Improvement in postural balance and mobility
Exercise for preventing falls in older people: systematic review and meta-analysis	– 5–120 weeks	– Reduction of fall rate (34%)
24-week program	– 3 times per week – Progressions: 2–5 sets, 7–12 repetitions	– Global exercise program (abdomen, lower and upper limbs with 7 exercises on the floor or under unstable surface)
Otago Exercise Programme	– 30 min, 3 times per week – Walk at least twice a week – Older adults must participate for at least 1 year, extendable for 2 years	– In the first 2 months, the older adult receives 4–5 visits from a physiotherapist or nurse – Older adults are always encouraged by the phone – It is planned to gradually increase the difficulty of the activities in the sixth month

(continued)

Table 16.2 (continued)

Multimodal program	Main topics of the organization	Overview
Falls Management Exercise (FaME)	Group exercises: – 36 weeks, for 1 h Exercises at home: – Twice a week – 30 min warm-up – 10 min for resistance exercises – Otago Exercise Programme – Flexibility and relaxation exercises – Recommendation for the older adult who is not able to get up from the floor alone: pre-training for 8 weeks	– Balance training – Compensatory step training – Lower limb muscle strength training – Functional training (squat, step, resistance exercises) – Flexibility exercises – Gait training – Floor exercises (crawling, rolling, lifting)

Case management program	Main topics of the organization	Overview
Prevention of Falls in Older People: American Geriatrics Society and British Geriatrics Society	– 12 weeks – 1–3 times per week – Individualized at home or in a group	– Monitoring risk factors for falls
Strategies for increasing independence, confidence, and energy (STRIDE)	– Individualized care plans – Home visit 6 months after the initial assessment and annually thereafter (reassessments) – Revisions to the care plan	Assessing risk factors: – Medications – Muscle strength, gait, and postural balance – Postural hypotension – Feet and footwear – Home security – Osteoporosis – Vitamin D – Visual impairment
Multifactor program	– 16 weeks – 32 sessions, each lasting 45 min – Home security	– Physical training – Home adaptations – Fear of falling
Multifactorial program for the prevention of falls in older people (Prevquedas Brazil)	– 12 weeks – Individualized assessment of modifiable risk factors – Multimodal physical activity once a week – Behavioral education	– Improvement in motor variables (e.g., muscle strength, postural balance)
Multidisciplinary and assistance program for the management of falls for older fallers (Magic)	– 16 weeks – Individualized assessment of modifiable risk factors – 3 times per week of multimodal physical activity – Cognitive activity—APG protocol – Case management – Individualized progression for physical exercises	– Reduce incidence of falls – Improvement in interpersonal relationships (WHODAS) – Long-term cognitive improvement – Greater adherence to the program

Final Considerations

Postural control is essential for the majority of daily motor activities. Degradation of this system over the years may be related to the increased risk of falls in the older population. Neural activation and sensorimotor coupling seem altered in older people, leading to poor postural responses to the environment. The practice of regular physical exercises results in benefits for postural control in neurologically healthy older adults, improving balance and reducing the risk of falls. Although the mechanisms underlying the improvements in the postural control system are not entirely known, many countries have developed fall prevention programs to reduce the incidence of falls and public costs from hospitalizations and morbidities in the older population.

References

1. Instituto Brasileiro de Geografia e Estatística. Censo demográfico 2022. Brasília, DF: IBGE; 2023.
2. Panel on Prevention of Falls in Older Persons. American Geriatrics Society and British geriatrics society. Summary of the updated American Geriatrics Society/British geriatrics society clinical practice guideline for prevention of falls in older persons. J Am Geriatr Soc. 2011;59(1):148–57.
3. Silva RB, Eslick GD, Duque G. Exercise for falls and fracture prevention in long term care facilities: a systematic review and meta-analysis. J Am Med Dir Assoc. 2013;14(9):685–9.
4. Ganz SB, Peterson MG, Russo PW, Guccione A. Functional recovery after hip fracture in the subacute setting. HSS J. 2007;3(1):50–7.
5. Gregg EW, Pereira MA, Caspersen CJ. Physical activity, falls, and fractures among older adults: a review of the epidemiologic evidence. J Am Geriatr Soc. 2000;48(8):883–93.
6. Brasil. Ministério da Saúde. DATASUS: Departamento de Informática do SUS. Brasília, DF: Ministério da Saúde; 2023.
7. GBD 2019 Diseases and Injuries Collaborators. GBD 2019 diseases and injuries collaborators. Global burden of 369 diseases and injuries in 204 countries and territories, 1990-2019: a systematic analysis for the global burden of disease study 2019. Lancet. 2020;396(10258):1204–22.
8. Taguchi CK, Menezes PL, Melo ACS, Santana LS, Conceição WRS, Souza GF, et al. Frailty syndrome and risks for falling in the elderly community. Codas. 2022;34(6):e20210025. https://doi.org/10.1590/2317-1782/20212021025pt.
9. Camargos FF, Dias RC, Dias JM, Freire MT. Cross-cultural adaptation and evaluation of the psychometric properties of the falls efficacy scale-international among elderly Brazilians (FES-I-Brazil). Rev Bras Fisioter. 2010;14(3):237–43.
10. Horak FB, Shupert CL, Mirka A. Components of postural dyscontrol in the elderly: a review. Neurobiol Aging. 1989;10:727–38.
11. Mackey DC, Robinovitch SN. Mechanisms underlying age-related differences in ability to recover balance with the ankle strategy. Gait Posture. 2006;23(1):59–68.
12. Rankin JK, Woollacott MH, Shumway-Cook A, Brown LA. Cognitive influence on postural stability: a neuromuscular analysis in young and older adults. J Gerontol A Biol Sci Med Sci. 2000;55(3):M112–M9.
13. Dault MC, Frank JS. Does practice modify the relationship between postural control and the execution of a secondary task in young and older individuals? Gerontology. 2004;50(3):157–64.
14. Seidler RD, Bernard JA, Burutolu TB, Fling BW, Gordon MT, Gwin JT, et al. Motor control and aging: links to age-related brain structural, functional, and biochemical effects. Neurosci Biobehav Rev. 2010;34(5):721–33.

15. Linortner P, Jehna M, Johansen-Berg H, Matthews P, Schmidt R, Fazekas F, et al. Aging associated changes in the motor control of ankle movements in the brain. Neurobiol Aging. 2014;35(10):2222–9.
16. St George RJ, Hinder MR, Puri R, Walker E, Callisaya ML. Functional near-infrared spectroscopy reveals the compensatory potential of pre-frontal cortical activity for standing balance in young and older adults. J Neurosci. 2021;452:208–18.
17. Rubega M, Formaggio E, Di Marco R, Bertuccelli M, Tortora S, Menegatti E, et al. Cortical correlates in upright dynamic and static balance in the elderly. Sci Rep. 2021;11(1):14132. https://doi.org/10.1038/s41598-021-93556-3.
18. Spedden ME, Beck MM, Christensen MS, Dietz MJ, Karabanov AN, Geertsen SS, et al. Directed connectivity between primary and premotor areas underlying ankle force control in young and older adults. NeuroImage. 2020;218:116982. https://doi.org/10.1016/j.neuroimage.2020.116982.
19. Noohi F, Kinnaird C, De Dios Y, Kofman I, Wood SJ, Bloomberg JJ, et al. Deactivation of somatosensory and visual cortices during vestibular stimulation is associated with older age and poorer balance. PLoS One. 2018;14(9):e0221954. https://doi.org/10.1371/journal.pone.0221954.
20. Cavanna AE, Trimble MR. The precuneus: a review of its functional anatomy and behavioural correlates. Brain. 2006;129(1):564–83.
21. Ioffe ME, Chernikova LA, Ustinova KI. Role of cerebellum in learning postural tasks. Cerebellum. 2007;6(1):87–94.
22. Horak FB, Macpherson JM. Postural orientation and equilibrium. In: Rowell LB, Shepherd JT, editors. Handbook of physiology: a critical, comprehensive presentation of physiological knowledge and concepts. New York, NY: Oxford University Press; 1996. p. 255–92.
23. Reed ES. Changing theories of postural development. In: Woollacott MH, Shumway-Cook A, editors. Development of posture and gait: across the life span. Columbia, SC: University of South Carolina Press; 1989. p. 3–24.
24. Polastri PF, Barela JA, Kiemel T, Jeka JJ. Dynamics of inter-modality re-weighting during human postural control. Exp Brain Res. 2012;223(1):99–108.
25. Alexander NB. Postural control in older adults. J Am Geriatr Soc. 1994;42(1):93–108.
26. Woollacott MH, Shumway-Cook A, Nashner LM. Aging and posture control: changes in sensory organization and muscular coordination. Int J Aging Hum Dev. 1986;23(2):97–114.
27. Melzer I, Kurz I, Oddsson LI. A retrospective analysis of balance control parameters in elderly fallers and non-fallers. Clin Biomech (Bristol, Avon). 2010;25(10):984–8.
28. Piirtola M, Era P. Force platform measurements as predictors of falls among older people - a review. Gerontology. 2006;52(1):1–16.
29. Muir JW, Kiel DP, Hannan M, Magaziner J, Rubin CT. Dynamic parameters of balance which correlate to elderly persons with a history of falls. PLoS One. 2013;8(8):e70566. https://doi.org/10.1371/journal.pone.0070566.
30. Oliveira MR, Vieira ER, Gil AWO, Fernandes KBP, Teixeira DC, Amorim CF, et al. One-legged stance sway of older adults with and without falls. PLoS One. 2018;13(9):e0203887. https://doi.org/10.1371/journal.pone.0203887.
31. Houk JC, Lehman S. Control systems: feedback, feedforward, and adaptative strategies. In: Adelman G, editor. Encyclopedia of neuroscience. Boston, MA: Birk Kauser; 1987. p. 275–7.
32. Gatev P, Thomas S, Kepple T, Hallett M. Feedforward ankle strategy of balance during quiet stance in adults. J Physiol. 1999;514(3):915–28.
33. Dufossé M, Hugon M, Massion J. Postural forearm changes induced by predictable in time or voluntary triggered unloading in man. Exp Brain Res. 1985;60:330–4.
34. Dault MC, de Haart M, Geurts AC, Arts IM, Nienhuis B. Effects of visual center of pressure feedback on postural control in young and elderly healthy adults and in stroke patients. Hum Mov Sci. 2003;22(3):221–36.
35. Woollacott MH, Manchester DL. Antecipatory postural adjustments in older adults: are changes in response characteristics due to changes in strategy ? J Gerontol. 1993;48(2):M64–70.

36. Kaewmanee T, Liang H, Madrid KC, Aruin AS. Older adults utilize less efficient postural adaptations when they are uncertain about the magnitude of a perturbation. Hum Mov Sci. 2022;85:102996. https://doi.org/10.1016/j.humov.2022.102996.
37. Duarte MB, da Silva Almeida GC, Costa KHA, Garcez DR, de Athay Decosta E silva A, da Silva Souza G, et al. Anticipatory postural adjustments in older versus young adults: a systematic review and meta-analysis. Syst Rev. 2022;11(1):251. https://doi.org/10.1186/s13643-022-02116-x.
38. Seidler RD, Noll DC, Thiers G. Feedforward and feedback processes in motor control. NeuroImage. 2004;22(4):1778–83.
39. Horak FB, Nashner LM. Central programming of postural movements: adaptation to altered support-surface configurations. J Neurophysiol. 1986;55(6):1369–81.
40. Winter DA. Human balance and posture control during standing and walking. Gait Posture. 1995;3:193–214.
41. Barrett RS, Lichtwark GA. Effect of altering neural, muscular and tendinous factors associated with aging on balance recovery using the ankle strategy: a simulation study. J Theor Biol. 2008;254(3):546–54.
42. Godoi D, Barela JA. Mecanismos de ajustes posturais feedback e feedforward em idosos. Revista Brasileira de Ciências do Esporte. 2002;23(3):9–22.
43. Arsenault D, Ivanova TD, Garland SJ. Postural control in response to unilateral and bilateral external perturbations in older adults. Gait Posture. 2022;94:26–31.
44. Mochizuki G, Boe S, Marlin A, McIlRoy W, E. Perturbation-evoked cortical activity reflects both the context and consequence of postural instability. J Neurosci. 2010;170(2):599–609.
45. Mochizuki G, Boe SG, Marlin A, McIlroy WE. Performance of a concurrent cognitive task modifies pre- and post-perturbation-evoked cortical activity. J Neurosci. 2017;348:143–52.
46. Varghese JP, Staines WR, McIlroy WE. Activity in functional cortical networks temporally associated with postural instability. J Neurosci. 2019;401:43–58.
47. Purohit R, Bhatt T. Mobile brain imaging to examine task-related cortical correlates of reactive balance: a systematic review. Brain Sci. 2022;12(11):1487. https://doi.org/10.3390/brainsci12111487.
48. Horak FB. Postural orientation and equilibrium: what do we need to know about neural control of balance to prevent falls? Age Ageing. 2006;35:ii7–ii11.
49. Posture GC. In: Kandel ER, Schwartz JH, Jessel TM, editors. Principles of neural science. 3rd ed. New York, NY: Elsevier; 1991. p. 596–607.
50. Nashner LM. Analysis of stance posture in humans. In: Towe AL, Luschei ES, editors. Motor coordination (handbook of behavioural neurology), vol. 5. New York, NY: Plenum Press; 1981. p. 527–64.
51. Oie KS, Kiemel T, Jeka JJ. Multisensory fusion: simultaneous re-weighting of vision and touch for the control of human posture. Cogn Brain Res. 2002;14:164–76.
52. Prioli AC, Freitas Júnior PB, Barela JA. Physical activity and postural control in the elderly: coupling between visual information and body sway. Gerontology. 2005;51(3):145–8.
53. Teasdale N, Simoneau M. Attentional demands for postural control: the effects of aging and sensory reintegration. Gait Posture. 2001;14:203–10.
54. Toledo DR, Barela JA. Age-related differences in postural control: effects of the complexity of visual manipulation and sensorimotor contribution to postural performance. Exp Brain Res. 2014;232(2):493–502.
55. Allison LK, Kiemel T, Jeka JJ. Multisensory reweighting of vision and touch is intact in healthy and fall-prone older adults. Exp Brain Res. 2006;175(2):342–52.
56. Allison LK, Kiemel T, Jeka JJ. Sensory-challenge balance exercises improve multisensory reweighting in fall-prone older adults. J Neurol Phys Ther. 2018;42(2):84–93.
57. Gianoudis J, Bailey CA, Ebeling PR, Nowson CA, Sanders KM, Hill K, et al. Effects of a targeted multimodal exercise program incorporating high-speed power training on falls and fracture risk factors in older adults: a community-based randomized controlled trial. J Bone Miner Res. 2014;29(1):182–91.

58. Barker AL, Bird M-L, Talevski J. Effect of Pilates exercise for improving balance in older adults: a systematic review with meta-analysis. Arch Phys Med Rehabil. 2015;66(4):715–23.
59. Gauchard GC, Jeandel C, Tessier A, Perrin PP. Beneficial effect of proprioceptive physical activities on balance control in elderly human subjects. Neurosci Lett. 1999;273:81–4.
60. Allin LJ, Brolinson PG, Beach BM, Kim S, Nussbaum MA, Roberto KA, et al. Perturbation-based balance training targeting both slip- and trip-induced falls among older adults: a randomized controlled trial. BMC Geriatr. 2020;20(1):205. https://doi.org/10.1186/s12877-020-01605-9.
61. Kuo CC, Chen SC, Chen TY, Ho TJ, Lin JG, Lu TW. Effects of long-term tai-chi Chuan practice on whole-body balance control during obstacle-crossing in the elderly. Sci Rep. 2022;12:2660.
62. Lee HC, Chang KC, Tsauo JY, Hung JW, Huang YC, Lin SI. Fall prevention initiatives in Taiwan (FPIT) investigators. Effects of a multifactorial fall prevention program on fall incidence and physical function in community-dwelling older adults with risk of falls. Arch Phys Med Rehabil. 2013;94(4):606–15.
63. Fernández-Argüelles EL, Rodríguez-Mansilla J, Antunez LE, Garrido-Ardila EM, Muñoz RP. Effects of dancing on the risk of falling related factors of healthy older adults: a systematic review. Arch Gerontol Geriatr. 2015;60(1):1–8.
64. Bruin ED, Murer K. Effect of additional functional exercises on balance in elderly people. Clin Rehabil. 2007;21(2):112–21.
65. Liu-Ambrose T, Davis JC, Best JR, Dian L, Madden K, Cook W, et al. Effect of a home-based exercise program on subsequent falls among community-dwelling high-risk older adults after a aall: a randomized clinical trial. J Am Med Assoc. 2019;321(21):2092–100.
66. Gschwind YJ, Kressig RW, Lacroix A, Muehlbauer T, Pfenninger B, Granacher U. A best practice fall prevention exercise program to improve balance, strength / power, and psychosocial health in older adults: study protocol for a randomized controlled trial. BMC Geriatr. 2013;13:105.
67. Balzer K, Bremer M, Schramm S, Lühmann D, Raspe H. Falls prevention for the elderly. GMS Health Technol Assess. 2012;8:Doc01. https://doi.org/10.3205/hta000099.
68. Ricci NA, Gonçalves DFF, Coimbra IB, Coimbra AMV. Fatores associados ao histórico de quedas de idosos assistidos pelo programa de saúde da família. Saúde e Sociedade. 2010;19(4):898–909.
69. Bherer L. Cognitive plasticity in older adults: effects of cognitive training and physical exercise. Ann N Y Acad Sci. 2015;1337:1–6.
70. Colcombe SJ, Erickson KI, Scalf PE, Kim JS, Prakash R, McAuley E, et al. Aerobic exercise training increases brain volume in aging humans. J Gerontol A Biol Sci Med Sci. 2006;61(11):1166–70.
71. Montero-Odasso M, van der Velde N, Martin FC, Petrovic M, Tan MP, Ryg J, Task Force on Global Guidelines for Falls in Older Adults, et al. World guidelines for falls prevention and management for older adults: a global initiative. Age Ageing. 2022;51(9):afac205. https://doi.org/10.1093/ageing/afac205.
72. Pau M, Leban B, Collu G, Migliaccio GM. Effect of light and vigorous physical activity on balance and gait of older adults. Arch Gerontol Geriatr. 2014;59(3):568–73.
73. Rodrigues IB, Ponzano M, Giangregorio LM. Practical tips for prescribing exercise for fall prevention. Osteoporos Int. 2019;30(10):1953–60.
74. Martínez-Amat A, Hita-Contreras F, Lomas-Vega R, Caballero-Martínez I, Alvarez PJ, Martínez-López E. Effects of 12-week proprioception training program on postural stability, gait, and balance in older adults: a controlled clinical trial. J Strength Cond Res. 2013;27(8):2180–8.
75. Bubela D, Sacharko L, Chan J, Brady M. Balance and functional outcomes for older community-dwelling adults who practice Tai Chi and those who do not: a comparative study. J Geriatr Phys Ther. 2019;42(2):209–15.
76. Duque G, Boersma D, Loza-Diaz G, Hassan S, Suarez H, Geisinger D, et al. Effects of balance training using a virtual-reality system in older fallers. Clin Interv Aging. 2013;8:257–63.

77. Sipilä S, Tirkkonen A, Savikangas T, Hänninen T, Laukkanen P, Alen M, et al. Effects of physical and cognitive training on gait speed and cognition in older adults: a randomized controlled trial. Scand J Med Sci Sports. 2021;31(7):1518–33.
78. Phu S, Vogrin S, Al Saedi A, Duque G. Balance training using virtual reality improves balance and physical performance in older adults at high risk of falls. Clin Interv Aging. 2019;14:1567–77.
79. Osti FR, Souza CR, Teixeira LA. Improvement of balance stability in older individuals by on-water training. J Aging Phys Act. 2018;26(2):222–6. https://doi.org/10.1123/japa.2017-0041.
80. Šarabon N, Kozinc Ž. Effects of resistance exercise on balance ability: systematic review and meta-analysis of randomized controlled trials. Life (Basel). 2020;10(11):284. https://doi.org/10.3390/life10110284.
81. Paillard T. The optimal method for improving postural balance in healthy young and older people: specific training for postural tasks encountered in personal physical practice. Front Physiol. 2023;14:1188496. https://doi.org/10.3389/fphys.2023.1188496.
82. Hess JA, Woollacott MH. Effect of high-intensity strength-training on functional measures of balance ability in balance-impaired older adults. J Manip Physiol Ther. 2005;28(8):582–90.
83. Kim Y, Vakula MN, Bolton DAE, Dakin CJ, Thompson BJ, Slocum TA, et al. Which exercise interventions can most effectively improve reactive balance in older adults? A systematic review and network meta-analysis. Front Aging Neurosci. 2022;13:764826. https://doi.org/10.3389/fnagi.2021.764826.
84. Perrin PP, Gauchard GC, Perrot C, Jeandel C. Effects of physical and sporting activities on balance control in elderly people. Br J Sports Med. 1999;33:121–6.
85. Rogge AK, Röder B, Zech A, Hötting K. Exercise-induced neuroplasticity: balance training increases cortical thickness in visual and vestibular cortical regions. NeuroImage. 2018;179:471–9.
86. World Health Organization. WHO global report on falls prevention in older age. Paris: WHO; 2007.
87. de Negreiros CK, Perracini MR, Soares AT, de Cristo SF, Sera CT, Tiedemann A, et al. Effectiveness of a multifactorial falls prevention program in community-dwelling older people when compared to usual care: study protocol for a randomised controlled trial (Prevquedas Brazil). BMC Geriatr. 2013;13:27. https://doi.org/10.1186/1471-2318-13-27.
88. Alberto SN, Ansai JH, Janducci AL, Florido JVB, Novaes ADC, Caetano MJD, et al. A case management program at home to reduce fall risk in older adults (the MAGIC study): protocol for a single-blind randomized controlled trial. JMIR Res Protoc. 2022;11(6):e34796. https://doi.org/10.2196/34796.

Fear and Anxiety in Older Adults and Its Impact on Postural Control

17

Mark G. Carpenter and Allan L. Adkin

Abstract

Recent evidence confirms that fear of falling is highly prevalent in older adults and represents an important contributing factor to future fall risk. The primary focus of this chapter is to examine current evidence derived from group comparisons and within-subject experimental designs to demonstrate how emotions such as fear and anxiety influence balance across different types of postural tasks in young and older adults. The results provide compelling evidence for an indirect and direct effect of fear and anxiety on all aspects of postural control, including changes in performance on clinical balance assessments and posturographic measures of static and dynamic balance control. Both young and older adults respond to threat and anxiety conditions in static and dynamic balance tasks with a combination of context-dependent protective strategies, and potentially maladaptive or inefficient neuro-muscular changes that are tightly coupled to anxiety and fear responses. The evidence of emotion-balance interactions in young and older adults provides important insight on the physiological, psychological, and social-cognitive interactions that contribute to human postural control and highlights the need to account for the potential confounding influence of anxiety and fear when performing balance assessments, and designing treatment and intervention solutions for age-related balance deficits.

M. G. Carpenter (✉)
School of Kinesiology, University of British Columbia, Vancouver, BC, Canada
e-mail: mark.carpenter@ubc.ca

A. L. Adkin
Department of Kinesiology, Brock University, St. Catharines, ON, Canada

F. A. Barbieri et al. (eds.), *Locomotion and Posture in Older Adults*,
https://doi.org/10.1007/978-3-031-74123-4_17

Introduction

Falls are a significant health issue for older adults, with approximately 30% of adults aged 65 years and older reporting a fall each year (for review, see Montero-Odessa et al. [1]). Falls in older adults result from a complex interaction between biological, behavioural, socioeconomic, and environmental risk factors (Seniors' Falls in Canada Second Report - Stinchcombe et al 2014 [2]). Historically, most clinical and research efforts have focussed primarily on the biological factors that contribute to age-related falls. However, more recent evidence has shown that emotional-behavioural changes, such as fear of falling, are also important contributors to fall risk in older adults. Prevalence rates of fear of falling vary considerably in the literature (for review, see Legters [3] and Mackay et al. [4]). In a systematic review, Scheffer et al. [5] reported that the prevalence of fear of falling in older adults ranged from 21% to 85%. Fear of falling prevalence is typically higher with advanced age [5] and with neurological balance deficits that predominantly affect older adults, such as Parkinson's disease [6, 7] and stroke [8, 9]. Fear of falling in older adults is associated with a wide range of behavioural changes, including balance and gait deficits (for review, see Hadjistavropoulos et al. [10]) and increased risk of falls [11–13]. Ultimately, fear of falling can lead to restriction of physical and social activities, decline in physical functioning, loss of independence, and reduced quality of life (for review, see Legters [3]).

Understanding the true effects of emotions, including fear and anxiety, on balance and gait control in older adults has been complicated by the diverse range of terms used in the literature to describe and categorize different emotional traits and states (for review, see Ellmers et al. [14]). Fear of falling was initially conceptualized as low perceived self-efficacy about falling that ultimately causes an individual to start to avoid activities that they can perform [15]. This term has been adopted by many to describe the broad psychological consequences of falling including emotionally based constructs (e.g., fear/anxiety/concerns/worry about falling) and cognitively based constructs (e.g., fall-related efficacy, balance efficacy, balance confidence). Although these constructs are interrelated, it is now established that they describe different phenomena and are related to different behavioural outcomes [10, 16–18].

Briefly, fear of falling refers to an intense emotional state triggered by an immediate real or perceived threat to balance, which elicits physiological and behavioural responses designed to avoid or escape imminent danger [14]. Fear of falling symptoms can vary widely in intensity and are only clinically diagnosed if distressing or functionally disabling [19]. This fearful emotional state is distinct from an individual's general sense of fear or concern about falling which has been defined as a "lasting feeling of dread and apprehension about situations that are believed to threaten or challenge balance" [14]. In contrast, anxiety is an emotional state of uneasiness or concern about a non-specific threat, which may or may not occur. Note that state anxiety is associated with a specific threat scenario, and remains distinct from an individuals' trait anxiety [19]. State anxiety involves somatic, cognitive and worry (ruminative) manifestations, and can occur in conjunction with, or independent from, sensations of fear [14]. Most somatic changes triggered by anxiety are attributed to an increase in arousal which refers to a general increase in physiological readiness, characterized by autonomic changes that affect blood pressure, heart rate, electrodermal activity, and pupil dilation [20]. However, arousal (excitement) can be increased in both positive and negative emotional states, and during physical exertion [19].

Another related, yet distinct term is balance efficacy/confidence, which refers to an individual's perceived capability to successfully perform a balance task [16, 21]. Balance efficacy/confidence requires a prediction of future performance, and therefore must be assessed in advance or anticipation of the balance task. Balance efficacy/confidence can be assessed within a specific context or state [22] or can be used to determine a general trait of balance efficacy/confidence [21].

Due to the varied definitions in the literature, there are several different tools that have been developed to assess these different constructs in older adults. As reviewed by Legters [3], many studies assess a trait characteristic or "generalized" fear of falling or balance confidence using questionnaires in the form of a) single questions (i.e., "Are you afraid of falling?", "Do you have a concern about falling"?), b) validated scales to assess trait balance efficacy/confidence (e.g., Falls Efficacy Scale; Falls Efficacy Scale-International, FES-I; Activities-specific Balance Confidence scale,) or anxiousness (e.g., State Trait Anxiety Inventory, STAI), or c) fear avoidance behaviour (e.g., Survey of Activities and Fear of Falling in the Elderly). Other tools assess the state-level fear, anxiety, or confidence of an individual within a specific context and moment in time, using either single item visual analogue scales or combinations of questions to assess different somatic/worry and concentration elements of anxiety (i.e., often modified from the STAI [23] or Sport-Specific Anxiety Scale [24]). Irrespective of the tool that is used, it is important to clearly distinguish trait and state measurements especially when trying to interpret the somewhat variable findings in the literature of reported associations between emotion and balance and gait performance in older adults [19]. Throughout this chapter, we have tried to maintain the original terminology used by individual studies as a means to highlight differences and maintain transparency. However, for consistency, when not specific to a particular study, we have relied on the general terms of fear and anxiety to reflect a general negative emotional state related to balance and falls.

The primary focus of this chapter is to examine the experimental evidence to date from cross-sectional and within-subject designs to understand the effects of emotional state (e.g., anxiety, fear) on balance control. This information provides critical insight into the mechanisms that may contribute to age-related balance decline and identifies potential new targets for treatments designed to improve balance and reduce falls in older adults. Most cross-sectional studies have compared older adults divided into groups based on trait measures of fear/confidence to observe potential balance differences between the groups. While these studies provide important insight into the possible effects of emotions on balance, the nature of the between-subject design limits any interpretation of a causal effect. For example, if altered balance performance is observed in a group that is fearful of falling compared to a non-fearful group, it cannot be ascertained whether balance changed as a result of the underlying fear, or if individuals with balance deficits have developed a corresponding fear of falling.

Approaches to Assess the Effects of Fear and Anxiety on Postural Control

More recent experiments have been designed to introduce a postural threat within a controlled lab environment to manipulate emotions in order to study the direct effect of these emotional changes on balance control (for review, see Adkin and Carpenter [25]). In these studies, there is an opportunity to compare balance performance with and without the postural threat within the same individual. Since the only change introduced in the experiment is the emotional response to the imposed postural threat, then any modifications in balance control can be more directly attributed to the altered emotional state.

Several different approaches have been used to experimentally manipulate postural threat to alter state anxiety and fear in order to observe any corresponding changes in balance. The most common source of threat used in balance experiments is the threat of falling from an elevated surface. In these experiments, participants perform postural tasks while standing on a surface that can be elevated from low/ground level, to heights varying from 0.5 to 3.2 m in a controlled lab environment. Studies using virtual heights as a manipulation can overcome physical barriers to achieve greater perceived standing heights [26, 27]. In all cases, a change in real or virtual height of at least 0.8 m in young adults has been shown to significantly increase self-reported anxiety and fear, decrease self-reported balance confidence or efficacy, and increase physiological arousal (for review, see Adkin and Carpenter [25]). While lower heights have also been used, primarily in older adults and individuals with balance deficits, the emotional response and/or physiological arousal changes may be less robust [28]. Alternatively, researchers have used the threat of an impending perturbation where individuals are required to stand with or without the threat of experiencing a sudden, unpredictable balance disturbance, including support surface translations or rotations [29–35] or push and pulls to the upper trunk [36]. Using the threat of multi-directional perturbations has the advantage of reducing the likelihood of individuals adopting any directionally specific strategies that are inherent to elevated surface paradigms [37]. Like height-induced threat, the threat of perturbation has been shown to significantly modify emotional state with increases in self-reported anxiety and fear and elevated physiological arousal observed (for review, see Adkin and Carpenter [25]).

Emotional state changes can also be achieved without increasing the likelihood, or consequences, of falling. For example, social anxiety has been used effectively to increase self-reported anxiety and fear and reduce self-reported balance confidence while performing postural tasks. Social anxiety has been manipulated by increasing the individual's perceived risk of negative evaluation when having to perform in front of others, particularly those considered to be in positions of authority like a clinician performing a balance assessment [38, 39]. Likewise, anxiety and arousal have been experimentally induced using affective pictures (for review, see Lelard and Stins [40]) or sounds [41, 42], or using mental stress associated with completing challenging cognitive tasks, particularly math tests [43–45].

The following sections examine current evidence derived from group comparisons and within-subject experimental designs to demonstrate how emotions influence balance across different types of balance tasks. Since most research involving threat manipulations has been conducted on healthy young adults [25], we present evidence from young adults first, followed by evidence of age-related changes specific to older adults, when applicable.

Fear and Anxiety Effects on Clinical Balance Measures

Fearful older adults have been shown to have significantly reduced limits of stability in both the anterior-posterior (AP) and medial-lateral (ML) directions, compared to non-fearful older adults, even when controlling for muscle strength [46]. One-leg stance time is also decreased in fearful compared to non-fearful older adults [47] and older adults with low compared to high balance confidence [48].

Using postural threat, Hauck et al. [49] observed that young adults had significantly shorter one-leg stance durations and reduced forward reach distance on a functional reach test (i.e., reduced stability limits) when standing on a high compared to low surface height. This work was extended to examine young and older adults performing clinical balance tests at ground level and on top of a 0.5 m high box with and without a secondary cognitive task [50]. When threatened, one-leg stance duration and functional reach distance were shorter, while the time to complete the 5-times sit-to-stand task was longer for both young and older adults, independent of the secondary cognitive task.

Geh et al. [38] used social anxiety as a source of threat to examine its effect on clinical balance performance measures in young and older female adults. Similar to the changes observed in older adults when the threat was evoked by a change in surface height, these researchers observed decreased one-leg stance durations in the older adults when performing the task in front of an expert evaluator (i.e., white-coat effect). During the functional reach task, older adults increased reach distance in the social anxiety condition. In contrast, no significant postural changes were observed in young adults despite having similar increases in anxiety and decreases in confidence to the presence of the evaluator as the older adults.

Fear and Anxiety Effects on Static Balance Control

Static balance control refers to maintaining balance during quiet stance. Quiet standing requires the sway of the centre of mass (COM) to be controlled within the base-of-support, using torques generated at the ankle and hip (ML only), which can be measured as displacements of the centre of pressure (COP) recorded with a force plate [51].

The effects of fear and anxiety on static balance control have been studied extensively in terms of changes in postural sway. Larger sway amplitude displacements during two leg standing tasks have been observed in more fearful older adults when standing without vision [47, 52]. Likewise, increases in sway amplitude have been reported in older adults with low compared to high balance confidence [48, 53, 54].

The effects of postural threat on static balance control in healthy young and older adults are well-established [25]. When standing on elevated surfaces, young adults consistently demonstrate a pattern of postural changes that includes decreased amplitude and increased frequency of COP and COM displacements and shifting the mean position of the COP and COM away from the platform edge (i.e., the direction of the perceived threat). The increase in frequency has been shown to result from a decrease in the lowest frequency band of COP displacements (0–0.05 Hz) and increases in higher frequency bands (0.5–1.8 Hz and 1.8–5.0 Hz), which under normal, non-threatening circumstances, usually contain little to no significant power [55, 56]. The increases in higher frequency COP displacement are highly correlated with increases in co-contraction between ankle dorsi-flexors and plantar-flexors [55]. Assuming the body is modelled as an inverted pendulum when standing quietly, the observed decrease in amplitude and increase in frequency of COP displacements has been used as evidence for an ankle stiffening strategy, with increased muscle activity around the ankle joints leading to increased ankle stiffness estimates, and restricted control of the COM within the limits of the base-of-support [51, 57, 58].

The threat of a possible perturbation (i.e., surface translation in the forward or backward direction) has been found to significantly increase the frequency as well as the amplitude of COP displacements, with a significant forward shift of the COP mean position [32, 34]. Similar increases in sway amplitude and frequency but no change in leaning has been observed when the threat is delivered in the ML direction [33]. Thus, standing balance changes appear to be highly specific to the context, direction, and nature of the perceived threat.

This context specific nature of some threat-related postural changes is also supported by unique adaptation patterns of postural responses to repeated threat exposure. Zaback et al. [55] exposed healthy young adults to repeated presentations of standing at the edge of a high surface. The initial threat-related increase in COP frequency and co-contraction was shown to significantly decrease in concert with decreasing levels of anxiety, fear, and arousal after repeated exposure to the height, with near-baseline frequency of sway achieved after full-adaptation. In contrast, decreased amplitude of sway, and backward leaning behaviours persisted and remained constant despite repeated exposure and the near complete adaptation of the emotional response. Similar observations were seen with repeated exposure to the threat of a postural perturbation, with frequency shown to adapt over time, yet amplitude and leaning behaviours appeared independent of waning fear and anxiety [33]. Thus, some threat-related postural changes are likely context dependent (i.e., mean position, sway amplitude) and have a protective role, whereas others (i.e., co-contraction, high-frequency sway) vary more closely with fear and arousal and may reflect more systemic changes that are potentially maladaptive [14, 25, 55]. Arousal specific changes are further corroborated by observations of increased COP frequencies observed in young adults standing at ground level while viewing affective pictures [40], which elicit an increase in arousal, independent of valence [59].

Healthy older adults demonstrate a similar ankle stiffening strategy to that of young adults when standing on elevated surfaces, with increased frequency of sway and either a decrease or no change in amplitude of sway observed [22, 60–63]. As highlighted in Table 17.1, some differences in age groups may be observed at more modest threat conditions, where older adults demonstrated a lower threshold to observe threat-related balance changes [28]. Most studies also show an ability to shift the COM away from the edge in older adults [22, 60]. Both young and older adults scale postural changes to height, with progressive decreases in sway amplitude and increases in sway frequency observed with increasing surface heights under real, and virtual height conditions [22, 26, 27, 64, 65]. However, there is some evidence that greater scaling may be observed with older adults [22].

Older adults also respond similarly to young adults when standing under the threat of perturbation delivered using a support surface translation. Increased anxiety and arousal are accompanied by increased amplitude and increased frequency of COP displacements when anticipating a postural perturbation, independent of age. The initial response to the threat adapts similarly to repeated threat exposure in both young and older adults [33], in concert with decreased anxiety. However, older adults respond differently compared to young adults when the threat of the

Table 17.1 —Summary of research utilizing postural threat manipulations to observe changes in static postural control in healthy older adults. (n.a. = not measured, OA = older adults)

Article	Group	Threat type	Sample duration	Mean position	Velocity/ frequency	Amplitude
Carpenter et al. [22]	13 OA	Height (1.6 m)	120 s	Back lean	MPF COP increased	COP decrease
Brown et al. [60]	15 OA	Height (1.4 m)	15 s	Back lean	MPF COP increased	COP decreased
Laufer et al. [28]	60 OA	Height (0.85 m)	60 s	n.a.	MPF COP increased	No effect
Pasman et al. [61]	14 OA	Height (1.6 m)	120 s	Back lean	MPF COP increased	No effect
Sturnieks et al. [63]	36 OA (non-anxious)	Height (0.65 m)	30 s	n.a.	MPF COP increased	COP decreased
Ellmers et al. [62]	44 OA	Height (0.60 m)	60 s	n.a.	MPF COP increased	No effect
Shaw et al. [36]	16 OA	Perturbation (trunk push/ pulls)	30 s	n.a	Trunk roll velocity decreased	Trunk roll decreased
Johnson et al. [32, 33]	27 OA	Perturbation (ML translations)	60 s	No effect	MPF COP increased	COP increased

perturbation is delivered in the form of a push or pull to the trunk. Young adults showed increased pitch and roll trunk sway while older adults had decreased trunk sway but only in the roll direction when threatened [36]. Likewise, increased frequency of COP displacement has been shown with "white-coat" effects in older women to a greater extent than young women when standing under the perceived threat of negative evaluation [38], even though they report similar levels of anxiety and efficacy changes when standing under evaluative conditions.

While changes in ankle stiffness may contribute to a perceived protection against a loss of balance by limiting body position and movement in the direction of the perceived risk associated with the threat, there may be unintended, negative consequences to this strategy, if the postural stiffness interferes with, or counters other postural requirements or voluntary actions. For example, Falk et al. [66] recently demonstrated that one of the key factors that distinguished older fallers from non-fallers in a dynamic balance paradigm was greater reliance on a stiffening strategy.

Fear and Anxiety Effects on Dynamic Balance Control

The ability to maintain balance and avoid falls depends on our ability to execute appropriate postural adjustments in anticipation of, and in response to, dynamically changing environments. Dynamic postural control is thus needed to counteract the different types of perturbations that we may experience during many of our daily tasks. The central nervous system (CNS) needs to predict and account for the destabilizing forces associated with expected external perturbations or disturbances that result from our own voluntary movements (e.g., pulling on a handle to open a door). In these cases, anticipatory postural adjustments (APAs) occur just before the perturbation or the initiation of the movement to counteract the forces associated with the expected perturbation or the upcoming movement [67]. Importantly, APAs also serve to assist movement initiation by acting to destabilize the body in the direction of the intended movement (e.g., initiating gait, rising to toes, transitioning from sitting to standing, [67]). When challenges to balance are unpredictable, such as an unexpected external perturbation (e.g., receiving a push to our upper body) the CNS implements rapid balance correcting and compensatory postural responses to the perturbation onset to counteract these external forces to maintain balance [68].

Anticipatory Postural Control

The spatial and temporal characteristics of APAs are critical for movement production. Alterations in the magnitude or timing of APAs can not only impact the ability to initiate the movement but also impact the stability and successful completion of the movement. Research has shown that APAs are influenced by age [69], which could be compounded through age-related effects of emotion.

Cross-sectional studies examining the effects of fear of falling on APAs in older adults are limited. Uemura et al. [70] examined the timing of APAs during visually cued gait initiation in single and dual task (i.e., counting backwards by 1 from 100 while waiting for the visual cue) conditions in fearful vs. non-fearful older adults. The results of this study revealed differences in APAs duration between the fearful and non-fearful groups but only in the dual task condition; APAs were significantly longer for individuals in the fearful vs. non-fearful group. The authors suggested that longer APAs in fearful older adults are likely initiated as a protective strategy to increase stability but could ultimately contribute to greater instability leading to future falls.

Most of our understanding of the effects of emotions on anticipatory postural control derives from studies that use different threats to balance in healthy young and older adults. Adkin et al. [71] first examined APAs associated with a rise-to-toes task performed at a low or high surface height in healthy young adults. To rise to the toes, APAs (i.e., backward COP displacement) propel the body forward towards the toes initiating the movement to the new position over the toes. When standing at the edge of a high platform, healthy young adults reduced the magnitude of the APAs, as evidenced by a smaller peak backward displacement of the COP and reduced tibialis anterior muscle activity, but did not change the duration of the APAs. Overall, as a result, the peak forward movement of the body was also reduced, and it took longer to reach this position in this most threatening condition, and a higher percentage of task failures was observed with increased threat. Converging evidence concerning APA magnitude changes has been reported in other studies; smaller APAs have been observed when performing rise to toes [72], leg raise [73, 74] or stepping [75] tasks towards the edge of a high compared to low platform. Threat-related changes in APA durations were also observed for leg raise tasks [73, 74].

Other studies have revealed that the effect of postural threat on anticipatory postural control varies depending on the threat context and the voluntary movement being performed. For example, when healthy young adults performed a rise-to-toes under the threat of a possible postural perturbation, larger and faster APAs were observed [30, 35], and this change in the APA was observed independent of the type or direction of the perturbation threat [35]. Ellmers et al. 2020, 2021 [76] investigated APAs during auditory cued gait initiation at a high compared to low surface height in healthy young adults. The results showed that there was no change in APA magnitude or direction when performing the task when threatened. However, given that the initial step was smaller in this condition, the APAs would be disproportionally larger when performing the task under threat.

Phanthanourak et al. [77] is the only study to date, to examine APAs in young as well as older adults using a postural threat model. Their participants performed handle pulls at different force levels with or without the threat of a postural perturbation. When pulling on a handle, the results revealed that both young and older adults had smaller APAs when threatened. The effect of postural threat on the ability to scale APAs to the force of the handle pull was less clear indicating that emotions may not contribute to the decreased ability to scale APAs in older adults.

Overall, this work shows that depending on the threat context and the voluntary movement task used, cautious movement strategies are adopted to preserve stability and/or adaptations are implemented to ensure the success of the voluntary movement. Further work is needed to better understand how emotional influences on APAs interact with age and determine if, and when, fear-related changes may begin to interfere with balance control.

Balance Correcting and Compensatory Postural Reactions

The first observation of a relationship between arousal and corrective responses to postural perturbations was made by Maki and Whitelaw [78]. To examine this relationship, they investigated changes in past experience with the perturbation and prior information about whether the perturbation was small (i.e., low threat) or large (i.e., high threat). Changes in arousal levels with perturbation experience were related to the postural response supporting the view that arousal could affect the corrective postural response.

Initial evidence for direct effects of fear and anxiety on dynamic balance responses was found by Brown and Frank [37], who had young adults respond to upper body perturbations when standing on low and high surfaces. They observed that postural threat contributed to a tighter control over the COM following controlled push forces applied to the back, accomplished with a more posterior initial COM position, and decreased range of COM displacement and time to peak COM velocity post-perturbation. Subsequently, Carpenter et al. [79] had young adults stand on elevated heights and respond to unpredictable, multi-directional support surface rotations in the AP and ML planes. Within this context, a number of distinct postural changes were observed when threatened that included: increased amplitude of balance correcting responses (120–220 ms) in all leg, trunk, and arm muscles and decreased onset latency of deltoid responses. These changes together likely contributed to the observed reduction in peak displacement of the COM during balance recovery. Cleworth et al. [80] replicated and extended the findings of Carpenter et al. [79], using a virtual height paradigm combined with a translating platform with unpredictable perturbation directions in the AP plane. Their results corroborated prior observations of increased amplitude of balance correcting responses and reduced magnitude of COM displacements when threatened. Their results also extended prior observations of early deltoid responses to other balance correcting response onset latencies in the lower leg.

Fear effects on dynamic postural control in older adults were first reported by Maki et al. [47]; reduced COP movement was observed in fearful vs. non-fearful elderly during eyes open continuous sinusoidal ML surface translations. Likewise, Baloh et al. [81] observed higher sway velocity in older adults reporting some fear of falling compared to no fear of falling during AP and ML sinusoidal platform tilts or translations. However, these dynamic postural stimuli were predictable (non-random), and thus rely on feed-forward control that is less relevant during reactions to unexpected perturbations.

Okada et al. [82] compared COP and muscular response changes to sudden acceleration-decelerations of the support surface (platform displacement of 1.5 cm), in older women with and without fear of falling. This study controlled for participants' level of physical function, given the potential for fear to indirectly influence balance through reductions in activities of daily living and physical capacity. No difference in onsets of the tibialis anterior and medial gastrocnemius were observed between groups, although a difference in onset latency between the antagonist ankle muscles was shorter in the fearful group, leading to significantly higher co-contraction. As a result, fearful older adults had significantly longer response times and initial displacement of the COP as a result of the platform deceleration.

To date, no studies have looked at age effects on compensatory postural responses specific to a known postural threat. However, Akinlosotu et al. [45] examined grasp reactions in older adults to dynamic perturbations under different levels of mental stress attributed to secondary cognitive task conditions. They observed that only in the stressful cognitive task condition, mental stress increased and resulted in an increase in grasp errors, characterized by missing or improperly contacting the supporting rail following the perturbation. Since this experiment was only performed in older adults, the extent to which this behaviour is unique to older adults is not known.

Summary

Overall, the results of this research have provided compelling evidence for an indirect and direct effect of fear and anxiety on balance. This includes changes in all aspects of postural control, including changes in performance on more subjective balance assessments used in the clinic, and more objective posturographic measures of static balance (quiet standing) and dynamic balance control. Both young and older adults respond to threat and anxiety conditions in both static and dynamic balance tasks with a combination of protective strategies that vary with the context, and neuro-muscular changes that are highly coupled to anxiety and fear responses that could be considered maladaptive or at least inefficient. Together these results are consistent with observations in other populations with known fear and anxiety issues [19, 83]. For example, recent work has demonstrated that individuals with panic disorder had shorter recovery times to support surface translations compared to healthy controls that were preceded by static sway that was consistent with a stiffening response (i.e., smaller amplitude and higher velocity COP displacement; [84]). These findings also fit within a broader range of known fear effects on human motor performance that includes changes in gait patterns of young and older adults that share many similar characteristics to changes in standing balance control (for review, see Ellmers et al. [14], and Staab et al. [19]).

Implications

Growing evidence of emotion-balance interactions in young and older adults has been critical in improving our understanding of the potential physiological, psychological, and social-cognitive factors that contribute to human postural control. Although not the primary focus of the chapter, there have been a number of proposed mechanisms contributing to emotionally-induced changes in balance behaviour in young and older adults [25]. These mechanisms include neural changes in sensorimotor control [29, 31, 85–92] that are likely influenced by strong neuroanatomical links between emotional processing areas of the brain and those responsible for volitional and reflexive balance control [19, 93, 94]. Potential cognitive-attentional mechanisms suspected of contributing to emotional-related changes in balance include selective processing of fall-related stimuli [95], increased perception of balance-relevant sensory signals [96, 97], and altered cognitive load and focus of attention [14, 62, 72, 98, 99]. These changes become problematic, and likely increase fall risk, when low perceived control of falling leads to an excessive fear response. In this case, protective strategies become too restrictive or inappropriate for a given context, or the reactive and compensatory changes interfere with other ongoing movements or actions resulting in a fall [14]. These mechanisms may also exaggerate existing age-related balance deficits and sensory deficits which can further impair mobility [19].

It is also becoming increasingly evident that accounting for an individual's anxiety and fear are critical factors for postural assessment [19]. Recently published "World guidelines for falls prevention and management for older adults" [1] strongly recommended that a standardized assessment of concern about falling, using the FES-I, should be incorporated into all future multifactorial falls risk assessment of older adults. While this is an important step, it does not account for the fact that trait measures of anxiety (such as the FES-I) are not designed to measure state-level emotional responses that vary with context and time, and likely have direct influences on postural performance in the clinic and lab, which may, or may not, interact with individual traits [19, 72]. Therefore, careful assessment of an individual's emotional state at the time of testing and specific to the testing environment is also crucial.

Thus, emotional state needs to be considered when interpreting postural control differences between groups of individuals that may have underlying levels of fear and anxiety at the time of testing, and could be confounded by factors such as the white-coat effect [38]. Likewise, measures of anxiety and fear are critical to accurately interpret changes in balance within a subject over repeated tests, both within a session, and across sessions, as confidence may increase, and fear and anxiety decrease accordingly [55, 56, 78, 100]. Otherwise, changes in balance observed over time, such as during treatment or intervention, cannot be attributed solely to the treatment due to potential confounds of fear and anxiety. To address this concern, study designs need to incorporate practice/adaptation trials, especially in the initial phase of the protocols, in order to ensure any anxiety effects linked to initial exposure to the testing environment, can be accounted for, and kept independent from, any effects linked to the specific treatment or intervention [100]. At present, there is no standardized assessment for state anxiety/fear that has been validated in older adults, although a modified state anxiety questionnaire has been shown to have good test-retest reliability in young adults [49]. Finally, it is important to consider how the use of medication and assistive devices may have effects on balance through secondary effects on an individual's fear, anxiety, and confidence.

Mounting evidence of fear and anxiety effects on balance control in older adults also highlights the need to reconsider how balance interventions are designed to address both emotional and physiological contributors to balance deficits in older adults. Early evidence in young adults suggests that repeated exposure to postural threat within the same session is highly effective in reducing state anxiety, fear and arousal and increasing balance confidence, with corresponding changes in some postural characteristics such as high-frequency sway and co-contraction that may be considered maladaptive. However, the carry-over adaptation to subsequent exposures is not complete [55], and the longer-term effectiveness has yet to be determined. Attempts to use distraction tasks to draw attention away from the perceived threat or restrict conscious motor processing have been effective in patient groups [101]. However, under postural threat conditions it has been shown to have minimal impact, with additional secondary tasks showing no effect, or a slight increase in threat-related postural changes in healthy young and older adults [34, 62]. This observation has been interpreted to suggest that some attentional focus is required to govern maladaptive changes due to fear, which, when interrupted by a secondary distraction task, leads to the emergence of the full anxiety and fear effects [62]. This has been supported by evidence of increases in sample entropy (more irregular sway) thought to reflect more automatic balance control when threatened [62, 102] with greater increases observed when distracted in this threatening condition [62].

Social support may offer some benefit to mitigating anxiety and fear in a clinical and experimental setting and could have modest effects on reducing anxiety-related postural changes [39]. However, further work is needed in this area to understand the extent to which this has a significant benefit to balance control. Likewise, evidence suggests that exercise interventions can decrease anxiety and fear, with exercise interventions that include a cognitive/emotional component being more effective in reducing fall risk than those that do not include such elements (for review, see Montero-Odasso et al. [1]).

As an alternative to trying to reduce/eliminate an individual's natural anxiety and fear towards the postural threat, interventions could focus on strengthening an individual's perceived control of falling, defined as "one's perceived ability to control situations that threaten or challenge balance, with respect to both the behavioural (i.e., perceived ability to control their balance and prevent a fall) and emotional response (i.e., perceived ability to harness the emotional response in helpful ways)" [14]. In this way, normal responses to the perceived threat are maintained within an optimal/beneficial range, in order to preserve protective strategies that are appropriate for the specific context, while limiting maladaptive strategies from becoming detrimental/intrusive. This view underscores the idea that fear and anxiety are important, and appropriate, emotions under certain contexts, and only when perceived control is lacking does the fear-response spiral into states that may have negative consequences to balance, where strategies become prohibitive or counter to intended movements and activities.

References

1. Montero-Odasso M, van der Velde N, Martin FC, Petrovic M, Tan MP, Ryg J, et al. World guidelines for falls prevention and management for older adults: a global initiative. Age Ageing. 2022;51(9):afac205. https://doi.org/10.1093/ageing/afac205.
2. Stinchcombe A, Kuran N, Powell S. Report summary. Seniors' falls in Canada: second Report: key highlights. Chronic Dis Inj Can. 2014;34(2–3):171.
3. Legters K. Fear of falling. Phys Ther. 2002;82:264–72. https://doi.org/10.1093/ptj/82.3.264.
4. MacKay S, Ebert P, Harbidge C, Hogan DB. Fear of falling in older adults: a scoping review of recent literature. Can Geriatr J. 2021;24(4):379. https://doi.org/10.5770/cgj.24.521.
5. Scheffer AC, Schuurmans MJ, Van Dijk N, Van Der Hooft T, De Rooij SE. Fear of falling: measurement strategy, prevalence, risk factors and consequences among older persons. Age Ageing. 2008;37:19–24. https://doi.org/10.1093/ageing/afm169.
6. Bloem BR, Grimbergen YA, Cramer M, Willemsen M, Zwinderman AH. Prospective assessment of falls in Parkinson's disease. J Neurol. 2001;248:950–8. https://doi.org/10.1007/s004150170047.
7. Adkin AL, Frank JS, Jog MS. Fear of falling and postural control in Parkinson's disease. Mov Disord. 2003;18:496–502. https://doi.org/10.1002/mds.10396.
8. Watanabe Y. Fear of falling among stroke survivors after discharge from inpatient rehabilitation. Int J Rehabil Res. 2005;28:149–52. https://doi.org/10.1097/00004356-200506000-00008.
9. Schmid AA, Van Puymbroeck M, Knies K, Spangler-Morris C, Watts K, Damush T, et al. Fear of falling among people who have sustained a stroke: A 6-month longitudinal pilot study. Am J Occup Ther. 2011;65:125–32. https://doi.org/10.5014/ajot.2011.000737.
10. Hadjistavropoulos T, Delbaere K, Fitzgerald TD. Reconceptualizing the role of fear of falling and balance confidence in fall risk. J Aging Health. 2011;23(1):3–23. https://doi.org/10.1177/0898264310378039.
11. Cumming RG, Salkeld G, Thomas M, Szonyi G. Prospective study of the impact of fear of falling on activities of daily living, SF-36 scores, and nursing home admission. J Gerontol A Biol Sci Med Sci. 2000;55:M299–305. https://doi.org/10.1093/gerona/55.5.M299.
12. Friedman SM, Munoz B, West SK, Rubin GS, Fried LP. Falls and fear of falling: which comes first? A longitudinal prediction model suggests strategies for primary and secondary prevention. J Am Geriatr Soc. 2002;50:1329–35. https://doi.org/10.1046/j.1532-5415.2002.50352.x.
13. Li F, Fisher KJ, Harmer P, McAuley E, Wilson NL. Fear of falling in elderly persons: association with falls, functional ability, and quality of life. J Gerontol B Psychol Sci Soc Sci. 2003;58(5):P283–90. https://doi.org/10.1093/geronb/58.5.P283.
14. Ellmers TJ, Wilson MR, Kal EC, Young WR. The perceived control model of falling: developing a unified framework to understand and assess maladaptive fear of falling. Age Ageing. 2023;52(7):afad093. https://doi.org/10.1093/ageing/afad093.
15. Tinetti ME, Richman D, Powell L. Falls efficacy as a measure of fear of falling. J Gerontol. 1990;45(6):P239–43. https://doi.org/10.1093/geronj/45.6.P239.
16. Bandura AV. Self-efficacy: the exercise of control. New York, NY: Freeman; 1981.
17. McAuley E, Mihalko SL, Rosengren K. Self-efficacy and balance correlates of fear of falling in the elderly. J Aging Phys Act. 1997;5:329–40.
18. Li F, McAuley E, Fisher KJ, et al. Self-efficacy as a mediator between fear of falling and functional ability in the elderly. J Aging Health. 2002;14:452–66. https://doi.org/10.1177/089826402237178.

19. Staab JP, Balaban CD, Furman JM. Threat assessment and locomotion: clinical applications of an integrated model of anxiety and postural control. Semin Neurol. 2013;33:297–306. https://doi.org/10.1055/s-0033-1356462.
20. Sibley KM, Mochizuki G, Lakhani B, McIlroy WE. Autonomic contributions in postural control: a review of the evidence. Rev Neurosci. 2014;25(5):687–97. https://doi.org/10.1515/revneuro-2014-0011.
21. Powell LE, Myers AM. The activities-specific balance confidence (ABC) scale. J Gerontol A Biol Sci Med Sci. 1995;50(1):M28–34. https://doi.org/10.1093/gerona/50a.1.m28.
22. Carpenter MG, Adkin AL, Brawley LR, Frank JS. Postural, physiological and psychological reactions to challenging balance: does age make a difference? Age Ageing. 2006;35:298–303. https://doi.org/10.1093/ageing/afl002.
23. Spielberger CD, Gorsuch RL, Lushene R, Vagg PR, Jacobs GA. Manual for the state-trait anxiety inventory. Palo Alto, CA: Consulting Psychologists Press; 1983.
24. Smith RE, Smoll FL, Schutz RW. Measurement and correlates of sport-specific cognitive and somatic trait anxiety: The sport anxiety scale. Anxiety Res. 1990;2:263–80.
25. Adkin AL, Carpenter MG. New insights on emotional contributions to human postural control. Front Neurol. 2018;9:789. https://doi.org/10.3389/fneur.2018.00789.
26. Wuehr M, Breitkopf K, Decker J, Ibarra G, Huppert D, Brandt T. Fear of heights in virtual reality saturates 20 to 40 m above ground. J Neurol. 2019;266(Suppl 1):80–7. https://doi.org/10.1007/s00415-019-09370-5.
27. Bzdúšková D, Marko M, Hirjaková Z, Kimijanová J, Hlavačka F, Riečanský I. The effects of virtual height exposure on postural control and psychophysiological stress are moderated by individual height intolerance. Front Hum Neurosci. 2022;15:773091. https://doi.org/10.3389/fnhum.2021.773091.
28. Laufer Y, Barak Y, Chemel I. Age-related differences in the effect of a perceived threat to stability on postural control. J Gerontol A Biol Sci Med Sci. 2006;61:500–4. https://doi.org/10.1093/gerona/61.5.500.
29. Horslen BC, Murnaghan CD, Inglis JT, Chua R, Carpenter MG. Effects of postural threat on spinal stretch reflexes: evidence for increased muscle spindle sensitivity? J Neurophysiol. 2013;110:899–906. https://doi.org/10.1152/jn.00065.2013.
30. Phanthanourak AL, Cleworth TW, Adkin AL, Carpenter MG, Tokuno CD. The threat of a support surface translation affects anticipatory postural control. Gait Posture. 2016;50:145–50. https://doi.org/10.1016/j.gaitpost.2016.08.031.
31. Lim SB, Cleworth TW, Horslen BC, Blouin JS, Inglis JT, Carpenter MG. Postural threat influences vestibular-evoked muscular responses. J Neurophysiol. 2017;117(2):604–11. https://doi.org/10.1152/jn.00712.2016.
32. Johnson KJ, Zaback M, Tokuno CD, Carpenter MG, Adkin AL. Exploring the relationship between threat-related changes in anxiety, attention focus, and postural control. Psychol Res. 2019a;83(3):445–58. https://doi.org/10.1007/s00426-017-0940-0.
33. Johnson KJ, Zaback M, Tokuno CD, Carpenter MG, Adkin AL. Repeated exposure to the threat of perturbation induces emotional, cognitive, and postural adaptations in young and older adults. Exp Gerontol. 2019b;122:109–15. https://doi.org/10.1016/j.exger.2019.04.015.
34. Johnson KJ, Watson AM, Tokuno CD, Carpenter MG, Adkin AL. The effects of distraction on threat-related changes in standing balance control. Neurosci Lett. 2020;716:134635. https://doi.org/10.1016/j.neulet.2019.134635.
35. Bax AM, Johnson KJ, Watson AM, Adkin AL, Carpenter MG, Tokuno CD. The effects of perturbation type and direction on threat-related changes in anticipatory postural control. Human Mov Sci. 2020;73:102674. https://doi.org/10.1016/j.humov.2020.102674.
36. Shaw JA, Stefanyk LE, Frank JS, Jog MS, Adkin AL. Effects of age and pathology on stance modifications in response to increased postural threat. Gait Posture. 2012;35:658–61. https://doi.org/10.1016/j.gaitpost.2011.12.020.

37. Brown LA, Frank JS. Postural compensations to the potential consequences of instability: kinematics. Gait Posture. 1997;6:89–97. https://doi.org/10.1016/S0966-6362(96)01106-X.
38. Geh CL, Beauchamp MR, Crocker PR, Carpenter MG. Assessed and distressed: white-coat effects on clinical balance performance. J Psychosom Res. 2011;70:45–51. https://doi.org/10.1016/j.jpsychores.2010.09.008.
39. Orcioli-Silva D, Pasman EP, Gobbi LT, Beauchamp MR, Carpenter MG. Effects of social anxiety on static and dynamic balance task assessment in older women. Gait Posture. 2021;86:174–9. https://doi.org/10.1016/j.gaitpost.2021.03.018.
40. Lelard T, Stins J. Mouras H Postural responses to emotional visual stimuli. Neurophysiol Clin. 2019;49(2):109–14. https://doi.org/10.1016/j.neucli.2019.01.005.
41. Ishida M, Saitoh J, Wada M, Nagai M. Effects of anticipatory anxiety and visual input on postural sway in an aversive situation. Neurosci Lett. 2010;474(1):1–4. https://doi.org/10.1016/j.neulet.2010.02.052.
42. Chen X, Qu X. Influence of affective auditory stimuli on balance control during static stance. Ergonomics. 2017;60(3):404–9. https://doi.org/10.1080/00140139.2016.1182649.
43. Maki BE, McIlroy WE. Influence of arousal and attention on the control of postural sway. J Vestib Res. 1996;6:53–9.
44. Doumas M, Morsanyi K, Young WR. Cognitively and socially induced stress affects postural control. Exp Brain Res. 2018;236:305–14. https://doi.org/10.1007/s00221-017-5128-8.
45. Akinlosotu RY, Alissa N, Waldstein SR, Creath RA, Wittenberg GF, Westlake KP. Examining the influence of mental stress on balance perturbation responses in older adults. Exp Gerontol. 2021;153:111495. https://doi.org/10.1016/j.exger.2021.111495.
46. Binda SM, Culham EG, Brouwer B. Balance, muscle strength, and fear of falling in older adults. Exp Aging Res. 2003;29(2):205–19. https://doi.org/10.1080/03610730303711.
47. Maki BE, Holliday PJ, Topper AK. Fear of falling and postural performance in the elderly. J Gerontol. 1991;46:M123–31. https://doi.org/10.1093/geronj/46.4.M123.
48. Lamarche L, Zaback M, Gammage KL, Klentrou P, Adkin AL. A method to investigate discrepancies between perceived and actual balance in older women. Gait Posture. 2013;38(4):888–93. https://doi.org/10.1016/j.gaitpost.2013.04.007.
49. Hauck LJ, Carpenter MG, Frank JS. Task-specific measures of balance efficacy, anxiety, and stability and their relationship to clinical balance performance. Gait Posture. 2008;27:676–82. https://doi.org/10.1016/j.gaitpost.2007.09.002.
50. Hauck LJ. Understanding the influence of fear of falling on clinical balance control -efforts in fall prediction and prevention. Waterloo, ON: University of Waterloo; 2011.
51. Winter DA. Human balance and posture control during standing and walking. Gait Posture. 1995;3:193–214. https://doi.org/10.1016/0966-6362(96)82849-9.
52. Maki BE, Holliday PJ, Topper AK. A prospective study of postural balance and risk of falling in an ambulatory and independent elderly population. J Gerontol. 1994;49(2):M72–84. https://doi.org/10.1093/geronj/49.2.m72.
53. Myers AM, Powell LE, Maki BE, Holliday PJ, Brawley LR, Sherk W. Psychological indicators of balance confidence: relationship to actual and perceived abilities. J Gerontol A Biol Sci Med Sci. 1996;51(1):M37–43. https://doi.org/10.1093/gerona/51a.1.m37.
54. Hughes MA, Duncan PW, Rose DK, Chandler JM, Studenski SA. The relationship of postural sway to sensorimotor function, functional performance, and disability in the elderly. Arch Phys Med Rehabil. 1996;77(6):567–72. https://doi.org/10.1016/s0003-9993(96)90296-8.
55. Zaback M, Adkin AL, Carpenter MG. Adaptation of emotional state and standing balance parameters following repeated exposure to height-induced postural threat. Sci Rep. 2019;9(1):12449. https://doi.org/10.1038/s41598-019-48722-z.
56. Zaback M, Luu MJ, Adkin AL, Carpenter MG. Selective preservation of changes to standing balance control despite psychological and autonomic habituation to a postural threat. Sci Rep. 2021a;11(1):384. https://doi.org/10.1038/s41598-020-79417-5.
57. Winter DA, Patla AE, Prince F, Ishac M, Gielo-Perczak K. Stiffness control of balance in quiet standing. J Neurophysiol. 1998;80:1211–21. https://doi.org/10.1152/jn.1998.80.3.1211.

58. Carpenter MG, Frank JS, Silcher CP, Peysar GW. The influence of postural threat on the control of upright stance. Exp Brain Res. 2001;138:210–8. https://doi.org/10.1007/s002210100681.
59. Horslen BC, Carpenter MG. Arousal, valence and their relative effects on postural control. Exp Brain Res. 2011;215:27. https://doi.org/10.1007/s00221-011-2867-9.
60. Brown LA, Polych MA, Doan JB. The effect of anxiety on the regulation of upright standing among younger and older adults. Gait Posture. 2006;24:397–405. https://doi.org/10.1016/j.gaitpost.2005.04.013.
61. Pasman EP, Murnaghan CD, Bloem BR, Carpenter MG. Balance problems with Parkinson's disease: are they anxiety-dependent? Neuroscience. 2011;177:283–91. https://doi.org/10.1016/j.neuroscience.2010.12.050.
62. Ellmers TJ, Kal EC, Young WR. Consciously processing balance leads to distorted perceptions of instability in older adults. J Neurol. 2021;268(4):1374–84. https://doi.org/10.1007/s00415-020-10288-6.
63. Sturnieks DL, Delbaere K, Brodie MA, Lord SR. The influence of age, anxiety and concern about falling on postural sway when standing at an elevated level. Hum Mov Sci. 2016;49:206–15. https://doi.org/10.1016/j.humov.2016.06.014.
64. Adkin AL, Frank JS, Carpenter MG, Peysar GW. Postural control is scaled to level of postural threat. Gait Posture. 2000;12:87–93. https://doi.org/10.1016/S0966-6362(00)00057-6.
65. Davis JR, Campbell AD, Adkin AL, Carpenter MG. The relationship between fear of falling and human postural control. Gait Posture. 2009;29:275–9. https://doi.org/10.1016/j.gaitpost.2008.09.006.
66. Falk J, Strandkvist V, Vikman I, Pauelsen M, Röijezon U. What explains successful or unsuccessful postural adaptations to repeated surface perturbations among older adults? Int J Environ Res Public Health. 2021;18(22):12069. https://doi.org/10.3390/ijerph182212069.
67. Yiou E, Caderby T, Hussein T. Adaptability of anticipatory postural adjustments associated with voluntary movement. World J Orthop. 2012;3(6):75. https://doi.org/10.5312/wjo.v3.i6.75.
68. Maki BE, McIlroy WE. Control of rapid limb movements for balance recovery: age-related changes and implications for fall prevention. Age Ageing. 2006;35(suppl_2):ii12–8. https://doi.org/10.1093/ageing/afl078.
69. Duarte MB, da Silva Almeida GC, Costa KHA, Garcez DR, de Athayde Costa e Silva A, da Silva Souza G, et al. Anticipatory postural adjustments in older versus young adults: a systematic review and meta-analysis. Syst Rev. 2022;11(1):1–14. https://doi.org/10.1186/s13643-022-02116-x.
70. Uemura K, Yamada M, Nagai K, Tanaka B, Mori S, Ichihashi N. Fear of falling is associated with prolonged anticipatory postural adjustment during gait initiation under dual-task conditions in older adults. Gait Posture. 2012;35(2):282–6. https://doi.org/10.1016/j.gaitpost.2011.09.100.
71. Adkin AL, Frank JS, Carpenter MG, Peysar GW. Fear of falling modifies anticipatory postural control. Exp Brain Res. 2002;143:160–70. https://doi.org/10.1007/s00221-001-0974-8.
72. Zaback M, Cleworth TW, Carpenter MG, Adkin AL. Personality traits and individual differences predict threat-induced changes in postural control. Hum Mov Sci. 2015;40:393–409. https://doi.org/10.1016/j.humov.2015.01.015.
73. Yiou E, Deroche T, Do MC, Woodman T. Influence of fear of falling on anticipatory postural control of medio-lateral stability during rapid leg flexion. Eur J Appl Physiol. 2011;111:611–20. https://doi.org/10.1007/s00421-010-1680-7.
74. Gendre M, Yiou E, Gélat T, Honeine J, Deroche T. Directional specificity of postural threat on anticipatory postural adjustments during lateral leg raising. Exp Brain Res. 2016;234:659–71. https://doi.org/10.1007/s00221-015-4471-x.
75. Coppens MJ, Carpenter MG, Inglis JT, Weerdesteyn V. Does height-induced threat modulate shortening of reaction times induced by a loud stimulus in a lateral stepping and a wrist extension task? Hum Mov Sci. 2021;80:102857. https://doi.org/10.1016/j.humov.2021.102857.

76. Ellmers TJ, Maslivec A, Young WR. Fear of falling alters anticipatory postural control during cued gait initiation. Neuroscience. 2020;438:41–9. https://doi.org/10.1016/j.neuroscience.2020.04.050.
77. Phanthanourak AL, Adkin AL, Carpenter MG, Tokuno CD. Effects of postural threat on the scaling of anticipatory postural adjustments in young and older adults. Front Hum Neurosci. 2023;17:1267093. https://doi.org/10.3389/fnhum.2023.1267093.
78. Maki BE, Whitelaw RS. Influence of expectation and arousal on center-of-pressure responses to transient postural perturbations. J Vestib Res. 1993;3(1):25–39.
79. Carpenter MG, Frank JS, Adkin AL, Paton A, Allum JHJ. Influence of postural anxiety on postural reactions to multi-directional surface rotations. J Neurophysiol. 2004;92:3255–65. https://doi.org/10.1152/jn.00724.2004.
80. Cleworth TW, Chua R, Inglis JT, Carpenter MG. Influence of virtual height exposure on postural reactions to support surface translations. Gait Posture. 2016;47:96–102. https://doi.org/10.1016/j.gaitpost.2016.04.006.
81. Baloh RW, Fife TD, Zwerling L, Socotch T, Jacobson K, Bell T, Beykirch K. Comparison of static and dynamic posturography in young and older normal people. J Am Geriatr Soc. 1994;42(4):405–12. https://doi.org/10.1111/j.1532-5415.1994.tb07489.x.
82. Okada S, Hirakawa K, Takada Y, Kinoshita H. Relationship between fear of falling and balancing ability during abrupt deceleration in aged women having similar habitual physical activities. Eur J Appl Physiol. 2001;85:501–6. https://doi.org/10.1007/s004210100437.
83. Redfern MS, Furman JM, Jacob RG. Visually induced postural sway in anxiety disorders. J Anxiety Disord. 2007;21:704–16. https://doi.org/10.1016/j.janxdis.2006.09.002.
84. Amiaz R, Kimel Naor S, Caspi A, Czerniak E, Noy S, Pelc T, et al. Responses to balance challenges in persons with panic disorder: A pilot study of computerized static and dynamic balance measurements. Brain Behav. 2022;12(1):e2411. https://doi.org/10.1002/brb3.2411.
85. Davis JR, Horslen BC, Nishikawa K, Fukushima K, Chua R, Inglis JT, et al. Human proprioceptive adaptations during states of height-induced fear and anxiety. J Neurophysiol. 2011;106(6):3082–90. https://doi.org/10.1152/jn.01030.2010.
86. Horslen BC, Dakin CJ, Inglis JT, Blouin JS, Carpenter MG. CrossTalk proposal: fear of falling does influence vestibular-evoked balance responses. J Physiol. 2015;593(14):2979–81. https://doi.org/10.1113/JP270269.
87. Horslen BC, Inglis JT, Blouin JS, Carpenter MG. Both standing and postural threat decrease Achilles' tendon reflex inhibition from tendon electrical stimulation. J Physiol. 2017;595(13):4493–506. https://doi.org/10.1113/JP273935.
88. Horslen BC, Zaback M, Inglis JT, Blouin JS, Carpenter MG. Increased human stretch reflex dynamic sensitivity with height-induced postural threat: increased stretch reflex dynamic sensitivity with postural threat. J Physiol. 2018;596(21):5251–65. https://doi.org/10.1113/JP276459.
89. Adkin AL, Campbell AD, Chua R, Carpenter MG. The influence of postural threat on the cortical response to unpredictable and predictable postural perturbations. Neurosci Lett. 2008;435(2):120–5. https://doi.org/10.1016/j.neulet.2008.02.018.
90. Sibley KM, Mochizuki G, Frank JS, McIlroy WE. The relationship between physiological arousal and cortical and autonomic responses to postural instability. Exp Brain Res. 2010;203(3):533–40. https://doi.org/10.1007/s00221-010-2257-8.
91. Zaback M, Adkin AL, Chua R, Inglis JT, Carpenter MG. Facilitation and habituation of cortical and subcortical control of standing balance following repeated exposure to a height-related postural threat. Neuroscience. 2022;487:8–25. https://doi.org/10.1016/j.neuroscience.2022.01.012.
92. Zaback M, Missen KJ, Adkin AL, Chua R, Inglis JT, Carpenter MG. Cortical potentials time-locked to discrete postural events during quiet standing are facilitated during postural threat exposure. J Physiol. 2023;601(12):2473–92. https://doi.org/10.1113/JP284055.
93. Balaban CD, Thayer JF. Neurological bases for balance-anxiety links. J Anxiety Disord. 2001;15:53–79. https://doi.org/10.1016/S0887-6185(00)00042-6.

94. Balaban CD. Neural substrates linking balance control and anxiety. Physiol Behav. 2002;77:469–75. https://doi.org/10.1016/S0031-9384(02)00935-6.
95. Brown LA, White P, Doan JB, de Bruin N. Selective attentional processing to fall-relevant stimuli among older adults who fear falling. Exp Aging Res. 2011;37(3):330–45. https://doi.org/10.1080/0361073X.2011.568833.
96. Cleworth TW, Adkin AL, Allum JHJ, Inglis JT, Chua R, Carpenter MG. Postural threat modulates perceptions of balance-related movement during support surface rotations. Neuroscience. 2019;404:413–22. https://doi.org/10.1016/j.neuroscience.2019.02.011.
97. Cleworth TW, Carpenter MG. Postural threat influences conscious perception of postural sway. Neurosci Lett. 2016;620:127–31. https://doi.org/10.1016/j.neulet.2016.03.032.
98. Huffman JL, Horslen BC, Carpenter MG, Adkin AL. Does increased postural threat lead to more conscious control of posture? Gait Posture. 2009;30(4):528–32. https://doi.org/10.1016/j.gaitpost.2009.08.001.
99. Zaback M, Carpenter MG, Adkin AL. Threat-induced changes in attention during tests of static and anticipatory postural control. Gait Posture. 2016;45:19–24. https://doi.org/10.1016/j.gaitpost.2015.12.033.
100. Zaback M, Reiter ER, Adkin AL, Carpenter MG. Initial experience of balance assessment introduces 'first trial'effects on emotional state and postural control. Gait Posture. 2021b;88:116–21. https://doi.org/10.1016/j.gaitpost.2021.05.013.
101. Wuehr M, Brandt T, Schniepp R. Distracting attention in phobic postural vertigo normalizes leg muscle activity and balance. Neurology. 2017;88(3):284–8. https://doi.org/10.1212/WNL.0000000000003516.
102. Fischer OM, Missen KJ, Tokuno CD, Carpenter MG, Adkin AL. Postural threat increases sample entropy of postural control. Front Neurol. 2023;14:1179237. https://doi.org/10.3389/fneur.2023.1179237.

18 Postural Control and Physical Function in Older Adults with Chronic Musculoskeletal Pain: Effects of the Physical Exercises and the Implications for Activities of Daily Living

Karina Gramani-Say, Daniela Godoi-Jacomassi, and Paula Fávaro Polastri

Abstract

Chronic pain is defined as an unpleasant sensory and emotional experience associated with or similar to actual or potential tissue damage. Chronic pain is a public health problem for individuals, families, and the healthcare system, affecting more than 30% of people worldwide. Chronic pain occupies the sixth position in individuals aged 50–74 years for years lived with a disability related to low back pain which demonstrates its negative functional impact in old age. It is believed that the speed in processing cognitive information, gait and postural control may be altered with the persistence of pain, but the association between chronic pain and cognitive function is still inconclusive. The objective of this chapter is to present evidence related to motor behavior and postural control in individuals with chronic pain. Some studies have shown that individuals with chronic pain have learning difficulties when compared to individuals without pain. Also, they present deficits in memory, attention, ability to plan actions,

K. Gramani-Say (✉)
LADORFE—Laboratory for the Study of Pain and Functionality in Aging, Department of Gerontology, Federal University of Sao Carlos—UFSCar, São Carlos, Brazil
e-mail: gramanisay@ufscar.br

D. Godoi-Jacomassi
Dinâmica—Motor Behavior Laboratory, Department of Physical Education, Federal University of Sao Carlos—UFSCar, São Carlos, Brazil
e-mail: danielagodoij@ufscar.br

P. F. Polastri
Laboratory of Information, Vision, and Action, Department of Physical Education, São Paulo State University – UNESP, Bauru, Brazil
e-mail: paula.polastri@unesp.br

F. A. Barbieri et al. (eds.), *Locomotion and Posture in Older Adults*,
https://doi.org/10.1007/978-3-031-74123-4_18

perception of faces, visuospatial orientation and emotional responses. The physical exercises contribute in reducing pain effects and associated symptoms such as: physical function, mood, sleep quality and quality of life.

Introduction

The International Association Study of Pain (IASP) defines chronic pain as an unpleasant sensory and emotional experience associated with or similar to actual or potential tissue damage [1]. Chronic pain can be influenced by social factors (e.g., social expectations, job satisfaction, past pain experiences, social support system, social and cultural barriers, among others), biological (e.g., genetic, age, sleep, lesion, sex, nervous system conditions) and psychological factors (e.g., depression, anxiety, cognitive beliefs, personality, fears, emotional stress, among others) [2]. Chronic pain can cause impairments in carrying out activities of daily living, reducing independence, mood swings, cognitive changes, changes in sleep quality, functional changes, social isolation, poorer mobility, and higher the risk of falls as well as damage to personal and occupational relationships.

Chronic pain is a public health problem for individuals, families, and the healthcare system, affecting more than 30% of people worldwide [3, 4], about 40% in the USA, 43.5% in England, and about 45.6% in Brazil. Moreover, this prevalence reaches up to 80% of institutionalized people when considering 20–40% of the older population who have chronic pain and frail older individuals [5].

The importance of healthy aging involves the maintenance of intrinsic capacity (physical and mental) and functional capacity (ability to carry out activities within the standard considered normal for the specific task). Thus, the variable of years lived with a disability becomes a marker to consider the impairment of a condition to the individual. Chronic pain occupies the sixth position in individuals aged 50–74 years for years lived with a disability related to low back pain which demonstrates its negative functional impact in old age [6]. However, despite the high prevalence, it is a mistake to consider that every person will have pain as they age. Studies show that staying physically and mentally active is a protective factor for pain chronification. Physical or psychosocial factors reduce the risk of developing chronic pain and are a crucial tool for chronic pain self-management. Continuous participation in vigorous weekly activity was protective against the development of chronic pain (odds ratio 0.74, standard error 0.07) when controlling for all identified socioeconomic, health, and social confounders. However, moderate weekly activity has no effect [7]. This finding shows the need to participate in physical activity programs with adequate professional monitoring so that the frequency of physical activity capable of generating protection for individuals is achieved. Regarding psychosocial factors, cultural engagement was also protective against the development of chronic pain (odds ratio 0.75, standard error 0.07). Many studies show that psychosocial and cultural factors improve pain severity and physical function besides the quality of life [7].

Based on the need to discuss and deeply understand this issue, the aim of this chapter is to demonstrate the effects of chronic musculoskeletal pain in postural control and physical function as well the implications for activities of daily living. In addition, we will discuss the effects of physical exercises to minimize the consequences of chronic pain in the individual life. First, aspects related to functional and cognitive changes will be discussed, after which, an overall view of the effects of exercise as an option to reduce pain and associated symptoms will be addressed.

Functional Changes and Pain

Chronic pain is severely disabling. Mechanisms underlying how chronic pain generates damage to individuals remain unknown as well as whether all types of chronic pain would cause these alterations or just in specific cases. In addition, chronic painful conditions can also cause changes in the perception of pain, and in functional and psychological disabilities, in addition to altering sensorimotor control, postural control, and gait.

Chronic pain can cause functional impairments in gait. Studies show differences in space-time variables between individuals with chronic low back pain and those without pain, and for those with chronic pain. Stride and step length, cadence, and step speed are reduced in individuals with chronic low back pain when they are compared to pain-free individuals [8]. In older people, however, all gait variables compared to individuals without pain showed worse performance, including shorter step width at the fast and self-speed selected, slower gait, in addition to the worst time of going up and down a step [9].

In a recent study, Pourahmadi and colleagues [10] organized a systematic review with meta-analysis in adults with chronic low back pain and dual-task activities associated with postural control. Only five studies matched the criteria, three of them of high methodological quality, with a control group, and three studies with moderate quality, without a control group. The results showed no difference in the performance of dual-task activities in adults with nonspecific chronic low back pain. However, these studies did not consider the older population with chronic pain. Therefore, the impact of the dual cognitive task on postural control in individuals with chronic pain remains controversial. Since 2008, Lacour and colleagues [11] have already proposed a model in which the burden of difficulty of the cognitive dual-task forces to impact postural control, with low degrees of cognitive difficulty allowing better attention to an efficient posture maintenance performance.

Regarding postural control, it is known that older people have a preference for using the strategy of compensatory postural adjustments to maintain postural balance when compared to young individuals [12]. However, there is little evidence that chronic pain is able to further influence these changes that occur in aging, which would further impact the safety and well-being of the elderly. This is because many studies on postural control strategies in pain conditions exclude the older population. Garcez and colleagues [13] demonstrated that older individuals with nonspecific chronic low back pain had impairments in anticipatory postural adjustments and had a less efficient feedforward mechanism for hip and ankle joints compared to individuals without low back pain. In this study, the authors found that the *rectus femoralis*, semitendinosus muscles, and the soleus muscle of the group with low back pain had an onset delay when compared to the control group. For the CoP variables, there was no difference between groups. In addition, Le Ge and colleagues [14] study showed that a load of cognitive activity is able to modulate the performance of older women with chronic low back pain, impairing the maintenance of their postural balance, and this finding is associated with a greater risk of falls in these women. Thus, it would be interesting to associate gradual cognitive loads with chronic low back pain rehabilitation in older women. In another study, the disturbance on a horizontal platform forward and sagittally was investigated in individuals with pain and without pain and with degeneration of the lumbar vertebral disc. It was found that anticipatory and compensatory postural adjustments differ in the group with pain and also for those with vertebral disc injury. In predictable forward perturbation, the group with vertebral disc injury with pain shows a change in the ankle strategy with a greater electromyographic activity to lateral gastrocnemius and anterior tibialis muscle than the group without pain and with this injury. Both groups with pain and without pain but with vertebral disc injury showed changes in hip strategy in predictable perturbation in both directions. All groups showed no differences in responses to unpredictable perturbation. These findings show that the injury leads to a change in the postural control strategy and the presence of pain should be considered as another factor that impacts anticipatory adjustments, and the assessment of postural control in these individuals and rehabilitation for pain management should be considered [15]. Hemmati and colleagues [16] showed that individuals with chronic nonspecific low back pain had changes with unpredictable perturbations and performing dual-tasks with attentional demands when compared to groups without pain. An increase in the electromyographic activity of the gastrocnemius and a delay in the activation of the tibialis anterior were found for the group with chronic nonspecific low back pain.

In the next section, the cognitive changes associated with chronic musculoskeletal pain as well the implications for activities of daily living are presented.

Cognitive Changes and Pain

Chronic pain can compromise cognitive performance since some cortical and subcortical structures, including the medial prefrontal cortex, thalamus, amygdala, and anterior cingulate cortex, involved in the modulation and perception of pain, are also related to cognitive processing [17]. Some studies suggest that cognitive information may be altered by the processing speed is increased with the persistence of pain [18]. However, it is still unclear which cognitive dimensions may be affected in individuals with chronic pain. The association between chronic pain and cognitive function was inconclusive. Some studies have shown that individuals with chronic pain have learning difficulties when compared with individuals without pain [19]. Also, they may alter memory, attention [19], ability to plan actions, perception of faces, visuospatial orientation, and emotional responses, but the results are controversial. The existence of some studies that show impairment of cognitive function in subjects with chronic pain generates a concern with older individuals with cognitive impairment, which requires long-term studies to verify whether there is a higher and more disabling impact.

In particular, studies show that cognitive demands can modulate postural control in older people with low back pain [14], and it highlights the need to assess the domains of cognition affected by the aging process and influenced by the chronification of pain. It might impact older individuals in their functional aspects, interpersonal relationships, and safety [20]. Chronic pain leads to functional alterations in the brain that can help in the persistence of painful symptoms as well as accentuate episodes of pain recurrence, pain intensity, and functional impacts on the individual's life. These brain changes lead to the presence of cognitive adaptations that are harmful to the individual, such as kinesiophobia, changes in sleep quality, catastrophizing, changes in the perception of pain itself, changes in beliefs and attitudes toward pain, hypervigilance, depression, anxiety [21, 22].

Several studies show the relationship between chronic pain and the impairment of carrying out activities of daily living. However, it was found that according to the pain intensity, we have different limitations in activities daily living. In addition, in the aging process, diffuse and intense pain reduces occupational activity and, because of this, the belief that pain negatively impacts interpersonal relationships was more associated with limitations for activities daily living, i.e., for the negative social effects of pain. It was indicated that the activities of daily living most compromised by chronic pain are sleep, occupational activities, taking public transport, performing physical activities, losing weight, squatting and kneeling, and going up and down stairs, among other activities [23].

Considering all the aforementioned changes observed in older adults with chronic musculoskeletal pain, how to proceed? What can be done? In this sense, physical exercise emerges as an option in the multimodal treatment for chronic pain.

Exercise and Chronic Pain

Exercise has been shown as forefront management for chronic pain (e.g., [24–27]. It is a non-invasive, non-pharmacological, and low-cost option [28, 29], which plays a role in pain reduction and associated symptoms such as physical function, mood, and quality of life [26, 27, 30–32]. It is important to point out that there is considerable variability across studies regarding pain conditions, characteristics of exercise programs, and outcomes [25–27, 30, 31, 33–44]. Table 18.1 displays an overview of the main pain conditions, exercise intervention parameters, type of exercise, and outcomes found in these studies. In summary, the main investigated pain conditions are low back pain [26, 27, 31, 33–41], fibromyalgia [25, 31, 37], and osteoarthritis [30, 31, 37, 40, 42–44]. Regarding the outcomes (primary and secondary), the most investigated ones have been, in addition to pain, physical function/disability (e.g., [31, 34, 39, 42, 44], and quality of life (e.g., [31, 39]).

Table 18.1 An overview of main pain conditions, exercise intervention parameters, type of exercise, and outcomes found in the literature

Chronic pain condition	Exercise intervention parameters (dose)	Type of exercise	Outcomes
Mainly with: • Low back pain • Osteoarthritis • Fibromyalgia	• Duration: Intervention duration: 1 session to 30 months (most often: 8–12 weeks) Session duration: 2–120 min (most often: 45–60 min) • Frequency: 1x/week à 2x/day (most often: 2-3x/week) • Intensity: Not always reported; when reported, is moderate intensity: 70–85% of maximum heart rate/11–13 Borg Scale (for aerobic exercises) 50–80% of 1 repetition maximum (for resistance exercises)	• Resistance exercises • Aerobic exercises • Flexibility exercises • Balance exercises • Mixed exercises ▪ Motor control ▪ Aquatic exercises ▪ Tai Chi ▪ Pilates ▪ Yoga	• Pain • Function • Quality of Life • Disability

Furthermore, there is a wide range of types of exercises (mainly aerobic exercises, resistance exercises, Tai Chi, Yoga, and Pilates) and exercise parameters (wide range of duration and frequency) reported in these studies. Thus, although exercise practice has a distinct place in the multimodal treatment for chronic pain, there is still limited evidence regarding the best type of exercise (if any) or the optimal exercise parameters (protocol/dose). Regarding the type of exercise, although studies have investigated whether some types of exercise are more effective than others (e.g., [33, 36, 38, 39, 42], the results have indicated little or no difference among different types of exercise. Therefore, overall results consistently support the benefits of exercise regardless of the type [34].

Despite the well-established importance of chronic pain, the mechanisms by which exercise improves chronic pain are not well understood [45]. It is known that the positive effects of exercise on chronic pain are multifactorial in nature and, consequently, difficult to define clearly [46]. However, some mechanisms were suggested to explain the effects of exercise practice in reducing pain and associated symptoms [47–50]. The mechanisms most frequently mentioned in the literature are those related to physiological aspects (e.g., [24, 47, 48, 50–55], but there are also underlying mechanisms related to general fitness [47, 56], neuromuscular aspects [47] and psychosocial factors [54].

The physiological mechanisms are based on evidence obtained not only from chronic pain populations but also from healthy adults or animals [50, 54]. Among the several processes included in these physiological mechanisms, it is possible to mention, for example, the release of endorphins and cytokines. Endorphins are neurotransmitters that act as natural painkillers; they bind to opioid receptors in the brain and spinal cord, which helps to reduce the perception of pain and promote a sense of well-being [48, 50, 51, 53, 57]. Cytokines are small proteins that may play a crucial role in cell signaling and communication within the immune system [53]. In general, pro-inflammatory cytokines are at elevated levels in patients with chronic pain (e.g., [55]). Furthermore, sedentary behavior results in the presence of fewer anti-inflammatory and more pro-inflammatory cytokines in both local and systemic circulation, and this disproportion contributes to the maintenance of chronic pain [48, 58]. On the other hand, studies with healthy subjects, animal models, and some with chronic pain patients show that exercise can increase the presence of anti-inflammatory cytokines and reduce the presence of pro-inflammatory cytokines [24, 50, 52, 54, 59, 60]. This cytokines production balance can reduce systemic inflammation and, consequently, may reduce chronic pain.

The mechanism related to general fitness focuses on the awareness that exercise contributes to weight loss, increased aerobic capacity, and increased self-efficacy [42, 51], which would help reduce pain and associated symptoms in the chronic pain population. The proposed mechanism related to neuromuscular aspects is based on the idea that exercise may contribute to the reduction of mechanical loads on the cartilage because of the effect of exercise on neuromuscular components such as muscles, energy absorbing capacity, proprioception, and stability [47]. Thus, physical exercises would contribute to the integrity of neuromuscular and intra-articular components and, as a result, may show a beneficial effect on pain and function. Therefore, studies suggest that these proposed mechanisms (physiological, general fitness, neuromuscular), adding to psychosocial factors [54], and other unknown mechanisms may explain the effects of exercise in reducing both pain and associated symptoms in the chronic pain population.

So, there is much to be learned about optimal exercise interventions (optimal dose and type of exercise). Based on the evidence in the studies, our clinical expertise, and the patient perspective, fueled by the evidence-based practice approach [61], some suggestions can be proposed. Considering that adherence is primordial to achieving the benefits of exercise [62], firstly, it is necessary to consider the patient's preferences. What would they like to do? What do they enjoy? What did they use to do in the past? From these answers, it is possible to have some tips on what to include in the exercise intervention.

Furthermore, taking into account the alterations in motor control associated with chronic pain (e.g., [63–65]) and the aforementioned mechanisms by which exercise improves chronic pain, exercise intervention should include exercises that combine physical abilities (resistance, strength, flexibility, speed) and motor skills (walking, sitting, throwing a ball, climbing steps, receiving a ball, etc.). In this way, it would be possible to take advantage of the physiological and general fitness mechanisms (mainly through the inclusion of exercises focused on physical abilities) and the mechanisms related to neuromuscular components as well as the motor control improvements (mainly through the insertion of exercises which include motor skills and variability of movements).

Moreover, it would be interesting not only to include already known motor skills but also new motor skills. It is well-established that the acquisition of new motor skills (motor learning) results in neuroplasticity [66–69]. So, since chronic pain is associated with cortical neuroplasticity [70–75], exercise programs should include novel motor skills practice in order to reduce the risk of further and unfavorable neuroplastic changes associated with pain [71]. Thus, neuroplasticity due to motor learning (favorable) could help in the process of minimizing or reversing the neuroplasticity due to chronic pain (unfavorable). Additionally, as this neuroplasticity can be optimized when the practice context is challenging [76] and studies have observed that random practice leads to different neural processes as compared to block practice [68, 76–78], exercise interventions should include random practice. Thus, the intervention involving exercises for chronic pain patients should not only include new motor skills but also organize them in a random schedule.

Another interesting suggestion is that exercise intervention should include situations that involve decision-making to increase the demand for motor control. As chronic pain results in motor control changes (e.g., [63–65]), promoting improvements in motor control is essential. Besides, a way to achieve success in decision-making performance is to enhance action-perception coupling by improving the detection and use of perceptual variables that inform which actions are possible or not to be performed [79]; that is, in short, to improve motor control. Therefore, including situations that involve decision-making is a two-way street that not only requires better motor control but also promotes improvements in motor control.

Finally, as kinesiophobia is common in chronic pain patients (e.g., [80, 81], exercise programs should include ludic activities to divert the focus from the movement itself. Thus, carrying out the activities in a playful way is a good strategy to obtain the benefits of exercise despite the fear or avoidance of movement. Taken together, an exercise intervention should include exercises of the patient's preference, which combine physical abilities and new motor skills, organized randomly, with situations that involve decision-making and, all this, in a playful way whenever possible.

Final Considerations

Chronic pain is a prevalent condition in aging and can become extremely disabling, affecting the individual's occupational, family, and functional relationships. Identifying the changes that chronic pain can cause to older individuals in their activities daily living is extremely important for healthy aging and their quality of life. Non-pharmacological strategies such as physical exercises have strong evidence in the literature for the management of chronic pain for older adults. In addition, it is more important than the involvement of patients and the public to promote research that can elucidate which mechanisms related to motor behavior and postural control are affected by chronic pain and have an impact on the functionality and well-being of the elderly. Studies are focused on chronic low back pain and osteoarthritis of the lower limbs, for example, but there are many other types of pain prevalent in the elderly population that deserve to be studied in order to develop better strategies for optimizing their functional capacity. Furthermore, the relationship between chronic pain and the risk of falls in the elderly is still controversial in the literature, indicating that musculoskeletal pain can actually increase the risk of falls, in addition to impairing gait performance and carrying out activities of daily living.

References

1. Raja SN, Carr DB, Cohen M, Finnerup NB, Flor H, Gibson S, et al. The revised International Association for the Study of Pain definition of pain: concepts, challenges, and compromises. Pain. 2020;161(9):1976–82.
2. Cohen SP, Vase L, Hooten WM. Chronic pain: an update on burden, best practices, and new advances. Lancet. 2021;397(10289):2082–97.
3. Hirase T, Kataoka H, Nakano J, Inokuchi S, Sakamoto J, Okita M. Impact of frailty on chronic pain, activities of daily living and physical activity in community-dwelling older adults: a cross-sectional study. Geriatr Gerontol Int. 2018;18(7):1079–84.
4. Viseux FJF, Simoneau M, Billot M. A comprehensive review of pain interference on postural control: from experimental to chronic pain. Medicina. 2022;58(6):812. https://doi.org/10.3390/medicina58060812.
5. Herr KA, Garand L. Assessment and measurement of pain in older adults. Clin Geriatr Med. 2001;17(3):457–78.
6. GBD 2019 Diseases and Injuries Collaborators. Global burden of 369 diseases and injuries in 204 countries and territories, 1990-2019: a systematic analysis for the global burden of disease study 2019. Lancet. 2020;396(10258):1204–22.
7. Fancourt D, Steptoe A. Physical and psychosocial factors in the prevention of chronic pain in older age. J Pain. 2018;19(12):1385–91.
8. Vickers J, Reed A, Decker R, Conrad BP, Olegario-Nebel M, Vincent HK. Effect of investigator observation on gait parameters in individuals with and without chronic low back pain. Gait Posture. 2017;53:35–40.
9. Hicks GE, Sions JM, Coyle PC, Pohlig RT. Altered spatiotemporal characteristics of gait in older adults with chronic low back pain. Gait Posture. 2017;55:172–6.
10. Pourahmadi M, Hegahban H, Koes BW, Fernández-de-Las-Peñas C, Takamjani IE, Bahramian M. The effect of dual-task conditions on postural control in adults with low back pain: a systematic review and meta-analysis. J Orthop Surg Res. 2023;18(1):555. https://doi.org/10.1186/s13018-023-04035-6.
11. Lacour M, Bernard-Demanze L, Dumitrescu M. Posture control, aging, and attention resources: models and posture-analysis methods. Neurophysiol Clin. 2008;38(6):411–21.
12. Polastri PF, Godoi D, Gramani-Say K. Falls and postural stability in older individuals: implications for activities of daily living. In: Barbieri F, Vitório R, editors. Locomotion and posture in older adults. New York, NY: Springer; 2017. p. 263–77.
13. Garcez DR, da Silva Almeida GC, Silva CFO, de Souza NT, de Athayde Costa e Silva A, AFR K, et al. Postural adjustments impairments in elderly people with chronic low back pain. Sci Rep. 2021;11(1):4783. https://doi.org/10.1038/s41598-021-83837-2.
14. Ge L, Yu Q, Wang C, Huang H, Li X, Zhang S, et al. How cognitive loads modulate the postural control of older women with low back pain? BMC Geriatr. 2021;21(1):82. https://doi.org/10.1186/s12877-021-02025-z.
15. Deane JA, Lim AKP, McGregor AH, Strutton PH. Understanding the impact of lumbar disc degeneration and chronic low back pain: a cross-sectional electromyographic analysis of postural strategy during predicted and unpredicted postural perturbations. PLoS One. 2021;16(4):e0249308. https://doi.org/10.1371/journal.pone.0249308.
16. Hemmatia L, Piroozib S, Rojhani-Shirazic S. Effect of dual tasking on anticipatory and compensatory postural adjustments in response to external perturbations in individuals with nonspecific chronic low back pain: Electromyographic analysis. J Back Musculoskelet Rehabil. 2017;31(3):489–97.

17. Moriarty O, McGuire BE, Finn DP. The effect of pain on cognitive function: a review of clinical and preclinical research. Prog Neurobiol. 2011;93(3):385–404.
18. Rusu AC, Gajsar H, Schlüter MC, Bremer YI. Cognitive biases toward pain: implications for a neurocognitive processing perspective in chronic pain and its interaction with depression. Clin J Pain. 2019;35(3):252–60.
19. Oosterman JM, Derksen LC, van Wijck AJ, Veldhuijzen DS, Kessels RP. Memory functions in chronic pain: examining contributions of attention and age to test performance. Clin J Pain. 2011;27(1):70–5.
20. Pereira Nery ECH, Rocha NP, Cruz VT, Silva AG. Systematic review and meta-analysis on the association between chronic low back pain and cognitive function. Pain Pract. 2023;23(4):399–408.
21. Larsson C, Ekvall Hansson E, Sundquist K, Jakobsson U. Kinesiophobia and its relation to pain characteristics and cognitive affective variables in older adults with chronic pain. BMC Geriatr. 2016;16:128. https://doi.org/10.1186/s12877-016-0302-6.
22. Malfliet A, Coppieters I, Van Wilgen P, Kregel J, De Pauw R, Dolphens M, et al. Brain changes associated with cognitive and emotional factors in chronic pain: a systematic review. Eur J Pain. 2017;21(5):769–86.
23. Dueñas M, Salazar A, de Sola H, Failde I. Limitations in activities of daily living in eople with chronic pain: identification of groups using clusters analysis. Pain Pract. 2020;20(2):179–87.
24. Chimenti RL, Frey-Law LA, Sluka KA. A mechanism-based approach to physical therapist management of pain. Phys Ther. 2018;98:302–14.
25. Ferro Moura Franco K, Lenoir D, Dos Santos Franco YR, Jandre Reis FJ, Nunes Cabral CM, Meeus M. Prescription of exercises for the treatment of chronic pain along the continuum of nociplastic pain: a systematic review with meta-analysis. Eur J Pain. 2021;25(1):51–70.
26. Hayden JA, Ellis J, Ogilvie R, Malmivaara A, van Tulder MW. Exercise therapy for chronic low back pain. Cochrane Database Syst Rev. 2021;9(9):CD009790. https://doi.org/10.1002/14651858.CD009790.pub2.
27. Wieland LS, Skoetz N, Pilkington K, Harbin S, Vempati R, Berman BM. Yoga for chronic non-specific low back pain. Cochrane Database Syst Rev. 2022;11:CD010671. https://doi.org/10.1002/14651858.CD010671.pub3.
28. Ambrose KR, Golightly YM. Physical exercise as non-pharmacological treatment of chronic pain: why and when. Best Pract Res Clin Rheumatol. 2015;29(1):120–30.
29. Mata Diz JB, de Souza JR, Leopoldino AA, Oliveira VC. Exercise, especially combined stretching and strengthening exercise, reduces myofascial pain: a systematic review. J Physiother. 2017;63(1):17–22.
30. Fransen M, McConnell S, Harmer AR, Van der Esch M, Simic M, Bennell KL. Exercise for osteoarthritis of the knee. Cochrane Database Syst Rev. 2015;1:1–130.
31. Geneen LJ, Moore RA, Clarke C, Martin D, Colvin LA, Smith BH. Physical activity and exercise for chronic pain in adults: an overview of Cochrane reviews. Cochrane Database Syst Rev. 2017;4:1–68.
32. IASP. International Association for the Study of Pain. Exercise and chronic low back pain [Fact sheet] 2021. Available from: https://www.iasp-pain.org/resources/fact-sheets/exercise-and-chronic-low-back-pain.
33. Demirel A, Oz M, Ozel YA, Cetin H, Ulger O. Stabilization exercise versus yoga exercise in non-specific low back pain: pain, disability, quality of life, performance: a randomized controlled trial. Complement Ther Clin Pract. 2019;35:102–8.
34. Grooten WJA, Boström C, Dedering Å, Halvorsen M, Kuster RP, Nilsson-Wikmar L, et al. Summarizing the effects of different exercise types in chronic low back pain - a systematic review of systematic reviews. BMC Musculoskelet Disord. 2022;23(1):801. https://doi.org/10.1186/s12891-022-05722-x.
35. Hall AM, Maher CG, Lam P, Ferreira M, Latimer J. Tai chi exercise for treatment of pain and disability in people with persistent low back pain: a randomized controlled trial. Arthritis Care Res. 2011;63(11):1576–83.

36. Hayden JA, Ellis J, Ogilvie R, Stewart SA, Bagg MK, Stanojevic S, et al. Some types of exercise are more effective than others in people with chronic low back pain: a network meta-analysis. J Physiother. 2021;67:252–62.
37. O'Connor SR, Tully MA, Ryan B, Bleakley CM, Baxter GD, Bradley JM, et al. Walking exercise for chronic musculoskeletal pain: systematic review and meta-analysis. Arch Phys Med Rehabil. 2015;96(4):724–34.
38. Nabavi N, Mohseni Bandpei MA, Mosallanezhad Z, Rahgozar M, Jaberzadeh S. The effect of 2 different exercise programs on pain intensity and muscle dimensions in patients with chronic low back pain: a randomized controlled trial. J Manip Physiol Ther. 2018;41(2):102–10.
39. Vanti C, Andreatta S, Borghi S, Guccione AA, Pillastrini P, Bertozzi L. The effectiveness of walking versus exercise on pain and function in chronic low back pain: a systematic review and meta-analysis of randomized trials. Disabil Rehabil. 2019;41(6):622–32.
40. Tan L, Cicuttini FM, Fairley J, Romero L, Estee M, Hussain SM, et al. Does aerobic exercise effect pain sensitisation in individuals with musculoskeletal pain? A systematic review. BMC Musculoskelet Disord. 2022;23(1):113. https://doi.org/10.1186/s12891-022-05047-9.
41. Wang XQ, Zheng JJ, Yu ZW, Bi X, Lou SJ, Liu J, et al. A meta-analysis of core stability exercise versus general exercise for chronic low back pain. PLoS One. 2012;7(12):e52082. https://doi.org/10.1371/journal.pone.0052082.
42. Alkatan M, Baker JR, Machin DR, Park W, Akkari AS, Pasha EP, et al. Improved function and reduced pain after swimming and cycling training in patients with osteoarthritis. J Rheumatol. 2016;43(3):666–72.
43. Kunduracilar Z, Guvenir Sahin H, Sonmezer E, Sozay S. The effects of two different water exercise trainings on pain, functional status and balance in patients with knee osteoarthritis. Complement Ther Clin Pract. 2018;31:374–8.
44. Rewald S, Lenssen AFT, Emans PJ, de Bie RA, van Breukelen G, Mesters I. Aquatic cycling improves knee pain and physical functioning in patients with knee osteoarthritis: a randomized controlled trial. Arch Phys Med Rehabil. 2020;101(8):1288–95.
45. Laubenstein S, Beissner K. Exercise and movement-based therapies in geriatric pain management. Clin Geriatr Med. 2016;32(4):737–62.
46. Pelland L, Brosseau L, Wells G, Macleay L, Lambert J, Lamothe C, et al. Efficacy of strengthening exercises for osteoarthritis (part I): a meta-analysis. Phys Ther Rev. 2004;9:77–108.
47. Beckwée D, Vaes P, Cnudde M, Swinnen E, Bautmans I. Osteoarthritis of the knee: why does exercise work? A qualitative study of the literature. Ageing Res Rev. 2013;12:226–36.
48. Borisovskaya A, Chmelik E, Karnik A. Exercise and chronic pain. In: Xiao J, editor. Physical exercise for human health. Advances in experimental medicine and biology. Singapure: Springer; 2020. p. 233–53.
49. Daenen L, Varkey E, Kellmann M, Nijs J. Exercise, not to exercise, or how to exercise in patients with chronic pain? Applying science to practice. Clin J Pain. 2015;31:108–14.
50. Sluka KA, Frey-Law LA, Bement MH. Exercise-induced pain and analgesia? Underlying mechanisms and clinical translation. Pain. 2018;159(9):S91–S7.
51. Naugle KM, Fillingim RB, Riley JL. A meta-analytic review of the hypoalgesic effects of exercise. J Pain. 2012;13(12):1139–50.
52. Petersen AMW, Pedersen BK. The anti-inflammatory effect of exercise. J Appl Physiol. 2005;98:1154–62.
53. Powers SK, Howley ET. Exercise physiology. Theory and application to fitness and performance. New York, NY: McGraw Hill; 2017.
54. Rice D, Nijs J, Kosek E, Wideman T, Hasenbring MI, Koltyn K, et al. Exercise-induced hypoalgesia in pain-free and chronic pain populations: state of the art and future directions. J Pain. 2019;20(11):1249–66.
55. Rodiguez-Pintó I, Agmon-Levin N, Howard A, Shoenfeld Y. Fibromyalgia and cytokines. Immunol Lett. 2014;161(2):200–3.
56. Mirtz TA, Greene L. Is obesity a risk factor for low back pain? An example of using the evidence to answer a clinical question. Chiropr Osteopat. 2005;13(2):1–6.

57. Bear MF, Connors BW, Paradiso MA. Neuroscience: exploring the brain. Burlington, MA: Jones & Barlett Learning; 2020.
58. Sluka KA, O'Donnell JM, Danielson J, Rasmussen LA. Regular physical activity prevents development of chronic pain and activation of central neurons. J Appl Physiol. 2013;114:725–33.
59. Cooper MA, Kluding PM, Wright DE. Emerging relationships between exercise, sensory nerves, and neuropathic pain. Front Neurosci. 2016;10:1–12.
60. Ortega E, Bote ME, Giraldo E, García JJ. Aquatic exercise improves the monocyte pro- and anti-inflammatory cytokine production balance in fibromyalgia patients. Sand J Med Sci Sports. 2012;22:104–12.
61. Steglitz T, Wright JD, Warnick JL, Hoffman SA, Johnston W, Spring B. Evidence-based practice. In: Wright JD, editor. International encyclopedia of social and behavioral sciences. 2nd ed. London: Oxford Elsevier; 2015. p. 332–8.
62. Ruegsegger GN, Booth FW. Health benefits of exercise. Cold Spring Harb Perspect Med. 2018;8(7):a029694. https://doi.org/10.1101/cshperspect.a029694.
63. Hodges PW. Pain and motor control: from the laboratory to rehabilitation. J Electromyogr Kinesiol. 2011;21:220–8.
64. Hodges PW, Tucker K. Moving differently in pain: a new theory to explain the adaptation to pain. Pain. 2011;152:S90–S8.
65. Hsu W-L, Chen CPC, Nikkhoo M, Lin C-F, Ching CT-S, Niu C-C, et al. Fatigue changes neck muscle control and deteriorates postural stability during arm movement perturbations in patients with chronic neck pain. Spine J. 2020;20(4):530–7.
66. Luft A, Buitrago MM. Stages of motor skill learning. Mol Neurobiol. 2005;32(3):205–16.
67. Park DC, Bischof GN. The aging mind: neuroplasticity in response to cognitive training. Dialogues Clin Neurosci. 2013;15(1):109–19.
68. Pauwels L, Chalavi S, Swinnen SP. Aging and brain plasticity. Aging. 2018;10(8):1789–90.
69. Phillips C. Lifestyle modulators of neuroplasticity: how physical activity, mental engagement, and diet promote cognitive health during aging. Neural Plast. 2017;2017:3589271. https://doi.org/10.1155/2017/3589271.
70. Bak MS, Park H, Kim SK. Neural plasticity in the brain during neuropathic pain. Biomedicines. 2021;9:1–17.
71. Boudreau SA, Farina D, Falla D. The role of motor learning and neuroplasticity in designing rehabilitation approaches for musculoskeletal pain disorders. Man Ther. 2010;15:410–4.
72. Hashmi JA, Baliki MN, Huang L, Baria AT, Torbey S, Hermann KM, et al. Shape shifting pain: chronification of back pain shifts brain representation from nociceptive to emotional circuits. Brain. 2013;136:2751–68.
73. Hiraga SI, Itokazu T, Nishibe M, Yamashita T. Neuroplasticity related to chronic pain and its modulation by microglia. Inflamm Regen. 2022;42(1):15. https://doi.org/10.1186/s41232-022-00199-6.
74. Kim W, Kim SK, Nabekura J. Functional and structural plasticity in the primary somatosensory cortex associated with chronic pain. J Neurochem. 2017;141:499–506.
75. Kuner R, Flor H. Structural plasticity and reorganisation in chronic pain. Nat Rev Neurosci. 2017;18:20–30.
76. Pauwels L, Chalavi S, Gooijers J, Maes C, Albouy G, Sunaert S, et al. Challenge to promote change: the neural basis of the contextual interference effect in young and older adults. J Neurosci. 2018;38(13):3333–45.
77. Lage GM, Ugrinowitsch H, Apolinário-Souza T, Vieira MM, Albuquerque MR, Benda RN. Repetition and variation in motor practice: a review of neural correlates. Neurosci Biobehav Rev. 2015;57:132–41.
78. Lage GM, Fernandes LA, Apolinário-Souza T, Nogueira NGHM, Ferreira BP. Mini-review: practice organization beyond memory processes. Braz J Mot Behav. 2021;15(5):333–41.
79. Travassos B, Araújo D, Davids K, Vilar L, Esteves P, Vanda C. Informational constraints shape emergent functional behaviours during performance of interceptive actions in team sports. Psychol Sport Exerc. 2012;13:216–23.

80. Bordeleau M, Vincenot M, Lefevre S, Duport A, Seggio L, Breton T, et al. Treatments for kinesiophobia in people with chronic pain: a scoping review. Front Behav Neurosci. 2022;16:933483. https://doi.org/10.3389/fnbeh.2022.933483.
81. Karayannis NV, Smeets RJEM, van den Hoorn W, Hodges PW. Fear of movement is related to trunk stiffness in low back pain. PLoS One. 2013;8(6):e67779. https://doi.org/10.1371/journal.pone.0067779.

Balance Control in People with Parkinson's Disease

19

Victor Spiandor Beretta, Gabriel Antonio Gazziero Moraca, and Lucas Simieli

Abstract

Adequate postural control is fundamental to performing the activities of daily living appropriately and safely. Postural control is a complex system based on the interaction of sensorimotor dynamic processes which have two main functional goals (i.e., postural orientation and equilibrium). Deficits in postural control increase the risk of falls, which is exacerbated by the presence of neurological diseases such as Parkinson's disease (PD). The loss of dopaminergic neurons in basal ganglia, characterized by PD, affects the functionality of several cortical and subcortical structures involved in postural control, increasing postural instability. People with PD demonstrate impairments in postural control during standing, dynamic conditions (e.g., walking), and postural responses to external perturbation. These impairments increase the risk of falls in people with PD and some of them are less responsive to PD medication. Thus, complementary therapies to improve postural control in PD have been explored. This chapter aims to describe postural control in people with PD and present some evidence regarding the effects of complementary therapies for balance rehabilitation in this population.

V. S. Beretta (✉)
School of Technology and Sciences, Physical Education Department, São Paulo State University (Unesp), Presidente Prudente, Brazil
e-mail: victor.beretta@unesp.br

G. A. G. Moraca
São Paulo State University (Unesp), Institute of Biosciences, Graduate Program in Movement Sciences, Posture and Gait Studies Laboratory (LEPLO), Rio Claro, Brazil

L. Simieli
São Paulo State University (Unesp), School of Sciences, Human Movement Research Laboratory (MOVI-LAB), Bauru, Brazil

F. A. Barbieri et al. (eds.), *Locomotion and Posture in Older Adults*,
https://doi.org/10.1007/978-3-031-74123-4_19

Introduction

The ability of the postural control system to recover body position and/or resist disturbance by the integration of sensory information, muscle activity, and proper center of mass (CoM) control is necessary for maintaining balance [1–3]. Adequate balance maintenance is fundamental to performing the activities of daily living appropriately and safely, such as moving around in different environments, cleaning the house, cooking, going shopping, and performing physical activities, among others.

Postural control is a complex system based on the interaction of sensorimotor dynamic processes [4], in which there is an interaction between individual, task, and environmental factors [1, 5]. The main functional goals of postural control are postural orientation and postural equilibrium [1, 4]. Postural orientation is related to the position of body segments in the environment. On the other hand, postural equilibrium is related to the internal and external forces that act on the body, trying to keep the CoM within the stability limit considering the expected and non-expected forces that act on the body [4]. Although postural orientation and postural equilibrium are different, these two main goals are interdependent (i.e., the impairments in one of these components can impact the performance of the other) [1].

In addition to the main objectives, there are several subcomponents involved in postural control and required for balance maintenance. These subcomponents may be grouped into the following domains [2]: biomechanical constraints, movement strategies, sensory strategies, orientation in space, control of dynamics, and cognitive processing [2]. The support base, limits of stability, and muscle strength/balance are some biomechanical constraints involved in postural control [2, 4] and their impairments could impact balance performance. The movement strategies domain includes the postural adjustment in situation with expected and non-expected perturbation, such as reactive, anticipatory, and voluntary adjustments. The domain regarding sensory strategies involves the integration of the different sensory information and its reweighting considering the relevance to maintaining the balance according to the task characteristics. The orientation in space domain is related to the individual capacity to perceive the sensory information, control the standing considering the gravity, and maintain adequate verticality. In addition, the control of dynamics involves the resources required to maintain balance during dynamics tasks such as gait. Lastly, the cognitive processing domain is related to the performance of attention and executive functions. Changes in any of these subcomponents may impact the postural control performance and may increase the risk of falls as evidenced in people with Parkinson's disease (PD) [2, 4].

PD is characterized by the progressive degeneration of dopaminergic neurons in the substantia nigra pars compacta [6–8]. Decreased dopaminergic levels in the basal ganglia inhibit thalamocortical and brainstem motor systems [8], which impair brain activity [7, 9] and cause several motor deficits [6, 7], such as postural instability. The specific impairments in postural control during standing, dynamic, and postural adjustment in situations with perturbation are demonstrated in the following section of this chapter. The exacerbated postural instability increases the risk of falls in people with PD.

Falls occurrence can be two to three times higher than in neurologically healthy older adults [10, 11]. Approximately, 70% of people with PD fall at least once time during a year [12, 13] and ~ 50% of them reports the recurrence of the falls [12]. The occurrence of falls can lead to a decrease in the individual's ability to perform activities of daily living and independence [14] and is the third leading cause of hospitalization in people with PD [15]. In addition, complications resulting from falls increase the cost of healthcare systems [16].

In the past, postural control was considered a reflex activity [1]. However, after several research studies over time, postural control is now considered a sensorimotor skill that is learned during motor development [1]. As a characteristic of a skill, postural control can be improved by practice. Thus, the participation of several cortical and subcortical structures in postural control has been highlighted. This chapter will present cortical and subcortical structures involved in postural control and how neurodegeneration impairs the neural control of balance and hence, impairs balance capacity in PD.

In this context, this chapter aims to describe the postural control in people with PD. Regarding the neural control of balance, we will focus mainly on how the nervous system (i.e., structures and pathways) acts to maintain balance in different conditions and how PD neurodegeneration impacts this control. In addition, we will discuss some biomechanics and motor behavior components of postural control in people with PD. Lastly, we will present the changes in postural control in people with PD during standing and dynamic balance and the postural responses in situations with external perturbation.

Neural Control of Balance in PD

Several cortical, subcortical, and brainstem areas, such as frontal and temporal-parietal areas, thalamus, cerebellum, and basal ganglia seem to be involved during postural control in several domains (i.e., postural sway, anticipatory postural adjustments—APAs, and reactive postural adjustments) [1, 17]. Cortical and subcortical structures involved in the integration of sensory information are important to create an adequate body schema (internal model) and generate adequate postural sway control [1, 18]. In summary, the brainstem, cerebellum, thalamus, and cerebral cortex are involved in receiving and integrating the sensory information from sensory systems (i.e., vestibular, visual, and somatosensory) to create an internal model of the body and to generate adequate motor programs and muscle activity to control the postural balance to keep the CoM within the stability limit [18]. However, as mentioned earlier, the decreased dopaminergic levels in the basal ganglia result in hypoactivation of the thalamocortical and brainstem areas that are involved in the sensory information integration and control of muscle synergy, respectively [1, 8]. This imbalanced activity in cortico-basal pathways and the dysfunctional brainstem activity contributes to muscle rigidity and hypokinesia which contributes to postural instability during standing, walking, and postural adjustments in situations with perturbation evidenced in people with PD.

Neurophysiological aspects of PD may elucidate the delayed gait initiation observed. Loss of dopaminergic neurons in PD leads to diminished dopamine levels in the suplementary motor area and basal ganglia, whereas goal-directed movement is generated by a circuit that includes dorsolateral premotor cortex and primary motor cortex [19]. In PD, the output nuclei of the basal ganglia send excessive inhibitory signaling to several brain areas [19]. A less excitable circuitry in PD necessitates extended temporal intervals and heightened input to accomplish tasks compared to normally functioning circuitry. This challenge extends to the initiation of voluntary movements, including gait initiation. Impairments may also arise from perturbations in supplementary motor and premotor regions, which play pivotal roles in APAs generation. Reduced activity in the premotor cortices, stemming from the loss of dopaminergic neurons, may disrupt motor programming essential for precise gait control. In more complex settings, such as concurrent motor or cognitive task execution, additional brain regions may become involved in gait initiation control. Impaired information processing could lead to APA errors and gait freezing.

Postural responses seem to be generated mainly from the subcortical structures such as pedunculopontine nucleus and reticular formation [20]. In addition to pedunculopontine nucleus and reticular formation, other brain structures are involved in postural responses, highlighting areas of the cerebral cortex (e.g., motor and prefrontal cortices), the basal ganglia, and the cerebellum [17, 18, 21]. Deficits in cortico-basal pathways are evidenced in people with PD [18, 22], affecting the neural control of postural response in situation with external perturbation. People with PD demonstrate a hypoactivation of the pedunculopontine nucleus and reticular formation as a consequence from the lower excitatory activity of the thalamus on primary motor cortex and higher inhibitory activity of the basal ganglia on these structures (i.e., pedunculopontine nucleus and reticular formation) [8]. A growing body of evidence suggests the involvement of cortical areas (i.e., primary motor cortex, supplementary motor area, and prefrontal cortex) during postural responses to perturbation [8, 17, 21, 23, 24].

Cortical activity is important for anticipation and planning, optimizing postural responses by changes in commands in the central-set [17, 25, 26], which is impaired in PD [27, 28]. Two main postural and locomotor pathways have been highlighted using mobile techniques that analyze cortical activity, such as electroencephalography and functional near-infrared spectroscopy: direct and indirect postural pathway [24, 29]. Direct postural pathway is activated in less challenging situations and reflects an automatic postural control; it involves the participation of the primary motor cortex [24, 29]. On the other hand, the indirect postural pathway is activated when compensatory executive-attentional resources are required for postural control by increasing the activation of the prefrontal cortex and supplementary motor area [24, 29–32]. The compensatory resources are required when automaticity is reduced by the presence of pathologies or lower intrinsic subject balance ability such as PD, and in challenging situations, such as the presence of external perturbation [24, 29–32]. Thus, as a consequence of reduced automaticity due to deficits in cortico-basal pathways, people with PD compensate by activating the indirect pathway to control the postural response after perturbation [33].

Postural Control in PD During Standing

People with PD show impairments in postural control during standing considering both main functional goals proprieties (i.e., postural orientation and equilibrium). Regarding the postural orientation, people with PD demonstrate a stooped posture with some bending of the knees and trunk [34]. Furthermore, lateral flexion of the trunk is also common and may appear later in PD course [34]. Other postural abnormalities may include extreme neck flexion, Pisa syndrome, and camptocormia [35]. It is worth highlighting that studies on the effects of levodopa intake on camptocormia and Pisa syndrome are still scarce [36].

Regarding postural equilibrium, previous studies demonstrated that, when compared with neurologically healthy older adults, people with PD showed a reduced limit of stability, larger center of pressure (CoP) oscillation area, and CoP displacement in both anteroposterior and mediolateral axes [37, 38]. These impairments demonstrated in postural control are more prominent with visual system deprivation, such as in eyes closed conditions [37, 38]. However, Feller and colleagues [39] evidenced that individuals with PD can reweight proprioceptive, visual and vestibular information for postural control when sensory conditions changed.

The postural sway in people with PD can be abnormal since before the start of treatment based on levodopa intake. Mancini and colleagues [40] demonstrated, by use of accelerometry, that measures of postural sway were able to identify impairments in postural control prematurely in PD progression. In addition, they demonstrated that mediolateral sway is more sensitive in identifying the impairments than anteroposterior sway [40]. It is worth mentioning that postural sway seems to increase according to the severity of PD [41]. Regarding the effect of levodopa medication on postural sway, this treatment seems to help postural sway early in the disease but worsens it later in the disease progression [36].

Postural Control in PD During Dynamic Balance

Balance during dynamic situations (i.e., walking) is impaired in people with PD. Balance impairments during walking impact the performance in activities of daily life and the quality of life in this population. People with PD demonstrates lower margin of stability during walking and more unstable gait than healthy older adults [42]. In addition, deficits in gait initiation and APAs are also evidenced in people with PD, which impact the dynamic balance [43].

Gait initiation represents a critical phase in human locomotion, entailing a complex interplay of postural and muscular adjustments as individual's transition from a static standing posture to the initiation of walking. This phase culminates in the toe-off event, marking the onset of the initial step [44]. Successful gait initiation hinges on the precise orchestration of APAs to maintain equilibrium and propel the CoM forward [19]. The execution of APAs requires the integration of motor commands and sensory inputs [19, 44, 45]. This section explores the impact of PD on APAs and spatial-temporal parameters during gait initiation (Fig. 19.1), delving into the modulating roles of factors such as dual tasking, cueing, and medication.

Eight studies have systematically investigated the alterations in APAs among people with PD, consistently revealing notable differences [19, 44, 46–51]. These findings collectively illustrate that people with PD exhibit slower CoP movements and reduced CoP displacements compared to their healthy counterparts [44, 48, 50]. Healthy controls typically exhibit a stereotypical CoP movement during gait initiation, progressing toward the leading limb before transitioning to the trailing limb. Conversely, people with PD demonstrate delayed CoP movements, characterized by diminished and decelerated CoP shifts in both anterior–posterior and mediolateral directions. This delay coincides with a protracted interval between APA onset and step initiation [44, 46, 49, 52]. People with PD also demonstrate diminished step velocity and step length during the initial step [45, 47, 49, 50]. Additionally, they manifest prolonged intervals between the onset of muscle activity and observable foot movement compared to controls [19, 44, 46–51].

Previous studies have investigated the influence of concurrent tasks during gait initiation [44, 46, 49, 50, 52]. One study assessed the influence of a secondary cognitive task during gait initiation, while four others explored the effects of sensory cueing. In the context of gait initiation with concurrent cognitive task execution, people with PD exhibited reduced CoP displacement in the mediolateral direction and slower CoP velocity in both mediolateral and anterior–posterior directions compared to healthy controls. Interestingly, the secondary cognitive task did not

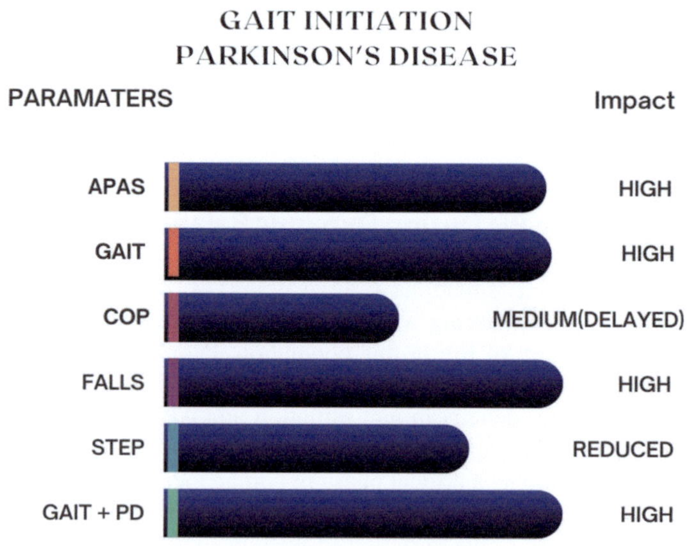

Fig. 19.1 Summary of gait initiation changes in people with PD

exert additional effects on APA displacement or gait initiation velocity when juxtaposed with single-task gait initiation in people with PD. Regarding cueing, auditory cues positively influenced gait initiation in both people with PD and healthy older individuals. Attentional cues, provided as specific instructions, improved gait initiation by serving as triggers. However, it is noteworthy that people with PD who experienced freezing exhibited superfluous APAs in 63% of trials during cued gait initiation. Those without freezing displayed similar APA patterns in 51% of trials, while healthy older adults exhibited this behavior in 48% of trials. A study by McCandless and colleagues [45] examined various cue types during gait initiation, revealing that visual cues enhanced CoP displacements in both directions and reduced freezing episodes in people with PD.

A single study investigated the influence of medication on gait initiation in people with PD (we only considered here those studies in which the subjects must performed more than three steps before stop), comparing the OFF-state (absence of medication) to the ON state and neurologically healthy older individuals. In the ON state, people with PD exhibited more pronounced mediolateral CoP displacements during the transition phase [from inertial position (standing to walking)] from cued to compensatory stepping compared to the OFF-state. However, for other analyzed parameters, no significant disparities were observed between the ON and OFF states [46].

In general, this section has explored the impact of PD on gait initiation, with a particular emphasis on APAs and spatial-temporal parameters associated with the initial step. Individuals with PD demonstrate APAs marked by reduced COP displacements, decelerated movement, and a slower, shorter initial step compared to healthy counterparts during gait initiation. These effects are further exacerbated by concurrent task engagement but are partially mitigated by cueing and exhibit limited response to medication (L-Dopa) during gait initiation. It is plausible that the basal ganglia deficits induced by PD underlie these impairments during gait initiation in this population [53].

Visual cues appear to mitigate the consequences of basal ganglia dysfunction, enhancing gait initiation in people with PD. Basal ganglia malfunction is associated with decreased supplementary motor area activity, contributing to difficulties in movement preparation. In this context, cues may elevate supplementary motor area activation through augmented sensory input. Additionally, individuals with PD tend to rely more on visual information, potentially due to dopamine depletion in the retina and compromised perception. To ensure secure and stable gait initiation, accurate information about foot placement and environmental factors is crucial. Thus, visual cues represent an effective strategy for enhancing gait initiation in people with PD.

Postural Responses in PD in Situations with External Perturbation

Unexpected external perturbations are present in activities of daily living, such as crossing an obstacle, breaking a moving vehicle (i.e., standing in a bus moving), tripping and/or slipping while walking, etc. These unexpected perturbations increase the risk of falls in people with PD, since their postural responses are inadequate [3, 54]. Reactive responses have been analyzed by studies that carried out perturbations triggered by rotation and translation movements of the support surface [55–61]. Reactive adjustment occurs after the postural perturbation [3, 55, 62, 63], are triggered by sensory signals, and the main objective is recovery of body position and stability after the perturbation [3, 64, 65]. Some types of responses are evidenced after situations with external perturbation such as ankle, hip, and step strategies [2, 3, 5].

Reactive responses in people with PD have revealed a decrease in the flexibility of the central nervous system to control muscles appropriately in situations of external perturbation [3, 60, 66]. People with PD demonstrate difficulty in changing postural response patterns and difficulty in adequately controlling muscles in situations with external perturbation [5, 60, 66], evidenced by excessive muscle coactivation and greater activity of the antagonist muscle [3, 28, 56, 66–68]. These impairments are evidenced even after the ingestion of Levodopa and increase the risk of falls [3, 69].

The effects of the medication on the postural responses in people with PD are controversial [64, 70–72]. The medication seems to improve the protective postural responses that require stepping, and this response is important to prevent a backward fall [72]. Also, the medication alleviates bradykinesia and muscle coactivation in people with PD [3]. However, other studies have shown that the use of the drug does not seem to contribute to postural responses in people with PD [3, 56], with weaker and slower responses and difficulty in changing postural responses in situations with external perturbation [3, 64, 70, 71]. Also, the medication may be related to the increase in the occurrence of falls in this population [3]. The greater number of falls in the ON state may be due to the medication decreasing bradykinesia and rigidity and not contributing to the magnitude of the postural response, which allows the patient to move faster through space without adequate balance control [3]. Thus, complementary therapies have been explored for postural responses in people with PD, such as transcranial direct current stimulation (tDCS) [33, 73, 74].

Our meta-analysis demonstrated small to moderate effect of tDCS on improving balance (i.e., during standing, dynamic balance, and postural responses) in adults with neurological disorders, such as stroke, cerebellar ataxia and PD [73]. Thus, tDCS is a promising complementary therapy for balance rehabilitation in several neurological disorders [73]. tDCS is a technique that generates low-intensity electrical currents (generally 1–4 mA) through the scalp that changes the membrane potential of neuronal cells, leading to an increase or decrease in the excitability of the target brain area [75, 76]. tDCS effects can be observed also in the subcortical structures beyond the cerebral cortex [20, 77]. In addition to modifying excitability, anodal tDCS increase dopamine release, decrease GABAergic neurotransmitters [78–80] and promotes behavioral changes (e.g., improve balance and locomotion) [81]. Thus, these possible effects promoted by tDCS are relevant for people with PD considering the characteristics the disease impairments.

Specifical for postural responses in people with PD, we demonstrated that a single session of anodal tDCS over M1 for 20 min, mainly with 2 mA, improves postural control [33]. The positive changes obtained with tDCS included faster activation of the medial gastrocnemius muscle (MG) and shorter time to recover balance after the external perturbation [33]. Kaski et al. (2014) demonstrated that people with PD recover balance in less time after perturbation when tDCS was combined with physical exercise. However, postural responses were not benefited by tDCS performed alone (i.e., without physical exercise) [74]. Thus, although promising, future studies are needed in order to identify the factors that can optimize/enhance the use of this technique for the rehabilitation of postural responses in people with PD.

In addition to the deficits in reactive adjustments described previously, there is evidence that people with PD present a delay in habituation to postural perturbations, highlighting the difficulty these individuals have in changing the patterns of postural responses [82, 83]. This impairment in postural control seems to be related to deficits in the functioning of the cortico-basal pathways, which are altered by PD [84–87]. During the habituation process to perturbations, there is a decrease in activity in the supplementary motor area, which suggests greater adaptation and less need for cortical resources to respond to the perturbation [23, 88]. Also, the basal ganglia participate in postural control by acting in the pre-selection of a response and in its optimization according to the characteristics of the perturbation [17]. In addition, the basal ganglia receive sensory input and try to automate the selection and execution of a postural response based on the specific context [22, 89]. Thus, due to the impairment in its functionality caused by the disease (i.e., increase in inhibitory projections due to the increase in GABAergic neurotransmitters), it is reasonable to assume that people with PD need to increase cortical activity to respond to the perturbation [22]. However, they have lower thalamic excitatory activity on primary motor cortex, resulting in hypoactivation of this cortical region [8]. Thus, people with PD need more trials to habituate to the perturbation and recruit additional areas for control [82, 83].

Final Considerations

This chapter covers evidence about postural control in people with PD, highlighting the neural control of balance and how PD neurodegeneration impacts this control. Also, we presented some impairments in postural control in people with PD during standing and dynamic balance and during postural responses in situations with external perturbation.

Several cortical and subcortical areas are involved in postural control. The loss of dopaminergic neurons in the basal ganglia affects the functionality of these structures and leads to several impairments in postural control. In general, people with PD demonstrate greater postural sway during standing. Also, people with Parkinson's disease PD show reduced margin of stability during walking, and deficits in the gait initiation and APAs, which impact the dynamic balance [90]. In addition, impaired postural response after external perturbation are evidenced in people with PD by difficulties in changing postural response patterns and difficulties in adequately controlling muscles (excessive muscle coactivation and greater activity of the antagonist muscle) [3, 28, 56, 66–68].

We presented studies that investigated the effects of PD medication on postural control in people with PD and studies that explored possible complementary therapies to benefit the balance in this population. Although promising results have been evidenced, such as positive changes in postural control after the application of tDCS, future studies are needed to identify the factors that can optimize/enhance the use of this technique for the rehabilitation of balance in people with PD.

References

1. Mancini M, Nutt JG, Horak FB. Chapter 1—How is balance controlled by the nervous system? In: Mancini M, Nutt JG, Horak FB, editors. Balance dysfunction in Parkinson's disease [internet]. Academic Press; 2020. p. 1–24. Available from: http://www.sciencedirect.com/science/article/pii/B9780128138748000015.
2. Gandolfi M, Valè N, Filippetti M, Dimitrova EK, Geroin C, Picelli A, et al. Postural control in individuals with Parkinson's disease. In: IntechOpen. IntechOpen; 2018. p. 1–18.
3. Mancini M, Nutt JG, Horak FB. Chapter 4—How are postural responses to external perturbations affected by PD? In: Mancini M, Nutt JG, Horak FB, editors. Balance dysfunction in Parkinson's disease [internet]. Academic Press; 2020. p. 63–81. https://doi.org/10.1016/C2017-0-00054-X.
4. Horak FB. Postural orientation and equilibrium: what do we need to know about neural control of balance to prevent falls? Age Ageing [Internet]. 2006;35(Suppl 2):ii7–11. Available from: http://www.ncbi.nlm.nih.gov/pubmed/16926210.
5. Horak FB, Henry SM, Shumway-Cook A. Postural perturbations: new insights for treatment of balance disorders. Phys Ther. 1997;77(5):517–33.
6. Takakusaki K, Saitoh K, Harada H, Kashiwayanagi M. Role of basal ganglia-brainstem pathways in the control of motor behaviors. Neurosci Res [Internet]. 2004;50(2):137–51. Available from: http://www.ncbi.nlm.nih.gov/pubmed/15380321.
7. Wichmann T, DeLong MR. Núcleos da Base. In: Kandel ER, Schwarts JH, Jessell TM, Siegelbaum SA, Hudspeth AJ, editors. Princípios de neurociências. Porto Alegre: AMGH; 2014. p. 811–32.
8. Peterson DS, Horak FB. Neural control of walking in people with parkinsonism. Physiol [Internet]. 2016;31(2):95–107. Available from: http://www.ncbi.nlm.nih.gov/pubmed/26889015.
9. Obeso JA, Rodriguez-Oroz MC, Benitez-Temino B, Blesa FJ, Guridi J, Marin C, et al. Functional organization of the basal ganglia: therapeutic implications for Parkinson's disease. Mov Disord [Internet]. 2008;23(Suppl 3):S548–59. Available from: http://www.ncbi.nlm.nih.gov/pubmed/18781672.
10. Bloem BR, Hausdorff JM, Visser JE, Giladi N. Falls and freezing of gait in Parkinson's disease: a review of two interconnected, episodic phenomena. Mov Disord [Internet]. 2004;19(8):871–84. Available from: http://www.ncbi.nlm.nih.gov/pubmed/15300651.

11. Pickering RM, Grimbergen YA, Rigney U, Ashburn A, Mazibrada G, Wood B, et al. A meta-analysis of six prospective studies of falling in Parkinson's disease. Mov Disord [Internet]. 2007;22(13):1892–900. Available from: http://www.ncbi.nlm.nih.gov/pubmed/17588236.
12. Wood BH, Bilclough JA, Bowron A, Walker RW. Incidence and prediction of falls in Parkinson's disease: a prospective multidisciplinary study. J Neurol Neurosurg Psychiatry. 2002 Jun;72(6):721–5.
13. Shen X, Wong-Yu ISK, Mak MKY. Effects of exercise on falls, balance, and gait ability in Parkinson's disease: a meta-analysis. Neurorehabil Neural Repair. 2016 Jul;30(6):512–27.
14. Schoneburg B, Mancini M, Horak F, Nutt JG. Framework for understanding balance dysfunction in Parkinson's disease. Mov Disord. 2013 Sep;28(11):1474–82.
15. Okunoye O, Kojima G, Marston L, Walters K, Schrag A. Factors associated with hospitalisation among people with Parkinson's disease—a systematic review and meta-analysis. Parkinsonism Relat Disord. 2020;71:66–72.
16. Stevens JA, Corso PS, Finkelstein EA, Miller TR. The costs of fatal and non-fatal falls among older adults. Inj Prev. 2006 Oct;12(5):290–5.
17. Jacobs JV, Horak FB. Cortical control of postural responses. J Neural Transm [Internet]. 2007;114(10):1339–48. Available from: http://www.ncbi.nlm.nih.gov/pubmed/17393068.
18. Takakusaki K. Functional neuroanatomy for posture and gait control. J Mov Disord [Internet]. 2017;10(1):1–17. Available from: http://www.ncbi.nlm.nih.gov/pubmed/28122432.
19. Delval A, Tard C, Defebvre L. Why we should study gait initiation in Parkinson's disease. Neurophysiol Clin Neurophysiol [Internet]. 2014;44(1):69–76. Available from: https://linkinghub.elsevier.com/retrieve/pii/S0987705313003249.
20. Nonnekes J, Arrogi A, Munneke MAM, Van Asseldonk EHF, Nijhuis LBO, Geurts AC, et al. Subcortical structures in humans can be facilitated by transcranial direct current stimulation. PLoS One [Internet]. 2014;9(9):e107731. https://doi.org/10.1371/journal.pone.0107731.
21. Mihara M, Miyai I, Hatakenaka M, Kubota K, Sakoda S. Role of the prefrontal cortex in human balance control. Neuroimage [Internet]. 2008;43(2):329–36. Available from: http://www.ncbi.nlm.nih.gov/pubmed/18718542.
22. Takakusaki K, Oohinata-Sugimoto J, Saitoh K, Habaguchi T. Role of basal ganglia-brainstem systems in the control of postural muscle tone and locomotion. Prog Brain Res. 2004;143:6.
23. Mierau A, Hulsdunker T, Struder HK. Changes in cortical activity associated with adaptive behavior during repeated balance perturbation of unpredictable timing. Front Behav Neurosci [Internet]. 2015;9:272. Available from: http://www.ncbi.nlm.nih.gov/pubmed/26528154.
24. Solis-Escalante T, van der Cruijsen J, de Kam D, van Kordelaar J, Weerdesteyn V, Schouten AC. Cortical dynamics during preparation and execution of reactive balance responses with distinct postural demands. NeuroImage. 2019 Mar;188:557–71.
25. Horak FB, Diener HC. Cerebellar control of postural scaling and central set in stance. J Neurophysiol. 1994;72(2):479–93.
26. Bastian AJ. Learning to predict the future: the cerebellum adapts feedforward movement control. Curr Opin Neurobiol [Internet]. 2006;16(6):645–9. Available from: http://www.ncbi.nlm.nih.gov/pubmed/17071073.
27. Lee RG, Tonolli I, Viallet F, Aurenty R, Massion J. Preparatory postural adjustments in parkinsonian patients with postural instability. Can J Neurol Sci. 1995;22(2):126–35.
28. Chong RK, Jones CL, Horak FB. Postural set for balance control is normal in Alzheimer's but not in Parkinson's disease. J Gerontol Ser A Biol Sci Med Sci. 1999;54(3):M129–35.
29. Herold F, Wiegel P, Scholkmann F, Thiers A, Hamacher D, Schega L. Functional near-infrared spectroscopy in movement science: a systematic review on cortical activity in postural and walking tasks. Neurophotonics [Internet]. 2017;4(4):041403. Available from: http://www.ncbi.nlm.nih.gov/pubmed/28924563.
30. Mahoney JR, Holtzer R, Izzetoglu M, Zemon V, Verghese J, Allali G. The role of prefrontal cortex during postural control in Parkinsonian syndromes a functional near-infrared spectroscopy study. Brain Res [Internet]. 2016;1633:126–38. Available from: http://www.ncbi.nlm.nih.gov/pubmed/26551767.

31. Payne AM, Ting LH. Worse balance is associated with larger perturbation-evoked cortical responses in healthy young adults. Gait Posture [Internet]. 2020;80:324–30. Available from: http://www.sciencedirect.com/science/article/pii/S0966636220302198.
32. Al-Yahya E, Mahmoud W, Meester D, Esser P, Dawes H. Neural substrates of cognitive motor interference during walking; peripheral and central mechanisms. Front Hum Neurosci. 2019;12:536.
33. Beretta VS, Vitório R, Nóbrega-Sousa P, Conceição NR, Orcioli-Silva D, Pereira MP, et al. Effect of different intensities of transcranial direct current stimulation on postural response to external perturbation in patients with Parkinson's disease. Neurorehabil Neural Repair [Internet]. 2020;34(11):1009–19. https://doi.org/10.1177/1545968320962513.
34. Benatru I, Vaugoyeau M, Azulay JP. Postural disorders in Parkinson's disease. Neurophysiol Clin =Clin Neurophysiol. 2008;38(6):459–65.
35. Vaugoyeau M, Hakam H, Azulay JP. Proprioceptive impairment and postural orientation control in Parkinson's disease. Hum Mov Sci [Internet]. 2011;30(2):405–14. Available from: https://linkinghub.elsevier.com/retrieve/pii/S0167945710001740.
36. Mancini M, Nutt JG, Horak FB. Chapter 2—Why is balance so important in Parkinson disease? In: Mancini M, Nutt JG, Horak FB, editors. Balance dysfunction in Parkinson's disease [internet]. Academic Press; 2020. p. 25–36. Available from: http://www.sciencedirect.com/science/article/pii/B9780128138748000027.
37. Doná F, Aquino CC, Gazzola JM, Borges V, Silva SMCA, Ganança FF, et al. Changes in postural control in patients with Parkinson's disease: a posturographic study. Physiotherapy [Internet]. 2016;102(3):272–9. Available from: https://pubmed.ncbi.nlm.nih.gov/26582134/.
38. Błaszczyk JW, Orawiec R, Duda-Kłodowska D, Opala G. Assessment of postural instability in patients with Parkinson's disease. Exp Brain Res. 2007 Oct;183(1):107–14.
39. Feller KJ, Peterka RJ, Horak FB. Sensory re-weighting for postural control in Parkinson's disease. Front Hum Neurosci [Internet]. 2019;13:126. Available from: https://www.frontiersin.org/article/10.3389/fnhum.2019.00126.
40. Mancini M, Carlson-Kuhta P, Zampieri C, Nutt JG, Chiari L, Horak FB. Postural sway as a marker of progression in Parkinson's disease: a pilot longitudinal study. Gait Posture [Internet]. 2012;36(3):471–6. Available from: https://pubmed.ncbi.nlm.nih.gov/22750016/.
41. Frenklach A, Louie S, Koop MM, Bronte-Stewart H. Excessive postural sway and the risk of falls at different stages of Parkinson's disease. Mov Disord [Internet]. 2009;24(3):377–85. Available from: https://onlinelibrary.wiley.com/doi/10.1002/mds.22358.
42. Mancini M, Nutt JG, Horak FB. Chapter 6—How is dynamic balance during walking affected by PD? In: Mancini M, Nutt JG, Horak FB, editors. Balance dysfunction in Parkinson's disease: basic mechanisms to clinical management. Academic Press; 2020. p. 99–122. Available from: https://www.sciencedirect.com/science/article/pii/B9780128138748000064.
43. Bonora G, Mancini M, Carpinella I, Chiari L, Horak FB, Ferrarin M. Gait initiation is impaired in subjects with Parkinson's disease in the OFF state: evidence from the analysis of the anticipatory postural adjustments through wearable inertial sensors. Gait Posture [Internet]. 2017;51:218–21. Available from: https://linkinghub.elsevier.com/retrieve/pii/S0966636216306208.
44. Nocera JR, Roemmich R, Elrod J, Altmann LJP, Hass CJ. Effects of cognitive task on gait initiation in Parkinson disease: evidence of motor prioritization? J Rehabil Res Dev [Internet]. 2013;50(5):699. Available from: http://www.rehab.research.va.gov/jour/2013/505/pdf/nocera505.pdf.
45. McCandless PJ, Evans BJ, Janssen J, Selfe J, Churchill A, Richards J. Effect of three cueing devices for people with Parkinson's disease with gait initiation difficulties. Gait Posture [Internet]. 2016;44:7–11. Available from: https://linkinghub.elsevier.com/retrieve/pii/S096663621500942X.
46. Delval A, Moreau C, Bleuse S, Tard C, Ryckewaert G, Devos D, et al. Auditory cueing of gait initiation in Parkinson's disease patients with freezing of gait. Clin Neurophysiol [Internet]. 2014;125(8):1675–81. Available from: https://linkinghub.elsevier.com/retrieve/pii/S1388245713013588.

47. Rocchi L, Chiari L, Mancini M, Carlson-Kuhta P, Gross A, Horak FB. Step initiation in Parkinson's disease: influence of initial stance conditions. Neurosci Lett. 2006;406(1–2):128–32.
48. Mancini M, Zampieri C, Carlson-Kuhta P, Chiari L, Horak FB. Anticipatory postural adjustments prior to step initiation are hypometric in untreated Parkinson's disease: an accelerometer-based approach. Eur J Neurol. 2009;16(9):1028–34.
49. Tard C, Dujardin K, Bourriez JL, Destée A, Derambure P, Defebvre L, et al. Attention modulates step initiation postural adjustments in Parkinson freezers. Park Relat Disord. 2014;20(3):284–9.
50. Schlenstedt C, Mancini M, Horak F, Peterson D. Anticipatory postural adjustment during self-initiated, cued, and compensatory stepping in healthy older adults and patients with Parkinson disease. Arch Phys Med Rehabil. 2017;98(7):1316–1324.e1.
51. Martin M, Shinberg M, Kuchibhatla M, Ray L, Carollo JJ, Schenkman ML. Gait initiation in community-dwelling adults with Parkinson disease: comparison with older and younger adults without the disease. Phys Ther. 2002;82(6):566–77.
52. Vallabhajosula S, Buckley TA, Tillman MD, Hass CJ. Age and Parkinson's disease related kinematic alterations during multi-directional gait initiation. Gait Posture [Internet]. 2013;37(2):280–6. Available from: https://linkinghub.elsevier.com/retrieve/pii/S0966636212002883.
53. Massion J. Movement, posture and equilibrium: interaction and coordination. Prog Neurobiol [Internet]. 1992;38(1):35–56. Available from: http://www.sciencedirect.com/science/article/pii/030100829290034C.
54. Visser JE, Carpenter MG, van der Kooij H, Bloem BR. The clinical utility of posturography. Clin Neurophysiol [Internet]. 2008;119(11):2424–36. Available from: http://www.ncbi.nlm.nih.gov/pubmed/18789756.
55. Henry SM, Fung J, Horak FB. EMG responses to maintain stance during multidirectional surface translations. J Neurophysiol. 1998;80(4):1939–50.
56. Chong RK, Horak FB, Woollacott MH. Parkinson's disease impairs the ability to change set quickly. J Neurol Sci. 2000;175(1):57–70.
57. Dimitrova D, Nutt J, Horak FB. Abnormal force patterns for multidirectional postural responses in patients with Parkinson's disease. Exp Brain Res [Internet]. 2004;156(2):183–95. Available from: http://www.ncbi.nlm.nih.gov/pubmed/14991211.
58. Dimitrova D, Horak FB, Nutt JG. Postural muscle responses to multidirectional translations in patients with Parkinson's disease. J Neurophysiol. 2003;91(1):489–501.
59. Smith BA, Jacobs JV, Horak FB. Effects of amplitude cueing on postural responses and preparatory cortical activity of people with Parkinson disease. J Neurol Phys Ther [Internet]. 2014;38(4):207–15. Available from: http://www.ncbi.nlm.nih.gov/pubmed/25198870.
60. Horak FB, Dimitrova D, Nutt JG. Direction-specific postural instability in subjects with Parkinson's disease. Exp Neurol [Internet]. 2005;193(2):504–21. https://doi.org/10.1016/j.expneurol.2004.12.008.
61. Smith BA, Jacobs JV, Horak FB. Effects of magnitude and magnitude predictability of postural perturbations on preparatory cortical activity in older adults with and without Parkinson's disease. Exp Brain Res [Internet]. 2012;222(4):455–70. Available from: http://www.ncbi.nlm.nih.gov/pubmed/22936099.
62. Maki BE, McIlroy WE, Clin GM. Postural control in the older adult. Clin Geriatr Med. 1996;12(4):635–58.
63. Macpherson JM, Horak FB. Postura. In: Kandel ER, Schwartz JH, Jessel TM, Siegelbaum SA, Hudspeth AJ, editors. Princípios de neurociências. Porto Alegre: AMGH; 2014. p. 811–32.
64. Park JH, Kang YJ, Horak FB. What is wrong with balance in Parkinson's disease? J Mov Disord [Internet]. 2015;8(3):109–14. Available from: http://www.ncbi.nlm.nih.gov/pubmed/26413237.
65. Alexandrov AV, Frolov AA, Horak FB, Carlson-Kuhta P, Park S. Feedback equilibrium control during human standing. Biol Cybern [Internet]. 2005;93(5):309–22. Available from: http://www.ncbi.nlm.nih.gov/pmc/articles/PMC1430400/.

66. Horak FB, Nutt JG, Nashner LM. Postural inflexibility in parkinsonian subjects. J Neurol Sci. 1992;111(1):46–58.
67. Bloem BR. Postural instability in Parkinson's disease. Clin Neurol Neurosurg. 1992;94(Suppl):S41–5.
68. Lang KC, Hackney ME, Ting LH, McKay JL. Antagonist muscle activity during reactive balance responses is elevated in Parkinson's disease and in balance impairment. PLoS One. 2019;14(1):e0211137.
69. Curtze C, Nutt JG, Carlson-Kuhta P, Mancini M, Horak FB. Levodopa is a double-edged sword for balance and gait in people with Parkinson's disease. Mov Disord [Internet]. 2015;30(10):1361–70. Available from: http://www.ncbi.nlm.nih.gov/pubmed/26095928.
70. Horak FB, Diener HC, Nashner LM. Influence of central set on human postural responses. J Neurophysiol [Internet]. 1989;62(4):841–53. https://doi.org/10.1152/jn.1989.62.4.841.
71. Horak FB, Frank J, Nutt J. Effects of dopamine on postural control in parkinsonian subjects: scaling, set, and tone. J Neurophysiol. 1996 Jun;75(6):2380–96.
72. Peterson DS, Horak FB. The effect of levodopa on improvements in protective stepping in people with Parkinson's disease. Neurorehabil Neural Repair. 2016;30(10):931–40.
73. Beretta VS, Santos PCR, Orcioli-Silva D, Zampier VC, Vitório R, Gobbi LTB. Transcranial direct current stimulation for balance rehabilitation in neurological disorders: a systematic review and meta-analysis. Ageing Res Rev [Internet]. 2022;81:101736. Available from: https://linkinghub.elsevier.com/retrieve/pii/S1568163722001787.
74. Kaski D, Dominguez RO, Allum JH, Islam AF, Bronstein AM. Combining physical training with transcranial direct current stimulation to improve gait in Parkinson's disease: a pilot randomized controlled study. Clin Rehabil. 2014;28(11):1115–24.
75. Nitsche MA, Paulus W. Excitability changes induced in the human motor cortex by weak transcranial direct current stimulation. J Physiol. 2000;527(3):6.
76. Nitsche MA, Liebetanz D, Tergau F, Paulus W. Modulation of cortical excitability by transcranial direct current stimulation. Nervenarzt. 2002;73(4):332–5.
77. Bolzoni F, Pettersson LG, Jankowska E. Evidence for long-lasting subcortical facilitation by transcranial direct current stimulation in the cat. J Physiol [Internet]. 2013;591(13):3381–99. Available from: http://www.ncbi.nlm.nih.gov/pubmed/23507876.
78. Fonteneau C, Redoute J, Haesebaert F, Le Bars D, Costes N, Suaud-Chagny MF, et al. Frontal transcranial direct current stimulation induces dopamine release in the ventral striatum in human. Cereb Cortex [Internet]. 2018;28(7):2636–46. https://doi.org/10.1093/cercor/bhy093.
79. Fukai M, Bunai T, Hirosawa T, Kikuchi M, Ito S, Minabe Y, et al. Endogenous dopamine release under transcranial direct-current stimulation governs enhanced attention: a study with positron emission tomography. Transl Psychiatry. 2019;9(1):115. https://doi.org/10.1038/s41398-019-0443-4.
80. Bunai T, Hirosawa T, Kikuchi M, Fukai M, Yokokura M, Ito S, et al. tDCS-induced modulation of GABA concentration and dopamine release in the human brain: a combination study of magnetic resonance spectroscopy and positron emission tomography. Brain Stimul [Internet]. 2021;14(1):154–60. Available from: https://linkinghub.elsevier.com/retrieve/pii/S1935861X20303132.
81. Beretta VS, Conceição NR, Nóbrega-Sousa P, Orcioli-Silva D, Dantas LKBF, Gobbi LTB, et al. Transcranial direct current stimulation combined with physical or cognitive training in people with Parkinson's disease: a systematic review. J Neuroeng Rehabil [Internet]. 2020;17(1):74. Available from: https://jneuroengrehab.biomedcentral.com/articles/10.1186/s12984-020-00701-6.
82. Nanhoe-Mahabier W, Allum JH, Overeem S, Borm GF, Oude Nijhuis LB, Bloem BR. First trial reactions and habituation rates over successive balance perturbations in Parkinson's disease. Neuroscience [Internet]. 2012;217:123–9. Available from: http://www.ncbi.nlm.nih.gov/pubmed/22542872.
83. Beretta VS, Carpenter MG, Barbieri FA, Santos PCR, Orcioli-Silva D, Pereira MP, et al. Does the impaired postural control in Parkinson's disease affect the habituation to non-sequential external perturbation trials? Clin Biomech (Bristol, Avon). 2021;85:105363.

84. Jahn K, Deutschländer A, Stephan T, Kalla R, Hüfner K, Wagner J, et al. Chapter 4.20—Supraspinal locomotor control in quadrupeds and humans. In: Kennard C, Leigh RJ, editors. Progress in brain research [internet]. Elsevier; 2008. p. 353–62. Available from: http://www.sciencedirect.com/science/article/pii/S0079612308006523.
85. Fling BW, Cohen RG, Mancini M, Nutt JG, Fair DA, Horak FB. Asymmetric pedunculopontine network connectivity in parkinsonian patients with freezing of gait. Brain [Internet]. 2013;136(8):2405–18. https://doi.org/10.1093/brain/awt172.
86. Peterson DS, Dijkstra BW, Horak FB. Postural motor learning in people with Parkinson's disease. J Neurophysiol [Internet]. 2016;263(8):1518–29. Available from: http://www.ncbi.nlm.nih.gov/pubmed/27193311.
87. Van Ooteghem K, Frank JS, Horak FB. Postural motor learning in Parkinson's disease: the effect of practice on continuous compensatory postural regulation. Gait Posture [Internet]. 2017;57:299–304. Available from: http://www.ncbi.nlm.nih.gov/pubmed/28688367.
88. Payne AM, Hajcak G, Ting LH. Dissociation of muscle and cortical response scaling to balance perturbation acceleration. J Neurophysiol. 2019;121(3):867–80.
89. Grillner S, Hellgren J, Menard A, Saitoh K, Wikstrom MA. Mechanisms for selection of basic motor programs—roles for the striatum and pallidum. Trends Neurosci [Internet]. 2005;28(7):364–70. Available from: http://www.ncbi.nlm.nih.gov/pubmed/15935487.
90. Simieli L. Gait initiation and Parkinson's disease: influence of an obstacle, a cognition task and sensory information [Internet]. São Paulo State University (Unesp); 2021. Available from: http://hdl.handle.net/11449/216204.

Postural Control and Somatosensory Information: Effects of Aging and Parkinson's Disease

20

Ellen Lirani-Silva, Victor Spiandor Beretta, Alejandra Maria Franco Jimenez, and Lilian Teresa Bucken Gobbi

Abstract

Sensory information from visual, vestibular, and somatosensory systems plays an important role in postural control. Deficits in postural control performance are the primary cause of the increased number of falls during aging. Postural instability in older adults is related to a decline in sensory and motor function and this can be more evident when associated with Parkinson's disease (PD). Among the declines in the sensory systems, deficits in the somatosensory function have been identified in older adults and these appear to be even higher in people with PD. Evidence supporting the importance of the somatosensory system in postural control comes from experiments that artificially reduced sensitivity in the soles of the feet and studies involving individuals with compromised plantar sensation. In an attempt to improve somatosensory input, previous research has shown that artificially enhancing cutaneous information can improve postural control. This chapter aims to describe the postural control of neurologically healthy older adults and people with PD and highlight the importance of

E. Lirani-Silva (✉)
Translational and Clinical Research Institute, Faculty of Medical Sciences, Clinical Ageing Research Unit, Newcastle University, Newcastle upon Tyne, UK
e-mail: ellenlirani@gmail.com

V. S. Beretta
School of Technology and Sciences, Physical Education Department, São Paulo State University (Unesp), Presidente Prudente, Brazil

A. M. Franco Jimenez
Department of Physical Education and Sports, Universidad Industrial de Santander, Bucaramanga, Colombia

L. T. B. Gobbi (Deceased)
São Paulo State University (Unesp), Institute of Biosciences, Graduate Program in Movement Sciences, Posture and Gait Studies Laboratory (LEPLO), Rio Claro, Brazil

F. A. Barbieri et al. (eds.), *Locomotion and Posture in Older Adults*,
https://doi.org/10.1007/978-3-031-74123-4_20

somatosensory information to postural control in both populations. In addition, we will discuss some therapies using enhanced somatosensory information to improve postural control and, consequently, prevent or reduce falls.

Introduction

Falls have been reported as one of the primary causes of hospitalization of older adults and are the main consequence of changes in postural control [1, 2]. Postural control is a complex motor system based on the interaction of sensorimotor dynamic processes [3]. To maintain balance in static and dynamic activities, it is necessary to maintain the center of mass (CoM) of the body within the area of the supporting base, which is determined by the distance between the feet. Another strong influence factor for balance is the stability limit, which varies between individuals and relates to the oscillation of the CoP within the support base, and the larger the oscillation without imbalance, the greater the stability of the individual [4, 5]. The relation between the sensorial and motor systems is extremely important for individuals to demonstrate appropriate orientation and postural balance. However, significant alterations in these systems are observed during the aging process [6].

Older adults can present functional and structural changes, and these can interfere directly with the posture and position of body segments, setting the body in a forward posture position called stooped posture [7]. In addition, changes in kinetic parameters related to postural control are observed, such as an increase in the frequency and amplitude of center of pressure (CoP) in the anteroposterior and mediolateral directions [8].

Added to problems due to the aging process, diseases such as Parkinson's disease (PD) can further highlight motor and sensory deficits and, consequently, greater losses in postural control are observed. Postural instability is one of the main signs of PD and its causes are multifactorial. Changes in the integration of sensory information are suggested as one of the possible causes [9]. As older adults, people with PD can present a forward posture (stooped posture), causing a displacement in CoP to near the anterior boundary of the support base. Also, other symptoms such as rigidity and bradykinesia can be related to the physiopathology present in postural instability.

Besides those already mentioned, changes in the integration of sensory information from visual, somatosensory, and vestibular systems can negatively impact the postural control [6] of neurologically healthy older adults and people with PD. Specifically concerning the somatosensory system, mechanoreceptors in the sole of the foot play an important role in postural control. Research with artificial decreases in plantar sensitivity demonstrates this importance [10].

Alterations in plantar sensitivity have been commonly related to aging and PD [11, 12]. These changes have an important impact on postural instability and an increase in the number of falls [13]. Based on this, some studies have investigated the increase in somatosensory information of the sole of the foot in the postural control of older adults and people with PD [14, 15]. These studies are based on the fact that increased sensorial input could promote greater feedback to motor output.

In this way, this chapter aimed to describe the main alterations in postural control due to the aging process and the presence of PD. Regarding the somatosensory systems, we will focus specifically on the importance of the somatosensory system, in particular the role of the receptors in the sole of the feet, to postural control in both populations, older adults and people with PD. In addition, we will present changes in plantar sensitivity and their relationship to postural control. We will demonstrate intervention strategies with a focus on increased sensory input through stimulation of the sole of the foot, aiming to improve postural control, specifically through insoles.

Postural Control in Neurologically Healthy Older Adults

In the age group 18–60 years, postural control presents a stabilization phase. At this stage, improvements can be observed depending on the stimulus provided, where individuals who are more exposed to balance activities or orientation of posture may present better postural control. After this age and due to genetic (primary aging) and environmental factors (secondary aging) [6, 16], structural and functional alterations are observed [1, 17]. These factors determine changes in the nervous and musculoskeletal systems, among others, directly affecting postural control [16, 18, 19] and reflecting in an increased risk of falls and musculoskeletal complaints [1].

Postural control is defined as the body's position of dominance in space in order to maintain the proper relationship between body segments and the environment (orientation and postural alignment) and the ability to maintain the body in balance (postural stability) through the complex interaction between neural and musculoskeletal components [3, 20]. In postural control, guidance and stability are two distinct sensorimotor processes and act depending on the type of activity, performance, or biomechanical needs; some aspects can be common to both [6].

The neuronal component of motor, sensory, and integrative processes is affected by age, which is essential to ensure the anticipation and adaptation of postural control [20]. Visual and vestibular changes and even multi-sensory deficits (loss of more than one important sense for stability and mobility) are observed in the somatosensory system, resulting in adjustments to the senses in the postural control needed for sensory and motor selection strategies for a given task or environment [6, 21].

The somatosensory system is one of the systems affected by the aging process. Among the alterations observed is decreased tactile sensitivity mediated by Meissner's corpuscles and Pacinian corpuscles, due to a decrease in the number of receptors [21, 22]. These receptors are responsible for information on the distribution of the fast power during balance activities. Another system that presents alterations is the visual system, which is affected by multiple changes in the structure of the eye (the eye threshold is lower for observing an object, due to the smaller quantity of light transmitted to the retina). As a result, there is a decrease in the visual field and in the perception of contrast (contour and depth) providing difficulties in detecting body movements (body position and center of mass (CoM) travel speed) for a specific environment and an increase in the body oscillation. In relation to the vestibular system, the decline in function causes the absolute reference system to become less reliable, resulting in difficulty for the nervous system to deal with the information coming from the visual and somatosensory systems. This degeneration in the vestibular system can lead to changes in automatic postural adjustments, endangering balance [20, 21, 23].

A musculoskeletal component of postural control can occur through a reduction in overall height due to changes in the intervertebral discs (such as dehydration of the nucleus pulpous) [24] and a decrease in flexibility of the spine. In older adults, flexibility is affected by the formation of cross-bridges between collagen fibers, decreasing the elastic muscle component (elastin fibers) and brittle, cracked, and hardened cartilage. This decrease represents around 20% between 20 and 65 years (increasing after this period). Associated with this, there is a decrease in joint mobility (50%) and neuromuscular coordination (90%) [25, 26]. The deterioration in muscle function is associated not only with reduced strength and endurance but also with maximum and rapid forces [22, 27] and the biomechanical relationships between body segments and the environment.

Postural control is important to the complex and dynamic relationship between sensory information (perception) and motor actions (action) which affect balance and postural orientation [21, 23]. Older adults may have difficulty in changing the weighting of the various sensory modalities, as well as accommodating variations in the environment and goals of the movement. For this reason, individuals on a firm, stable surface, who primarily depend on somatosensory information, or individuals on an unsteady airfoil, who depend more on vestibular and visual information, may struggle to judge which sensory modality is dominant, depending on the conditions of postural support and specific motor behavior [6].

All these declines induce the older adult to adopt, for example, a flexed or tilted forward position [16, 20], resulting from changes in kinematic parameters and difficulty in minimizing the spontaneous inclination of the vertical posture. In older adults, the change in position of body segments is especially pronounced in the sagittal plane, forming a characteristic postural pattern (stooped posture) often seen in older adults [7]. This postural pattern is characterized by a forward head, protruding shoulders, increased thoracic kyphosis, lumbar lordosis, and reduction in hip and knee flexion [19, 20, 28–30]. This posture may result in a larger displacement of the CoM and higher oscillation of the CoP, making it difficult to maintain stability (static or dynamic) or affecting functional performance [19, 31, 32].

Other issues affected by aging are the kinetic parameters, such as changes in the ability to respond effectively to threats to the balance of different magnitudes and velocities. In older adults, changes in the CoM occur, and these changes cause modifications in the ground reaction force (GRF) that influence the maintenance of balance. Regarding the kinetic analysis, impairments can be observed by the CoP parameters such as the increase in the frequency and amplitude of the oscillation in the anteroposterior and mediolateral directions, the mean speed of COP displacement, the total length of the COP path, and area of sway, among others [8]. Highlighting these changes, some studies indicate that older adults fluctuate more than young adults in maintaining an upright posture in both eyes open and eyes closed conditions [2, 21, 33, 34]. Furthermore, there are greater amplitudes of COP in the anteroposterior direction in older adults compared with young adults and physically active older adults compared to inactive older adults.

In postural control, some balance maintenance strategies are observed in response to unexpected (compensatory strategies) and expected disturbances (anticipatory strategies). The most frequently studied strategies in this population are the hip strategy, ankle strategy, and step strategy. These are characterized by muscle synergies that enable the maintenance of balance and/or regaining stability [6, 23], allowing repositioning of the body using the moment of inertia to oppose CoM, controlling the oscillation speed and COP [35, 36].

The hip strategy is one of the most used strategies in older adults. It is characterized by activation of the anterior and posterior muscles in a distal proximal sequence to seek relocation of the center of gravity (CoG) by extending and flexing the hip joint. In this strategy, the muscular action is associated with backward balance corrections, avoiding a fall in that direction. The hip strategy is used for rapid and long disturbances or when the support surface is small. Another strategy used is the ankle strategy, which is characterized by activation of the anterior and posterior muscles of the ankle, thigh, and trunk, proximal to the distal sequence. In this strategy, older adults swing an inverted pendulum and achieve a change in position of the CoG by rotating around the ankle joint with a minimum movement of the hip and knee. This strategy can be observed in small, slow disturbances and when the support surface is large and firm. Finally, the step strategy can be observed in situations where sufficiently strong disturbances move the CoG outside the support base. It is characterized by the body's response through lower limb flexion, displacing the CoG downward with forward displacement of the foot, reconfiguring a new support base. This strategy is used when the previous two strategies are ineffective or during very long and very fast disruptions [6, 22, 23, 35, 36].

As shown, changes in postural control can interfere directly in quality of life of older adults and the main problem caused by these changes is falling. Added to the normal aging process, diseases can emerge. The second most prevalent neurodegenerative disease in the older population is Parkinson's disease (PD). People with PD present some signs and symptoms, and one of these is postural instability. The next topic will present some of the alterations in postural control of people with PD and some explanations about the possible causes of these alterations.

Postural Control in People with Parkinson's Disease

Approximately 6 million people are affected by PD nowadays [37]. PD is considered the second most common neurodegenerative disease [38]. The number of people with Parkinson's disease PD is anticipated to rise significantly, driven by an aging population and increasing life expectancy. Projections indicate that by 2040, the number of individuals with PD worldwide will reach over 12 million [39]. PD occurs due to progressive degeneration of dopaminergic neurons in the substantia nigra pars compacta of the brain. Dopamine is a neurotransmitter that regulates the motor activity [20, 40]. Such a decrease in dopamine levels inhibits the thalamus-cortical motor systems and those located in the brainstem, compromising other brain structures [41] and causing motor damage [42]. PD is characterized by four cardinal symptoms: bradykinesia, resting tremor, rigidity, and postural instability [43–49].

Specifically, postural instability predominantly appears during the advanced stages of PD and can be affected by various causes. Other symptoms, such as rigidity and bradykinesia, can interfere with postural reactions, leading to a slower response to balance perturbation. In addition, other factors such as fear of falling and changes in sensory integration are possible causes of postural instability [42, 50]. Many individuals in moderate and advanced stages of PD present a posture with the upper body leaning forward and the head forward to the trunk, which is called the stooped posture. This position may be associated with postural instability as it moves the CoP near the limit of the support base [51].

Impairments in the integration of sensory information are the major reason for the changes in postural control. The proprioceptive system provides inside information on tensions and stretching of the muscle and joint positions and can contribute to the orientation of the body in relation to gravity. Thus, it is believed that the deficit in sensory-motor integration could be responsible for the stability deficit in PD [9]. Individuals with PD present a decline in the ability to adequately control the body orientation through failure in the integration of sensory information.

Another problem based on postural control in PD is hypometria, which can contribute to changes in balance recovery after a postural disorder [5]. This change can be observed even after the use of drugs for dopaminergic replacement, where the pharmacological treatment does not seem to reduce the postural instability of people with PD, as has been well described in the literature [52–54]. Based on the observations, it was hypothesized that the deficit in proprioceptive integration is primarily due to the degeneration of the supplementary motor area, which is crucial for planning and executing motor actions. This area has abundant dopaminergic innervation and is connected to the basal ganglia, which further supports this hypothesis. Among the additional evidence of proprioceptive integration in PD, it is the dependence on visual information for posture maintenance [55]. This greater dependence is evident from the fact that individuals cannot differentiate the importance of sensory information in the absence of vision, increasing the rigidity of the lower oscillation system by the CoP. In the absence of visual sensory integration, declines are more evident, demonstrating that individuals with PD have difficulty properly using proprioceptive information to create movement strategies [56].

Together with changes in the integration of sensory information, a lower limit of stability can be observed in individuals with PD, possibly caused by postures characteristic of the disease, such as hip, knee, and ankle flexion requiring greater antigravity forces for posture control [57]. In addition to the posture characteristic of the disease, other symptoms such as rigidity and bradykinesia may be related to the pathophysiology of postural instability. Bradykinesia is related to decreased dopamine in the basal ganglia caused by inhibition of the movement of the cerebral cortex [58]. This characteristic of slowness of movement [59–62] can be observed in individuals with postural control deficits, making it difficult for them to properly recruit muscle fibers for movement [63]. This slowness has an important influence on the musculoskeletal system and affects the reaction of postural responses. Due to the dysfunction of the basal ganglia caused by PD, changes are made in the automatic movements such as postural control, demanding more compensation from the cortex. Thus, there is a need for greater attention even in automatic movements, hindering the achievement of other concurrent tasks, both motor and cognitive. Despite the lack of knowledge on the pathophysiology of postural instability, postural control is due to the involvement of different afferent and efferent neural structures [64, 65]. The causes of postural control impairments are multifactorial for people with PD [66].

Studies on static and dynamic postural control in PD are very important for a better understanding of the changes caused by the disease, for example, the increase in asymmetry in postural control [67–71]. Beretta and colleagues [68] found increases in asymmetry in postural control in people with PD, mainly during challenging tasks. In addition to the complexity of the task, the stage of disease and the state of PD medication impact the asymmetry in postural control in this population (i.e., PD medication decreases the asymmetry of postural control in individuals with mild stage of disease) [69]. In addition, the asymmetry of postural control was positively associated with postural oscillation [70], which may increase the risk of falls in people with PD. Impaired postural control is a major cause of the increased risk of falls in this population [53, 54, 65, 66, 72, 73], the number of falls increases by two or three times in PD [74, 75], and complications of falls are the second leading cause of hospitalization [76]. Williams and colleagues [77] showed that 16.9% of falls in people with PD resulted in fractures.

Specifically for dynamic postural control, people with PD present inadequate responses to postural disturbances, an inability to modulate postural responses, delays or reduction in compensatory responses, inadequate arm movements to maintain balance, and deficits in somatosensory integration [53, 54, 72, 73]. Furthermore, inadequate muscular responses were found after posture disturbance [4, 72, 78, 79].

Older adults and people with PD can present changes in the integration of sensory information. Specifically in relation to the somatosensory system, some studies have shown that decreases in integrity of the receptors of the sole of the foot can influence postural control. The next topic will present changes in plantar sensibility caused by aging and PD and how these changes can negatively impact postural control. In addition, some somatosensory therapies will be presented, especially using insoles, with a focus on the benefits to postural control.

Somatosensory Information and Postural Control in Older Adults and People with PD: Role, Changes, and Therapies

As mentioned previously, changes in postural control can be multifactorial. Declines in the integration of sensory information from visual, somatosensory, and vestibular systems can play an important role in these changes. Specifically, regarding the somatosensory system, receptors in the sole of the foot play an important role in postural control. These receptors (mechanoreceptors) send information to the central nervous system on changes in pressure distribution, mainly in relation to vertical body position [80, 81].

In a study by Kennedy and Inglis [80], the authors evaluated the distribution and activity of the receptors of the sole of the foot and classified these mechanoreceptors according to the response of the stimuli and receptive field size. The authors were able to classify the receptors into four types: (a) slowly adapting type I; (b) slowly adapting type II; (c) fast adapting type I; and (d) fast adapting type II. Receptors of type I presented numerous receptive points and distribution in a small receptive field and receptors of type II presented a single receptive point, however, with large fields. The distribution of the receptors and the sensation they provide enable the somatosensory system to provide information of great importance for balance control, since in humans the feet are the only part in contact with the environment [82, 83]. This contact allows the plantar receptors to perceive information on temporal and spatial contact pressure of the feet with the ground, facilitating, for example, the control of compensatory reactions [84].

Considering the characteristics of the receptors of the sole of the foot and the importance of the information they provide, some studies have used a reduction in plantar sensory (mechanoreceptors) feedback, to highlight the role of these receptors for postural control. Billot and colleagues [10] investigated the effects of plantar sensitivity reduction, achieved through immersion of the feet in ice (cooling procedure), on balance control in neurologically healthy adults. For the cooling procedure, the feet of the participants were immersed in water between 0 °C and 2 °C for a total of 12 min. Next, the participants performed the balance control protocol on a force plate in the bipedal position. Seven trials of 30 s each were performed. The authors found that, after the cooling procedure, short-term changes were observed in balance control. There was an increase in CoP velocity and RMS of the velocity of CoP in the anterior–posterior and mediolateral directions. In addition to this study, findings of other studies in people with reduced somatosensation (e.g., diabetic neuropathy) also found changes in postural control [85]. As observed by Billot and colleagues [10], losses in somatosensory information could be the primary cause of these changes.

As shown so far, the integrity of the somatosensory system, especially in the sole of the foot, has an important role in postural control. However, due to the aging process, changes in the somatosensory system can be observed. Some studies show that older adults have higher thresholds of perception of vibratory stimulus and may experience difficulties in mild touch perception in some regions of the plantar surface when compared with young adults [11]. The main aspects that can influence these differences are: a) reduction in the total number of receptors; b) irregular distribution of receptors; c) morphological changes in receptors; d) reduction in skin elasticity, due to the smaller quantities of elastin and collagen [11, 86]. Specifically in relation to the age that changes can be accentuated, Perry [11] found that, from 70 years old, there is a sharp increase in vibration thresholds.

Based on the highlighted changes and considering the important role of mechanoreceptors of the sole of the foot in postural control, some studies have investigated the relation between changes in plantar sensibility, due to the aging process, and postural control. Menz and colleagues [87] verified that tactile plantar sensibility was strongly related to postural sway. In another study, Ueda and Carpes [88] verified a positive correlation between plantar sensitivity and postural control in older adults, specifically in the area and anteroposterior displacement of CoP. Individuals with less plantar sensitivity demonstrated a greater area and displacement of CoP. It is also important to highlight that changes in plantar sensitivity have been associated with an increased number of falls in older adults [13] and, in addition to this decrease in sensitivity, older adults have difficulty in processing and integrating sensory information [89].

As well as changes resulting from the aging process, older adults are more likely to have diseases that alter both sensitivity and integration of sensory information. Diseases such as atherosclerosis and diabetes can damage the somatosensory system and, consequently, reduce peripheral sensitivity [90]. Another disease that commonly affects older adults is PD. People with PD present more pronounced deficits in both sensory integration and peripheral sensory function when compared to healthy people [12]. Specifically in relation to plantar sensitivity of people with PD, Prätorius, Kimmeskamp & Milani [12] found that individuals with PD have higher sensitivity thresholds when compared with neurologically healthy individuals. The same authors also found a correlation between the somatosensory system and motor deficits in people with PD, where individuals with greater motor impairment presented higher plantar sensitivity thresholds. As in other studies, the authors highlight the fact that deficits in somatosensation can directly affect balance control in people with PD and individuals in later stages could present more pronounced deficits. In general, deficits in peripheral sensory function generate less sensory input. Due to this decreased input and added to the fact that people with PD have deficits in motor-sensory integration [91] less feedback to the motor output is generated, possibly explaining some deficits in the postural control.

Considering the impact of reduced plantar sensation on postural control, some studies have investigated the benefits of an increase in sensorial information of the sole of the foot on the postural control of neurologically healthy older adults and those with PD. These studies were based on the fact that an increase in sensory input would promote better feedback to the motor output and, consequently, benefit postural control.

Specifically in neurologically healthy older adults, Palluel, Nougier, and Oliver [14] verified the immediate and temporary benefits of increases in sensory input on postural control with eyes closed. To increase sensory input, the authors used sandals with an insole covered with an array of spikes. The evaluations of postural control with eyes closed were conducted immediately after the use of sandals and after two different protocols: (i) 5 min standing quietly in an upright position wearing sandals with the insole and 5 min without sensory stimulation; (ii) 5 min walking wearing sandals with the insole and 5 min walking without sensory stimulation. The authors did not find immediate effects of using the sandals with the insoles on healthy older adults. After 5 min of use while standing quietly in an upright position, a decrease in CoP area and anteroposterior RMS was verified. A decrease in CoP medium velocity and mediolateral RMS was also found for both the 5 min standing quietly in an upright position protocol and the 5 min walking protocol using an insole covered with an array of spikes. The authors suggest that the insole provides important tactile information about the corporal position in relation to verticality.

In another study, Qiu and colleagues [92] investigated the effects of different densities of insoles (barefoot, soft, and hard) with granulations on postural control of older adults. The older adults were evaluated in two different conditions of standing surface (firm and foam), with eyes open and closed. The authors verified a reduction in CoP area (especially on the foam surface using a soft insole), in path length and anteroposterior (both textured insoles on a foam surface), and mediolateral (both insoles on both surface conditions) sways. With eyes closed, older adults presented a decrease in mediolateral sway, path length, and CoP area, for both insoles on the foam surface. Based on these findings, the authors concluded that insoles with sensorial stimulation can reduce postural sway, especially in more challenging tasks, such as an unstable surface and eyes closed. As a possible explanation, Qiu and colleagues [92] showed that increased plantar pressure produced by textured insoles promoted higher stimulation of mechanoreceptors in this region. Consequently, there was an increase in feedback of cutaneous receptors to the central nervous system and, thus, an improvement in postural control.

Although some studies demonstrate the great potential of the use of additional somatosensory information on postural control of older adults, the use of this paradigm has been more restricted in research with people with PD. Qiu and colleagues [15] investigated postural control in people with PD and older adults in different insole conditions (barefoot, smooth insole, and textured insole), with and without visual information, on a firm and foam surface. The authors verified that for people with PD, there was a reduction in mediolateral sway when individuals were using the smooth insole or textured insole. Only the textured insole promoted a benefit to mediolateral sway and standard deviation during postural task on both firm and foam surfaces, with eyes open and closed. However, greater benefits were observed in people with PD when they used a textured insole, on a foam surface with eyes closed.

Nakano and colleagues [93] investigated the effects of insoles with a toe-grip bar on balance. Participants were included in two different groups: one wearing shoes without any extra plantar stimulation and another group wearing shoes having insoles with toe-grip bar. The intervention had a duration of 4 weeks. The center of gravity sway of standing posture (total trajectory length, envelope area, and maximum anterior–posterior center of pressure [AP-COP] distance) was measured pre- and post-intervention with participants being barefoot. The authors observed that the AP-COP distance was significantly improved in the intervention group compared to the control group, which indicates that insoles with a toe-grip bar may improve balance in people with PD.

As shown, neurologically healthy older adults present significant alterations in plantar sensibility and these changes directly affect postural control. Added to the aging process, the emergence of some diseases, such as PD, can further negatively affect the role of mechanoreceptors in the sole of the foot as well as the information processing coming from the somatosensory system. Strategies that offer an increase in somatosensory information, such as insole therapies, seem to be efficient and low cost for older people and people with PD. It is important to highlight that the results presented by the literature are encouraging in relation to applicability of insole therapy.

Final Considerations

This chapter provides important information about changes in postural control of neurologically healthy older adults and people with PD, highlighting the fact that the causes of the emergence of these changes are multifactorial. Deficits in processing and sensory integration are among the main causes and deficits in the somatosensory system explored in this chapter.

The role of plantar receptors and the importance of their integrity to postural control were evidenced. Both older adults and people with PD can present structural changes in mechanoreceptors distributed on the plantar surface, higher thresholds of stimuli perception, and difficulty in integration of information resulting from the somatosensory system. Based on these changes, some studies have investigated the relation between changes in plantar sensitivity and postural control in older adults and, especially for people with PD, changes in plantar sensibility and motor symptoms. It was verified that individuals with greater thresholds present changes in postural control and worse motor symptoms.

Considering the impact of decreased plantar sensitivity on postural control, we presented some studies that used additional somatosensory information in the sole of the foot (insole) as an intervention to benefit postural control in older adults and people with PD. Although some studies were found using this kind of intervention in neurologically healthy older adults, studies with people with PD are still limited. In both cases, the reported results are encouraging regarding the contributions of this type of intervention. The use of insoles seems to be an efficient, low cost and, principally, a simple intervention that can be easily used in the daily life of older adults and people with PD. However, further studies are necessary which explore the chronic use of insoles to detect possible adaptations of the receptors to continuous stimulus.

References

1. Farinatti PTV. Envelhecimento: Promoção da saúde e exercício. Barueri: Manole; 2013. p. 277.
2. Blaszczyk JW, Lowe DL, Hansen PD. Ranges of postural stability and their changes in the elderly. Gait Posture. 1994;2:11–7.
3. Horak FB. Postural orientation and equilibrium: what do we need to know about neural control of balance to prevent falls? Age Ageing. 2006;35(2):ii7–ii11.
4. Horak FB, Dimitrova D, Nutt JG. Direction-specific postural instability in subjects with Parkinson's disease. Exp Neurol. 2005;193(2):504–21.
5. Pollock AS, Durward BR, Rowe PJ, Paul JP. What is balance? Clin Rehabil. 2000;14(4):402–6.
6. Macpherson JM, Horak FB. Postura. In: Kandel E, Schwartz J, et al., editors. Princípios de Neurociências, vol. 5. Mc Graw Hill Education; 2014. p. 811–22.
7. Kendall FP, McCreary EK, Provance PG, Rodgers MM, Romani WA. Músculos Provas e Funções. Postura e Dor. 5th ed. Manole; 2007. p. 453.
8. Lemos LFC, Ribeiro JS, Mota CB. Correlações entre o centro de massa e o centro de pressão em idosos ativos. R Bras Ci e Mov. 2015;23(1):31–9.
9. Vaugoyeau M, Viel S, Assaiante C, Amblard B, Azulay JP. Impaired vertical postural control and proprioceptive integration deficits in Parkinson's disease. Neuroscience. 2007;146(2):852–63.
10. Billot M, Handrigana GA, Simoneaua M, Corbeila P, Teasdalea N. Short term alteration of balance control after a reduction of plantar mechanoreceptor sensation through cooling. Neurosci Lett. 2013;535:40–4.
11. Perry SD. Evaluation of age-related plantar-surface insensitivity and onset age of advanced insensitivity in older adults using vibratory and touch sensation tests. Neurosci Lett. 2006;392:62–7.
12. Prätorius B, Kimmeskamp S, Milani TL. The sensitivity of the sole of the foot in patients with Morbus Parkinson. Neurosci Lett. 2003;346:173–6.
13. Lord SR, Ward JA, Williams P, Anstey KJ. Physiological factors associated with falls in older community-dwelling women. J Am Geriatr Soc. 1994;42:1110–7.
14. Palluel E, Nougier V, Oliver I. Do spike insoles enhance postural stability and plantar–surface cutaneous sensitivity in the elderly? Age. 2008;30:53–61.
15. Qiu F, Cole MH, Davids KW, Henning EM, Silburn PA, Netscher H, Kerr GK. Effects of textured insoles on balance in people with Parkinson's disease. PLoS One. 2013;8:e83309.
16. Del Rosso, S. Fisiología del envejecimieto: cambios estructurales y funcionales EDICIÓN, P.: Grupo Sobre Entrenamiento 2010.
17. Okuma SS. O idoso e a atividade física: Fundamentos e pesquisa. Campinas: Papirus; 1998.
18. Redín, MI. Envejecimiento y entrenamiento de fuerza: adaptaciones neuromusculares y hormonales: Grupo Sobre Entrenamiento 2010.
19. Valduga R, Valduga LVA, Almeida JÁ, Carvalho GA. Relação entre o padrão postural e o nível de atividade física em idosas. R Bras Ci e Mov. 2013;21(3):5–12.
20. Shumway-Cook A, Woollacott MH. Controle Motor. Teoria e aplicações práticas. 2nd ed. Barueri: Manole; 2003.
21. Júnior PF, Barela JA. Alterações no funcionamento do sistema de controle postural de idosos. Uso da informação visual. Rev Port Cien Desp. 2006;6(1):94–105.
22. Sturnieks DL, George RST, Lord SR. Balance disorders in the elderly. Neurophysiol Clin. 2008;38(6):467–78.
23. Winter DA. Human balance and posture control during standing and walking. Gait Posture. 1995;3(4):193–214.
24. Brito, J. Efeitos de um programa de treino da força, a dois níveis de intensidade, na força máxima e na massa isenta de gordura de mulheres idosas. Lisboa. Dissertação (Mestrado em especialidade de Exercício e Saúde); faculdade de Motricidade Humana 1997.
25. American College of Sports Medicine, Chodzko-Zajko WJ, Proctor DN, Fiatarone Singh MA, Minson CT, Nigg CR, Salem GJ, Skinner JS. American College of Sports Medicine

position stand. Exercise and physical activity for older adults. Med Sci Sports Exerc. 2009;41(7):1510–30. Disponível em: http://www.ncbi.nlm.nih.gov/pubmed/19516148.
26. Coelho FG, Gobbi S, Costa JLR, Gobbi LTB. Exercício Físico no envelhecimento saudável e patológico: Da teoria à prática. Curitiba: CVR; 2013. p. 462.
27. Hunter GR, Mccarthy JP, Bamman MM. Effects of resistance training on older adults. Sports Med. 2004;34(5):329–48.
28. Guccione AA. Fisioterapia Geriátrica. Rio de Janeiro: Guanabara; 2002. p. 470.
29. Lamotte ACS. Contribuições da musculação na postura em portadores de escoliose estrutural [dissertação]. Brasilia: Universidade Catolica de Brasília.Mestrado em Educação Física; 2003.
30. Hinman MR. Comparison of thoracic kyphosis and postural stiffness in younger and older women. Spine J. 2004;4:413–7.
31. Faria JDC, Machala CC, Dias RC, Dias JMD. The importance of strength training programs for the rehabilitation of muscle function, equilibrium and mobility of the elderly. Acta Fisiátrica. 2003;10(3):133–7.
32. Da Silveira MM, Pasqualotti A, Colussi AE, Wibelinger LM. Human aging and body posture changes in the elderly. Revista Brasileira de Ciências da Saúde. 2010;8(26):52–8.
33. Blaszczyk J, Hansen P, Lowe D. Postural sway and perception of the upright stance stability borders. Perception. 1993;22:1333.
34. Collins JJ, De Luca CJ, Burrows A, Lipsitz LA. Age-related changes in open-loop and closed-loop postural control mechanisms. Exp Brain Res. 1995;104(3):480–92.
35. Bok SK, Lee TH, Lee SS. The effects of changes of ankle strength and range of motion according to aging on balance. Ann Rehabil Med. 2013;37(1):10–6.
36. Nagai K, Yamada M, Mori S, Tanaka B, Uemura K, Aoyama T, Ichihashi N, Tsuboyama T. Effect of the muscle coactivation during quiet standing on dynamic postural control in older adults. Arch Gerontol Geriatr. 2013;56(1):129–33.
37. GBD 2016 Neurology Collaborators. Global, regional, and national burden of neurological disorders, 1990-2016: a systematic analysis for the global burden of disease study 2016. Lancet Neurol. 2019;18(5):459–80. https://doi.org/10.1016/S1474-4422(18)30499-X. Epub 2019 Mar 14. PMID: 30879893; PMCID: PMC6459001.
38. De Lau LM, Breteler MM. Epidemiology of Parkinson's disease. Lancet Neurol. 2006;5(6):525–35.
39. Dorsey ER, Bloem BR. The Parkinson pandemic-a call to action. JAMA Neurol. 2018;75(1):9–10. https://doi.org/10.1001/jamaneurol.2017.3299. PMID: 29131880.
40. Saito M, Marayuama M, Ikeuchi K, Kondo H, Ishikawa A, Yuasa T, Tsuji S. Autosomal recessive juvenile parkinsonism. Brain and Development. 2000;22:S115–7.
41. Obeso JÁ, Rodriguez-Oroz MC, Rodriguez M, Lanciego JL, Artieda J, Gonzalo N, Olanow CW. Pathophysiology of the basal ganglia in Parkinson's disease. Trends Neurosci. 2000;23(10):S8–19.
42. Takakusaki K, Saitoh K, Harada H, Kashiwayanagi M. Role of basal ganglia-brainstem pathways in the control of motor behaviors. Neurosci Res. 2004;50(2):137–51.
43. Nutt GJ. Motor fluctuations and dyskinesia in Parkinson's disease. Parkinsonism Relat Disord. 2001;8(2):101–8.
44. Morris EM, Huxham F, McGinley J, Dodd K, Iansek R. The biomechanics and motor control of gait in Parkinson disease. Clin Biomech. 2001;16(6):459–70.
45. Morris M, Iansek R, McGinley J, Matyas T, Huxham F. Three-dimensional gait biomechanics in Parkinson's disease: evidence for a centrally mediated amplitude regulation disorder. Mov Disord. 2005;20:40–50.
46. Pieruccini-Faria F, Menuchi MRTP, Vitório R, Gobbi LTB, Stella F, Gobbi S. Parâmetros cinemáticos da marcha com obstáculos em idosos com doença de Parkinson, com e sem efeito da Levodopa: um estudo piloto. Rev Bras Fisioter. 2006;10(2):243–9.
47. Vitório R, Pieruccini-Faria F, Stella F, Gobbi S, Gobbi LTB. Effects of obstacle height on obstacle crossing in mild Parkinson's disease. Gait Posture. 2010;31:143–6.

48. Vitório R, Lirani-Silva E, Barbieri FA, Raile V, Stella F, Gobbi LTB. Influence of visual feedback sampling on obstacle crossing behavior in people with Parkinson's disease. Gait Posture. 2013;38(2):330–4.
49. Barbieri FA, Rinaldi NM, Santos PC, Lirani-Silva E, Vitorio R, Teixeira-Arroyo C, Stella F, Gobbi LTB. Functional capacity of Brazilian patients with parkinson's disease (PD): relationship between clinical characteristics and disease severity. Arch Gerontol Geriatr. 2012;54(2):83–8.
50. Jankovic J. Parkinson's disease: clinical features and diagnosis. J Neurol Neurosurg Psychiatry. 2008;79:368–76.
51. Jacobs JV, Dimitrova DM, Nutt JG, Horak FB. Can stooped posture explain multidirectional postural instability in patients with Parkinson's disease? Exp Brain Res. 2005;166:78–88.
52. Bloem BR, Beckley DJ, van Dijk JG, Zwinderman AH, Remler MP, Roos RA. Influence of dopaminergic medication on automatic postural responses and balance impairment in Parkinson's disease. Mov Disord. 1996;11(5):509–21.
53. Bloem BR, Grimbergen YAM, Cramer M. Prospective assessment of falls in Parkinson's disease. J Neurol. 2001a;248:950–8.
54. Bloem BR, Van Vugt JP, Beckley DJ. Postural instability and falls in Parkinson's disease. Adv Neurol. 2001b;87:209–23.
55. Brown LA, Cooper SA, Doan JB, Dickin DC, Whishaw IQ, Pellis SM, Suchowersky O. Parkinsonian deficits in sensory integration for postural control: temporal response to changes in visual input. Parkinsonism Relat Disord. 2006;12(6):376–81.
56. Tagliabue M, Ferrigno G, Horak F. Effects of Parkinson's disease on proprioceptive control of posture and reaching while standing. Neuroscience. 2009;158(4):1206–14.
57. Mancini M, Rocchi L, Horak FB, Chiari L. Effects of Parkinson's disease and levodopa on functional limits of stability. Clin Biomech. 2008;23(4):450–8.
58. Bergman J, Madras BK, Spealman RD. Behavioral effects of D1 and D2 dopamine receptor antagonists in squirrel monkeys. J Pharmacol ExpTher. 1991;258(3):910–7.
59. Flowers K. Ballistic and corrective movements on an aiming task. Intention tremor and parkinsonian movement disorders compared. Neurology. 1975;25(5):413–21.
60. Horak FB, Frank J, Nutt J. Effects of dopamine on postural control in parkinsonian subjects: scaling, set, and tone. J Neurophysiol. 1996;75(6):2380–96.
61. Pfann KD, Buchman AS, Comella CL, Corcos DM. Control of movement distance in Parkinson's disease. Mov Disord. 2001;16(6):1048–65.
62. Van Gemmert AW, Adler CH, Stelmach GE. Parkinson's disease patients undershoot target size in handwriting and similar tasks. J Neurol Neurosurg Psychiatry. 2003;74(11):1502–8.
63. Berardelli A, Dick JP, Rothwell JC, Day BL, Marsden CD. Scaling of the size of the first agonist EMG burst during rapid wrist movements in patients with Parkinson's disease. J Neurol Neurosurg Psychiatry. 1986;49(11):1273–9.
64. Boonstra TA, Van Der Kooij H, Munneke M, Bloem BR. Gait disorders and balance disturbances in Parkinson's disease: clinical update and pathophysiology. Curr Opin Neurol. 2008;21(4):461–71.
65. Błaszczyk JW, Orawiec R. Assessment of postural control in patients with Parkinson's disease: sway ratio analysis. Hum Mov Sci. 2011;30(2):396–404.
66. Benatru I, Vaugoyeau M, Azulay JP. Postural disorders in Parkinson's disease. Neurophysiol Clin. 2008;38:459–65.
67. Geurts AC, Boonstra TA, Voermans NC, Diender MG, Weerdesteyn V, Bloem BR. Assessment of postural asymmetry in mild to moderate Parkinson's disease. Gait Posture. 2011;33(1):143–5.
68. Beretta VS, Gobbi LTB, Lirani-Silva E, Simieli L, Orcioli-Silva D, Barbieri FA. Challenging postural tasks increase asymmetry in patients with Parkinson's disease. PLoS One. 2015;10:e0137722.
69. Barbieri FA, Polastri PF, Baptista AM, Lirani-Silva E, Simieli L, Orcioli-Silva D, Beretta VS, Gobbi LTB. Effects of disease severity and medication state on postural control asymmetry during challenging postural tasks in individuals with Parkinson's disease. Hum Mov Sci. 2016;46:96–103.

70. Boonstra TA, van Vugt JP, van der Kooij H, Bloem BR. Balance asymmetry in Parkinson's disease and its contribution to freezing of gait. PLoS One. 2014;9(7):e102493. https://doi.org/10.1371/journal.pone.0102493. PMID: 25032994; PMCID: PMC4102504.
71. Boonstra TA, Schouten AC, van Vugt JP, Bloem BR, van der Kooij H. Parkinson's disease patients compensate for balance control asymmetry. J Neurophysiol. 2014;112(12):3227–39.
72. Carpenter MG, Allum JH, Honegger F, Adkin AL, Bloem BR. Postural abnormalities to multidirectional stance perturbations in Parkinson's disease. J Neurol Neurosurg Psychiatry. 2004;75(9):1245–54.
73. Rocchi L, Chiari L, Horak FB. Effects of deep brain stimulation and levodopa on postural sway in Parkinson's disease. J Neurol Neurosurg Psychiatry. 2002;73:267–74.
74. Bloem BR, Hausdorff JM, Visser JE, Giladi N. Falls and freezing of gait in Parkinson's disease: a review of two interconnected, episodic phenomena. Mov Disord. 2004;19(8):871–84.
75. Pickering RM, Grimbergen YA, Rigney U, Ashburn A, Mazibrada G. Wood B.A meta-analysis of six prospective studies of falling in Parkinson's disease. Mov Disord. 2007;22:1892–900.
76. Temlett JA, Thompson PD. Reasons for admission to hospital for Parkinson's disease. Intern Med J. 2006;36(8):524–6.
77. Williams DR, Watt HC, Lees AJ. Predictors of falls and fractures in bradykinetic rigid syndromes: a retrospective study. J Neurol Neurosurg Psychiatry. 2006;77:468–73.
78. Dimitrova D, Horak FB, Nutt JG. Postural muscle responses to multidirectional translations in patients with Parkinson's disease. J Neurophysiol. 2004a;91(1):489–501.
79. Dimitrova D, Nutt JG, Horak FB. Abnormal force patterns for multidirectional postural responses in patients with Parkinson's disease. Exp Brain Res. 2004b;156:183–95.
80. Kennedy PM, Inglis JT. Distribution and behavior of glabrous cutaneous receptors in the human foot sole. J Physiol. 2002;538:995–1002.
81. Hijmans JM, Geertzen JHB, Dijkstra PU, Postema K. A systematic review of the effects of shoes and other ankle or foot appliances on balance in older people and people with peripheral nervous system disorders. Gait Posture. 2007;25:316–23.
82. Maki BE, Mcilroy WE. Postural control in the older adult. Clin Geriatr Med. 1996;12:635–58.
83. Eils E, Behrens S, Mers O, Thorwesten L, Völker K, Rosenbauma D. Reduced plantar sensation causes a cautious walking pattern. Gait Posture. 2004;20:54–60.
84. Perry SD, William E, Mcilroy WE, Makia BE. The role of plantar cutaneous mechanoreceptors in the control of compensatory stepping reactions evoked by unpredictable, multi-directional perturbation. Brain Res. 2000;877:401–6.
85. Kars HJ, Hijmans JM, Geertzen JH, Zijlstra W. The effect of reduced somatosensation on standing balance: a systematic review. J Diabetes Sci Technol. 2009;3:931–43.
86. Wells C, Ward LM, Chua R, Inglis JT. Regional variation and changes with ageing in vibrotactile sensitivity in the human footsole. J Gerontol A Biol Sci. 2003;58(8):680–6.
87. Menz HB, Morris ME, Lord SR. Foot and ankle characteristics associated with impaired balance and functional ability in older people. J Gerontol A Med Sci. 2005;60A:1546–52.
88. Ueda LS, Carpes FP. Relationship between foot sensibility and postural control in the young and elderly. Rev Bras Cineantropom Desempenho Hum. 2013;15:215–24.
89. Matsumura BA, Ambrose AF. Balance in the elderly. Clin Geriatr Med. 2006;22:395–412.
90. Konrad HR, Girardi M, Helfert R. Balance and aging. Laryngoscope. 1999;109:1454–60.
91. Abbruzzese G, BerardelliA. Sensorimotor integration in movement disorders. Mov Disord. 2003;18(3):231–40.
92. Qiu F, Cole MH, Davids KW, Henning EM, Silburn PA, Netscher H, Kerr GK. Enhanced somatosensory information decreases postural sway in older people. Gait Posture. 2012;35:630–5.
93. Nakano H, Murata S, Nakae H, Soma M, Isida H, Maruyama Y, Nagara H, Nagara Y. Effects of insole with toe-grip Bar on barefoot balance and walking function in patients with Parkinson's disease: a randomized controlled trial. Geriatrics (Basel). 2022;7(6):128. https://doi.org/10.3390/geriatrics7060128. PMID: 36412617; PMCID: PMC9680307.

New Insights for Identifying Dynamic Postural Instability in Early Stages of Parkinson's Disease

21

Ana Maria Forti Barela, Douglas Vicente Russo-Junior, Giovanna Athanásio Chaves Machado, and José Angelo Barela

Abstract

The goal of the present study was to analyze the dynamic postural instability of individuals in the early stages of Parkinson's disease (PD) in relation to non-disabled individuals using the statistical parametric mapping analysis. Sixteen individuals with PD (67.2 ± 4.4 years old, Hoehn and Yahr 1 and 2) and 16 non-disabled individuals (67.4 ± 4.8 years old) were assessed performing gait initiation. The distance between center of mass (CoM) and center of pressure (CoP), and ground reaction forces (GRF) components (i.e., vertical and horizontal mediolateral and anterior–posterior) were the main parameters investigated. Overall, the individuals with PD presented reduced distance between CoM and CoP and reduced GRF in the three components compared to their peers. These results suggest that postural instability is present in early stages of PD. Intervention protocols should comprise physical exercises that promote balance improvement even for individuals in early stages of PD.

A. M. F. Barela (✉) · D. V. Russo-Junior · G. A. C. Machado
Institute of Physical Activity and Sport Sciences, Cruzeiro do Sul University, São Paulo, SP, Brazil

J. A. Barela
Laboratory for Movement Studies, Department of Physical Education, Institute of Biosciences, São Paulo State University (UNESP), Rio Claro, SP, Brazil
e-mail: jose.barela@unesp.br

F. A. Barbieri et al. (eds.), *Locomotion and Posture in Older Adults*,
https://doi.org/10.1007/978-3-031-74123-4_21

Introduction

Contrary to standing still, in which the main task is to keep the body's center of mass (CoM) within the base of support in a safe way, when one starts to move forward, the criterion of balance is considerably altered [1]. The transition between standing still and walking is referred to gait initiation [2], a motor task commonly employed to investigate those with balance impairment, such as individuals with Parkinson's Disease (PD) [3]. One of the reasons to investigate gait initiation in PD is related to the fact that during gait initiation, the base of support diminishes (from double support to single support) as the CoM advances forward outside of it, and the first step is taken. Such fact increases postural instability, challenging the postural control system. Hence, gait initiation seems an appropriate motor task to investigate dynamic postural instability in individuals with PD.

It is important to note that PD is a multisystem neurodegenerative disorder with motor and nonmotor features [4], being the motor symptoms and signs mainly attributed to the loss of dopaminergic neurons [5]. Although these individuals also develop disturbances related to postural control and gait that are less dopamine-responsive [6], such disturbances are still caused by typical impairment in dopaminergic systems and its pathways [7]. The disorder leads to motor impairment and risk of falls, comprising their life quality.

Among different aspects of gait initiation that might be investigated in individuals with PD, the main focus of this chapter is on the relationship between the CoM and the center of pressure (CoP), as gait initiation cannot start without the separation of them [8], and in turns comprise the balance control of the whole body. Briefly, the CoM is an imaginary point that corresponds to the equilibrium of total body mass [9] that moves as a particle that is subject to external force [10]. The CoP, on the other hand, is the point of application of the total vertical component of ground reaction force acting on the support surface [9, 11]. The CoP is one of the main quantities used to infer the responses of the central nervous system to the total body movement and depicts the force that must be generated to return the CoM to an equilibrium point [12]. In this way, the distance between the CoM and CoP vertical projections in the transverse plane can indicate how effective the postural control system is in maintaining balance and stability in such a way that it should be more active as the distance between CoM and CoP increases [8, 12].

Although different investigations regarding gait initiation in individuals with PD have been conducted, the traditional statistical analysis of scalars (i.e., discrete values) from the CoP measurements, for example, are predominant [12–15]. And usually, gait initiation is not analyzed as a whole but either during postural phase [16, 17] or execution phase [18]. In this chapter, we employed the statistical parametric mapping (SPM) to analyze the time series of some selected measurements calculated from gait initiation. The SPM is a statistical procedure for analyzing typically smooth continua data [19]. It was originally developed for analyzing neuroimaging data [20], and nowadays it has been employed in different settings [e.g., 21–24].

Taking into consideration that postural instability is one of the most incapacitating disturbances in individuals with PD, it is important to investigate it in early stages of the disease to think about appropriate rehabilitation protocols for these individuals. Yet, as the separation of the CoM and CoP presents major implications on the whole-body balance control, it seems appropriate to analyze the whole cycle of gait initiation. Therefore, the goal of this study was to analyze dynamic postural instability of individuals with PD in the early stages of disease in relation to non-disabled individuals during the performance of gait initiation using the SPM analysis. We hypothesized that individuals with PD would present a reduced distance between CoM and CoP throughout most of gait initiation cycle and that such reduction would be due to the reduced ground reaction force generated by both swing and stance limbs.

Methods

Participants

Sixteen individuals with idiopathic PD, between 61 and 78 years old, who were in the initial stages of disease severity (Hoehn and Yahr scale 1 and 2) [25], and 16 non-disabled individuals (control group) matched by age and sex were selected for this study. The inclusion criteria for the participants with PD were idiopathic PD diagnosed by an experienced specialist, following the Movement Disorder Society criteria [26]; Hoehn and Yahr scale <3; no dyskinesia; no known musculoskeletal, visual, vestibular and/or neurologic impairments other than PD; able to follow simple verbal commands; under treatment of stable doses of levodopa; and no surgery in the last 6 months before participation in the study, including deep brain stimulation therapy. The inclusion criteria for the control group were absence of any known orthopedic and/or neurologic impairment and no use of any medication that could compromise balance and gait.

The Review Board of Cruzeiro do Sul University approved all procedures and all participants signed a written consent form before the experimental session. The individuals with PD were assessed during the "ON" state of medication. Table 21.1 presents the general characteristics of participants of both groups.

Table 21.1 General characteristics of individuals with Parkinson's disease (PD) and non-disabled individuals (Control)

	PD	*Control*
Age (years)*	67.2 ± 4.4	67.6 ± 4.8
Body mass (kg)*	78.6 ± 10.6	76.2 ± 11.9
Height (m)*	1.63 ± 0.09	1.68 ± 0.07
Sex (female/male)	2/14	2/14
Time of disease (years)*	7.5 ± 5.1	–
UPDRS motor score*	34 ± 11	–
Hoehn and Yahr classification		
1	n = 1	–
2	n = 15	–

Note: * Mean ± Standard deviation values; UPDRS=Unified Parkinson's Disease Rating Scale

Experimental Procedures

Based on the Vicon Plug-In Full Body gait model [27], 33 retro-reflective markers were placed on the body landmarks of each participant to define head, trunk, arms, hands, pelvis, legs, and feet. The participants were instructed to stand barefoot in an upright position with arms hanging aside for approximately 3 s, with each foot on a separate force plate (Kistler, model 9286BA), displayed side-by-side, and the body weight equally distributed between both feet. This initial stance position was traced on the top of the force plates to keep consistency throughout trials. After a verbal command, "get ready, go," they walked forward for approximately 4 m at a comfortable speed, without interruption, as the first step touched a third force plate. A thin rubber carpet covered the walkway, so the participants were not aware of the force plates' position. Figure 21.1 illustrates the cameras and force plates configuration for the experimental session. It is important to note that although the participants performed several steps, only the first step was considered for further analysis.

Prior to data acquisition, participants practiced the task three times, and the limb that initiated gait predominantly (i.e., left or right) was chosen as the leading limb. It is important to note that during gait initiation, each lower limb has a specific function [28]. The limb that takes the first step is referred to as the leading or swing limb, and the contralateral one is referred as the trailing or stance limb.

A minimum of five valid trials was acquired for each participant. A trial was valid if the leading foot made full contact with the third force plate during the first step and the participant walked, looking straight ahead with no interruption until the end of the walkway. All signals were acquired and synchronized using a computerized gait analysis system with eight cameras (VICON, Inc.), at a sample frequency of 100 Hz.

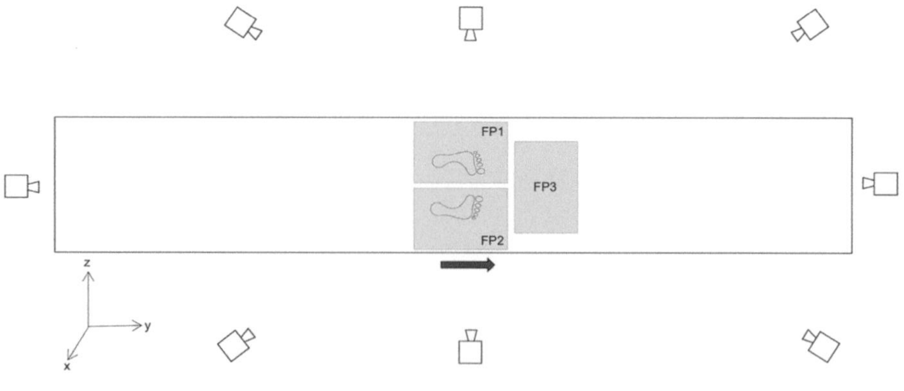

Fig. 21.1 Schematic representation of the walkway surrounded by the cameras with the three embedded force plates (FP1, FP2, and FP3) for the data acquisition during gait initiation and the illustration of the initial position. Note: the arrow indications the walking direction toward the walkway

All individuals with PD were clinically examined by an experienced physical therapist via the Unified Parkinson's Disease Rating Scale—part III (UPDRS-III) [29] and Freezing of Gait Questionnaire (FoG-Q) [30]. These data were used to characterize these participants (Table 21.1).

Data Analysis

We analyzed data for a total of five trials for each participant. The reconstruction of each marker trajectory and the calculation of CoM were performed using a commercial algorithm (Nexus, VICON, Inc.), and further analyses were performed with custom algorithms (MATLAB, MathWorks, Inc.). The ground reaction force (GRF) components in the vertical and horizontal (mediolateral and anterior–posterior) directions were calculated for each force plate, and the moments and CoP for the mediolateral and anterior–posterior directions were calculated for the three force plates from a global coordinate system, which considers all force plates as one. The GRF components and CoP were digitally filtered using a low-pass 2th order and zero-lag Butterworth filter with 10-Hz cut off.

The marker trajectories were digitally filtered using a low-pass 2th order and zero-lag Butterworth filter with 6-Hz cut off. From the markers placed on the calcaneus and metatarsal head, five events were identified: heel-off and toe-off for both limbs (swing and stance), and heel strike for the swing limb. This identification was obtained automatically, confirmed by visual inspection (Fig. 21.2). The onset of gait initiation (t0) was identified as the first dynamic phenomena of CoP in the mediolateral direction as the time when the trajectory increased more than two standard deviations of its mean value during the 3 s of quite standing [16]; heel-off was identified based upon the maximum acceleration of the calcaneus marker of each foot; toe-off was identified based upon the maximum vertical velocity of each foot [31] and the vertical component of ground reaction force (GRF); and the heel-strike was identified based upon the Fz and the minimum vertical velocity of swing foot [31]. Gait initiation cycle was defined from t0 to toe-off of stance limb [32].

Data from CoM and CoP in the mediolateral and anterior–posterior direction were first offset so they all presented common spatial origins [12], and then the distance between CoM and CoP was calculated using the following equation:

$$\text{Distance CoM} - \text{CoP} = \sqrt{\left[\left(\text{CoP}_{\text{ML}}\left(t_i\right) - \text{CoM}_{\text{ML}}\left(t_i\right)\right)^2 + \left(\text{CoP}_{\text{AP}}\left(t_i\right) - \text{CoM}_{\text{AP}}\left(t_i\right)\right)^2\right]}$$

where $\text{CoP}_{\text{ML/AP}}$ and $\text{CoM}_{\text{ML/AP}}$ correspond to center of pressure and center of mass in the mediolateral and anterior–posterior directions, respectively, and t_i corresponds to the specific time interval. Figure 21.3 depicts the CoP and CoM trajectories and the indication of CoM-CoP distance in specific gait initiation events for traditional statistical analysis of scalars [8, 12, 33], for example.

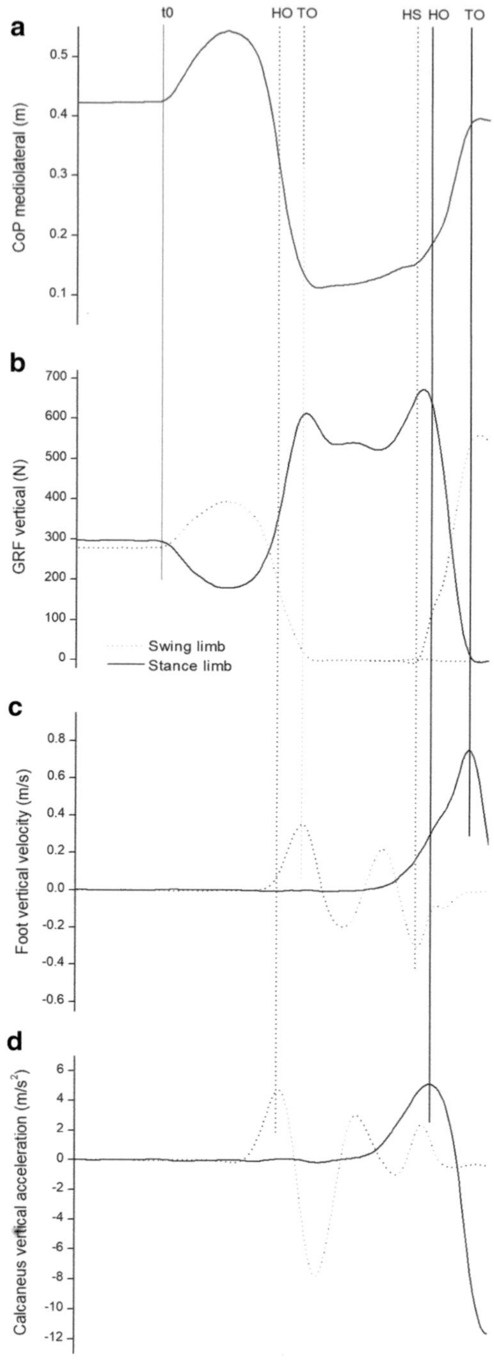

Fig. 21.2 Trajectories of center of pressure (CoP) in the mediolateral direction (**a**), ground reaction force (GRF) vertical component (**b**), foot vertical velocity (**c**), and calcaneus vertical acceleration (**d**). Vertical lines indicate the identification of gait initiation onset (t0) and the events heel-off (HO) and toe-off (TO) of swing/leading (dashed line) and stance/trailing (solid line) limbs, and heel strike (HS) of swing limb

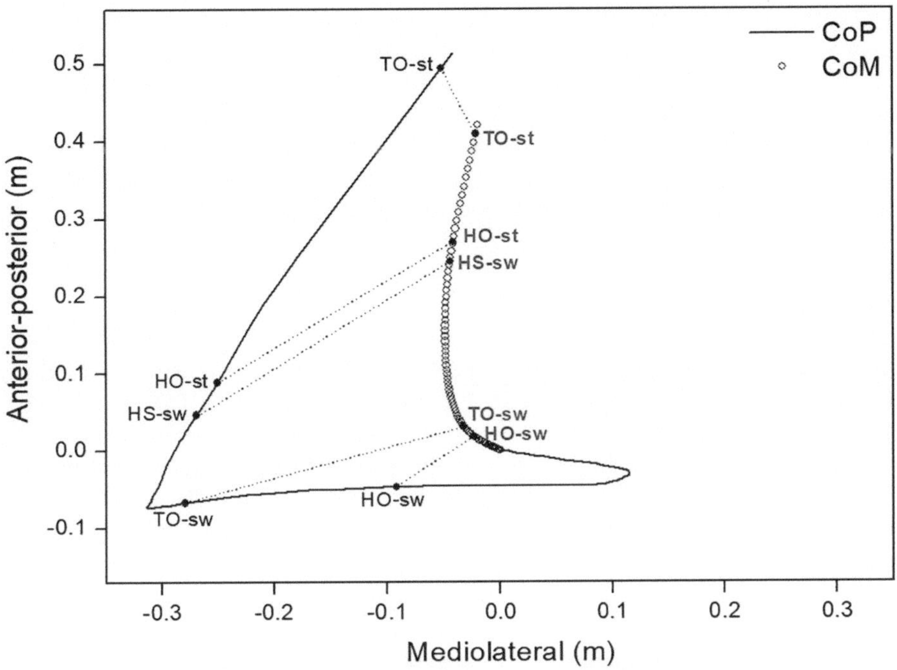

Fig. 21.3 Trajectories of center of pressure (CoP) and center of mass (CoM) in the mediolateral and anterior–posterior directions and the indication of the distance between CoP and CoM (dotted line) at heel-off (HO) and toe-off (TO) of swing (sw) and stance (st) limbs, and heel strike (HS) of swing limb

Gait initiation cycle duration was time normalized from 0% (t0) to 100% (toe-off of stance limb) and averaged to obtain the mean cycle for each participant. The primary variables for this study were the distance between CoM and CoP and the vertical and horizontal GRF components for each limb during the gait initiation cycle. The secondary variables were gait initiation duration, step length of the swing limb (distance between initial position of calcaneus marker and its final position at heel strike along the progression line), and the relative time of occurrence of swing limb heel-off, toe-off, and heel strike, and stance limb heel-off during gait initiation cycle (except the toe-off of stance limb, which as 100% for all participants).

Statistical Analysis

For all variables, the mean of five trials were obtained for each participant. We employed statistical parametric mapping (SPM) [20, 22] and conventional statistical procedures. One-way analyses of variance (ANOVA) were employed, having as factor group (Parkinson and control). More specifically, we performed ANOVAs for each data point of gait initiation cycle using custom algorithms (MATLAB, MathWorks, Inc.) [34]. The dependent variable for each ANOVA was the distance between CoM and CoP, and the vertical, mediolateral, and anterior–posterior components of GRF for both swing and stance limbs.

The conventional statistical procedures were performed with SPSS software, and we employed the ANOVAs, having as dependent variables, respectively, the duration of gait initiation, step length of the swing limb, and the relative time of occurrence of heel-off (swing and stance limbs), toe-off (swing limb), and heel strike (swing limb). An alpha level of 0.05 was set for all statistical tests.

Results

Seven individuals with PD were dignosed with FoG, but none of them presented any FoG episode during data acquisition. Three individuals with PD and six non-disabled individuals initiate gait with the left limb, and the remaining participants initiate gait with the right limb. Figure 21.4 depicts the mean (± standard deviation) values of the distance between CoM and CoP for both groups. The SPM ANOVA revealed that individuals with PD reduced the CoM-CoP distance compared to the non-disabled individuals ($F_{1,30}$ = 11.09) during 3–25% (p < 0.001), 38–54% (p < 0.001), and 95–98% (p = 0.04) of gait initiation cycle (Fig. 21.4).

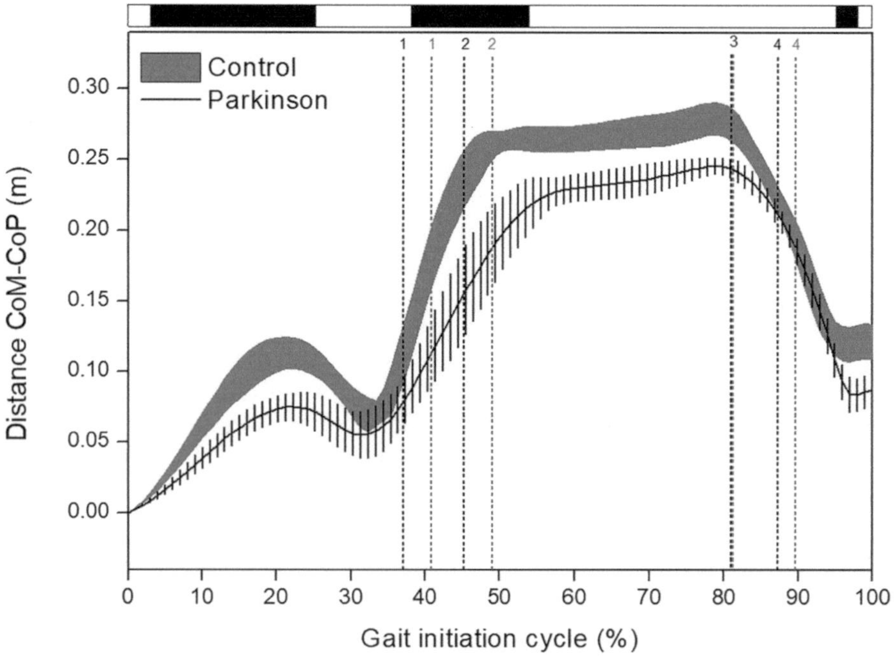

Fig. 21.4 Mean (± standard deviation) of the distance between center of mass (CoM) and center of pressure (CoP) during the normalized full gait initiation cycle for the control (gray area) and Parkinson (line) groups. The black shaded portions at the top of the figure indicate group effect. Note: black (Parkinson) and gray (Control) vertical lines indicate the events' instant of occurrence, with the numbers 1, 2, 3, and 4 corresponding, respectively, to swing limb heel-off, swing limb toe-off, swing limb heel-strike, and stance limb heel-off

Figure 21.5 depicts the mean (± standard deviation) values of GRF components of swing (Fig. 21.5a, c, e) and stance limbs (Fig. 21.5b, d, f) for both groups. The SPM ANOVAs revealed that the vertical GRF component of swing ($F_{1,30} = 8.54$) and stance ($F_{1,30} = 10.39$) limbs; mediolateral GRF component of swing ($F_{1,30} = 8.55$) and stance ($F_{1,30} = 9.77$) limbs; and anterior–posterior GRF component of swing ($F_{1,30} = 9.13$) and stance ($F_{1,30} = 10.27$) limbs were lower for individuals with PD compared to the non-disabled individuals (Fig. 21.5). More specifically, the vertical GRF component was lower for the swing (Fig. 21.5a) and stance limbs (Fig. 21.5b), respectively, during 9–23% ($p = 0.026$) and 40–56% ($p = 0.020$), and during 11–22% ($p = 0.005$), 41–51% ($p = 0.007$), and 76–82% ($p = 0.021$) of gait initiation cycle; the mediolateral GRF component was lower for the swing (Fig. 21.5c) and stance limbs (Fig. 21.5d), respectively, during 0–36% ($p < 0.001$), and during 35–53% ($p = 0.002$) and 69–87% ($p = 0.002$) of gait initiation cycle; and the anterior–posterior GRF component was lower for the swing (Fig. 21.5e) and stance limbs (Fig. 21.5f), respectively, during 11–33% ($p = 0.002$) and during 40–55% ($p = 0.001$) and 62–86% ($p < 0.001$) of gait initiation cycle.

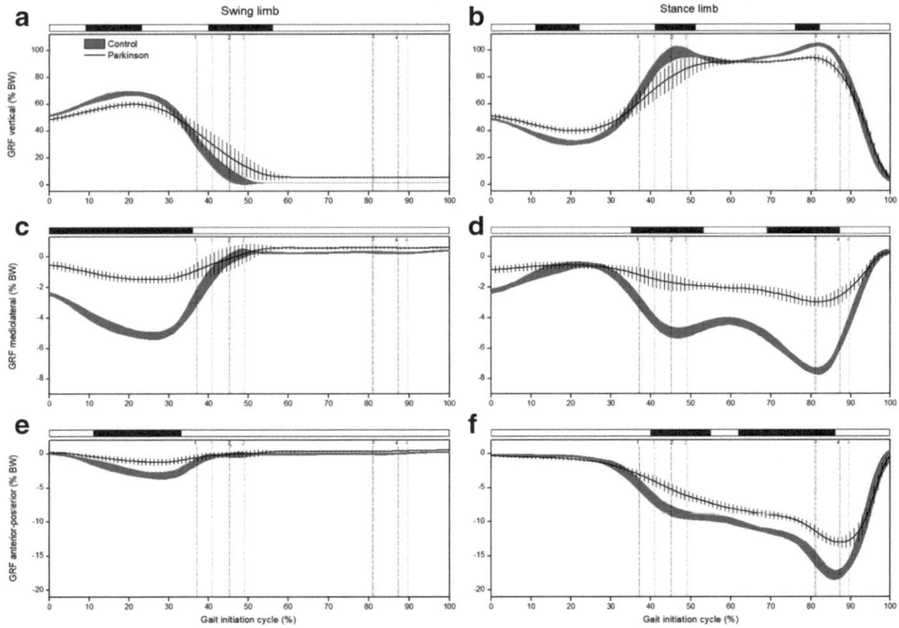

Fig. 21.5 Mean (± standard deviation) of ground reaction force (GRF) of the vertical (**a**, **b**) and horizontal mediolateral (**c**, **d**) and anterior–posterior (**e**, **f**) components for the swing (left panels) and stance (right panels) limbs, normalized by the body weight (BW) during the normalized full gait initiation cycle for the control (gray area) and Parkinson (line) groups. The black shaded portions at the top of the figure indicate group effect. Note: black (Parkinson) and gray (Control) vertical lines indicate the events' instant of occurrence with the numbers 1, 2, 3, and 4 corresponding, respectively, to swing limb heel-off, swing limb toe-off, swing limb heel-strike, and stance limb heel-off

Table 21.2 Mean (± standard deviation) of the secondary variables of gait initiation for the individuals with Parkinson's disease (PD) and non-disabled individuals (Control)

Variables	*PD*	*Control*	*p-value*
Gait initiation duration (s)	1.35 ± 0.15	1.22 ± 0.11	*0.002*
Step length (m)	0.54 ± 0.07	0.59 ± 0.07	*0.013*
Relative time of occurrence (%)			
Swing limb heel-off	41.8 ± 5.6	37.5 ± 3.5	*0.014*
Swing limb toe-off	49.3 ± 5.0	45.3 ± 3.0	*0.011*
Swing limb heel-strike	81.4 ± 3.8	81.2 ± 1.7	0.837
Stance limb heel-off	89.6 ± 3.1	87.4 ± 3.6	0.073

Table 21.2 presents the mean (± standard deviation) values of the gait initiation duration, step length of the swing limb, and the relative time of occurrence of the feet events from both limbs. The first two ANOVAs revealed that individuals with PD presented longer duration ($F_{1,30} = 11.70$) and shorter step ($F_{1,30} = 6.95$) during the gait initiation performance compared to the non-disabled individuals. The remaining ANOVAS revealed group effect for the heel-off ($F_{1,30} = 6.77$) and toe-off ($F_{1,30} = 7{,}0.29$) of swing limb, and did not reveal any group effect for the heel-strike of swing limb ($F_{1,30} = 0.04$) and heel-off of stance limb ($F_{1,30} = 3.46$) (Table 21.2).

Discussion

We analyzed dynamic postural instability of individuals in the early stages of PD in relation to non-disabled individuals during the performance of gait initiation using the SPM analysis. Overall, the results revealed that individuals with PD presented postural instability, revealed by the reduced distance between CoM and CoP. This reduction was mainly at the beginning of the task, before swing limb hell-off (i.e., "postural phase"), and during the preparation and beginning of swing limb forward movement (Fig. 21.4). The individuals with PD also presented reduced GRF in the three components (i.e., vertical, mediolateral, and anterior–posterior), with the mediolateral presenting the broadest difference between both groups (Fig. 21.5c and d). These results are in accordance with our hypothesis, revealing postural instability in the early stages of PD. We also recognized that SPM analysis is suitable for analyzing gait initiation as it lies in the continuum data.

Previous investigations have identified the distance between CoM and CoP in individuals with PD [12, 14, 33] using traditional statistical analysis. Those investigations found that individuals with PD presented reduced CoM-CoP distance compared to non-disabled individuals. More specifically, individuals with PD presented reduced CoM-CoP distance at the instant of maximum CoP toward swing limb [12, 33], at heel-off and toe-off of swing and stance limbs, and heel-strike of swing limb [33]. Hass et al. [14], on the other hand, investigated only individuals with PD at different stages of the disease, and found that less disabled individuasl presented greater CoM-CoP distance at the end of single support phase than the more disabled ones. Contrary to previous investigations, the present study investigated individuals with PD classified up to stage 2 of Hoehn and Yahr [25], over 60 years old, and a control group, matched by age and sex, revealing that older individuals at early stages of PD present postural instability compared to their peers.

The SPM analysis allowed us to identify the difference between both groups, before the heel-off of the swing limb, in the preparation period (3–25% of gait initiation cycle). During this period, the main task is to transfer the body weight toward the stance limb and generate forward motion [8]. Our results revealed a remarkable reduction of the mediolateral GRF component in the swing limb (Fig. 21.5c) of the individuals with PD before the heel-off, as well as a reduced anterior–posterior GRF component (Fig. 21.5e). The group difference remained during the transition between the preparation and swing limb movement (hell-off and toe-off) (Fig. 21.5, right panels). Such difference may affect the temporal organization between both groups, revealed by the relative time of occurrence for the swing limb heel-off and toe-off (Table 21.2). The postural instability identified for the individuals with PD in this study might be attributed to the reduction of these two GRF components, which is in accordance with previous investigations that revealed reduced lateral [33] and forward [13, 33] impulses for individuals with PD.

It is important to note that the anterior–posterior GRF component corresponds to the impulse that propels the whole body forward. We can observe in the Fig. 21.5f the reduction of this component for the individuals with PD during the period that corresponds to the swing limb forward motion (40–80% approximately of gait initiation cycle), which also corroborates to the postural instability, as well as the shorter step length and longer gait initiation duration of individuals with PD compared to the non-disabled individuals.

This was a first attempt to employ a new tool to analyze the gait initiation cycle in individuals with PD. Although we found important results related to postural instability in early stages of PD, this study presents some limitations. For example, we assessed a reduced number of individuals and in only one experimental condition. We also selected a reduced number of variables for investigation. Future studies should investigate additional variables, such as muscle activation, joint angles. Also, it would be important to analyze individuals with PD diagnosed with FoG separately to advance the knowledge regarding this specific impairment that many individuals with PD present. Finally, studies aiming to examine the effects of intervention protocols specific to balance impairment based upon the results presented in this study could improve their dynamic balance, avoid falls, and yield better life quality.

Altogether, the results from this study advance our knowledge regarding postural instability of individuals with PD, revealing that even in early stages of the disease they present impairment in the postural control system. The analysis of gait initiation using the SPM analysis seems to be a suitable way to investigate postural instability, and further studies could examine the effects of specific intervention protocols for improving balance control during transition tasks.

References

1. Winter DA. A.B.C. (Anatomy, Biomechanics and Control) of balance during standing and walking. Waterloo, ON: Graphic Services, University of Waterloo; 1995. p. 56.
2. Breniere Y, Do MC. When and how does steady state gait movement induced from upright posture begin? J Biomech. 1986;19(12):1035–40.
3. Delval A, Tard C, Defebvre L. Why we should study gait initiation in Parkinson's disease. Neurophysiol Clin. 2014;44(1):69–76.
4. Archibald N, Miller N, Rochester L. Neurorehabilitation in Parkinson disease. In: Barnes MP, Good DC, editors. Handb Clin Neurol. 110. Edinburgh: Elsevier; 2013. p. 435–42.
5. Hughes AJ, Daniel SE, Kilford L, Lees AJ. Accuracy of clinical diagnosis of idiopathic Parkinson's disease: a clinico-pathological study of 100 cases. J Neurol Neurosurg Psychiatry. 1992;55(3):181–4.
6. Sethi K. Levodopa unresponsive symptoms in Parkinson disease. Mov Disord. 2008;23 Suppl 3:S521–33.
7. Takakusaki K. Functional neuroanatomy for posture and gait control. J Mov Disord. 2017;10(1):1–17.
8. Jian Y, Winter DA, Ishac MG, Gilchrist L. Trajectory of the body COG and COP during initiation and termination of gait. Gait Posture. 1993;1(1):9–22.
9. Winter DA. Human balance and posture control during standing and walking. Gait Posture. 1995;3:193–214.
10. Rodgers MM, Cavanagh PR. Glossary of biomechanical terms, concepts, and units. Phys Ther. 1984;64(12):1886–902.
11. Duarte M, Freitas SM. Revision of posturography based on force plate for balance evaluation. Rev Bras Fisioter. 2010;14(3):183–92.
12. Martin M, Shinberg M, Kuchibhatla M, Ray L, Carollo JJ, Schenkman ML. Gait initiation in communitydwelling adults with Parkinson disease: comparison with older and younger adults without the disease. Phys Ther. 2002;82(6):566–77.
13. Halliday SE, Winter DA, Frank JS, Patla AE, Prince F. The initiation of gait in young, elderly, and Parkinson's disease subjects. Gait Posture. 1998;8(1):8–14.
14. Hass CJ, Waddell DE, Fleming RP, Juncos JL, Gregor RJ. Gait initiation and dynamic balance control in Parkinson's disease. Arch Phys Med Rehabil. 2005;86(11):2172–6.
15. Naugle KM, Hass CJ, Bowers D, Janelle CM. Emotional state affects gait initiation in individuals with Parkinson's disease. Cogn Affect Behav Neurosci. 2012;12(1):207–19.
16. Mancini M, Zampieri C, Carlson-Kuhta P, Chiari L, Horak FB. Anticipatory postural adjustments prior to step initiation are hypometric in untreated Parkinson's disease: an accelerometer-based approach. Eur J Neurol. 2009;16(9):1028–34.
17. Schlenstedt C, Mancini M, Horak F, Peterson D. Anticipatory postural adjustment during self-Initiated, cued, and compensatory stepping in healthy older adults and patients with Parkinson disease. Arch Phys Med Rehabil. 2017;98(7):1316–24 e1.
18. Roemmich RT, Nocera JR, Vallabhajosula S, Amano S, Naugle KM, Stegemoller EL, et al. Spatiotemporal variability during gait initiation in Parkinson's disease. Gait Posture. 2012;36(3):340–3.
19. Pataky TC, Vanrenterghem J, Robinson MA, Liebl D. On the validity of statistical parametric mapping for nonuniformly and heterogeneously smooth one-dimensional biomechanical data. J Biomech. 2019;91:114–23.
20. Friston KJ, Holmes AP, Worsley KJ, Poline J-B, Frith CD, Frackowiak RSJ. Statistical parametric maps in functional imaging: a general linear approach. Hum Brain Mapp. 1995;2:189–210.
21. De Ridder R, Willems T, Vanrenterghem J, Robinson M, Pataky T, Roosen P. Gait kinematics of subjects with ankle instability using a multisegmented foot model. Med Sci Sports Exerc. 2013;45(11):2129–36.
22. Pataky TC. Generalized n-dimensional biomechanical field analysis using statistical parametric mapping. J Biomech. 2010;43(10):1976–82.

23. Robinson MA, Vanrenterghem J, Pataky TC. Statistical parametric mapping (SPM) for alpha-based statistical analyses of multi-muscle EMG time-series. J Electromyogr Kinesiol. 2015;25(1):14–9.
24. Toro IS, Weir G, Amado A, Emmerik RV, Ervilha U, Hamill J. Is coordination variability using vector coding different in overground and treadmill walking and running? Gait Posture. 2022;92:413–20.
25. Hoehn MM, Yahr MD. Parkinsonism: onset, progression and mortality. Neurology. 1967;17(5):427–42.
26. Postuma RB, Poewe W, Litvan I, Lewis S, Lang AE, Halliday G, et al. Validation of the MDS clinical diagnostic criteria for Parkinson's disease. Mov Disord. 2018;33(10):1601–8.
27. Vicon. Vicon plug-in-gait product guide - foundation notes revision 2.0 March 2010. Vicon Motion System: Vicon Motion System Limited; 2010.
28. Tokuno CD, Eng JJ. Gait initiation is dependent on the function of the paretic trailing limb in individuals with stroke. Gait Posture. 2006;24(4):424–8.
29. Goetz CG, Tilley BC, Shaftman SR, Stebbins GT, Fahn S, Martinez-Martin P, et al. Movement Disorder Society-sponsored revision of the Unified Parkinson's Disease Rating Scale (MDS-UPDRS): scale presentation and clinimetric testing results. Mov Disord. 2008;23(15):2129–70.
30. Giladi N, Tal J, Azulay T, Rascol O, Brooks DJ, Melamed E, et al. Validation of the freezing of gait questionnaire in patients with Parkinson's disease. Mov Disord. 2009;24(5):655–61.
31. O'Connor CM, Thorpe SK, O'Malley MJ, Vaughan CL. Automatic detection of gait events using kinematic data. Gait Posture. 2007;25(3):469–74.
32. Nissan M, Whittle MW. Initiation of gait in normal subjects: a preliminary study. J Biomed Eng. 1990;12(2):165–71.
33. Machado G, Russo-Junior D, Doná F, Barela J, Ferraz H, Silva S, et al. Effects of mild impairment in Parkinson's disease on balance control. Arch Physiother Rehabil. 2019;2(2):18–27.
34. Pataky T. One-dimensional statistical parametric mapping in Matlab 2019 [June 19th, 2022]. Available from: https://github.com/0todd0000/spm1dmatlab.

Part IV

Technology and Rehabilitation Applied to Locomotion and Posture

Mobility and Cognitive Function in Older Adults with Multiple Sclerosis: Physical Activity and Exercise Training as Rehabilitation Therapy

22

Emerson Sebastião, Vitor Antonio Assis Alves Siqueira, Felipe Balistieri Santinelli, Christopher Mark Hill, and Ana Rodriguez Larrad

Abstract

Multiple sclerosis (MS) is an inflammatory, progressive, often disabling, and neurodegenerative disease of the central nervous system that affects approximately 2.8 million people worldwide. Currently, there is a greater number of older adults living with MS than ever before. This growing number of older adults with MS undergoes age-related declines in physical and cognitive functioning that appear to be compounded by the disease and its progression. This chapter aims at describing: (i) the first line of treatment for MS; (ii) mobility and cognitive function in older adults with MS; (iii) physical activity and exercise training as adjuvant rehabilitative therapy to improve mobility and cognitive function in older adults with MS; and (iv) common tests used to assess mobility/walking ability and cognitive function in MS. To accomplish these goals, the current scientific literature was reviewed, analyzed, and summarized.

E. Sebastião (✉) · V. A. A. A .Siqueira
Department of Health and Kinesiology, University of Illinois Urbana-Champaign, Urbana, IL, USA
e-mail: esebast2@illinois.edu; vitoras2@illinois.edu

F. B. Santinelli
REVAL – Rehabilitation Research Center, Hasselt University University, Hasselt, Belgium
e-mail: felipe.balistierisantinelli@uhasselt.be

C. M. Hill
School of Kinesiology, Louisiana State University, Baton Rouge, LA, USA
e-mail: chrishill@lsu.edu

A. R. Larrad
Department of Physiology, Faculty of Medicine and Nursing, University of the Basque Country, Leioa, Spain
e-mail: ana.rodriguez@ehu.eus

F. A. Barbieri et al. (eds.), *Locomotion and Posture in Older Adults*,
https://doi.org/10.1007/978-3-031-74123-4_22

Introduction

Multiple sclerosis (MS) is an inflammatory, often disabling, progressive and neurodegenerative disease of the central nervous system (CNS) [1, 2]. Although the exact cause of MS is unknown, research shows that interactions between the environment and genetic factors trigger an immune-mediated cascade leading the immune system to attack the CNS and destroy the myelin sheath of nerve cells [3]. The degeneration of the myelin sheath—the layer of fat that surrounds the nerve cell—negatively affects the conduction of the nerve impulse along the neural pathway in the CNS [2] interrupting the traffic of information in the brain and between the brain and the body. Such degeneration reduces nerve signal conduction velocity and subsequently interferes with movement coordination. MS is unpredictable in presentation and course. Researchers have defined different clinical courses of the disease: relapsing-remitting MS, primary progressive MS, and secondary progressive MS [4]. Relapsing-remitting MS is the most common manifestation of the disease, accounting for about 85% of cases [4]. Although MS remains a challenge, there currently appears to be a better understanding of the underlying genetic and environmental factors that drive the condition [1, 5].

The prevalence of MS has increased substantially across the globe since 1990. According to a recent published MS Atlas, it is estimated that there are approximately 2.8 million people living with MS worldwide [6] with high prevalence being observed in countries like Canada, the USA, and Northern European countries. Researchers have shown that MS is more prevalent among women than men (ratio 1:3), and it is usually diagnosed in individuals between the ages of 20 and 50 years old. Although some studies have found that MS can shorten patients' lives by 6–10 years [7, 8], survival in people with MS (pwMS) has significantly improved over the past decades, with most patients having a life expectancy equivalent or moderately reduced compared to unaffected peers and live to old ages [9, 10]. Thus, similar to the demographic transition observed in the general population, the population of pwMS is undergoing an aging process. For example, in the USA, an epidemiological study collecting data on adults with MS in the USA between 2008 and 2010 indicates that the majority of pwMS were over 45 years old, with the highest prevalence being in the 55–64 years old age group [11]. There are over one million people living with MS in the USA [11] and a "greying" of this population based on both increased life expectancy after MS diagnosis and the shifting demographic landscape worldwide [12, 13]. Of the over one million adults living with MS in the USA, estimates indicate that one in four Americans with MS are now over the age of 60 years [14].

The demyelination, axonal injury, and neurodegenerative processes occurring in the CNS produce neurologic deficits typical of MS, and this includes sensory, motor, and cognitive dysfunction. Reduced mobility and gait dysfunction are the most noticeable signs of MS, with 85% of pwMS reporting difficulty in walking after 10 years of disease onset [15]. Cognitive impairment is further a concern among pwMS. A recent review study observed that the prevalence of cognitive impairment varied by MS phenotype (i.e., Relapsing-Remitting MS and Secondary Progressive

MS), with the prevalence ranging from 31% to 83% [16]. In addition, fatigue and postural control impairment also appear ubiquitous over the course of MS [17, 18]. Consequently, MS disease progression can negatively impact employment, participation in everyday activities and quality of life. Regarding mobility cognitive function, the growing number of older adults with MS have worsened mobility and cognitive function compared to age-matched controls without MS [19–21] and undergo a faster rate of disability. This is a concern as mobility and cognitive function are paramount for independent living, and continued loss of functionality is one of the most common concerns raised by those aging with MS [22]. Older adults with MS who have increased mobility limitations and cognitive difficulties may become more isolated and less able to leave home than younger pwMS [23], which can negatively impact the quality of life and participation [24].

Disease Modifying Therapy (DMT) constitutes the first line of treatment for MS. These drugs focus on reducing MS progression and are not appropriate to treat disease symptoms. Thus, non-pharmacological therapies such as physical activity (PA) and exercise training are potential approaches to manage disease symptoms (e.g., mobility and cognitive impairment) and progression in pwMS—including older adults with MS [25–28]; corroborating the global exercise is medicine movement [29]. Acknowledging the growing population of older adults with MS, the challenges associated with drug treatment, and the benefits of PA and exercise training for managing and treating MS-related symptoms, this chapter: (1) describes two ubiquitous symptoms of MS, namely mobility and cognitive impairment in older adults with MS (2) describes the first line of treatment for MS (i.e., drugs) and general benefits of PA and exercise training for pwMS; (3) describes PA and exercise training as adjuvant rehabilitation therapy to maintain and/or restore mobility and cognitive function in older adults with MS; and (4) provides examples of common tests used to measure mobility/walking ability and cognitive function in older adults with MS.

To accomplish these goals the current scientific literature was reviewed, analyzed, and summarized. This chapter is organized into seven distinct but interconnected subsections: (1) Mobility in older adults with MS; (2) Cognitive function in older adults with MS; (3) MS: first line of treatment; (4) PA and exercise training as rehabilitation therapy for MS; (5) The role of PA and exercise training in improving mobility in older adults with MS; (6) The role of PA and exercise training in improving cognitive function in older adults with MS; (7) Measuring mobility/walking ability and cognitive function in MS. Therefore, by the end of this chapter the reader will gain an understanding of mobility and cognitive impairment in older adults with MS, drug treatment for MS, the importance of PA and exercise training in restoring or maintaining mobility and cognitive function in the growing population of older adults with MS and will learn about common tests used to measure mobility/walking ability and cognitive function in this population.

Mobility in Older Adults with Multiple Sclerosis

Mobility is a domain where pwMS, including older adults with MS experience impairments [30, 31] and significantly affect independence. In fact, one of the major consequences of MS is a loss of independent mobility, with 93% of pwMS experiencing difficulty walking 10 years after diagnosis [32]. Declines in mobility function are associated with loss of social connections, reduced participation, and altered abilities to perform self-care, productivity, and leisure occupations. Overall, research has found that older adults with MS are more physically disabled than younger individuals [33, 34]. Older adults with MS undergo age-related declines in ambulation, balance, and muscular function (weakness) that may be further compounded by the disease and its association. For instance, Finlayson and van Denend [35] conducted a study to develop an understanding of the experience and meaning of mobility loss among older adults with MS. The authors observed that loss of balance was the most common of the symptoms that may influence mobility in older adults with MS, with 96% of the participants enrolled in the study (n = 26) reporting such a problem. In general, studies have suggested a faster rate of disability progression among older adults with MS [20, 36, 37]. In fact, older age is a significant predictor of reaching disability milestones in MS. For example, previous work found that the median age for adopting unilateral assistance during walking is nearly 65 years of age [38]. However, a recent study observed that a great portion of pwMS require assistive device around the age of 40 years [39].

Several studies have been conducted aiming at understanding mobility, in older adults with MS. In a study using baseline data of 2156 pwMS [where 169 (7.8%) were over 65 years] from the *Sonya Slifka Longitudinal Multiple Sclerosis Study*, the authors examined demographic and clinical characteristics of participants over and under 65 years of age and observed that disability was significantly higher in older versus younger adults [36]. As physical function declines, older adults with MS presenting with mobility impairments are faced with the decision to utilize assistive technology or continue to attempt activities without aid. Minden and colleagues [36] observed that a higher percentage of pwMS over 65 years of age required a cane or bilateral support to walk 25 feet or were completely wheelchair or scooter dependent [36]. Consistent with the reported level of disability, a significantly higher percentage of those aged 65 years and older needed help from a person or assistive device with one or more basic or instrumental activities of daily living except for eating, managing finances, preparing meals, or doing housework. However, because of their health condition, about 57% of the study participants reported to be unable to leave their flat or house and only 15% were able to use public transportation. Bollaert and colleagues [20] compared physical function between 40 older adults with MS (60 years and older) and 40 age- and sex-matched healthy older adults using a collection of mobility and walking ability measures. After a comprehensive data analysis, the authors observed that older adults with MS performed significantly worse on all measures compared with their healthy control counterparts, providing evidence of reduced mobility function in older adults with MS.

Klewer and colleagues [40] conducted a survey study to investigate specific disease problems of older adults with MS. The authors evaluated a total of 53 older adults from the Berlin Section of the German Multiple Sclerosis Association. Forty-four participants were females and nine were males, with an average age of 73 years, and about 25 years of average of course of the disease. The authors observed that all participants reported problems with mobility [40]. As disability often increases with age, this same study reported average disability level measured using the Expanded Disability Status Scale (EDSS) scores to be above 6.0—requiring ambulatory assistance, in about 96% of participants, and about 70% required wheelchairs for their mobility (EDSS score > 6.5). Due to the high prevalence of assistive device use in older adults and high levels of disability, the risk of falling is also more common in older adults [41].

Based on the aforementioned, we noted that mobility impairment is ubiquitous to MS and researchers have shown a faster rate of disability progression in older adults with MS compared to young and middle-aged counterparts [33, 34]. This has a significant impact on this population as mobility impairment drastically reduces independence to perform activities of daily living, negatively impacting quality of life.

Cognitive Function in Older Adults with Multiple Sclerosis

There is a plethora of evidence that pwMS experience deficits in cognitive function. Similarly, to mobility impairment, cognitive impairment is very detrimental in pwMS and can have a significant impact on activities of daily living [42]. Cognitive impairment is a highly prevalent and life-changing outcome in pwMS that is present in an estimated 45–65% of those affected by this disease [43]. Similarly, older adults (60 years and over) often experience changes to cognitive function due to age related brain changes. Decreases in working memory, reaction time, and cognitive flexibility are widely reported after the sixth decade of life [44–46]. As a result, the aging process adds a new dimension to the experience of pwMS, as they navigate the intersection of disease progression and growing old. With this growing demographic within the disease, researchers have attempted to document changes in cognition for older adults with MS, with researchers demonstrating that the prevalence of cognitive impairment in older adults with MS is higher than the observed in younger pwMS [47].

A study conducted by Branco and colleagues [48] described the prevalence and profile of cognitive impairment in older adults with MS. The authors observed that about 77% of older adults with MS (55 years and over) demonstrate impairment in two or more cognitive domains. Detailed results from this study demonstrated that information processing speed was the most impaired domain (68.8%), followed by verbal learning (49.5%), executive function (47.7%), and visuospatial learning (26.6%). Similarly, a group of researchers from New York and Wisconsin in the USA [49] examined cognitive impairment in older adults with MS (mean age:

62 years) and observed that approximately 47% of older adults with MS presented with cognitive impairment.

Researchers have observed that older adults with MS demonstrate significant impairments in cognitive function compared to young and middle-aged adults with MS [50] with further evidence suggesting that older adults with MS have potentially worse cognitive function compared to their older adult counterparts without MS [20]. The next paragraphs briefly focus on previous studies that successfully identified domains of cognitive function where significant changes have been observed in older adults with MS.

Cognitive processing speed (CPS) is defined as the rate of processing perceptual information and time to perform automatic cognitive operations in response to cued stimuli [51]. A common task used in prior research to access CPS is the Symbol Digits Modality Test (SDMT). In a large-scale longitudinal study, age and MS disease duration were significant predictors of SDMT scores [52], with higher age and MS disease duration being correlated with lower SDMT scores. This was further confirmed within a battery of cognitive functional tests performed by Jakubowski and colleagues [49] in a cross-sectional study with older adults with MS and age matched health controls. They found significant differences between groups with a large effect (Cohen's $d = 0.91$). Subsequent modeling performed in this study found SDMT scores to be a significant predictor of diagnosis of MS [53]. Despite the common usage of SDMT, other CPS tests have also been used like the Stroop task—a measure of selective attention (inhibitory control). For example, Bodling and colleagues [54] examined the Stroop task in a cross-sectional study with young adults, older adults, and older adults with MS. The authors found a lack of differences between older adults with MS and age matched controls, suggesting that lack of differences may stem from the simplicity of the task. This means that the simple conflict monitoring (i.e., saying the color of a word rather than reading it) did not provide enough cognitive challenge to differentiate health and MS disease states [54].

Verbal fluency and memory are often measured in the assessment of cognition in older adults with MS. The California Verbal Learning Test (CVLT-II), where a list of 16 words is recalled immediately after being read aloud, is often used to clinically access this domain [55]. Branco and colleagues [48] demonstrated an inverse relationship between level of verbal fluency/working memory and age with MS. In other words, as the age of an individual with MS increased there was a decrease in verbal cognition. Some of these decreases in verbal cognition have been related to cortical changes within the brain. In a set of longitudinal studies using magnetic resonance imaging, identified higher amounts of atrophy to white and grey matter (overall decrease in brain volume) was associated with lower verbal working memory and fluency scores in older adults with MS [56, 57].

Deficits in visuospatial learning and memory are another common cognitive symptom that results from MS and partially stems from the known motor deficits associated with MS disease. Moreover, decreases in visuospatial learning and memory are the most reported deficit across the literature studying older adults with MS [49, 50, 52]. Recent studies examining visuospatial learning and memory used the Brief Visuospatial Memory Test (BVMT–R), where patients are presented briefly with six figures on screen and then asked to draw them from memory in the order they appeared [58]. Baird and colleagues [50] found that BVMT-R score linearly decreased with age in pwMS, with the oldest having the lowest scores, which contrasts other forms of cognitive tests such as the SDMT and CVLT-II which saw abrupt decreases in those over the age of 60. This suggests visuospatial learning and memory are affected differently in older adults with MS in comparison to other forms of cognition and should be given special consideration in comparison to other domains of cognition [50].

Despite the research outlined above, the impact of the concurrent effects of aging and the disease progression on cognitive function remains understudied in MS, as research in this area has concentrated on younger and middle-aged populations [57, 59]. Given the emerging nature of this area of research there lacks a consensus on the nature of cognition in older adults with MS. This is especially true given more recent differences found in clinical symptoms between early onset (between ages 20 and 40) and late onset (after age 50) MS [60, 61]. Moreover, some evidence suggests cognitive reserve moderates the rate of cognitive decline in MS, like Alzheimer's disease [57]. Further research is needed to determine the factors that predict cognitive decline in older adults with MS and the impact of disease onset age.

Multiple Sclerosis: First Line of Treatment

Despite significant advancement in the disease understanding, currently, there is no cure for MS. The first line of treatment for the disease consists of the use of medicines (i.e., DMTs), which are commonly prescribed following disease diagnosis. There are over 17 approved DMTs for the treatment of different types of MS, with the majority being for the relapsing forms of MS. These drugs focus on reducing both the number and severity of relapses (exacerbations) by targeting latent immune dysregulation of cytokines and lymphocytes and, therefore, slowing the progression of the disease [62, 63]. However, DMTs are not appropriate for treating disease symptoms or curing MS. For instance, these medications seem to not positively affect common disease symptoms such as fatigue and cognition.

DMTs may further cause significant side effects, which may compromise medication adherence. For symptoms management, pwMS are often prescribed numerous medications for alleviating the numerous symptoms and therefore improving their quality of life [64]. Consequently, polypharmacy may have serious side effects, such as the increased risk of adverse drug events, drug interactions, reduced functional capacity, and medication non-adherence [65, 66]. To this end, non-pharmacological therapies that result in minimal side effects are of particular interest to the MS population, particularly for older adults as there is, at best, modest evidence of DMTs' effect in older adults with MS [67]. A non-pharmacological therapy with potential beneficial effects in a wide array of MS-related symptoms, including physical and cognitive function, with minimal to almost no side-effects is PA and exercise training [26, 68, 69]. Figure 22.1 displays detailed information about MSMS's first line of treatment (i.e., drugs) and the general benefits associated

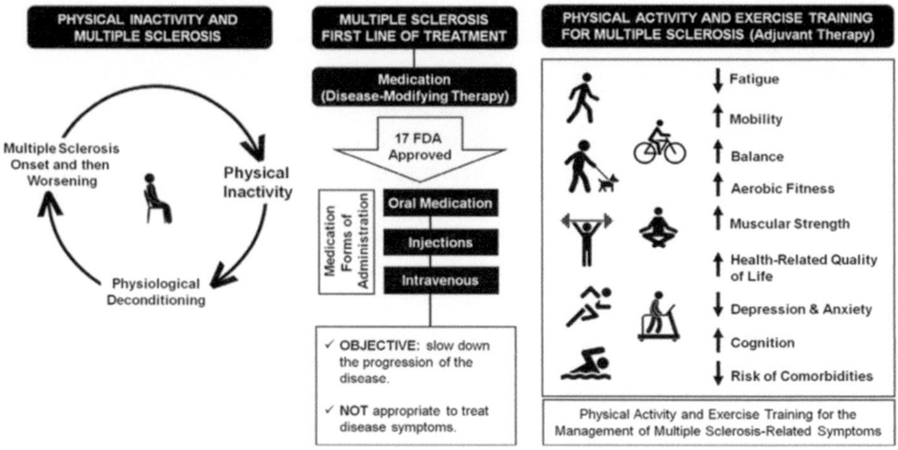

Fig. 22.1 Schematic illustration of multiple sclerosis first line of treatment and overall benefits of PA and exercise training in people with multiple sclerosis. Adapted with permission from Sebastião and colleagues [25]

with PA and/or exercise training participation for pwMS. In the next part, we talk about the importance of PA and exercise training for pwMS and current recommendations for this population.

Overview of Physical Activity and Exercise Training as Rehabilitation Therapy for People with Multiple Sclerosis

There is available evidence supporting PA and exercise training in pwMS as an important component of rehabilitation therapy. A plethora of studies conducted in countries like the USA, Canada, and several European countries, where the prevalence of MS is high, have demonstrated that both PA and exercise training are safe and result in positive effects in many relevant outcomes for this population [26, 27], with researchers stating that exercise is indeed medicine for pwMS [70].

In 2020, the United States National MS Society convened clinical and research experts in the field of MS, exercise, rehabilitation, and PA to discuss and develop exercise and PA consensus for pwMS across the disability spectrum (0–9 in the EDSS) [27]. The document published in *Multiple Sclerosis Journal* recognizes that wellness is a priority for pwMS, and that wellness can be achieved through healthy behavior such as PA and exercise. Table 22.1 highlights the exercise and PA recommendations from the National MS Society, which was endorsed by the Consortium of Multiple Sclerosis Centers [27] for pwMS.

In addition to being essential to general health and well-being, PA and exercise are important to help pwMS manage many MS symptoms, with researchers demonstrating that PA and exercise is a safe and effective means of rehabilitation in pwMS. For instance, there is evidence demonstrating that supervised and

Table 22.1 Summary of the exercise and physical activity recommendations from the National Multiple Sclerosis Society for people with multiple sclerosis across the disability spectrum

National Multiple Sclerosis Society Recommendations for Lifestyle physical activity and Exercise	
1.	Healthcare providers should endorse and promote the benefits/safety of exercise and lifestyle PA for every person with MS.
2.	Early evaluation by a physical or occupational therapist or exercise or sport scientist, experienced in MS (hereafter referred to as "specialists"), is recommended to establish an individualized exercise and/or lifestyle PA plan.
3.	Considering comorbidities and symptom fluctuations, healthcare providers should encourage $\geq$ 150 min/week of exercise and/or $\geq$ 150 min/week of lifestyle PA.
4.	Progress toward these targets should be gradual, based on the person's abilities, preferences, and safety.
5.	If disability increases and exercise/PA becomes more challenging, referrals to specialists are essential to ensure safe and appropriate prescriptions.
6.	When physical mobility is very limited, exercise should be facilitated by a trained assistant.

individualized exercise programs improve fitness, functional capacity, and quality of life as well as modifiable impairments (e.g., impaired balance and mobility) in pwMS [26, 71]. In fact, PA and appropriate exercise programs (e.g., aerobic or resistance training) for pwMS can result in important and positive improvement in cardiovascular fitness, muscular strength, flexibility, fatigue, physical and cognitive function [72].

As the MS population ages, integrative general preventive and geriatric care for MS must focus on physical functional rehabilitation (e.g., mobility), cognitive health, and maximizing quality of life [24], something that can be achieved with regular PA and exercise training [70].

The Role of Physical Activity and Exercise Training in Improving Mobility in Older Adults with Multiple Sclerosis

As previously mentioned, mobility impaired is highly prevalent among pwMS. Several studies have demonstrated the potential of PA, particularly exercise training, to improve mobility in the MS population. However, it is important to note that most of the PA and exercise studies have been conducted in young and middle-aged adults with MS.

Considered a fundamental aspect of mobility, balance problems (static and dynamic) are common in pwMS, and addressing balance-related challenges in pwMS is an important aspect for managing mobility and walking problems in this population. Arik and colleagues [73] recently conducted a systematic review and meta-analysis to determine the effects of Pilates exercises on balance in pwMS. Although their search yielded 246 relevant records, only eight articles evaluated Pilates. According to the authors, significant advantages of Pilates on balance in pwMS were observed when compared to the control group in the Berg Balance

Scale (a measure of a person's ability to safely balance), Activities-Specific Balance Confidence Scale (a measure of a person's confidence in performing activities) and Timed Up and Go Test (a measure of mobility, balance, and walking ability). The authors concluded that Pilates exercises might be an optional method for improving balance in pwMS. Using a similar approach to the previous study, Hao and colleagues [74] conducted a network meta-analysis of randomized controlled trial to investigate the effects of seven different exercise therapies (i.e., aquatic exercise, aerobic exercise, yoga, Pilates, virtual reality exercise, whole-body vibration exercise, and resistance exercise) on balance and walking ability of pwMS. The authors included a total of 31 randomized controlled trial studies with a pool of 904 pwMS. Based on their analysis, the authors concluded that although each type of exercise is useful, yoga, virtual reality training, and aerobic training were more effective in improving balance, while aquatic exercise, virtual reality training, and aerobic training were more effective in improving the walking ability in pwMS. In a systematic literature review with meta-analysis, Pearson and colleagues [75] investigated the literature to quantify the expected benefits of exercise on mobility (quantified as walking ability) in pwMS. The authors compiled data from 13 randomized controlled trials of exercise training in pwMS and observed significant improvements in walking speed (measured by the 10-meter Walking Test) and walking endurance (measured by the 6-min and 2-min Walking Test) in pwMS who exercised, but no improvements in the Timed Up and Go test—a measure of functional mobility.

There is a paucity of studies looking at the benefits of PA and exercise training on mobility in older adults with MS. McAuley and colleagues [76] conducted a pilot study to examine the effects of a Digital Versatile Disc (DVD) exercise intervention targeting lower-extremity function, flexibility, strength, and balance in older adults with MS with the goal of generating effect sizes to power a larger trial. Forty-eight older adults with MS (mean age: ~60 years old) were randomly assigned to a six-month DVD exercise intervention (n = 24) or a healthy aging DVD control condition (n = 24). The intervention group (DVD—exercise intervention—FlexToBa) comprised three DVDs, two resistance bands (one light and one moderate intensity), a yoga mat, and a FlexToBa handbook. The first DVD introduced the program while the remaining two disks consisted of six progressive exercise sessions with each session containing two sets of 11–12 different exercises focusing on balance, strength, and flexibility. Modifications of each exercise were modeled by the leader exercise trainer for those who required an easier task and for those preferring a more challenging version of the activity. For the first 2 weeks of each month, participants were instructed to complete one to two sets of eight to ten repetitions at a rating of perceived exertion of 10–12 (i.e., fairly light), and for the last 2 weeks of the month, the prescription advised participants to complete two sets of 10–12 repetitions at 13–15 Rate of Perceived Exertion (RPE; i.e., somewhat hard). The authors observed that the DVD exercise intervention (FlexToBa) was well received with no adverse events. Effects sizes ranged from small to modest reflecting improved lower-extremity function, balance, and upper and lower-body flexibility) compared to the control condition. In addition, it was noted that the absolute adjusted difference between the Short Physical Performance Battery (SPPB) scores—a measure of lower-extremity function, approximated the lower-bound threshold for a small clinically meaningful difference.

The results observed by McAuley and colleagues [76] are similar to those observed by Sebastião and colleagues [77]. In their study, the authors conducted a feasibility study of a 12-week, home-based Square-Stepping Exercise (SSE) program in older adults with MS. Part of the study also examined the preliminary efficacy of the SSE to improve aspects of mobility function in older adults with MS. Twenty-five older adults with MS (mean age: 64.3 ± 4.5 years) were randomly allocated into the SSE (n = 15) or stretching control condition (n = 10). The SSE intervention was performed on a thin mat of 250 × 100 cm, partitioned into 40 smaller squares (25 cm per side). The program provides sequences of stepping patterns wherein participants learn and practice specific stepping routines by progressively stepping along the mat length direction and avoid treading on the lines of the squares. The exercise intervention started with sessions being performed twice a week with a duration between 10 and 15 min and progressed to five sessions per week with a duration between 25 and 30 min per session. Participants started with basic step patterns that focused on walking-like movements and gradually progressed to more complex step patterns requiring forward, lateral, diagonal, and backward movement. The control condition was a light intensity stretching and minimal muscle strengthening program based on an illustrated manual for persons with MS developed by the National MS Society that involves major muscle groups of the upper and lower body stretching. The authors observed small-to-moderate effect sizes for all mobility parameters between the intervention and the control conditions, thereby providing preliminary evidence that participation in the SSE program may improve mobility function in older adults with MS. The results support the feasibility, acceptability, and possible efficacy of a home-based SSE intervention for older adults with MS.

As briefly described above, there is preliminary evidence demonstrating the importance and the benefits of PA, particularly exercise training, to improve mobility or important elements directly associated with mobility (e.g., balance) in older adults with MS.

The Role of Physical Activity and Exercise Training in Improving Cognitive Function in Older Adults with Multiple Sclerosis

As previously stated, the first line of treatment for MS is DMTs (i.e., drugs); however, DMTs are not suitable for improving or managing symptoms of the disease. On the other hand, non-pharmacological approaches such as PA and exercise training are key elements not only to maintain or restore mobility but also to preserve or avoid cognitive impairment in pwMS.

The focus on preserving or recovering cognition through PA and exercise in pwMS has increased in the last years. A quick search on PubMed—a free search engine accessing primarily the MEDLINE database of references and abstracts on life sciences and biomedical topics—using the terms "exercise OR physical activity AND cognition AND multiple sclerosis," yielded 99 studies 2012 compared to 14 back in 1997. However, when including the term "older adults" in the search, only one randomized controlled trial investigated the impact of home-based exercise (i.e., square-stepping exercise) on this population [77]. The paucity of studies addressing the PA and exercise in older adults with MS warrant studies as this subpopulation of MS undergoes common age-related declines in addition to a neurological progressive disease (i.e., MS), which can impact cognitive function severely [48]. Therefore, the role of PA and exercise training on cognitive function here in described use data from studies conducted in young and middle-aged adults with MS. Additionally, we discuss how PA and exercise can influence different cognitive domains affected by MS: information processing speed, attention, executive function, working memory and learning.

Researchers have shown the potential of PA and exercise to improve cognitive function in pwMS. For example, Sandroff and Motl [78] showed in a large sample of pwMS (mean age: 50 years) that higher levels of PA were associated with better performance on the cognitive processing speed (measured using the SDMT). Similarly, Motl and colleagues [79] showed that moderate-to-vigorous PA was significantly associated with cognitive processing speed but not learning and memory in cognitive impaired pwMS. By contrast, Vanner and colleagues [80] conducted a cross-sectional survey with a convenience sample of 43 people with severe disability level (i.e., EDSS 6–8) to explore clinical and non-clinical correlates of PA. Regarding cognitive function, the authors observed that higher levels of PA were associated with better learning and memory functions in their sample. Importantly, the association between PA and cognitive function, mainly cognitive processing speed, seem to not happen in cognitively impaired and people with progressive MS [81].

The effect of PA and exercise on cognition seems to be contradictory in pwMS. This is exemplified by two recent systematic reviews and meta-analyses [82, 83]. For example, Gharakhanlou and colleagues [82] demonstrated that physical exercise does not support improvements in cognitive function in pwMS. On the other hand, Li and colleagues [83] demonstrated that physical exercise is able to improve cognitive function in pwMS but only in the domain of memory, with no effects on cognitive processing speed or learning. Potentially, the difference on the findings between the previous studies, and highlighted by the Li and colleagues [83], lies in the inclusion of eight new studies from 2021 to 2023 and only randomized controlled studies. Recently, DeLuca and colleagues [84] highlighted that studies investigating the effects of exercise on cognition in pwMS were lacking in methodological strength (lack of adaptation and specificity in the intervention studies), which are the basis of exercise principles and that could have been addressed by the new eight studies included and analyzed by Li and colleagues [83]. Despite the equivocal findings, PA and exercise are still encouraged to improve cognitive function in pwMS [85].

Different exercise modalities have been used as strategies to improve cognitive function in pwMS. For instance, aerobic and resistance training, Pilates, functional exercises, core stability, balance, yoga, stretching endurance and coordination exercises have all been applied in randomized controlled studies to improve cognitive function in pwMS [83]. For example, Feys and colleagues [86] observed that after 12 weeks of remotely supervised aerobic training, memory and visuospatial perception improved. Improved physical fitness, after 12 weeks of health promotion by telephone, was associated with improvement in working memory [87]. A large randomized controlled trial, multicenter study in 11 countries is being conducted to improve cognitive function (focus on cognitive processing speed), in progressive and cognitively impaired pwMS, combining cognitive rehabilitation with aerobic exercise [88]. In the only study with older adults with MS investigating a 12-week home-based exercise program to improve cognition, Sebastião and colleagues [77] observed a small-to-moderate improvement in the cognitive memory domain. Thus, exercise training seems to be beneficial for cognitive performance in pwMS (including older adults) and could be explained by the effects of the exercise on different brain regions.

PA and exercise can promote brain health and neuroplasticity, which may explain the effects on cognitive function in pwMS. Higher PA levels are associated with higher hippocampus volume [89], an important region for memory and learning. In a pilot study conducted by Leavit and colleagues [90] observed an increase in hippocampus volume, followed by improvement in memory after 12 weeks of aerobic cycling exercise. Physical exercise can also produce neurotrophic factors such as the brain-derived neurotrophic factor [91], which can assist in neuroplasticity [89] and is moderately correlated with cognitive processing speed [92] in pwMS. A conceptual framework named **PR**ocessing, **I**ntegration of **M**ultisensory **E**xercise-**R**elated **S**timuli (PRIMERS) was proposed by Sandroff and colleagues [93] to set the stage for the systematic examination of the effects of exercise on brain connectivity, brain structure, and molecular/cellular mechanisms that explain improvements in mobility and cognition in the general population and pwMS. According to the framework, the multisensory input and complexity of motor output of physical exercise, there is an adaptation in the networks of cortical and subcortical brain structures through neuroplasticity, which would induce improvements in physical and cognition performance.

Improving cognitive function through exercise requires the right choice of several components: frequency, duration, volume, and modality [84]. In a recent literature review, Li and colleagues [83] underscore important aspects to consider when targeting cognitive performance as a primary outcome. The authors suggested the following to improve cognitive function in pwMS: (a) multicomponent training, (b) 8–10 weeks, (c) three times or more per week, (d) duration of up to 60 min per session, totalizing at least 180 min per week. Lastly, the baseline status should be considered as the exercise has an effect on cognition in pwMS older than 45, while no effect is observed under 45 years old [83]. However, no evidence is given to older adults with MS (>65 years old) [83], which underscores the need for randomized controlled trials in this growing subgroup of the MS population.

Measuring Mobility and Cognitive Function in Multiple Sclerosis

Table 22.2 provides examples of common tests used to evaluate mobility and walking ability in pwMS in general, including older adults with MS and the respective domain assessed.

Table 22.3 displays examples of common tests used to measure cognitive function in pwMS in general, including older adults with MS and the respective domain assessed.

Final Considerations

As a neurological, often disabling, progressive disease affecting the CSN, MS causes a large array of symptoms that include but are not limited to mobility and cognitive impairment. Although more common in young ages (20–40 years), advances in the understanding of the disease and treatment have allowed pwMS to live into old age. In fact, there is a "greying" of the MS population with evidence suggesting that older adults with MS present with worse mobility and cognitive function compared to older adults without MS, and that this subpopulation of MS experiences a faster rate of disability. To date, MS has no cure, and DMTs constitute the first line of treatment to slowdown the disease progression. However, there is evidence suggesting no to modest effect of DMT in older adults with MS. Further, DMTs are not appropriate to treat disease symptoms. Thus, non-pharmacological therapies such as PA and exercise training have been highly recommended for pwMS in general to treat a wide range of MS-related symptoms including physical and cognitive impairment. There is solid evidence of the benefits of PA and exercise training in young and middle-aged adults with MS; however, studies examining the effects of such behaviors in older adults with MS are somehow incipient. The limited literature on this topic suggests that similarly to young and middle-aged adults with MS, older adults with MS can improve mobility and cognitive function (mainly in the domain of memory) with regular participation in PA and exercise. However, further research into this niche of the MS population is important because older

Table 22.2 Examples of valid and reliable tests to assess mobility/walking ability in people with multiple sclerosis

	Test	Domain assessed
1.	Timed up and go (TUG) [94]	Functional mobility
2.	Timed 25-foot walk (T25FW) [95, 96]	Walking speed
3.	Six-minute walk (6 MW) [97]	Walking endurance
4.	Six-step spot test (SSST) [98]	Ambulation and lower-extremity coordination
5.	Short physical performance battery (SPPB) [99]	Lower-extremity function
6.	Four-square step test [100, 101]	Dynamic balance and coordination

Table 22.3 Examples of valid and reliable tests to assess cognitive function in people with multiple sclerosis

	Test	Domain assessed
1.	Brief international cognitive assessment in MS (BICAMS) [102]	
	• Brief visuospatial memory test (BVMT-R).	Visuospatial memory
	• California verbal learning test (CVLT-II).	Verbal learning
	• Symbol digits modalities test (SDMT).	Information processing speed
2.	Paced auditory serial addition test (PASAT) [95]	Information processing speed

adults with MS undergo the normal age-related declines that are compounded by the disease and its progression.

References

1. Cree BAC, Oksenberg JR, Hauser SL. Multiple sclerosis: two decades of progress. Lancet Neurol. 2022;21(3):211–4. https://doi.org/10.1016/S1474-4422(22)00040-0.
2. Compston A, Coles A. Multiple sclerosis. Lancet. 2008;372(9648):1502–17. https://doi.org/10.1016/S0140-6736(08)61620-7.
3. Baranzini SE, Oksenberg JR. The genetics of MS: from 0 to 200 in 50 years. Trends Genet. 2017;33:960–70. https://doi.org/10.1016/j.tig.2017.09.004.
4. Lublin FD, Reingold SC, Cohen JA, et al. Defining the clinical course of multiple sclerosis: the 2013 revisions. Neurology. 2014;83(3):278–86. https://doi.org/10.1212/WNL.0000000000000560.
5. Oh J, Vidal-Jordana A, Montalban X. Multiple sclerosis: clinical aspects. Curr Opin Neurol. 2018;31(6):752–9. https://doi.org/10.1097/WCO.0000000000000622.
6. Walton C, King R, Rechtman L, et al. Rising prevalence of multiple sclerosis worldwide: insights from the atlas of MS, third edition. Mult Scler J. 2020;26(14):1816–21. https://doi.org/10.1177/1352458520970841.
7. Scalfari A, Neuhaus A, Daumer M, et al. Age and disability accumulation in multiple sclerosis. Neurology. 2011;77(13):1246–52. https://doi.org/10.1212/WNL.0b013e318230a17d.
8. Sadovnick AD, Yee IM, Guimond C, et al. Age of onset in concordant twins and other relative pairs with multiple sclerosis. Am J Epidemiol. 2009;170(3):289–96. https://doi.org/10.1093/aje/kwp143.
9. Koch-Henriksen N, Laursen B, Stenager E, Magyari M. Excess mortality among patients with multiple sclerosis in Denmark has dropped significantly over the past six decades: a population based study. J Neurol Neurosurg Psychiatry. 2017;88(8):626–31. https://doi.org/10.1136/jnnp-2017-315907.
10. Lunde HMB, Assmus J, Myhr KM, et al. Survival and cause of death in multiple sclerosis: a 60-year longitudinal population study. J Neurol Neurosurg Psychiatry. 2017;88(8):621–5. https://doi.org/10.1136/jnnp-2016-315238.
11. Wallin MT, Culpepper WJ, Campbell JD, et al. The prevalence of MS in the United States: a population-based estimate using health claims data. Neurology. 2019;92(10):e1029–40. https://doi.org/10.1212/WNL.0000000000007035.
12. Marrie RA, Elliott L, Marriott J, et al. Effect of comorbidity on mortality in multiple sclerosis. Neurology. 2015;85(3):240–7. https://doi.org/10.1212/WNL.0000000000001718.

13. Marrie RA, Yu N, Blanchard J, et al. The rising prevalence and changing age distribution of multiple sclerosis in Manitoba. Neurology. 2010;74(6):465–71. https://doi.org/10.1212/WNL.0b013e3181cf6ec0.
14. NARCOMS. Aging with multiple sclerosis. NARCOMS NOW. 2020;9:4–8.
15. LaroccaNG. Impact of walking impairment in multiple sclerosis: perspectives of patients and care partners. Patient. 2011;4(3):189–201. https://doi.org/10.2165/11591150-000000000-00000.
16. Brochet B, Ruet A. Cognitive impairment in multiple sclerosis with regards to disease duration and clinical phenotypes. Front Neurol. 2019;10:261. https://doi.org/10.3389/fneur.2019.00261.
17. Van Emmerik REA, Remelius JG, Johnson MB, et al. Postural control in women with multiple sclerosis: effects of task, vision and symptomatic fatigue. Gait Posture. 2010;32:608–14. https://doi.org/10.1016/j.gaitpost.2010.09.002.
18. Oliva Ramirez A, Keenan A, Kalau O, et al. Prevalence and burden of multiple sclerosis-related fatigue: a systematic literature review. BMC Neurol. 2021;21:468. https://doi.org/10.1186/s12883-021-02396-1.
19. Motl RW, Chaparro G, Hernandez ME, et al. Physical function in older adults with multiple sclerosis: an application of the short physical performance battery. J Geriatr Phys Ther. 2018;41(3):155–60. https://doi.org/10.1519/JPT.0000000000000115.
20. Bollaert RE, Motl RW. Physical and cognitive functions, physical activity, and sedentary behavior in older adults with multiple sclerosis. J Geriatr Phys Ther. 2017;42(4):304–12. https://doi.org/10.1519/JPT.0000000000000163.
21. Bollaert RE, Balto JM, Sandroff BM, et al. Preliminary evidence for the effects of aging and multiple sclerosis on cognitive performance: an analysis based on effect size estimates. Exp Aging Res. 2017;43(4):346–54. https://doi.org/10.1080/0361073X.2017.1333820.
22. DalMonte J, Finlayson M, Helfrich C. In their own words: coping processes among women aging with multiple sclerosis. Occup Ther Heal Care. 2003;17(3–4):115–37. https://doi.org/10.1080/J003v17n03_08.
23. Cattaneo D, Lamers I, Bertoni R, et al. Participation restriction in people with multiple sclerosis: prevalence and correlations with cognitive, walking, balance, and upper limb impairments. Arch Phys Med Rehabil. 2017;98(7):1308–15. https://doi.org/10.1016/j.apmr.2017.02.015.
24. Buhse M. The elderly person with multiple sclerosis: clinical implications for the increasing life-span. J Neurosci Nurs. 2015;47(6):333–9; quiz E1. https://doi.org/10.1097/JNN.0000000000000172.
25. Sebastião E, Wood T, Motl RW, et al. The importance of promoting physical activity and exercise training as adjuvant therapy for people with multiple sclerosis. Motriz. 2022;28:1–5. https://doi.org/10.1590/S1980-657420220016021.
26. Motl RW, Pilutti LA. The benefits of exercise training in multiple sclerosis. Nat Rev Neurol. 2012;8:487–97. https://doi.org/10.1038/nrneurol.2012.136.
27. Kalb R, Brown TR, Coote S, et al. Exercise and lifestyle physical activity recommendations for people with multiple sclerosis throughout the disease course. Mult Scler. 2020;26(12):1459–69. https://doi.org/10.1177/1352458520915629.
28. Horton S, MacDonald DJ, Erickson K. MS, exercise, and the potential for older adults. Eur Rev Aging Phys Act. 2010;7:49–57. https://doi.org/10.1007/s11556-010-0062-9.
29. Pedersen BK, Saltin B. Exercise as medicine—evidence for prescribing exercise as therapy in 26 different chronic diseases. Scand J Med Sci Sport. 2015;25(Suppl 3):1–72. https://doi.org/10.1111/sms.12581.
30. Gustavsen S, Olsson A, Søndergaard HB, et al. The association of selected multiple sclerosis symptoms with disability and quality of life: a large Danish self-report survey. BMC Neurol. 2021;21(1):317. https://doi.org/10.1186/s12883-021-02344-z.
31. Dilorenzo T. Aging with multiple sclerosis. Clinical bulletin: information for health professionals. New York, NY: National Multiple Sclerosis Society; 2011.

32. van der Feen FE, de Haan GA, van der Lijn I, et al. Independent outdoor mobility of persons with multiple sclerosis—a systematic review. Mult Scler Relat Disord. 2020;37:101463. https://doi.org/10.1016/j.msard.2019.101463.
33. Baird JF, Cederberg KLJ, Sikes EM, et al. Physical activity and walking performance across the lifespan among adults with multiple sclerosis. Mult Scler Relat Disord. 2019;35:36–41. https://doi.org/10.1016/j.msard.2019.07.003.
34. Jeng B, Šilić P, Bollaert RE, et al. Physical function across the lifespan in adults with multiple sclerosis: an application of the short physical performance battery. Mult Scler Relat Disord. 2023;73:104624. https://doi.org/10.1016/j.msard.2023.104624.
35. Finlayson M, van Denend T. Experiencing the loss of mobility: perspectives of older adults with MS. Disabil Rehabil. 2003;25(20):1168–80. https://doi.org/10.1080/09638280310001596180.
36. Minden SL, Frankel D, Hadden LS, et al. Disability in elderly people with multiple sclerosis: an analysis of baseline data from the Sonya Slifka longitudinal multiple sclerosis study. NeuroRehabilitation. 2004;19(1):55–67. https://doi.org/10.3233/nre-2004-19107.
37. Cortese M, Bjornevik K, Chitnis T, et al. Aging with multiple sclerosis: a longitudinal study of physical function, mental health, and memory in two cohorts of US women. Mult Scler J. 2022;28(1):121–31. https://doi.org/10.1177/13524585211007739.
38. Confavreux C, Vukusic S. Age at disability milestones in multiple sclerosis. Brain. 2006;129(Pt 3):595–605. https://doi.org/10.1093/brain/awh714.
39. Berriozabalgoitia R, Bidaurrazaga-Letona I, Otxoa E, Urquiza M, Irazusta J, Rodriguez-Larrad A. Overground robotic program preserves gait in individuals with multiple sclerosis and moderate to severe impairments: a randomized controlled trial. Arch Phys Med Rehabil. 2021;102(5):932–9. https://doi.org/10.1016/j.apmr.2020.12.002.
40. Klewer J, Pohlau D, Nippert I, Haas JKJ. Problems reported by elderly patients with multiple sclerosis. J Neurosci. 2001;33(3):167–71. https://doi.org/10.1097/01376517-200106000-00009.
41. Nilsagård Y, Lundholm C, Denison E, Gunnarsson L-G. Predicting accidental falls in people with multiple sclerosis—a longitudinal study. Clin Rehabil. 2009;23(3):259–69. https://doi.org/10.1177/0269215508095087.
42. Kalmar JH, Gaudino EA, Moore NB, et al. The relationship between cognitive deficits and everyday functional activities in multiple sclerosis. Neuropsychology. 2008;22(4):442–9. https://doi.org/10.1037/0894-4105.22.4.442.
43. Benedict RH, Zivadinov R. Risk factors for and management of cognitive dysfunction in multiple sclerosis. Nat Rev Neurol. 2011;7(6):332–42. https://doi.org/10.1038/nrneurol.2011.61.
44. Bopp KL, Verhaeghen P. Aging and verbal memory span: a meta-analysis. J Gerontol B Psychol Sci Soc Sci. 2005;60(5):P223–33. https://doi.org/10.1093/geronb/60.5.p223.
45. Fozard JL, Vercruyssen M, Reynolds SL, et al. Age differences and changes in reaction time: the Baltimore longitudinal study of aging. J Gerontol. 1994;49(4):P179–89. https://doi.org/10.1093/geronj/49.4.p179.
46. Head D, Kennedy KM, Rodrigue KM, Raz N. Age-differences in perseveration: cognitive and neuroanatomical mediators of performance on the Wisconsin card sorting test. Neuropsychologia. 2009;47(4):1200–3. https://doi.org/10.1016/j.neuropsychologia.2009.01.003.
47. Chiang HS, Khera A, Stopschinski BE, et al. Cognitive decline in older people with multiple sclerosis—a narrative review of the literature. Geriatr. 2022;7(3):61. https://doi.org/10.3390/geriatrics7030061.
48. Branco M, Ruano L, Portaccio E, Goretti B, Niccolai C, Patti F, Chisari C, et al. Aging with multiple sclerosis: prevalence and profile of cognitive impairment. Neurol Sci. 2019;40(8):1651–7. https://doi.org/10.1007/s10072-019-03875-7.
49. Jakimovski D, Weinstock-Guttman B, Roy S, et al. Cognitive profiles of aging in multiple sclerosis. Front Aging Neurosci. 2019;11:105. https://doi.org/10.3389/fnagi.2019.00105.

50. Baird JF, Cederberg KLJ, Morghen Sikes E, et al. Changes in cognitive performance with age in adults with multiple sclerosis. Cogn Behav Neurol. 2019;32:201. https://doi.org/10.1097/WNN.0000000000000200.
51. Salthouse TA. Aging and measures of processing speed. Biol Psychol. 2000;54(1–3):35–54. https://doi.org/10.1016/s0301-0511(00)00052-1.
52. Roy S, Frndak S, Drake AS, et al. Differential effects of aging on motor and cognitive functioning in multiple sclerosis. Mult Scler. 2017;23(10):1385–93. https://doi.org/10.1177/1352458516679036.
53. Jakimovski D, Weinstock-Guttman B, Roy S, et al. Cognitive profiles of aging in multiple sclerosis. Front Aging Neurosci. 2019;11:105. https://doi.org/10.3389/FNAGI.2019.00105/BIBTEX.
54. Bodling AM, Denney DR, Lynch SG. Cognitive aging in patients with multiple sclerosis: a cross-sectional analysis of speeded processing. Arch Clin Neuropsychol. 2009;24(8):761–7. https://doi.org/10.1093/arclin/acp076.
55. Yi A. California verbal learning test (California verbal learning test-II). In: Kreutzer JS, DeLuca J, Caplan B, editors. Encyclopedia of clinical neuropsychology. New York, NY: Springer; 2011. https://doi.org/10.1007/978-0-387-79948-3_1112.
56. Rocca MA, Riccitelli GC, Meani A, Pagani E, Del Sette P, Martinelli V, Comi G, et al. Cognitive reserve, cognition, and regional brain damage in MS: a 2-year longitudinal study. Mult Scler J. 2019;25(3):372–81.
57. Amato MP, Razzolini L, Goretti B, et al. Cognitive reserve and cortical atrophy in multiple sclerosis: a longitudinal study. Neurology. 2013;80(19):1728–33. https://doi.org/10.1212/WNL.0b013e3182918c6f.
58. Tam JW, Schmitter-Edgecombe M. The role of processing speed in the brief visuospatial memory test—revised. Clin Neuropsychol. 2013;27:962. https://doi.org/10.1080/13854046.2013.797500.
59. Prakash RS, Snook EM, Lewis JM, et al. Cognitive impairments in relapsing-remitting multiple sclerosis: a meta-analysis. Mult Scler. 2008;14:1250. https://doi.org/10.1177/1352458508095004.
60. Alexandra T, Kim C, Estefania B, et al. The effects of aging and disease duration on cognition in multiple sclerosis. Brain Cogn. 2020;146:105650. https://doi.org/10.1016/j.bandc.2020.105650.
61. Butler Pagnotti R, Hua LH, Miller JB. Cognition and disease characteristics in adult onset versus late onset multiple sclerosis. Mult Scler. 2021;28(6):933–41. https://doi.org/10.1177/13524585211039112.
62. Galetta SL, Markowitz C. US FDA-approved disease-modifying treatments for multiple sclerosis: review of adverse effect profiles. CNS Drugs. 2005;19(3):239–52. https://doi.org/10.2165/00023210-200519030-00005.
63. Coalition M (2017) The use of disease-modifying therapies in multiple sclerosis: principles and current evidence summary.
64. Frahm N, Hecker M, Zettl UK. Polypharmacy among patients with multiple sclerosis: a qualitative systematic review. Expert Opin Drug Saf. 2020;19(2):139–45. https://doi.org/10.1080/14740338.2020.1720646.
65. Maher RL, Hanlon J, Hajjar ER. Clinical consequences of polypharmacy in elderly. Expert Opin Drug Saf. 2014;13(1):57–65. https://doi.org/10.1517/14740338.2013.827660.
66. Kołtuniuk A, Rosińczuk J. Adherence to disease-modifying therapies in patients with multiple sclerosis. Patient. 2018;12:1557–66. https://doi.org/10.2147/PPA.S175095.
67. Shirani A, Zhao Y, Petkau J, et al. Multiple sclerosis in older adults: the clinical profile and impact of interferon Beta treatment. Biomed Res Int. 2015;2015:451912. https://doi.org/10.1155/2015/451912.
68. Motl RW, Sandroff BM, Kwakkel G, et al. Exercise in patients with multiple sclerosis. Lancet Neurol. 2017;16(10):848–56. https://doi.org/10.1016/S1474-4422(17)30281-8.
69. Motl RW. Lifestyle physical activity in persons with multiple sclerosis: the new kid on the MS block. Mult Scler J. 2014;20(8):1025–9. https://doi.org/10.1177/1352458514525873.

70. Dalgas U, Langeskov-Christensen M, Stenager E, et al. Exercise as medicine in multiple sclerosis—time for a paradigm shift: preventive, symptomatic, and disease-modifying aspects and perspectives. Curr Neurol Neurosci Rep. 2019;19(11):88. https://doi.org/10.1007/s11910-019-1002-3.
71. Platta ME, Ensari I, Motl RW, Pilutti LA. The effect of exercise training on fitness in multiple sclerosis: a meta-analysis. Arch Phys Med Rehabil. 2016;97(9):1564–72. https://doi.org/10.1016/j.apmr.2016.01.023.
72. Halabchi F, Alizadeh Z, Sahraian MA, Abolhasani M. Exercise prescription for patients with multiple sclerosis; potential benefits and practical recommendations. BMC Neurol. 2017;17(1):185. https://doi.org/10.1186/s12883-017-0960-9.
73. Arik MI, Kiloatar HSI. Do Pilates exercises improve balance in patients with multiple sclerosis? A systematic review and meta-analysis. Mult Scler Relat Disord. 2022;57:103410. https://doi.org/10.1016/j.msard.2021.103410.
74. Hao Z, Zhang X, Chen P. Effects of different exercise therapies on balance function and functional walking ability in multiple sclerosis disease patients—a network meta-analysis of randomized controlled trials. Int J Environ Res Public Health. 2022;19(12):7175. https://doi.org/10.3390/ijerph19127175.
75. Pearson M, Dieberg GSN. Exercise as a therapy for improvement of walking ability in adults with multiple sclerosis: a meta-analysis. Arch Phys Med Rehabil. 2015;96(7):1339–1348.e7. https://doi.org/10.1016/j.apmr.2015.02.011.
76. McAuley E, Wojcicki TR, Learmonth YC, et al. Effects of a DVD-delivered exercise intervention on physical function in older adults with multiple sclerosis: a pilot randomized controlled trial. Mult Scler J—Exp Transl Clin. 2015;1:2055217315584838. https://doi.org/10.1177/2055217315584838.
77. Sebastião E, McAuley E, Shigematsu R, et al. Home-based, square-stepping exercise program among older adults with multiple sclerosis: results of a feasibility randomized controlled study. Contemp Clin Trials. 2018;73:136–44. https://doi.org/10.1016/j.cct.2018.09.008.
78. Sandroff BM, Motl R. Device-measured physical activity and cognitive processing speed impairment in a large sample of persons with multiple sclerosis. J Int Neuropsychol Soc. 2020;6(8):798–805. https://doi.org/10.1017/S1355617720000284.
79. Motl RW, Sandroff BM, Benedict RHB. Moderate-to-vigorous physical activity is associated with processing speed, but not learning and memory, in cognitively impaired persons with multiple sclerosis. Mult Scler Relat Disord. 2022;63:103833. https://doi.org/10.1016/j.msard.2022.103833.
80. Vanner EA, Block P, Christodoulou CC, Horowitz BP, Krupp LB. Pilot study exploring quality of life and barriers to leisure-time physical activity in persons with moderate to severe multiple sclerosis. Disabil Health J. 2008;1(1):58–65. https://doi.org/10.1016/j.dhjo.2007.11.001.
81. Sandroff BM, Motl RW, Amato MP, Brichetto G, Chataway J, Chiaravalloti ND, Cutter GR, Dalgas U, DeLuca J, Farrell R, Feys P, Filippi M, Freeman J, Inglese M, Meza C, Rocca MA, Salter A, Feinstein A. Cardiorespiratory fitness and free-living physical activity are not associated with cognition in persons with progressive multiple sclerosis: baseline analyses from the CogEx study. Mult Scler. 2022;28(7):1091–100. https://doi.org/10.1177/13524585211048397.
82. Gharakhanlou R, Wesselmann L, Rademacher A, Lampit A, Negaresh R, Kaviani M, Oberste M, Motl RW, Sandroff BM, Bansi J, Baker JS, Heesen C, Zimmer F, Javelle F. Exercise training and cognitive performance in persons with multiple sclerosis: a systematic review and multilevel meta-analysis of clinical trials. Mult Scler. 2021;27(13):1977–93. https://doi.org/10.1177/1352458520917935.
83. Li G, You Q, Hou X, Zhang S, Liwen D, Yuanyuan Lv LY. The effect of exercise on cognitive function in people with multiple sclerosis: a systematic review and meta-analysis of randomized controlled trials. J Neurol. 2023;270(6):2908–23. https://doi.org/10.1007/s00415-023-11649-7.

84. DeLuca J, Chiaravalotti ND, Sandroff BM. Treatment and management of cognitive dysfunction in patients with multiple sclerosis. Nat Rev Neurol. 2020;16(6):319–32. https://doi.org/10.1038/s41582-020-0355-1.
85. Kalb R, Beier M, Benedict RHB, et al. Recommendations for cognitive screening and management in multiple sclerosis care. Mult Scler J. 2018;24(13):1665–80. https://doi.org/10.1177/1352458518803785.
86. Feys P, Moumdjian L, Halewyck FV, Wens I, Eijnde BO, Van Wijmeersch B, Popescu VA. Effects of an individual 12-week community-located "start-to-run" program on physical capacity, walking, fatigue, cognitive function, brain volumes, and structures in persons with multiple sclerosis. Mult Scler. 2019;25(1):92–103. https://doi.org/10.1177/1352458517740211.
87. Beier M, Bombardier CH, Hartoonian N, et al. Improved physical fitness correlates with improved cognition in multiple sclerosis. Arch Phys Med Rehabil. 2014;95(7):1328–34. https://doi.org/10.1016/j.apmr.2014.02.017.
88. Feinstein A, Amato MP, Brichetto G, et al. Study protocol: improving cognition in people with progressive multiple sclerosis: a multi-arm, randomized, blinded, sham-controlled trial of cognitive rehabilitation and aerobic exercise (COGEx). BMC Neurol. 2020;20(1):204. https://doi.org/10.1186/s12883-020-01772-7.
89. Kalron A, Menascu S, Hoffmann C, Anat A. The importance of physical activity to preserve hippocampal volume in people with multiple sclerosis: a structural MRI study. J Neurol. 2020;267:3723–30. https://doi.org/10.1007/s00415-020-10085-1.
90. Leavitt VM, Cirnigliaro C, Cohen A, et al. Aerobic exercise increases hippocampal volume and improves memory in multiple sclerosis: preliminary findings. Neurocase. 2014;20(6):695–7. https://doi.org/10.1080/13554794.2013.841951.
91. Shobeiri P, Karimi A, Momtazmanesh S, et al. Exercise-induced increase in blood-based brain-derived neurotrophic factor (BDNF) in people with multiple sclerosis: a systematic review and meta-analysis of exercise intervention trials. PLoS One. 2022;17(3):e0264557. https://doi.org/10.1371/journal.pone.0264557.
92. Santinelli FB, Sebastião E, Simieli L, Antunes BM, Vieira LHP, Kalron A, Barbieri FA. Is BDNF related to spatial-temporal gait parameters in people with multiple sclerosis? An observational study. Mult Scler Relat Disord. 2022;66:104064. https://doi.org/10.1016/j.msard.2022.104064.
93. Sandroff BM, Motl RW, Reed WR, et al. Integrative CNS plasticity with exercise in MS: the PRIMERS (PRocessing, Integration of Multisensory Exercise-Related Stimuli) conceptual framework. Neurorehabil Neural Repair. 2018;32(10):847–62. https://doi.org/10.1177/1545968318798938.
94. Sebastião E, Sandroff BM, Learmonth YC, Motl RW. Validity of the timed up and go as a measure of functional mobility in persons with multiple sclerosis. Arch Phys Med Rehabil. 2016;97(7):1072–7. https://doi.org/10.1016/j.apmr.2015.12.031.
95. Fischer JS, Rudick RA, Cutter GR, Reingold SC. The multiple sclerosis functional composite measure (MSFC): an integrated approach to MS clinical outcome assessment. National MS Society clinical outcomes assessment task force. Mult Scler. 1999;5(4):244–50. https://doi.org/10.1177/135245859900500409.
96. Kaufman M, Moyer D, Norton J. The significant change for the timed 25-foot walk in the multiple sclerosis functional composite. Mult Scler J. 2000;6(4):286–90. https://doi.org/10.1177/135245850000600411.
97. Goldman MD, Marrie RA, Cohen JA. Evaluation of the six-minute walk in multiple sclerosis subjects and healthy controls. Mult Scler. 2008;14(3):383–90. https://doi.org/10.1177/1352458507082607.
98. Sandroff BM, Motl RW, Sosnoff JJ, Pula JH. Further validation of the six-spot step test as a measure of ambulation in multiple sclerosis. Gait Posture. 2015;41(1):222–7. https://doi.org/10.1016/j.gaitpost.2014.10.011.

99. Motl RW, Learmonth YC, Wójcicki TR, et al. Preliminary validation of the short physical performance battery in older adults with multiple sclerosis: secondary data analysis. BMC Geriatr. 2015;15:157. https://doi.org/10.1186/s12877-015-0156-3.
100. Wagner JM, Norris RA, Van Dillen LR, et al. Four square step test in ambulant persons with multiple sclerosis: validity, reliability, and responsiveness. Int J Rehabil Res. 2013;36(3):253–9. https://doi.org/10.1097/MRR.0b013e32835fd97f.
101. Kalron A, Givon U. Construct validity of the four square step test in multiple sclerosis. Arch Phys Med Rehabil. 2016;97(9):1496–501. https://doi.org/10.1016/j.apmr.2016.04.012.
102. Benedict RHB, Amato MP, Boringa J, et al. Brief international cognitive assessment for MS (BICAMS): international standards for validation. BMC Neurol. 2012;12:55. https://doi.org/10.1186/1471-2377-12-55.

Effects of Physical Activity on Walking in Individuals with Parkinson's Disease

23

Diego Orcioli-Silva, Vinicius Cavassano Zampier, Gabriel Antonio Gazziero Moraca, Victor Spiandor Beretta, and Paulo Henrique Silva Pelicioni

Abstract

Gait impairments are common and disabling symptoms of Parkinson's disease (PD) and are associated with the risk of falls. Non-pharmacological interventions, such as physical exercise, may efficiently complement PD treatment and may mitigate the gait problems in people with PD. In this chapter, we bring to light different types of exercises that have shown positive results for gait parameters in people with PD. Because of the large number of findings, initially, we will present an overview of the effects of different exercises on walking, and, later, the chapter will focus mainly in two topics widely discussed recently: (i) gait adaptation (due to its close relationship with falls) and (ii) exercise combined with transcranial direct current stimulation (tDCS; as it is a potential tool to optimize the benefits of exercise in gait parameters). Overall, physical exercise is an effective method to treat gait problems in PD.

D. Orcioli-Silva (✉) · V. C. Zampier · G. A. G. Moraca
Department of Physical Education, Institute of Biosciences, São Paulo State University (UNESP), Rio Claro, SP, Brazil

V. S. Beretta
School of Technology and Sciences, Physical Education Department, São Paulo State University (Unesp), Presidente Prudente, Brazil
e-mail: victor.beretta@unesp.br

P. H. S. Pelicioni
School of Health Sciences, University of New South Wales, Sydney, NSW, Australia
e-mail: paulo.silvapelicioni@unsw.edu.au

F. A. Barbieri et al. (eds.), *Locomotion and Posture in Older Adults*,
https://doi.org/10.1007/978-3-031-74123-4_23

Introduction

Gait impairments are common and disabling symptoms of Parkinson's disease (PD) [1] and are associated with tripping and body imbalance, which increase fall episodes [2, 3]. The number of fall episodes in people with PD is approximately two or even threefold bigger than their healthy peers [2, 4] and is the second major cause of hospitalization [5], mainly due to fractures [6, 7]. In addition to fractures, the consequences of a fall episode are related to physical, psychological, and functional impairments such as fear of falling, decrease in mobility, and loss of independence to perform activities of daily living [8–10]. Therefore, researchers all over the world have focused on investigating disease-related locomotor behavior and developing interventions to alleviate gait impairments and prevent fall episodes.

Gait patterns of people with PD include shorter step length, slower gait velocity, and greater gait variability and gait asymmetry [1, 11–14]. These deficits are exacerbated when the locomotor control of people with PD are challenging as walking over uneven terrain or dual-task condition. Previous studies have consistently reported that dual-task walking further reduces gait speed and step length, and increases gait variability [15–19]. Walking over uneven terrain requires constant adaptations in gait parameters. Since people with PD also face uneven terrain in their everyday lives, a recent and large set of studies has been published on obstacle avoidance describing the walking behavior by means of kinematic parameters [11, 13, 20–27]. The results of these studies revealed that two major disease features (bradykinesia and hypometria) could be seen in both the approaching and the crossing phases: reduction in stride length and stride velocity, decreased distances between the leading foot and the obstacle before and after crossing and similar toe clearance when people with PD were compared with their age-matched healthy controls. Also, such results have shown an increase in gait asymmetry and variability; consequently, the risk of falls increases in this population.

People with PD rely on executive resources to compensate for gait problems, especially due to loss of gait automaticity (demonstrated by increased gait variability). Studies involving functional near-infrared spectroscopy (fNIRS) reported increased oxygenated hemoglobin (HbO_2) concentration (i.e., a proxy for greater cortical activation) in the prefrontal cortex (PFC) in people with PD during usual walking [28–30] compared to healthy older adults. In addition, people with PD further increased PFC HbO_2 during obstacle avoidance [21, 28, 31], and dual task [17, 32–34]. The PFC is part of the executive locomotor pathway [35, 36] and is argued to become activated when the automatic execution of walking is reduced [35, 37, 38]. Therefore, PD may lead to a shift from automatic gait control (i.e., direct locomotor pathway) to a more attentional, executive control (i.e., indirect locomotor pathway) [39], as a compensatory mechanism for gait impairments [35, 40].

Dopaminergic medications are the gold standard treatment for people with PD and their effects on motor function, mobility, and postural instability have been established [41–43]. Specifically related to gait parameters, dopamine replacement improves step length and velocity [17, 21, 41, 42]. In addition, dopaminergic medication facilitates the recruitment of PFC during challenging walking, which may increase the available cognitive resources during walking [17, 21]. However, long-term levodopa administration reduces its effectiveness, increases the tolerance for some symptoms, and causes side effects such as motor fluctuations and dyskinesias (involuntary movements) [44]. Thus, the inclusion of non-pharmacological interventions, such as physical exercise, may efficiently complement PD treatment and improve the quality of life for people with PD. Due to the importance of interventions to improve the locomotor pattern, we have carried out a literature review of the effects of exercise on the locomotion of people with PD. Because of the large number of findings, initially, we will present an overview of the effects of different exercises on walking, and, later, the chapter will focus mainly in two topics widely discussed recently: (i) gait adaptation (due to its close relationship with falls [3, 45]) and (ii) exercise combined with transcranial direct current stimulation (tDCS; as it is a potential tool to optimize the benefits of exercise in gait parameters [46–48]).

Walking and Exercise in Parkinson's Disease

Physical exercise is a non-invasive and low-cost method of intervention and has been employed as an effective complementary therapy to improve PD signs and symptoms such as walking, postural instability, freezing of gait, cognitive impairment, and depression [49–54]. In addition, physical exercise, when combined with dopaminergic treatment, holds the potential to elevate dopaminergic levels [55], modify gray matter [56], and enhance cerebral connectivity [57]. Also, previous studies have suggested that physical exercise can retard the disease progression and induce plastic effects in the patients' brains [58–60].

Walking, a seemingly simple daily activity, takes a great significance in the context of PD. Gait disturbances are a prevalent motor symptom, leading to compromised mobility, increased risk of falls, and reduced quality of life. Protas et al. [61] recognized the pivotal role of gait training in reducing falls among people with PD. Their study demonstrated that targeted training interventions could improve gait stability, thereby contributing to fall prevention. Herman et al. [62] conducted a mini-review that underscored the positive impact of treadmill training on gait parameters in people with PD. Treadmill-based interventions were found to enhance stride length and velocity, potentially ameliorating the motor deficits associated with PD [62].

Cueing techniques provided another avenue for gait improvement. A meta-analysis revealed that auditory and visual cues substantially improved gait performance in people with PD [63]. These cues act as external rhythmic stimuli, facilitating movement initiation and regulation. Expanding upon traditional walking, Nordic walking emerged as a novel intervention. Van Eijkeren et al. [64] investigated the effects of Nordic walking in people with PD, demonstrating improvements in both mobility and psychological well-being. This multidimensional benefit underscores the potential of walking interventions to address diverse aspects of PD. Recent research by Zampier et al. [65] further enhances our understanding about auditory instructions on motor symptoms in PD. The study revealed an intriguing relationship between arm swing during walking and gait bradykinesia. It was found that after people with PD received verbal instructions to increase their arm swing amplitude and frequency, gait bradykinesia and hypometria decreased. This finding not only sheds light on the intricate interplay between upper and lower body movements but also opens possibilities for targeted interventions that leverage arm swing modulation to address specific motor symptoms in PD.

A spectrum of exercise modalities has been explored to improve locomotion in people with PD. Dance-based interventions, including Argentine tango and American ballroom, have gained attention for their potential to enhance movement control and motor function in individuals with PD [66–69]. Dance involves complex and varied movements that challenge motor planning, coordination, and balance. This can be particularly beneficial for individuals with PD, as it encourages adaptive strategies and engages different neural circuits [66–69]. Tai Chi, a mind-body exercise that involves slow and controlled movements, has emerged as a potential intervention for enhancing postural stability, mobility, cognition, reducing fall risk, and improving overall motor function in people with PD [70, 71]. Tai Chi's emphasis on controlled movements and balance challenges aligns with the motor deficits seen in PD, making it a suitable exercise modality [70, 71]. Additionally, Tai Chi incorporates mindfulness and relaxation techniques, which could potentially alleviate non-motor symptoms such as anxiety and depression [54, 72].

Despite the consensus regarding the benefits of physical exercise for people with PD, the appropriate exercise intensity for this population is still debated. The investigation by van der Kolk et al. [73] explored the effectiveness of home-based and remotely supervised aerobic exercises, revealing comparable improvements in aerobic capacity and cognitive function regardless of exercise intensity. Similarly, a meta-analysis conducted by Shu et al. [51] corroborated these findings, indicating that both moderate and light-intensity aerobic exercises exhibit significant benefits in managing PD symptoms (e.g. increasing gait velocity), without distinct superiority of one intensity over the other. These studies challenge the notion that higher intensity exercise necessarily yields greater therapeutic outcomes for individuals with PD. Additionally, the meta-analysis suggests that any intensity level, when integrated into a structured exercise regimen, can substantially contribute to ameliorating both motor and non-motor symptoms of PD, underscoring the importance of personalized exercise programs tailored to individual needs and capacities [51]. Although the optimal exercise intensity is not conclusive, current evidence continues to suggest that it is not solely about the exercise intensity, but rather the consistent engagement in tailored exercises that plays a pivotal role in enhancing the quality of life of people with PD.

Recent technological advancements have led to the application of virtual reality and robotics to enhance locomotor behavior in people with PD [74–76]. Virtual reality has shown promise in promoting motor learning through multisensory inputs and repetitive movement practice [77]. Robotic resources, in combination with treadmill training, have demonstrated positive effects on the gait parameters of people with PD, such as increased stride length and velocity [78, 79]. Technological advancements have also allowed the combination of physical exercise with other types of interventions, such as tDCS [46, 80]. The information regarding the effect of tDCS combined with exercise for walking in people with PD are described in the section "Transcranial Direct Current Stimulation and Physical Exercise on Walking".

As evidenced in this section, a diverse range of physical interventions have been employed to enhance walking behavior in people with PD. However, consensus is lacking regarding the optimal type, frequency, intensity, and duration of physical exercise for this purpose [81]. Nonetheless, the diversity of exercise options allows individuals to choose activities they find enjoyable, as motivation is crucial for sustained participation in intervention programs [82, 83]. It is important to highlight that a combination of medication and physical exercise is essential to improve locomotion and reduce fall incidents [84].

Effects of Physical Exercise on Adaptive Gait

In the first edition of this book [85], we investigated the effects of "physical exercise and walking over uneven terrain." In this new version, we are currently examining the effects of physical exercise on adaptive gait since humans are constantly adapting our gait due to environmental constraints [86–88]. Pathologies affecting motor control also modify how humans adapt their gait; PD is an example. Using a gait adaptation paradigm [86–88], Caetano et al. [89, 90] and Pelicioni et al. [91] examined how people with PD adapt their gait when required to step on targets or avoid obstacles. Compared to healthy subjects, people with PD had difficulties adapting their gait in response to targets, showing poor stepping accuracy [89]. This poor stepping accuracy was associated with poor executive function and reactive balance [90]. People with PD had more difficulties when dealing with obstacle avoidance, taking more steps to deal with obstacles [89]. Also, limited cognitive capacity was associated with leg adjustments to avoid obstacles [90]. In a further examination, we investigated the cortical activity of the dorsolateral PFC, supplementary motor area and premotor cortex concurrently with the performance of the gait adaptability test [91]. These areas involve cognitive processing, executive functioning, and motor planning. People with PD demonstrated having no cortical capacity beyond what they require for simple walking; therefore, they performed a more conservative adaptive gait, slowing down and taking short steps to deal with obstacles. In summary, the association between cognition, executive function, balance, limited neural resources, and adaptive gait in PD help us understand the best strategies to prevent falls in this group.

Overall, physical activity has many benefits for people with PD [92]. Physical activity programs were proven to attenuate symptoms related to poor gait adaptability. In cognitive features, for example, a 6-month intervention (twice a week, 60 min each session) with a focus on locomotor and cognitive exercises maintained cognitive degeneration in people with mild-to-moderate PD assessed via different cognitive domains [93]. In a different study, participants with mild-to-moderate PD performed multimodal exercises for 6 months (three times a week, 60 min each session), and the effects of exercises were assessed via diverse executive functioning assessments. Similarly, participants had benefits of exercises on their executive functioning [94]. In a protocol including resistance training with instability (twice a week, 60 min each session for 12 weeks), people with mild-to-moderate PD have overall improved their balance and concern of falling [95].

Even though physical activity can improve parameters associated with adaptive gait, other studies have investigated the direct effects of exercise on adaptive gait outcomes. Landers et al. [96] investigated the effects of 4 weeks of balance intervention on 49 people with PD. The study participants were divided into four groups that undertook (i) balance exercise with external attentional focus, (ii) balance exercise with internal attentional focus, (iii) balance exercises without attentional focus, and (iv) a control group. These exercises were undertaken three times per week, 45 min for each session. The investigators examined the time to complete an obstacle course where participants had to adapt their gait. All groups completed the course, and the authors did not observe any discrepancy between groups at reassessment. In two different studies, the authors investigated the accuracy of negotiating with obstacles. First, Song et al. [97] investigated the effects of 12 weeks of exergame stepping interventions on 60 people with PD (Hoehn and Yahr stages from I to III). The study participants were divided into two groups: the exercise and control groups. The exergames were played three times per week, 15 min for each session. The investigators used the accuracy in the gait adaptability paradigm [86–88, 91] measured as a foot placement in a target or fully avoidance when an obstacle was presented as outcomes. The authors did not observe any effects of the intervention on the adaptive gait of the participants. On the other hand, Wang et al. [98] observed a positive effect of augmented reality training using a treadmill on adaptive gait. These authors investigated the effects of 7 days of intervention, 30 min each session, in 52 people with PD, divided into PIGD and non-PIGD subtypes. The participants undertook augmented reality training using the C-Mill treadmill protocol. The success of adapting participants' gait on virtual objects projected on the treadmill was used as an outcome. The authors observed that regardless of the PD subtype, participants were more successful in adapting their gait when virtual objects were projected on their way.

When examining more robust measurements of adaptive gait, positive effects of the intervention were observed. Mirelman et al. [77] investigated the effects of 6 weeks of progressive treadmill intervention with virtual obstacles performed three times per week, 45 min each session, on 20 people with PD (Hoehn and Yahr stages from I to III). The authors observed a positive effect of an intervention on gait speed and stride length during obstacle negotiation at both immediate reassessment and follow-up 4 weeks after the end of the intervention. Similarly, Liao et al. [99] examined the effect of two different interventions on obstacle crossing in comparison to a control group: (i) virtual reality Wii-fit, combining Yoga, strengthening and balance exercise; (ii) traditional strengthening and balance exercises. Thirty-six participants with PD (Hoehn and Yahr stages from I to III) were divided into three groups. The authors observed that participants in the virtual reality training group showed better performance in immediate post-assessment and follow-up (1 month) on crossing velocity and stride length for obstacle crossing compared to the control group. It seems that when a more robust measurement of obstacle crossing is used to measure individuals' performance, such as kinematic analysis of gait (gait speed, crossing velocity, and stride length), the authors were able to observe positive effects of their planned interventions in comparison to the studies above [96, 97], which the authors just adopted the time to complete an obstacle course as an outcome. In addition, virtual reality protocols seem to be a good exercise modality to enhance adaptive gait in PD, as its use has been previously discussed [100]. The effect of different exercises on adaptive gait was also examined when analyzing the kinetic characteristics of gait. Kim et al. [101] investigated the effect of Tai Chi (12 weeks, 3 sessions per week, each session lasting 60 min) on the center of pressure on the swing and stance phases during obstacle negotiation. The authors observed an increased anteroposterior and mediolateral displacement during foot placement during obstacle negotiation when participants were reassessed. The results are suggestive of the use of more degrees of freedom to cope with such complex tasks, allowing participants to use their biomechanics to compensate for task constraints (e.g. obstacle negotiation). Tai chi has been considered an important physical activity modality, and the activities that participants perform balancing over their limits of stability can explain such important results [72].

Finally, Maidan et al. [102] examined concurrent PFC activity with obstacle negotiation as an outcome for treadmill interventions. Sixty-four people with PD were allocated to a group undertaking virtual reality associated with a treadmill, while another group performed only treadmill training (for 6 weeks, 3 times per week, 45 min each session for both groups). The authors observed a reduction in right PFC activity during obstacle negotiation in participants who were part of the virtual reality and treadmill training group. These results, in addition to reduced falls, suggest that the use of a virtual reality protocol and treadmill training might lead to more efficient use of prefrontal cortical resources due to enhancing the use of the striatal-thalamic-cortical-motor circuit, therefore leading to a more automatic process during walking.

Transcranial Direct Current Stimulation and Physical Exercise on Walking

Despite the benefits of physical exercise on walking in people with PD, complementary therapies associated with the exercise have been investigated to optimize such benefits, such as tDCS. tDCS is a non-invasive brain stimulation technique that applies weak electric current through electrodes on the scalp [103, 104]. In general, anodal tDCS increases the excitability of the target cortical area, and cathodic decreases the excitability of the target cortical area. This technique stands out for its safety and ease of use [105], the low cost when compared to other brain stimulation techniques (e.g., transcranial magnetic stimulation), and the possibility of clinical application combined with another intervention, such as physical exercise/therapy. tDCS is considered safe because the most common adverse effects are mild tingling and itching that disappear few minutes after the stimulation ending. A previous demonstrates that tDCS with ≤4 mA applied up to 40 min does not to cause serious adverse effects or irreversible damage in human brain [105]. This study considered across over 33,200 sessions and 1000 subjects with repeated sessions with conventional tDCS (i.e., protocols characteristics described above). On the other hand, seizure is the main concern (adverse effect) in the transcranial magnetic stimulation. Although this concern spread to tDCS application, it should be highlighted that tDCS produce weak static electric fields in the brain and not pulsed as evidenced in repetitive transcranial magnetic stimulation [105].

tDCS application may promote several neurophysiological effects, such as decreased GABAergic neurotransmitters and increased dopamine levels in the striatum [106]. Furthermore, tDCS application may also favor neuroplasticity [107], and modulate brain functional connectivity [108] and blood flow, increasing the supply of oxygen to cortical and subcortical areas [109]. tDCS prolonged the cortical excitability caused by walking training with visual cues, suggesting that the combination of stimulation with physical exercise causes superior effects in cortical excitability [110]. In addition to the neurophysiological improvement, the benefits of intervention that combined tDCS with physical exercise on motor symptoms in people with PD have been demonstrated in recent years, such as the improvements in walking [111, 112].

The synergistic effects of a single session of tDCS combined with physical exercise are still mixed in the literature. In the study of Kaski and colleagues [111], an experimental group performed physical training (focused on walking and balance) concomitantly with the tDCS application (15 min) on the primary motor and premotor cortices, while the other group only received the tDCS. They found that the combined intervention generated improvements in walking velocity when compared to the tDCS application alone. Moreover, the combined intervention improved walking velocity more than only gait training, suggesting that tDCS can act as a technique that enhances the effects of physical exercise [111]. In this sense, Conceição et al. [112] observed that 20 min of aerobic physical exercise combined with tDCS applied over PFC may improve gait parameters of people with PD by decreasing step time variability. Also, the author observed an increase in PFC activity in the stimulated hemisphere while walking. This last result is particularly interesting as it denotes that the combination was able to increase the use of PFC resources in gait control, facilitating the compensatory mechanism used by people with PD (greater use of the indirect locomotor pathway) [113]. On the other hand, other studies did not show synergistic effects after only one session of physical exercise combined with tDCS application [114, 115].

The effects of multiple sessions of physical exercise combined with tDCS application on walking have also been studied. For example, Costa-Ribeiro and colleagues [116] carried out 10 sessions of cueing gait training in combination with tDCS application on the supplementary motor area. tDCS did not optimize the positive effects on walking generated by cueing gait training, but it was able to prolong the improvements in functional mobility (i.e., performance in the timed up and go test), assessed 4 weeks after the last training session. Schabrun and colleagues [117] combined tDCS application with dual-task gait training for 9 sessions and found improvements in walking velocity, cadence, step length, and double support time independent of stimulation. Other study evidenced results similar in walking parameters, with the positive effects and positive effects being maintained up to 8 weeks after the end of the intervention [118]. Due to the heterogeneity of tDCS protocols and the mixed results shown by studies in walking, some systematic reviews have been published.

A recent meta-analysis investigated the effects of tDCS on walking from two perspectives: short-term and long-term effects [119]. This study found a significant effect only in short-term treatment (effect size = 0.359), suggesting that tDCS slightly improved post-test locomotion within 24 h. Another systematic review reinforces that stimulation in motor areas is promising (showing improvements in the gait parameters), while stimulation in the PFC has been less explored and its results have been more heterogeneous [120]. Both reviews considered studies that applied tDCS as a stand-alone intervention or combined with another intervention, such as physical exercise. To our knowledge, just one systematic review involved only studies that applied tDCS in combination with physical and/or cognitive intervention and it supports that synergistic effects of combination may be obtained for walking, mainly after an intervention with multiple sessions [80].

In summary, the synergistic effects of combined tDCS application with other motor intervention needs to be more understood, and there is a need for more studies that specifically analyze the effects of combining physical exercise and tDCS. Many recent systematic reviews point to the need to establish an ideal tDCS protocol for improving the walking of people with PD [80, 119, 120]. Future studies in this field must focus on establishing the duration, area, moment (before or during the training), and intensity ideal of stimulation and verify what kind of exercise (gait training, aerobic, among others) can be more beneficial by applying tDCS.

Final Remarks

Figure 23.1 summarizes the benefits of physical exercise for walking in people with PD. Overall, physical exercise is an effective method to improve gait impairments (e.g. increasing gait velocity and step/stride length) of people with PD, especially during adaptive gait. However, designing an intervention with physical exercise in order to improve gait parameters in people with PD is still a challenge. There is no consensus in the literature with respect to better intervention characteristics (type, frequency, intensity, and duration of physical exercises) to promote effects on the walking behavior of people with PD. In addition, although new methods have emerged, such as a combination of tDCS and motor/non-motor intervention, the results are still controversial. In this sense, new research is needed to optimize the benefits of physical exercise for walking problems in people with PD. However, it is a fact that there is a large amount of evidence that shows the most important thing is to encourage people with PD to adopt and maintain an active lifestyle to improve gait patterns, hence reducing the risk of falls.

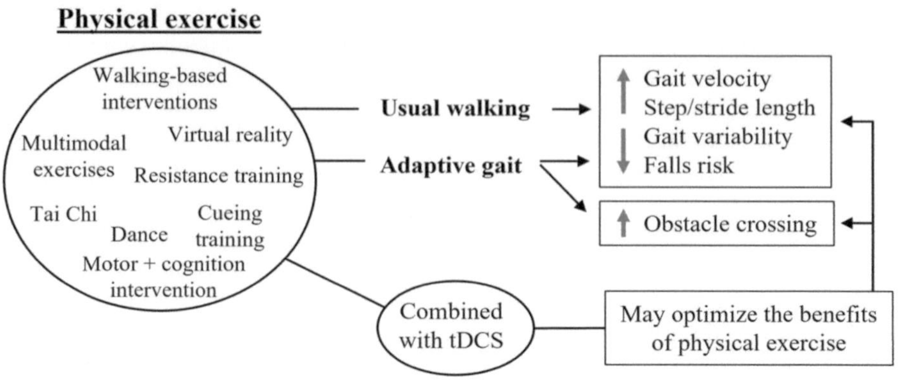

Fig. 23.1 In summary, different types of physical exercise improve gait parameters in both usual walking and adaptive gait. Moreover, complementary therapies, such as transcranial direct current stimulation (tDCS), when associated with exercise, may optimize the benefits of exercise on gait parameters

References

1. Mirelman A, Bonato P, Camicioli R, Ellis TD, Giladi N, Hamilton JL, et al. Gait impairments in Parkinson's disease. Lancet Neurol. 2019;18(7):697–708. https://doi.org/10.1016/S1474-4422(19)30044-4.
2. Bloem BR, Hausdorff JM, Visser JE, Giladi N. Falls and freezing of gait in Parkinson's disease: a review of two interconnected, episodic phenomena. Mov Disord. 2004;19:871–84. https://doi.org/10.1002/mds.20115.
3. Stolze H, Klebe S, Zechlin C, Baecker C, Friege L, Deuschl G. Falls in frequent neurological diseases. J Neurol. 2004;251:79–84. https://doi.org/10.1007/s00415-004-0276-8.
4. Pickering RM, Grimbergen YAM, Rigney U, Ashburn A, Mazibrada G, Wood B, et al. A meta-analysis of six prospective studies of falling in Parkinson's disease. Mov Disord. 2007;22:1892–900. https://doi.org/10.1002/mds.21598.
5. Temlett JA, Thompson PD. Reasons for admission to hospital for Parkinson's disease. Intern Med J. 2006;36:524–6. https://doi.org/10.1111/j.1445-5994.2006.01123.x.
6. Johnell O, Melton LJ 3rd, Atkinson EJ, O'Fallon WM, Kurland LT. Fracture risk in patients with parkinsonism: a population-based study in Olmsted County, Minnesota. Age Ageing. 1992;21:32–8. https://doi.org/10.1093/ageing/21.1.32.
7. Williams DR. Predictors of falls and fractures in bradykinetic rigid syndromes: a retrospective study. J Neurol Neurosurg Psychiatry. 2006;77:468–73. https://doi.org/10.1136/jnnp.2005.074070.
8. Adkin AL, Frank JS, Jog MS. Fear of falling and postural control in Parkinson's disease. Mov Disord. 2003;18:496–502. https://doi.org/10.1002/mds.10396.
9. Bloem BR, Grimbergen YAM, Cramer M, Willemsen M, Zwinderman AH. Prospective assessment of falls in Parkinson's disease. J Neurol. 2001;248:950–8. https://doi.org/10.1007/s004150170047.
10. Pelicioni PHS, Menant JC, Latt MD, Lord SR. Falls in Parkinson's disease subtypes: risk factors, locations and circumstances. Int J Environ Res Public Health. 2019;16:2216. https://doi.org/10.3390/ijerph16122216.
11. Orcioli-Silva D, Barbieri FA, Simieli L, Vitorio R, dos Santos PCR, Beretta VS, et al. Walking behavior over multiple obstacles in people with Parkinson's disease. Gait Posture. 2017;58:510–5. https://doi.org/10.1016/j.gaitpost.2017.09.021.

12. Barbieri FA, Simieli L, Orcioli-Silva D, Baptista AM, Borkowske Pestana M, Spiandor Beretta V, et al. Obstacle avoidance increases asymmetry of crossing step in individuals with Parkinson's disease and neurologically healthy individuals. J Mot Behav. 2018;50:17–25. https://doi.org/10.1080/00222895.2016.1271303.
13. Simieli L, Gobbi LTB, Orcioli-Silva D, Beretta VS, Santos PCR, Baptista AM, et al. The variability of the steps preceding obstacle avoidance (approach phase) is dependent on the height of the obstacle in people with Parkinson's disease. PLoS One. 2017;12(9):e0184134. https://doi.org/10.1371/journal.pone.0184134.
14. Orcioli-Silva D, Barbieri FA, dos Santos PCR, Beretta VS, Simieli L, Vitorio R, et al. Double obstacles increase gait asymmetry during obstacle crossing in people with Parkinson's disease and healthy older adults: a pilot study. Sci Rep. 2020;10:2272. https://doi.org/10.1038/s41598-020-59266-y.
15. Rochester L, Galna B, Lord S, Burn D. The nature of dual-task interference during gait in incident Parkinson's disease. Neuroscience. 2014;265:83–94. https://doi.org/10.1016/j.neuroscience.2014.01.041.
16. Raffegeau TE, Krehbiel LM, Kang N, Thijs FJ, Altmann LJP, Cauraugh JH, et al. A meta-analysis: Parkinson's disease and dual-task walking. Park Relat Disord. 2019;62:28–35. https://doi.org/10.1016/j.parkreldis.2018.12.012.
17. Orcioli-Silva D, Vitório R, Nóbrega-Sousa P, da Conceição NR, Beretta VS, Lirani-Silva E, et al. Levodopa facilitates prefrontal cortex activation during dual task walking in Parkinson disease. Neurorehabil Neural Repair. 2020;34:589–99. https://doi.org/10.1177/1545968320924430.
18. Plotnik M, Dagan Y, Gurevich T, Giladi N, Hausdorff JM. Effects of cognitive function on gait and dual tasking abilities in patients with Parkinson's disease suffering from motor response fluctuations. Exp Brain Res. 2011;208:169–79. https://doi.org/10.1007/s00221-010-2469-y.
19. Kelly VE, Eusterbrock AJ, Shumway-Cook A. A review of dual-task walking deficits in people with Parkinson's disease: motor and cognitive contributions, mechanisms, and clinical implications. Parkinsons Dis. 2012;2012:918719. https://doi.org/10.1155/2012/918719.
20. Vitório R, Lirani-Silva E, Baptista AM, Barbieri FA, Dos Santos PCR, Teixeira-Arroyo C, et al. Disease severity affects obstacle crossing in people with Parkinson's disease. Gait Posture. 2014;40:266–9. https://doi.org/10.1016/j.gaitpost.2014.03.003.
21. Orcioli-Silva D, Vitório R, Nóbrega-Sousa P, Beretta VS, da Conceição NR, Oliveira AS, et al. Cortical activity underlying gait improvements achieved with dopaminergic medication during usual walking and obstacle avoidance in Parkinson disease. Neurorehabil Neural Repair. 2021;35(5):406–18. https://doi.org/10.1177/15459683211000736.
22. Vitório R, Pieruccini-Faria F, Stella F, Gobbi S, Gobbi LTB. Effects of obstacle height on obstacle crossing in mild Parkinson's disease. Gait Posture. 2010;31:143–6. https://doi.org/10.1016/j.gaitpost.2009.09.011.
23. Orcioli-Silva D, Vitório R, Lirani-Silva E, Santos PCR, Beretta VS, Gobbi LTB. Objective measures of unobstructed walking and obstacle avoidance in Parkinson's disease subtypes. Gait Posture. 2018;62:405–8. https://doi.org/10.1016/j.gaitpost.2018.03.046.
24. Galna B, Peters A, Murphy AT, Morris ME. Obstacle crossing deficits in older adults: a systematic review. Gait Posture. 2009;30(3):270–5. https://doi.org/10.1016/j.gaitpost.2009.05.022.
25. Galna B, Murphy AT, Morris ME. Obstacle crossing in people with Parkinson's disease: foot clearance and spatiotemporal deficits. Hum Mov Sci. 2010;29:843–52. https://doi.org/10.1016/j.humov.2009.09.006.
26. Pieruccini-Faria F, Jones JA, Almeida QJ. Motor planning in Parkinson's disease patients experiencing freezing of gait: the influence of cognitive load when approaching obstacles. Brain Cogn. 2014;87:76–85. https://doi.org/10.1016/j.bandc.2014.03.005.
27. Simieli L, Barbieri FA, Orcioli-Silva D, Lirani-Silva E, Beretta VS, Santos PCRD, Gobbi LTB. Author correction: variability of crossing phase in older people with Parkinson's disease is dependent of obstacle height. Sci Rep. 2018;8:14852. https://doi.org/10.1038/s41598-018-33312-2.

28. Maidan I, Nieuwhof F, Bernad-Elazari H, Reelick MF, Bloem BR, Giladi N, et al. The role of the frontal lobe in complex walking among patients with Parkinson's disease and healthy older adults: an fNIRS study. Neurorehabil Neural Repair. 2016;30:963–71. https://doi.org/10.1177/1545968316650426.
29. Maidan I, Bernad-Elazari H, Giladi N, Hausdorff JM, Mirelman A. When is higher level cognitive control needed for locomotor tasks among patients with Parkinson's disease? Brain Topogr. 2017;30:531–8. https://doi.org/10.1007/s10548-017-0564-0.
30. Stuart S, Belluscio V, Quinn JF, Mancini M. Pre-frontal cortical activity during walking and turning is reliable and differentiates across young, older adults and people with Parkinson's disease. Front Neurol Switzerland. 2019;10:536. https://doi.org/10.3389/fneur.2019.00536.
31. Orcioli-Silva D, Vitório R, Beretta VS, da Conceição NR, Nóbrega-Sousa P, Oliveira AS, et al. Is cortical activation during walking different between Parkinson's disease motor subtypes? Le Couteur D, editor. J Gerontol Ser A United States. 2021;76:561–7. https://doi.org/10.1093/gerona/glaa174.
32. Pelicioni PHS, Tijsma M, Lord SR, Menant J. Prefrontal cortical activation measured by fNIRS during walking: effects of age, disease and secondary task. PeerJ United States. 2019;7:e6833. https://doi.org/10.7717/peerj.6833.
33. Nieuwhof F, Reelick MF, Maidan I, Mirelman A, Hausdorff JM, Olde Rikkert MGM, et al. Measuring prefrontal cortical activity during dual task walking in patients with Parkinson's disease: feasibility of using a new portable fNIRS device. Pilot Feasibility Stud. 2016;2:59. https://doi.org/10.1186/s40814-016-0099-2.
34. Al-Yahya E, Mahmoud W, Meester D, Esser P, Dawes H. Neural substrates of cognitive motor interference during walking; peripheral and central mechanisms. Front Hum Neurosci. 2019;12:536. https://doi.org/10.3389/fnhum.2018.00536.
35. Herold F, Wiegel P, Scholkmann F, Thiers A, Hamacher D, Schega L. Functional near-infrared spectroscopy in movement science: a systematic review on cortical activity in postural and walking tasks. Neurophotonics. 2017;4:41403. https://doi.org/10.1117/1.NPh.4.4.041403.
36. la Fougère C, Zwergal A, Rominger A, Förster S, Fesl G, Dieterich M, et al. Real versus imagined locomotion: a [18F]-FDG PET-fMRI comparison. NeuroImage. 2010;50:1589–98. https://doi.org/10.1016/j.neuroimage.2009.12.060.
37. Vitorio R, Stuart S, Rochester L, Alcock L, Pantall A. fNIRS response during walking — artefact or cortical activity? A systematic review. Neurosci Biobehav Rev. 2017;83:160–72. https://doi.org/10.1016/j.neubiorev.2017.10.002.
38. Stuart S, Vitorio R, Morris R, Martini DN, Fino PC, Mancini M. Cortical activity during walking and balance tasks in older adults and in people with Parkinson's disease: a structured review. Maturitas. 2018;113:53–72. https://doi.org/10.1016/j.maturitas.2018.04.011.
39. Wu T, Hallett M, Chan P. Motor automaticity in Parkinson's disease. Neurobiol Dis. 2015;82:226–34. https://doi.org/10.1016/j.nbd.2015.06.014.
40. Reuter-Lorenz PA, Cappell KA. Neurocognitive aging and the compensation hypothesis. Curr Dir Psychol Sci. 2008;17(3):177–82. https://doi.org/10.1111/j.1467-8721.2008.00570.x.
41. Curtze C, Nutt JG, Carlson-Kuhta P, Mancini M, Horak FB. Levodopa is a double-edged sword for balance and gait in people with Parkinson's disease. Mov Disord. 2015;30:1361–70. https://doi.org/10.1002/mds.26269.
42. Smulders K, Dale ML, Carlson-Kuhta P, Nutt JG, Horak FB. Pharmacological treatment in Parkinson's disease: effects on gait. Park. Relat. Disord. 2016;31:3–13. https://doi.org/10.1016/j.parkreldis.2016.07.006.
43. Armstrong MJ, Okun MS. Diagnosis and treatment of Parkinson disease. JAMA. 2020;323:548. https://doi.org/10.1001/jama.2019.22360.
44. Nonnekes J, Timmer MHM, de Vries NM, Rascol O, Helmich RC, Bloem BR. Unmasking levodopa resistance in Parkinson's disease. Mov Disord. 2016;31(11):1602–9. https://doi.org/10.1002/mds.26712.
45. Gazibara T, Pekmezovic T, Tepavcevic DK, Tomic A, Stankovic I, Kostic VS, et al. Circumstances of falls and fall-related injuries among patients with Parkinson's disease in

an outpatient setting. Geriatr Nurs (Minneap). 2014;35:364–9. https://doi.org/10.1016/j.gerinurse.2014.05.001.
46. Beretta VS, Santos PCR, Orcioli-Silva D, Zampier VC, Vitório R, Gobbi LTB. Transcranial direct current stimulation for balance rehabilitation in neurological disorders: a systematic review and meta-analysis. Ageing Res Rev. 2022;81:101736. https://doi.org/10.1016/j.arr.2022.101736.
47. de Oliveira PCA, de Araújo TAB, DGDS M, Rodrigues AC, Bikson M, Andrade SM, Okano AH, Simplicio H, Pegado R, Morya E. Transcranial direct current stimulation on Parkinson's disease: systematic review and meta-analysis. Front Neurol. 2022;12:2378.
48. Liu X, Liu H, Liu Z, Rao J, Wang J, Wang P, et al. Transcranial direct current stimulation for Parkinson's disease: a systematic review and meta-analysis. Front Aging Neurosci. 2021;13:691.
49. Ernst M, Folkerts AK, Gollan R, Lieker E, Caro-Valenzuela J, Adams A, et al. Physical exercise for people with Parkinson's disease: a systematic review and network meta-analysis. Cochrane Database Syst Rev. 2023;1(1):CD013856. https://doi.org/10.1002/14651858.CD013856.PUB2.
50. Ni M, Hazzard JB, Signorile JF, Luca C. Exercise guidelines for gait function in Parkinson's disease: a systematic review and meta-analysis. Neurorehabil Neural Repair. United States. 2018;32:872–86. https://doi.org/10.1177/1545968318801558.
51. Shu HF, Yang T, Yu SX, Huang HD, Jiang LL, Gu JW, et al. Aerobic exercise for Parkinson's disease: a systematic review and meta-analysis of randomized controlled trials. PLoS One. 2014;9(7):e100503. https://doi.org/10.1371/journal.pone.0100503.
52. Ji X, Lu D, Yang Q, Xiao L, Wang J, Wang G. Physical therapy for at least 6 months improves motor symptoms in Parkinson's patients: a meta-analysis. Comput Math Methods Med. 2022;2022:3393191. https://doi.org/10.1155/2022/3393191.
53. da Silva FC, da Silva FC, RDR I, de Oliveira LC, Boll AM, de Alvarenga JGS, PJB GF, de Melo LMAB, Xavier AJ, da Silva R. Effects of physical exercise programs on cognitive function in Parkinson's disease patients: a systematic review of randomized controlled trials of the last 10 years. PLoS One. 2018;13:e0193113. https://doi.org/10.1371/journal.pone.0193113.
54. Wu P-L, Lee M, Huang T-T. Effectiveness of physical activity on patients with depression and Parkinson's disease: a systematic review. PLoS One. 2017;12:e0181515. https://doi.org/10.1371/journal.pone.0181515.
55. Fisher BE, Li Q, Nacca A, Salem GJ, Song J, Yip J, et al. Treadmill exercise elevates striatal dopamine D2 receptor binding potential in patients with early Parkinson's disease. Neuroreport. 2013;24:509–14. https://doi.org/10.1097/WNR.0b013e328361dc13.
56. Sehm B, Taubert M, Conde V, Weise D, Classen J, Dukart J, et al. Structural brain plasticity in Parkinson's disease induced by balance training. Neurobiol Aging. 2014;35:232–9. https://doi.org/10.1016/j.neurobiolaging.2013.06.021.
57. Beall EB, Lowe MJ, Alberts JL, Frankemolle AMM, Thota AK, Shah C, et al. The effect of forced-exercise therapy for Parkinson's disease on motor cortex functional connectivity. Brain Connect United States. 2013;3:190–8. https://doi.org/10.1089/brain.2012.0104.
58. Paillard T, Rolland Y, de Souto BP. Protective effects of physical exercise in Alzheimer's disease and Parkinson's disease: a narrative review. J Clin Neurol. 2015;11:212. https://doi.org/10.3988/jcn.2015.11.3.212.
59. Hirsch MA, Iyer SS, Sanjak M. Exercise-induced neuroplasticity in human Parkinson's disease: what is the evidence telling us? Parkinsonism Relat Disord. 2016;22:S78–81. https://doi.org/10.1016/j.parkreldis.2015.09.030.
60. Angelucci F, Piermaria J, Gelfo F, Shofany J, Tramontano M, Fiore M, et al. The effects of motor rehabilitation training on clinical symptoms and serum BDNF levels in Parkinson's disease subjects. Can J Physiol Pharmacol. 2016;94:455–61. https://doi.org/10.1139/cjpp-2015-0322.
61. Protas EJ, Mitchell K, Williams A, Qureshy H, Caroline K, Lai EC. Gait and step training to reduce falls in Parkinson's disease. Neuro Rehabilitation Netherlands. 2005;20:183–90.

62. Herman T, Giladi N, Hausdorff JM. Treadmill training for the treatment of gait disturbances in people with Parkinson's disease: a mini-review. J Neural Transm Austria. 2009;116:307–18. https://doi.org/10.1007/s00702-008-0139-z.
63. Spaulding SJ, Barber B, Colby M, Cormack B, Mick T, Jenkins ME. Cueing and gait improvement among people with Parkinson's disease: a meta-analysis. Arch Phys Med Rehabil. 2013;94:562–70. https://doi.org/10.1016/j.apmr.2012.10.026.
64. van Eijkeren FJM, Reijmers RSJ, Kleinveld MJ, Minten A, ter Bruggen JP, Bloem BR. Nordic walking improves mobility in Parkinson's disease. Mov Disord. 2008;23:2239–43. https://doi.org/10.1002/mds.22293.
65. Zampier VC, Vitório R, Beretta VS, Jaimes DAR, Orcioli-Silva D, Santos PCR, et al. Gait bradykinesia and hypometria decrease as arm swing frequency and amplitude increase. Neurosci Lett. 2018;687:248–52. https://doi.org/10.1016/j.neulet.2018.09.051.
66. Ismail SR, Lee SWH, Merom D, Megat Kamaruddin PSN, Chong MS, Ong T, et al. Evidence of disease severity, cognitive and physical outcomes of dance interventions for persons with Parkinson's disease: a systematic review and meta-analysis. BMC Geriatr. 2021;21:503. https://doi.org/10.1186/s12877-021-02446-w.
67. Lötzke D, Ostermann T, Büssing A. Argentine tango in Parkinson disease—a systematic review and meta-analysis. BMC Neurol. 2015;15:226. https://doi.org/10.1186/s12883-015-0484-0.
68. McNeely ME, Mai MM, Duncan RP, Earhart GM. Differential effects of tango versus dance for PD in Parkinson disease. Front Aging Neurosci. 2015;7:239. https://doi.org/10.3389/fnagi.2015.00239.
69. Sharp K, Hewitt J. Dance as an intervention for people with Parkinson's disease: a systematic review and meta-analysis. Neurosci Biobehav Rev. 2014;47:445–56. https://doi.org/10.1016/j.neubiorev.2014.09.009.
70. Aras B, Seyyar GK, Fidan O, Colak E. The effect of tai chi on functional mobility, balance and falls in Parkinson's disease: a systematic review and meta-analysis of systematic reviews. Explore (NY). 2022;18:402–10. https://doi.org/10.1016/j.explore.2021.12.002.
71. Pan ZJ, Su XW, Fang Q, Hou LJ, Lee YH, Chen CC, et al. The effects of tai chi intervention on healthy elderly by means of neuroimaging and EEG: a systematic review. Front Aging Neurosci. 2018;10:110. https://doi.org/10.3389/fnagi.2018.00110.
72. Li F, Harmer P, Fitzgerald K, Eckstrom E, Stock R, Galver J, et al. Tai chi and Postural stability in patients with Parkinson's disease. N Engl J Med. 2012;366:511–9. https://doi.org/10.1056/NEJMoa1107911.
73. van der Kolk NM, de Vries NM, Kessels RPC, Joosten H, Zwinderman AH, Post B, et al. Effectiveness of home-based and remotely supervised aerobic exercise in Parkinson's disease: a double-blind, randomised controlled trial. Lancet Neurol. 2019;18:998–1008. https://doi.org/10.1016/S1474-4422(19)30285-6.
74. Truijen S, Abdullahi A, Bijsterbosch D, van Zoest E, Conijn M, Wang Y, et al. Effect of home-based virtual reality training and telerehabilitation on balance in individuals with Parkinson disease, multiple sclerosis, and stroke: a systematic review and meta-analysis. Neurol Sci. 2022;43:2995–3006. https://doi.org/10.1007/s10072-021-05855-2.
75. Dockx K, Bekkers EM, Van den Bergh V, Ginis P, Rochester L, Hausdorff JM, et al. Virtual reality for rehabilitation in Parkinson's disease. Cochrane Database Syst Rev. 2016;2016:CD010760. https://doi.org/10.1002/14651858.CD010760.pub2.
76. Sarasso E, Gardoni A, Tettamanti A, Agosta F, Filippi M, Corbetta D. Virtual reality balance training to improve balance and mobility in Parkinson's disease: a systematic review and meta-analysis. J Neurol. 2022;269:1873–88. https://doi.org/10.1007/s00415-021-10857-3.
77. Mirelman A, Maidan I, Herman T, Deutsch JE, Giladi N, Hausdorff JM. Virtual reality for gait training: can it induce motor learning to enhance complex walking and reduce fall risk in patients with Parkinson's disease? J Gerontol Ser A Biol Sci Med Sci. 2011;66A:234–40. https://doi.org/10.1093/gerona/glq201.
78. Picelli A, Melotti C, Origano F, Waldner A, Fiaschi A, Santilli V, et al. Robot-assisted gait training in patients with Parkinson disease. Neurorehabil Neural Repair. 2012;26:353–61. https://doi.org/10.1177/1545968311424417.

79. Picelli A, Melotti C, Origano F, Waldner A, Gimigliano R, Smania N. Does robotic gait training improve balance in Parkinson's disease? A randomized controlled trial. Parkinsonism Relat Disord. 2012;18:990–3. https://doi.org/10.1016/j.parkreldis.2012.05.010.
80. Beretta VS, Conceição NR, Nóbrega-Sousa P, Orcioli-Silva D, Dantas LKBF, Gobbi LTB, et al. Transcranial direct current stimulation combined with physical or cognitive training in people with Parkinson's disease: a systematic review. J Neuroeng Rehabil. 2020;17:74. https://doi.org/10.1186/s12984-020-00701-6.
81. Abbruzzese G, Marchese R, Avanzino L, Pelosin E. Rehabilitation for Parkinson's disease: current outlook and future challenges. Parkinsonism Relat Disord. 2016;22:S60–4. https://doi.org/10.1016/j.parkreldis.2015.09.005.
82. Cano-de-la-Cuerda R, Molero-Sánchez A, Carratalá-Tejada M, Alguacil-Diego IM, Molina-Rueda F, Miangolarra-Page JC, et al. Teorías y modelos de control y aprendizaje motor. Aplicaciones clínicas en neurorrehabilitación. Neurología. 2015;30:32–41. https://doi.org/10.1016/j.nrl.2011.12.010.
83. Ene H, McRae C, Schenkman M. Attitudes toward exercise following participation in an exercise intervention study. J Neurol Phys Ther. 2011;35:34–40. https://doi.org/10.1097/NPT.0b013e31820cb917.
84. Shen X, Wong-Yu ISK, Mak MKY. Effects of exercise on falls, balance, and gait ability in Parkinson's disease. Neurorehabil Neural Repair. 2016;30:512–27. https://doi.org/10.1177/1545968315613447.
85. Gobbi LTB, Lahr J, Jaimes DAR, Pestana MB, Pelicioni PHS. Effects of physical activity on walking in individuals with Parkinson's disease. Locomot posture older adults. Cham: Springer International Publishing; 2017. p. 177–93. https://doi.org/10.1007/978-3-319-48980-3_12.
86. Caetano MJD, Lord SR, Schoene D, Pelicioni PHS, Sturnieks DL, Menant JC. Age-related changes in gait adaptability in response to unpredictable obstacles and stepping targets. Gait Posture. 2016;46:35–41. https://doi.org/10.1016/j.gaitpost.2016.02.003.
87. Caetano MJD, Menant JC, Schoene D, Pelicioni PHS, Sturnieks DL, Lord SR. Sensorimotor and cognitive predictors of impaired gait adaptability in older people. J Gerontol Ser A Biol Sci Med Sci. 2017;72(9):1257–63. https://doi.org/10.1093/gerona/glw171.
88. Caetano MJD, Lord SR, Brodie MA, Schoene D, Pelicioni PHS, Sturnieks DL, et al. Executive functioning, concern about falling and quadriceps strength mediate the relationship between impaired gait adaptability and fall risk in older people. Gait Posture. 2018;59:188–92. https://doi.org/10.1016/j.gaitpost.2017.10.017.
89. Caetano MJD, Lord SR, Allen NE, Brodie MA, Song J, Paul SS, et al. Stepping reaction time and gait adaptability are significantly impaired in people with Parkinson's disease: implications for fall risk. Parkinsonism Relat Disord. 2018;47:32–8. https://doi.org/10.1016/j.parkreldis.2017.11.340.
90. Caetano MJD, Lord SR, Allen NE, Song J, Paul SS, Canning CG, et al. Executive functioning, muscle power and reactive balance are major contributors to gait adaptability in people with Parkinson's disease. Front Aging Neurosci. 2019;11:154. https://doi.org/10.3389/fnagi.2019.00154.
91. Pelicioni PHS, Lord SR, Okubo Y, Menant JC. Cortical activation during gait adaptability in people with Parkinson's disease. Gait Posture. 2022;91:247–53. https://doi.org/10.1016/j.gaitpost.2021.10.038.
92. Tsukita K, Sakamaki-Tsukita H, Takahashi R. Long-term effect of regular physical activity and exercise habits in patients with early Parkinson disease. Neurology. 2022;98:e859–71. https://doi.org/10.1212/WNL.0000000000013218.
93. Gobbi LTB, Pelicioni PHS, Lahr J, Lirani-Silva E, Teixeira-Arroyo C, dos Santos PCR. Effect of different types of exercises on psychological and cognitive features in people with Parkinson's disease: a randomized controlled trial. Ann Phys Rehabil Med. 2021;64:101407. https://doi.org/10.1016/j.rehab.2020.05.011.
94. Tanaka K, de Quadros AC, Santos RF, Stella F, Gobbi LTB, Gobbi S. Benefits of physical exercise on executive functions in older people with Parkinson's disease. Brain Cogn. 2009;69:435–41. https://doi.org/10.1016/j.bandc.2008.09.008.

95. Silva-Batista C, Corcos DM, Kanegusuku H, Piemonte MEP, Gobbi LTB, de Lima-Pardini AC, et al. Balance and fear of falling in subjects with Parkinson's disease is improved after exercises with motor complexity. Gait Posture. 2018;61:90–7. https://doi.org/10.1016/j.gaitpost.2017.12.027.
96. Landers MR, Hatlevig RM, Davis AD, Richards AR, Rosenlof LE. Does attentional focus during balance training in people with Parkinson's disease affect outcome? A randomised controlled clinical trial. Clin Rehabil. 2016;30:53–63. https://doi.org/10.1177/0269215515570377.
97. Song J, Paul SS, Caetano MJD, Smith S, Dibble LE, Love R, et al. Home-based step training using videogame technology in people with Parkinson's disease: a single-blinded randomised controlled trial. Clin Rehabil. 2018;32:299–311. https://doi.org/10.1177/0269215517721593.
98. Wang Y, Gao L, Yan H, Jin Z, Fang J, Qi L, et al. Efficacy of C-mill gait training for improving walking adaptability in early and middle stages of Parkinson's disease. Gait Posture. 2022;91:79–85. https://doi.org/10.1016/j.gaitpost.2021.10.010.
99. Liao Y-Y, Yang Y-R, Cheng S-J, Wu Y-R, Fuh J-L, Wang R-Y. Virtual reality–based training to improve obstacle-crossing performance and dynamic balance in patients with Parkinson's disease. Neurorehabil Neural Repair. 2015;29:658–67. https://doi.org/10.1177/1545968314562111.
100. Canning CG, Allen NE, Nackaerts E, Paul SS, Nieuwboer A, Gilat M. Virtual reality in research and rehabilitation of gait and balance in Parkinson disease. Nat Rev Neurol. 2020;16:409–25. https://doi.org/10.1038/s41582-020-0370-2.
101. Kim H-D, Jae HD, Jeong JH. Tai chi exercise can improve the obstacle negotiating ability of people with Parkinson's disease: a preliminary study. J Phys Ther Sci. 2014;26:1025–30. https://doi.org/10.1589/jpts.26.1025.
102. Maidan I, Nieuwhof F, Bernad-Elazari H, Bloem BR, Giladi N, Hausdorff JM, et al. Evidence for differential effects of 2 forms of exercise on prefrontal plasticity during walking in Parkinson's disease. Neurorehabil Neural Repair. 2018;32:200–8. https://doi.org/10.1177/1545968318763750.
103. Nitsche MA, Paulus W. Excitability changes induced in the human motor cortex by weak transcranial direct current stimulation. J Physiol England. 2000;527(Pt 3):633–9. https://doi.org/10.1111/j.1469-7793.2000.t01-1-00633.x.
104. Nitsche MA, Liebetanz D, Tergau F, Paulus W. Modulation of cortical excitability by transcranial direct current stimulation. Nervenarzt. 2002;73:332–5. https://doi.org/10.1007/s00115-002-1272-9.
105. Bikson M, Grossman P, Thomas C, Zannou AL, Jiang J, Adnan T, et al. Safety of transcranial direct current stimulation: evidence based update 2016. Brain Stimul. 2016;9:641–61. https://doi.org/10.1016/j.brs.2016.06.004.
106. Fonteneau C, Redoute J, Haesebaert F, Le Bars D, Costes N, Suaud-Chagny M-F, et al. Frontal transcranial direct current stimulation induces dopamine release in the ventral striatum in human. Cereb Cortex. 2018;28:2636–46. https://doi.org/10.1093/cercor/bhy093.
107. Nitsche MA, Cohen LG, Wassermann EM, Priori A, Lang N, Antal A, et al. Transcranial direct current stimulation: state of the art 2008. Brain Stimul. 2008;1:206–23. https://doi.org/10.1016/j.brs.2008.06.004.
108. Morya E, Monte-Silva K, Bikson M, Esmaeilpour Z, Biazoli CE, Fonseca A, et al. Beyond the target area: an integrative view of tDCS-induced motor cortex modulation in patients and athletes. J Neuroeng Rehabil. 2019;16:141. https://doi.org/10.1186/s12984-019-0581-1.
109. Zheng X, Alsop DC, Schlaug G. Effects of transcranial direct current stimulation (tDCS) on human regional cerebral blood flow. Neuroimage United States. 2011;58:26–33. https://doi.org/10.1016/j.neuroimage.2011.06.018.
110. Costa-Ribeiro A, Maux A, Bosford T, Tenório Y, Marques D, Carneiro M, et al. Dopamine-independent effects of combining transcranial direct current stimulation with cued gait training on cortical excitability and functional mobility in Parkinson's disease. J Rehabil Med Sweden. 2016;48:819–23. https://doi.org/10.2340/16501977-2134.

111. Kaski D, Dominguez RO, Allum JH, Islam AF, Bronstein AM. Combining physical training with transcranial direct current stimulation to improve gait in Parkinson's disease: a pilot randomized controlled study. Clin Rehabil England. 2014;28:1115–24. https://doi.org/10.1177/0269215514534277.
112. Conceição NR, Gobbi LTB, Nóbrega-Sousa P, Orcioli-Silva D, Beretta VS, Lirani-Silva E, et al. Aerobic exercise combined with transcranial direct current stimulation over the prefrontal cortex in Parkinson disease: effects on cortical activity, gait, and cognition. Neurorehabil Neural Repair. 2021;35(8):717–28. https://doi.org/10.1177/15459683211019344.
113. Nóbrega-Sousa P, Gobbi LTB, Orcioli-Silva D, da Conceição NR, Beretta VS, Vitório R. Prefrontal cortex activity during walking: effects of aging and associations with gait and executive function. Neurorehabil Neural Repair United States. 2020;34:915–24. https://doi.org/10.1177/1545968320953824.
114. Fernández-Lago H, Bello O, Mora-Cerdá F, Montero-Cámara J, Fernández-Del-Olmo MÁ. Treadmill walking combined with anodal transcranial direct current stimulation in Parkinson disease: a pilot study of kinematic and neurophysiological effects. Am J Phys Med Rehabil United States. 2017;96:801–8. https://doi.org/10.1097/PHM.0000000000000751.
115. Criminger C, Swank C, Almutairi S, Mehta J. Transcranial direct current stimulation plus concurrent activity may influence task prioritization during walking in people with Parkinson's disease—initial findings. J Park Restless Legs Syndr. 2018;8:25–32. https://doi.org/10.2147/JPRLS.S161740.
116. Costa-Ribeiro A, Maux A, Bosford T, Aoki Y, Castro R, Baltar A, et al. Transcranial direct current stimulation associated with gait training in Parkinson's disease: a pilot randomized clinical trial. Dev Neurorehabil England. 2017;20:121–8. https://doi.org/10.3109/17518423.2015.1131755.
117. Schabrun SM, Lamont RM, Brauer SG. Transcranial direct current stimulation to enhance dual-task gait training in Parkinson's disease: a pilot RCT. PLoS One United States. 2016;11:e0158497. https://doi.org/10.1371/journal.pone.0158497.
118. Yotnuengnit P, Bhidayasiri R, Donkhan R, Chaluaysrimuang J, Piravej K. Effects of transcranial direct current stimulation plus physical therapy on gait in patients with Parkinson disease: a randomized controlled trial. Am J Phys Med Rehabil. United States. 2018;97:7–15. https://doi.org/10.1097/PHM.0000000000000783.
119. Lee HK, Ahn SJ, Shin YM, Kang N, Cauraugh JH. Does transcranial direct current stimulation improve functional locomotion in people with Parkinson's disease? A systematic review and meta-analysis. J Neuroeng Rehabil England. 2019;16:84. https://doi.org/10.1186/s12984-019-0562-4.
120. Pol F, Salehinejad MA, Baharlouei H, Nitsche MA. The effects of transcranial direct current stimulation on gait in patients with Parkinson's disease: a systematic review. Transl Neurodegener. 2021;10:22. https://doi.org/10.1186/s40035-021-00245-2.

Split-Belt Treadmill to Treat Gait Disorders

24

Christian Schlenstedt, Jana Seuthe, and Nicholas D'Cruz

Abstract

A split-belt treadmill not only offers possibilities for studying neural control of gait and motor learning, it can also be used as a therapeutic tool to address complex gait disorders, particularly gait asymmetry, and gait adaptation deficits. These gait deficits have been linked to falls and often occur in individuals post-stroke or people with Parkinson's disease. This chapter will first describe motor control mechanisms when walking on a split-belt treadmill and will then summarize the effectiveness of repeated split-belt treadmill training in different populations. It will be shown that split-belt treadmill training has proven to be effective for reducing gait asymmetry in stroke and improving gait adaptation and overall gait quality in Parkinson's disease. Different options of how to adjust a split-belt treadmill to reach training progression will be presented. Finally, neurophysiological aspects of split-belt treadmill walking will be discussed.

Introduction

To treat gait disorders is highly relevant as gait impairments often lead to falls and a loss of mobility. In this chapter, we are going to focus on two more complex gait disorders, namely gait asymmetry and gait adaptation deficits, and how the use of a split-belt treadmill may potentially improve these impairments.

C. Schlenstedt (✉) · J. Seuthe
Institute of Interdisciplinary Exercise Science and Sports Medicine, Medical School Hamburg, Hamburg, Germany
e-mail: christian.schlenstedt@medicalschool-hamburg.de; jana.seuthe@medicalschool-hamburg.de

N. D'Cruz
Department of Rehabilitation Sciences, KU Leuven, Leuven, Belgium
e-mail: Nicholas.dcruz@kuleuven.be

F. A. Barbieri et al. (eds.), *Locomotion and Posture in Older Adults*,
https://doi.org/10.1007/978-3-031-74123-4_24

Gait asymmetry particularly plays a role in stroke or Parkinson's disease (PD), where gait asymmetry is imposed by the lateral position of the lesion or the laterality of the disease [1, 2]. Gait asymmetry also occurs in healthy older people and has been linked to falls [1] and the likelihood of slips [3]. Gait asymmetry can present in different components of gait, such as temporal or spatial gait parameters [1, 4] as well as joint kinematics [5]. Different methods exist to calculate the degree of asymmetry and have been summarized in detail previously [6]. Gait asymmetry can further deteriorate when adding a cognitive task [1].

Another complex gait feature is the ability to adapt gait to changing walking conditions such as obstacle avoidance, on-target and reactive stepping or a change in surface [7, 8]. Motor adaptation is defined as a gradual and continuous modification of a movement, which keeps the overall pattern of the original movement, and which is retained [9]. More specifically, gait adaptation is highly relevant for daily life mobility given the various and consistent changes when we move in the environment. Gait adaptation has been shown to be reduced in healthy older adults [8] and there is some evidence that older adults who experience falls also show significantly more difficulty in adapting their gait pattern to a challenging situation, e.g. stepping onto a curb [10]. Gait adaptation deficits are also present in people with PD, particularly with freezing of gait [11].

A *split-belt treadmill* has two belts which can run at individual speeds for the left and right legs. This allows to introduce a novel asymmetric walking condition with one belt running faster or slower than the other. Generally, split-belt paradigms start out with the *tied-baseline* where both belts run at the same speed. This is followed by the *split-adaptation* where one belt is manipulated to run faster or slower than previously. During that phase, gait needs to be adapted to the novel condition. The phase where both belts return to the same speed again is the so-called *tied-adaptation*, as the walking pattern needs to be readjusted back to its original state and we can see after effects of the *split-adaptation* phase. Optionally, a *washout* (tied-belt) and a *re-adaptation* (repeated split-adaptation) can be added to the paradigm. The common structure of split-belt paradigms is visualized in Fig. 24.1.

Split-belt treadmills have been used for either studying motor learning and motor control or as a therapeutic tool. We will first briefly summarize the literature with regard to the motor control mechanisms when walking on a split-belt treadmill and then focus on studies conducted to investigate prolonged split-belt treadmill training interventions.

Split-Belt Treadmill to Study Motor Learning and Motor Control

Split-belt treadmills have been used to introduce new gait patterns to study motor learning and motor control in humans but also in spinal cats [12–14]. The split-belt treadmill offers a way to study gait in a novel context and investigate how a new gait pattern is adopted upon first exposure to the split-belt treadmill. Generally, on immediate exposure to a split-belt treadmill condition, healthy adults adjust their

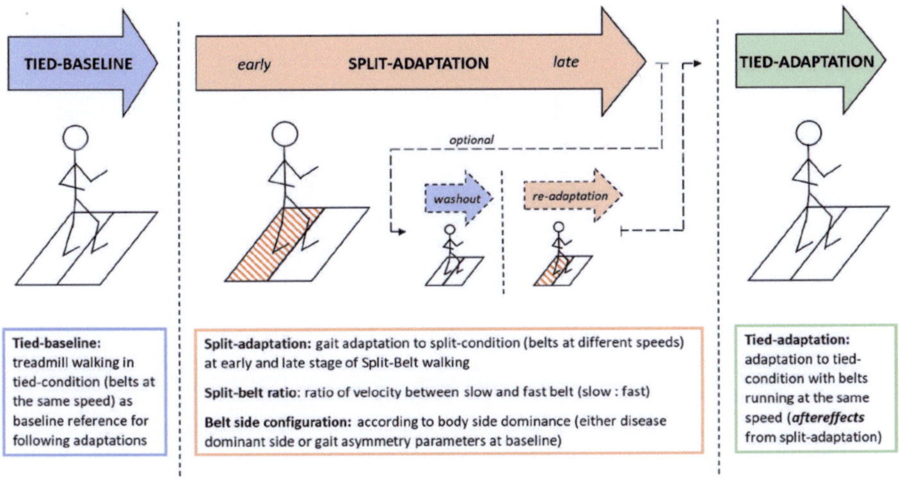

Fig. 24.1 Typical split-belt paradigm with different phases. From "Split-belt treadmill walking in patients with Parkinson's disease: A systematic review" by Seuthe et al., 2019, Gait & posture, 69, 187–194. Copyright 2019 by Elsevier

walking by increasing the stance time of the leg on the slow belt [15]. This adjustment is reactive in its nature and persists over the split-adaptation phase. In parallel, there is an increase in step length asymmetry. Gradually, over time, this initial asymmetry of step length slowly reduces through the feedforward adaptation [15]. When the belts return to the same speed, short-term aftereffects are present for the step length asymmetry [15]. These adjustment and adaptation processes are depicted in Fig. 24.2.

It was shown that the adaptive capacity of older adults to split-belt treadmill walking does not differ significantly compared to young individuals, although older adults may use a different adaptation strategy [16]. Furthermore, there were some age-related differences in the storage of the newly learned gait pattern upon second exposure after a rest-break [17]. In older adults with neurological disease, however, adaptation upon first exposure can be altered. For people with PD, this means slower adaptation and adaptation to a lesser degree and for people post-stroke, this means difficulty adapting when the paretic leg is placed on the slow belt [18]. Adaptation on the split-belt treadmill is usually measured using asymmetry indexes of temporal or spatial gait parameters. The outcomes commonly used are step length asymmetry and stance time asymmetry [11] and more recently asymmetry indexes of join kinematics have been used [19]. Different methods how to calculate asymmetry indexes for the split-belt treadmill have been summarized previously [6].

The second aspect that the split-belt treadmill has been used for in research is in the context of therapeutic interventions, which will be elaborated in the following.

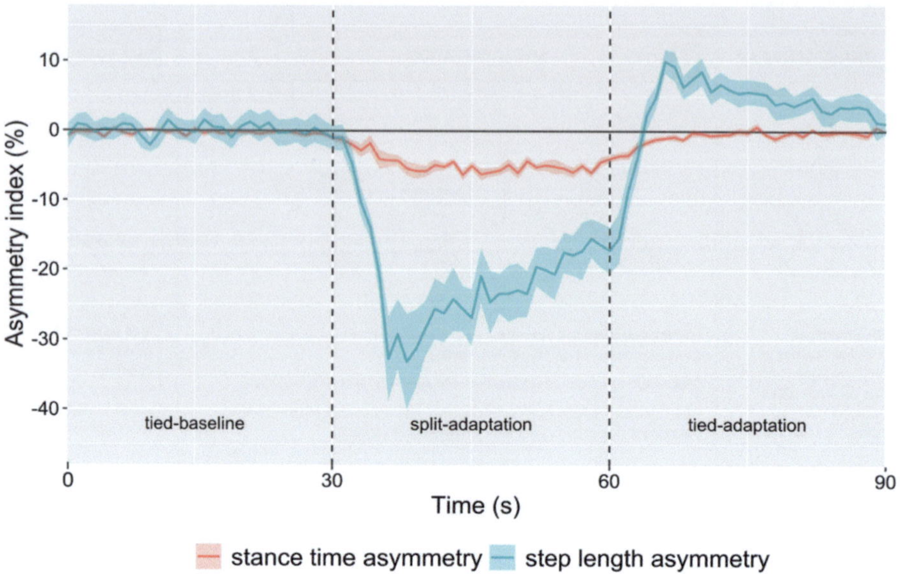

Fig. 24.2 Step length asymmetry and stance time asymmetry in healthy controls (n = 38) during a 90 s gait adaptation on the split-belt treadmill (own data). Dashed lines represent the switches from the belts running at the same speed (tied-baseline) to the belts running at different speeds (split-adaptation, 50% reduction on one side) and back (tied-adaptation). The colored lines represent the mean and the shaded areas around the lines represent the standard error. A value of zero represents perfect symmetry

Split-Belt Treadmill as a Therapeutic Tool

Despite much research regarding perturbation treadmill training in healthy older adults, which has some overlap with split-belt treadmill, interventional studies using split-belt treadmill training are scarce. Only one study has investigated prolonged split-belt treadmill training in healthy older people with a rehabilitative aim. Wade, Baudendistel [20] found in their study that split-belt treadmill training was not effective to improve mobility outcomes compared to traditional treadmill training in healthy older individuals.

Clinical studies using split-belt treadmills as a therapeutic tool in diseased older populations mainly focus on two neurological conditions which are stroke and PD. Given the lateral nature of both diseases, the use of a split-belt treadmill might be more promising for these populations.

Split-Belt Treadmill Training in Individuals Post-Stroke

People with post-stroke can present with marked gait asymmetry with a shorter step length for the non-paretic leg and reduced propulsive forces for the paretic leg [21].

Gait asymmetry in stroke is related to reduced walking speed [22], a loss of bone density [23], dynamic postural control [24], and increased energy consumption [25], making gait asymmetry one of the most important targets for rehabilitation for people post-stroke.

Many split-belt treadmill studies have investigated the short-term effects of a single training session. Those interventions were summarized in a recent review and meta-analysis [26], showing with large effect sizes that a single split-belt treadmill training session has the potential to reduce step length asymmetry in individuals post-stroke. More specifically, the authors summarized that training with the leg with a longer step length on the slower belt was the most effective strategy to reduce step length asymmetry. This strategy is called "error augmentation," as asymmetry is first exaggerated when walking with the leg with the longer step length on the slower belt, thus driving the nervous system to correct the gait deviation. The error augmentation strategy is particularly important for individuals post-stroke, as there is some evidence that spatiotemporal gait asymmetry is not perceived as abnormal in this population [27]. Regarding adaptation, it was found that asymmetry at baseline was not significantly different from the late phase of split-belt treadmill adaptation, indicating that adaptation was successful [26].

Only few studies have implemented a prolonged split-belt treadmill training intervention to investigate the retention effects of repeated split-belt treadmill training sessions [28–30]. They found that after as little as six training sessions post-stroke participants could significantly reduce their step length asymmetry and retain those improvements for a month [28]. Similar results were found for step length asymmetry after a 4-week split-belt treadmill intervention using the error augmentation strategy [30]. Lewek, Braun [29] found that irrespective of the split-belt treadmill setting (error augmentation or error minimization), verbal feedback was helpful for reducing step length asymmetry.

Future research needs to confirm those findings in large-scale randomized-controlled trials. Additionally, determining which belt side to reduce in speed can also be one of the pitfalls in people post-stroke. Many studies have reported if the non-paretic or the paretic side was placed on the faster belt. However, although usually the paretic side presents with the longer step length, according to Chen, Patten [31] this is not consistently the case, hence assessment of step length asymmetry could be useful at baseline.

Split-Belt Treadmill Training in People with Parkinson's Disease

People with PD show increased gait asymmetry due to the laterality of the disease [32]. Additionally, gait adaptation is compromised in individuals with PD [33, 34]. Both, gait asymmetry and gait adaptation deficits have been associated with falls in this population [32, 33]. The research of split-belt treadmill training in people with PD has developed based on some of the previous findings in people post-stroke given some overlapping gait impairments despite different neurophysiological mechanisms at play. A recent review summarized the effects of short-term split-belt treadmill interventions for people with PD and found that individuals with mild to moderate PD are generally able to walk on a split-belt treadmill and adapt to split-belt treadmill conditions in the same manner but slower as healthy older people [6]. One of the first studies in this field aimed to investigate the differences in aftereffects of reducing the speed on the body side with the longer or with the shorter step length within a single session of split-belt treadmill walking [35]. According to their results, the reduction of speed on the side with the longer step length ("best side reduction") produced larger aftereffects. Another study investigated the efficacy of different speed ratios of the left and right belts in people with PD and this study specifically targeted gait adaptation deficits by introducing a condition with changing belt speed ratios to introduce more challenge to the training [36, 37]. The results showed that the condition with changing ratios was not only effective in ameliorating gait adaptation but also most effective in enhancing gait symmetry [36].

Based on those findings, the first study with repeated split-belt treadmill training was conducted to compare the effects of 4 weeks of progressive split-belt treadmill training with regular treadmill training on gait adaptability in people with PD [38]. The group of split-belt treadmill trained with changing belt speed differences in the range of 1:2 to 1:1. The study showed that while both training modes were equally effective to improve gait speed and step length with clinically meaningful effects, split-belt treadmill training was more effective to improve gait adaptability during an adaptation test on the split-belt treadmill compared to regular treadmill training and effects were retained after 4 weeks without training. Additionally, only the split-belt treadmill group had clinically meaningful improvements in motor signs of PD. However, neither of the training modes showed any effects on turning. Another recent pilot study has addressed the lack of comparison to real-world walking by applying an individualized split-belt treadmill training program with an immersive virtual reality component [39]. They found that walking with an additional cognitive dual task improved significantly after a 4-week intervention, compared to the control group, however, they also measured gait in-laboratory only [39]. There is a strong need for implementing gait assessment outside the laboratory within the home-environment into future intervention studies.

Split-Belt Treadmill to Treat Freezing of Gait in Parkinson's Disease

Split-belt treadmill has been of special interest as an approach to treat Freezing of Gait (FOG) in people with PD. The transient gait dysfunction is characterized by the inability to produce an effective stepping [40]. FOG has been linked to asymmetry as FOG often occurs during asymmetric movements such as gait initiation or turning and people with PD with FOG show increased gait asymmetry [41, 42]. Additionally, people with PD with FOG show motor- (and cognitive) switching deficits [43, 44]. Therefore, researchers suspect that targeting gait asymmetry and gait adaptation deficits by using a split-belt treadmill could potentially be effective for reducing FOG [45]. There is some evidence that people with PD with FOG have an impaired perception of belt speed differences and adapt slower to split-belt treadmill conditions compared to those without FOG [44, 46]. Another study found freezers adapted differently to split-belt treadmill walking compared to non-freezers [47]. A recent study has investigated how cognition affects adaptation and aftereffects on split-belt treadmill in PD with FOG and found that impaired cognition and more specifically reduced working memory can negatively influence adaptation and aftereffects [45].

There is some evidence that split-belt treadmill walking might be beneficial to treat FOG. The study by Fasano, Schlenstedt [35] found that walking on a split-belt treadmill had some positive after effects on the sequence effect, which is the progressive shortening of the step length which may lead to a FOG episode. Another positive short-term effect was shown by D'cruz, Seuthe [37], in terms of improvements during walking and turning with an additional cognitive task. This is especially clinically relevant as cognition plays a major role in the occurrence of FOG [48]. In a prolonged split-belt treadmill training intervention (as described above), there was no effect on subjective and objective FOG despite overall positive effects on gait and gait adaptation [38].

Split-Belt Treadmill in Other Age-Related Diseases

Regarding other diseases that occur mostly in older adults split-belt treadmill training is almost unresearched. One proof-of-concept study has investigated the potential of split-belt treadmill training for older women with unilateral hip osteoarthritis [19] and did not find a clear benefit of a single training session. Another study has looked into how people with multiple sclerosis can improve their gait asymmetry using split-belt treadmill [49], showing that they could walk more symmetrically after one session of split-belt treadmill. Due to the cross-sectional design of these studies, they only deliver very preliminary results.

How to Adjust Training Progression in Split-Belt Treadmill Interventions

Many factors should be considered when designing a split-belt treadmill training intervention, including how to reach optimal training progression during the course of the intervention. For regular treadmill training, progression can be reached by increasing the intensity (e.g., increasing treadmill speed or adding incline), by increasing the length of the block/session/intervention-duration or by decreasing rest periods. These adjustments primarily target cardiovascular load and can obviously also be used for split-belt treadmill training. However, as for split-belt treadmill training, the primary aim usually is to improve coordination of gait, split-belt treadmill specific adjustments to challenge the sensorimotor integration should be considered. This can be done by (i) changing the belt speed ratios, (ii) the number of switches (switch = change in the belt speed ratio), and/or (iii) introducing

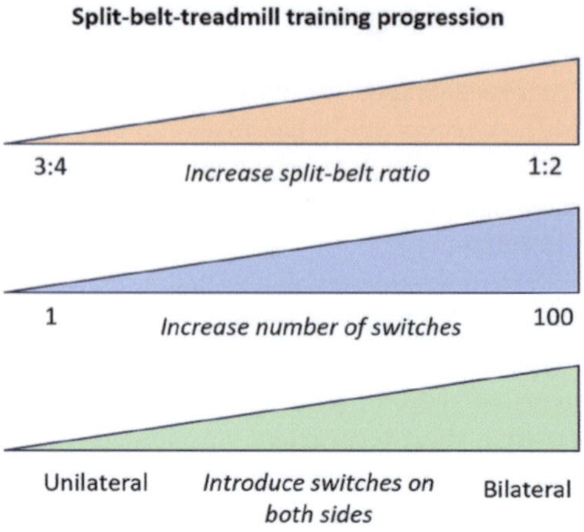

Fig. 24.3 Different options which can be combined to increase training progression in split-belt-treadmill training

unilateral or bilateral switches (Fig. 24.3) [38]. Usually, belt speed ratios of 3:4 up to 1:2 are used in the current literature, indicating that one belt is running at 75% [3, 4] or 50% [1, 2] of speed compared to the other belt. Larger ratios usually lead to better generalization [50] and larger training effects [37]. Furthermore, the number of switches can be used to add progression to the training. By introducing more switches in the belt speed participants have to adjust their gait pattern more often, requiring more gait flexibility and adaptability [36]. For additional challenge, belt speed can be decreased (or increased) only on one side (unilateral) or on both sides (bilateral). To target gait adaptability, changes in the ratios should be implemented in a randomized order.

Generally, when designing a split-belt treadmill intervention the overall strategy regarding split-belt ratios and switches should match the target of the training. If the training aims to reduce pronounced gait asymmetry using steady split-belt treadmill ratios without switching sides would be more adequate. If the training wants to focus on improving gait adaptability, a strategy with more switches and especially switches between sides should be adopted [51]. Interestingly, one study in healthy young adults showed that including multiple washout periods within a split-belt treadmill training session led to gains in adaptation similar to multiple days of training [52]. This strategy has not yet been tested out in older adults or clinical populations, and its therapeutic value is yet to be explored.

However, given the limited amount of literature in this field, it must be noted that no clear disease-specific recommendation for training progression in split-belt treadmill exist so far. Furthermore, it is unclear whether components of overground walking should be implemented in the split-belt training interventions to increase the effect of transfer to overground walking or daily life mobility.

Neurophysiological Aspects

Regarding neurophysiological aspects, split-belt treadmill has been used to investigate which factors facilitate and which aggravate adequate gait adaptation. In one of the first studies, investigating locomotor adaptations to split-belt treadmill Morton and Bastian [13] found that cerebellar damage disrupted predictive feedforward motor adaptation. Thus, they conclude that this brain area is important for the step-by-step adjustments during split-belt treadmill adaptation. Hinton, Conradsson and Paquette [53] summarized previous split-belt treadmill studies with regard to neurophysiological aspects and found that especially the initial adjustments during split-belt treadmill walking are made based on proprioceptive feedback providing input to central pattern generators, whereas proprioceptive and visual feedback will inform supraspinal centers for motor planning and motor output later on during adaptation. The authors also found that brain injuries such as stroke or cerebellar lesions reduce but do not take away adaptation during split-belt treadmill walking and concluded that different brain areas (central pattern generators, cerebellum, basal ganglia) are involved in split-belt adaptation [53]. This approach was confirmed by results from a study using brain imaging techniques in healthy young adults [54]. The authors found increased activity in the supplementary motor areas, the posterior parietal cortex, the anterior cingulate cortex, and the anterior lateral cerebellum and decreased activity of the posterior cingulate and medial prefrontal cortex during split-belt treadmill walking. Recent work has shown that people with cognitive impairment show reduced ability to adapt to split-belt treadmill conditions [55]. Similar results have been found in individuals with PD where cognitive impairment and specifically reduced working memory were associated with less adaptation [45]. Those results suggest that a certain level of cognition is involved and required to adjust gait to changing environmental demands.

Final Remarks

Split-belt treadmill is an attractive therapeutic tool as it offers a unique way to modulate gait asymmetry and gait adaptation deficits—two aspects which have been linked to falls. Findings from studies investigating repeated split-belt treadmill training in individuals post-stroke and in people with PD are promising. However, strategies and investigations of how to better transfer effects to daily life mobility are still lacking and should be addressed in future studies.

References

1. Yogev G, Plotnik M, Peretz C, Giladi N, Hausdorff JM. Gait asymmetry in patients with Parkinson's disease and elderly fallers: when does the bilateral coordination of gait require attention? Exp Brain Res. 2007;177(3):336–46.

2. Patterson KK, Parafianowicz I, Danells CJ, Closson V, Verrier MC, Staines WR, et al. Gait asymmetry in community-ambulating stroke survivors. Arch Phys Med Rehabil. 2008;89(2):304–10.
3. Kim S, Lockhart T, editors. Gait asymmetry: factors influencing slip severity and tendency among older adults. Proceedings of the human factors and ergonomics society annual meeting. Los Angeles, CA: SAGE Publications; 2006.
4. Plotnik M, Giladi N, Balash Y, Peretz C, Hausdorff JM. Is freezing of gait in Parkinson's disease related to asymmetric motor function? Ann Neurol. 2005;57(5):656–63.
5. Arippa F, Leban B, Monticone M, Cossu G, Casula C, Pau M. A study on lower limb asymmetries in Parkinson's disease during gait assessed through kinematic-derived parameters. Bioengineering. 2022;9(3):120.
6. Seuthe J, Nicholas DC, Ginis P, Weisser B, Berg D, Deuschl G, et al. Split-belt treadmill walking in patients with Parkinson's disease: a systematic review. Gait Posture. 2019;69:187–94. https://doi.org/10.1016/j.gaitpost.2019.01.032.
7. Fettrow T, Hupfeld K, Hass C, Pasternak O, Seidler R. Neural correlates of gait adaptation in younger and older adults. Sci Rep. 2023;13(1):3842.
8. Caetano MJD, Lord SR, Schoene D, Pelicioni PH, Sturnieks DL, Menant JC. Age-related changes in gait adaptability in response to unpredictable obstacles and stepping targets. Gait Posture. 2016;46:35–41.
9. Martin T, Keating J, Goodkin H, Bastian A, Thach W. Throwing while looking through prisms: I. Focal olivocerebellar lesions impair adaptation. Brain. 1996;119(4):1183–98.
10. Van Andel S, Cole MH, Pepping G-J. Associations between gait-related falls and gait adaptations when stepping onto a curb: a prospective falls study. J Aging Phys Act. 2019;27(3):309–15.
11. Roemmich RT, Nocera JR, Stegemoller EL, Hassan A, Okun MS, Hass CJ. Locomotor adaptation and locomotor adaptive learning in Parkinson's disease and normal aging. Clin Neurophysiol. 2014;125(2):313–9.
12. Kuczynski V, Telonio A, Thibaudier Y, Hurteau MF, Dambreville C, Desrochers E, et al. Lack of adaptation during prolonged split-belt locomotion in the intact and spinal cat. J Physiol. 2017;595(17):5987–6006.
13. Morton SM, Bastian AJ. Cerebellar contributions to locomotor adaptations during splitbelt treadmill walking. J Neurosci. 2006;26(36):9107–16.
14. Dietz V, Zijlstra W, Duysens J. Human neuronal interlimb coordination during split-belt locomotion. Exp Brain Res. 1994;101(3):513–20.
15. Reisman DS, Bastian AJ, Morton SM. Neurophysiologic and rehabilitation insights from the split-belt and other locomotor adaptation paradigms. Phys Ther. 2010;90(2):187–95.
16. Vervoort D, Den Otter AR, Buurke TJ, Vuillerme N, Hortobágyi T, Lamoth CJ. Effects of aging and task prioritization on split-belt gait adaptation. Front Aging Neurosci. 2019;11:10.
17. Malone LA, Bastian AJ. Age-related forgetting in locomotor adaptation. Neurobiol Learn Mem. 2016;128:1–6.
18. Reisman DS, Wityk R, Silver K, Bastian AJ. Locomotor adaptation on a split-belt treadmill can improve walking symmetry post-stroke. Brain. 2007;130(Pt 7):1861–72.
19. Huang C-H, Aydemir B, Foucher KC. Split-Belt treadmill training improves mechanical energetics and metabolic cost in women with unilateral hip osteoarthritis: a proof-of-concept study. Biomechanics. 2023;3(2):220–30.
20. Wade F, Baudendistel S, Stone A, Roper J, Raffegeau T, Terza M, et al. Locomotor adaptation training to prevent mobility disability. Biomechanics. 2022;2(3):395–420.
21. Balasubramanian CK, Bowden MG, Neptune RR, Kautz SA. Relationship between step length asymmetry and walking performance in subjects with chronic hemiparesis. Arch Phys Med Rehabil. 2007;88(1):43–9.
22. Bowden MG, Balasubramanian CK, Neptune RR, Kautz SA. Anterior-posterior ground reaction forces as a measure of paretic leg contribution in hemiparetic walking. Stroke. 2006;37(3):872–6.

23. Jorgensen L, Crabtree NJ, Reeve J, Jacobsen BK. Ambulatory level and asymmetrical weight bearing after stroke affects bone loss in the upper and lower part of the femoral neck differently: bone adaptation after decreased mechanical loading. Bone. 2000;27(5):701–7.
24. Lewek MD, Bradley CE, Wutzke CJ, Zinder SM. The relationship between spatiotemporal gait asymmetry and balance in individuals with chronic stroke. J Appl Biomech. 2014;30(1):31–6.
25. Awad LN, Palmer JA, Pohlig RT, Binder-Macleod SA, Reisman DS. Walking speed and step length asymmetry modify the energy cost of walking after stroke. Neurorehabil Neural Repair. 2015;29(5):416–23.
26. Dzewaltowski AC, Hedrick EA, Leutzinger TJ, Remski LE, Rosen AB. The effect of split-belt treadmill interventions on step length asymmetry in individuals poststroke: a systematic review with meta-analysis. Neurorehabil Neural Repair. 2021;35(7):563–75.
27. Wutzke CJ, Faldowski RA, Lewek MD. Individuals Poststroke do not perceive their spatiotemporal gait asymmetries as abnormal. Phys Ther. 2015;95(9):1244–53.
28. Betschart M, McFadyen BJ, Nadeau S. Repeated split-belt treadmill walking improved gait ability in individuals with chronic stroke: a pilot study. Physiother Theory Pract. 2018;34(2):81–90.
29. Lewek MD, Braun CH, Wutzke C, Giuliani C. The role of movement errors in modifying spatiotemporal gait asymmetry post stroke: a randomized controlled trial. Clin Rehabil. 2018;32(2):161–72.
30. Reisman DS, McLean H, Keller J, Danks KA, Bastian AJ. Repeated Split-Belt treadmill training improves Poststroke step length asymmetry. Neurorehabil Neural Repair. 2013;27(5):460–8. https://doi.org/10.1177/1545968312474118.
31. Chen G, Patten C, Kothari DH, Zajac FE. Gait differences between individuals with post-stroke hemiparesis and non-disabled controls at matched speeds. Gait Posture. 2005;22(1):51–6.
32. Lord S, Galna B, Yarnall AJ, Coleman S, Burn D, Rochester L. Predicting first fall in newly diagnosed Parkinson's disease: insights from a fall-naive cohort. Mov Disord. 2016;31(12):1829–36.
33. Caetano MJD, Lord SR, Allen NE, Brodie MA, Song J, Paul SS, et al. Stepping reaction time and gait adaptability are significantly impaired in people with Parkinson's disease: implications for fall risk. Parkinsonism Relat Disord. 2018;47:32–8.
34. Zijlstra W, Rutgers AW, Van Weerden TW. Voluntary and involuntary adaptation of gait in Parkinson's disease. Gait Posture. 1998;7(1):53–63.
35. Fasano A, Schlenstedt C, Herzog J, Plotnik M, Rose FEM, Volkmann J, et al. Split-belt locomotion in Parkinson's disease links asymmetry, dyscoordination and sequence effect. Gait Posture. 2016;48:6–12.
36. Seuthe J, D'Cruz N, Ginis P, Becktepe JS, Weisser B, Nieuwboer A, et al. The effect of one session Split-Belt treadmill training on gait adaptation in people with Parkinson's disease and freezing of gait. Neurorehabil Neural Repair. 2020;34(10):954–63.
37. D'cruz N, Seuthe J, Ginis P, Hulzinga F, Schlenstedt C, Nieuwboer A. Short-term effects of single-session Split-Belt treadmill training on dual-task performance in Parkinson's disease and healthy elderly. Front Neurol. 2020;11:560084.
38. Hulzinga F, Seuthe J, D'Cruz N, Ginis P, Nieuwboer A, Schlenstedt C. Split-Belt treadmill training to improve gait adaptation in Parkinson's disease. Mov Disord. 2023;38(1):92–103. https://doi.org/10.1002/mds.29238.
39. Lau J, Regis C, Burke C, Kaleda M, McKenna R, Muratori LM. Immersive Technology for Cognitive-Motor Training in Parkinson's disease. Front Hum Neurosci. 2022;16:863930.
40. Nieuwboer A, Giladi N. Characterizing freezing of gait in Parkinson's disease: models of an episodic phenomenon. Mov Disord. 2013;28(11):1509–19.
41. Frazzitta G, Pezzoli G, Bertotti G, Maestri R. Asymmetry and freezing of gait in parkinsonian patients. J Neurol. 2013;260(1):71–6.
42. Plotnik M, Giladi N, Hausdorff JM. Bilateral coordination of walking and freezing of gait in Parkinson's disease. Eur J Neurosci. 2008;27(8):1999–2006.
43. Smulders K, Esselink RA, Bloem BR, Cools R. Freezing of gait in Parkinson's disease is related to impaired motor switching during stepping. Mov Disord. 2015;30(8):1090–7.

44. Mohammadi F, Bruijn SM, Vervoort G, van Wegen EE, Kwakkel G, Verschueren S, et al. Motor switching and motor adaptation deficits contribute to freezing of gait in Parkinson's disease. Neurorehabil Neural Repair. 2015;29(2):132–42.
45. Sasikumar S, Sorrento G, Lang AE, Strafella AP, Fasano A. Cognition affects gait adaptation after split-belt treadmill training in Parkinson's disease. Neurobiol Dis. 2023;181:106109.
46. Bekkers EMJ, Hoogkamer W, Bengevoord A, Heremans E, Verschueren SMP, Nieuwboer A. Freezing-related perception deficits of asymmetrical walking in Parkinson's disease. Neuroscience. 2017;364:122–9.
47. Nanhoe-Mahabier W, Snijders AH, Delval A, Weerdesteyn V, Duysens J, Overeem S, et al. Split-belt locomotion in Parkinson's disease with and without freezing of gait. Neuroscience. 2013;236:110–6.
48. Nutt JG, Bloem BR, Giladi N, Hallett M, Horak FB, Nieuwboer A. Freezing of gait: moving forward on a mysterious clinical phenomenon. Lancet Neurol. 2011;10(8):734–44.
49. Hagen AC, Acosta JS, Geltser CS, Fling BW. Split-Belt treadmill adaptation improves spatial and temporal gait symmetry in people with multiple sclerosis. Sensors. 2023;23(12):5456.
50. Aucie Y, Harket HM, Sombric CJ, Torres-Oviedo G. Older adults generalize their movements across walking contexts more than young during gradual and abrupt split-belt walking. bioRxiv. 2021:2021.08. 06.455403.
51. Seuthe J, Hulzinga F, D'Cruz N, Ginis P, Nieuwboer A, Schlenstedt C. The potential of Split-Belt treadmill walking as a therapeutic tool in Parkinson's disease: a narrative review. Dtsch Z Sportmed. 2021;72:344–50. https://doi.org/10.5960/dzsm.2021.509.
52. Day KA, Leech KA, Roemmich RT, Bastian AJ. Accelerating locomotor savings in learning: compressing four training days to one. J Neurophysiol. 2018;119(6):2100–13.
53. Hinton DC, Conradsson DM, Paquette C. Understanding human neural control of short-term gait adaptation to the Split-belt treadmill. Neuroscience. 2020;451:36–50.
54. Hinton DC, Thiel A, Soucy J-P, Bouyer L, Paquette C. Adjusting gait step-by-step: brain activation during split-belt treadmill walking. NeuroImage. 2019;202:116095.
55. Pottorf TS, Nocera JR, Eicholtz SP, Kesar TM. Locomotor adaptation deficits in older individuals with cognitive impairments: a pilot study. Front Neurol. 2022;13:800338. https://doi.org/10.3389/fneur.2022.800338.

One Plus One Is More Than Two: Enhanced Physical, Motor, and Cognitive Gains from Simultaneous Multicomponent Training in Older Adults

25

Luis Augusto Teixeira

Abstract

Regular aging is associated with declines in multiple organismic dimensions, including aerobic capacity, muscular resistance, motor fitness, and cognitive functions. These multiple age-related declines are interconnected and bring negative, sometimes dramatic, consequences for life quality in older ages. I scrutinize encouraging data indicating that training approaches aiming to improve multiple dimensions simultaneously rather than training each dimension separately may be more effective for functional improvements in older individuals. Training programs combining simultaneous multidimensional components, such as aerobic capacity, muscular resistance, dual-tasking exercises, exergames, and dancing, have been shown to induce greater attenuation or even reversal of age-related declines at the behavioral and neural levels in comparison with isolated training of each behavioral dimension. To conclude, I propose applied translational principles for training programs for older individuals aiming to reach the highest achievements in the physical, motor, and cognitive dimensions.

Age-Related Organismic Multidimensional Decline

With the increasing life expectancy in modern times, the proportion of older individuals in the global population is on the rise. Particularly in western countries, the percentage of people aged 60 and above is projected to reach approximately 20% across all age groups by 2025. Furthermore, the proportion of older individuals in the population residing in these countries is expected to increase by an additional 10% by 2060 [1]. These statistics are a matter of both individual and societal

L. A. Teixeira (✉)
School of Physical Education and Sport, University of São Paulo, São Paulo, SP, Brazil
e-mail: lateixei@usp.br

F. A. Barbieri et al. (eds.), *Locomotion and Posture in Older Adults*,
https://doi.org/10.1007/978-3-031-74123-4_25

concern, as longer life expectancy has been accompanied by various health issues that negatively affect the quality of life in older individuals. Some of the most significant declines associated with aging are observed in aerobic capacity, body balance, muscular resistance, and cognitive functions. The Baltimore Longitudinal Study of Aging, conducted in the USA, provides representative data on functional declines associated with aging. In this study, aerobic (cardiovascular) capacity was measured in a sample of healthy independent community-dwelling women ($n = 375$) and men ($n = 435$) aged between 21 and 87 years [2]. The results revealed a nonlinear decline in aerobic capacity across different age groups, with a more pronounced acceleration in successive decades of life.

Large national studies have provided normative data documenting the decline in physical and motor dimensions associated with aging. Dodds and colleagues [3] analyzed grip strength data from 12 studies in Great Britain, including 60,803 observations from 49,964 participants aged 4–90 years. The results revealed that manual strength begins to decline around the age of 40, with a more accelerated decline from the age of 60 onwards. Similarly, the Canadian Longitudinal Study on Aging assessed healthy community-dwelling individuals aged 45–85 years on various tests of muscular resistance, mobility, and dynamic balance [4]. The findings showed performance decline across all tests, including grip strength, lower limb power (five-repetition chair rise), gait speed, quiet body balance (single leg stance), mobility and dynamic body balance (timed up and go test). This multiple performance decline was equivalent between men and women. Comparable results were found in the 10-year prospective population-based longitudinal Malmo study conducted in Sweden, revealing progressive performance decline in grip strength, body balance, and gait velocity among individuals aged 50–80 years [5]. The decline in physical and motor dimensions associated with aging is clinically concerning, as low scores on body balance and leg muscular resistance tests have been identified as major predictors of fall risk [6], while reduced grip strength, limb strength, and gait speed have been associated with an increased likelihood of physical disability [7] in older adults.

Decline of cognitive functions is another crucial aspect for achieving an independent and high quality of life in older adults. Cognitive functions encompass various mental abilities underling our daily activities, including executive functions (inhibition control, working memory, and cognitive flexibility, see [8]), planning, decision-making, processing speed, and visuospatial abilities [9]. In the Cardiovascular Health Study, conducted in the USA, 5888 participants aged over 65 years underwent clinical evaluations, with 3608 of them further assessed through magnetic resonance imaging. The results revealed concerning rates of unhealthy cognitive aging, including about 16% of cases of mild cognitive impairment, 13% of incident dementia, and 6% of prevalent dementia, while only about 65% of this group were rated as having normal cognitive functioning for their age [10]. Memory appears to be the cognitive function that declines earliest among several cognitive functions [11, 12]. In a study examining diverse cognitive functions in a sample of 350 participants aged 10–86 years, Ferguson and colleagues [13] found that decline of working memory and inhibitory control started from the age of 30–40 years and continued to decline further in more advanced ages. The mixing costs of cognitive flexibility were also found to decline across the evaluated age span. Assessing cognitive flexibility during a walking task, Kim and colleagues [14] observed that older compared to young participants exhibited more stepping errors and increased between-task interference when the rules of stepping *on* versus *off* markers on a rolling treadmill surface changed. In a study conducted in an ecologically valid context, Hennah and Doumas [15] compared adaptive behavior between older and young individuals while walking on outdoor paths with smooth (asphalt) or irregular (grass) surfaces associated with a concurrent or absent cognitive task. The findings revealed that older adults showed less adaptation of step width and height when performing dual-task walking, suggesting an increased susceptibility of older individuals to tripping in real-world environments. Functional cognitive declines with aging can be attributed to structural changes in the aging brain, such as reduced brain volume, thinning of the cerebral cortex [16], and smaller hippocampal volumes [17]. Rates of prefrontal cortex and hippocampus atrophy in regular aging have been estimated to be about 1–2% per year in individuals over the age of 55 [18], with higher rates of cerebral shrinkage observed in people experiencing some degree of cognitive impairment [19]. Age-related declines in cognitive functioning, and likely in other dimensions as well, have also been shown to be influenced by diminished neural connectivity between the prefrontal and posterior regions of the cerebral cortex [12].

Interdimensional Relationships

A notable aspect of the aging process is the complex interplay between various organismic dimensions involving aerobic capacity, body balance, muscular resistance, and cognitive functions. Spirduso showed earlier evidence for the association between aerobic fitness and motor performance. It was found that continuous engagement in aerobic training during the lifespan by older individuals was associated with shorter reaction time [20], in addition to increased manual dexterity and coordination [21], when compared to sedentary older adults. McGregor and colleagues [22] further explored the relationship between physical fitness and motor performance, showing that increased aerobic fitness in middle-aged individuals was associated with better performance on manual motor tasks, including hand strength, dexterity, and psychomotor speed. In a longitudinal study on the association between aerobic fitness and cognitive function in healthy older people, Barnes and colleagues [23] showed that older individuals with low fitness levels at the baseline assessment experienced steeper cognitive decline in a follow-up assessment conducted 6 years later. Middleton and colleagues [24] reported that older women engaged in physical activity at different periods of life had a reduced risk of cognitive deficits. Additionally, in a representative population-based cross-sectional study conducted in Madeira, Portugal, Gouveia and colleagues [25] found that aerobic fitness accounted for a significant portion of the variance in body balance and gait performance. Overall, these results indicate that aerobic fitness is a protective factor against cognitive and motor dysfunctions in older adults (see also [9, 26, 27]).

Examining the bidirectional relationship between cognition and body balance, Biasin and colleagues [28] tested performance of older individuals with impairment of global cognitive functioning, as indexed by the Mini Mental State Examination and Montreal Cognitive Assessment, and used stability measures of the Biodex Balance System, Short Physical Performance Battery test, and Tinetti scale to evaluate body balance. Results indicated that scores from the Mini Mental State Examination correlated with scores from the Biodex Balance System, while scores from the Montreal Cognitive Assessment test correlated with the Short Physical Performance Battery and Tinetti scores. Based on these results, the authors suggest a bidirectional relationship between the cognitive and motor dimensions, so that training focused on the motor dimension can be thought to lead to cognitive gains, while cognitive training could potentially lead to improvements of motor performance. Examining a more complex association among aerobic capacity, motor performance, and cognition, Voelcker-Rehage and colleagues [29] evaluated older people on respective tests for each targeted dimension and associated cortical activation. At the behavioral level, they found that both physical fitness (aerobic fitness and muscular resistance) and motor fitness (movement speed, balance and motor coordination) showed high correlations with the evaluated cognitive functions (executive control and perceptual speed). These findings reinforce the notion of a bidirectional relationship between cognition and motor fitness. At the neural level, functional brain imaging data showed that physical and motor fitness were differentially associated with cortical activation. Older individuals with higher physical fitness were found to activate frontal areas related to executive control in a specific and focal way, while older individuals with higher motor fitness showed increased activation of posterior cortical areas related to visuospatial processing. Investigation of effects of physical fitness on structural changes in the aging brain in about 300 older adults from the Cardiovascular Health Cognition Study, conducted in the USA, showed evidence that longer walked distances in preceding years correlates with increased gray matter volume and reduced risk of cognitive deficits [30].

In a comprehensive review of literature, Hayes and colleagues [31] showed a noticeable association of aerobic fitness with cerebral structure and function. The revised studies employed magnetic resonance imaging and showed consistent evidence of a relationship between aerobic fitness and brain volume in different cortical regions comprising the anterior cingulate, lateral prefrontal, and lateral parietal cortices. Review of findings from investigations employing functional magnetic resonance imaging revealed that aerobic fitness in older individuals correlates with activation of similar cortical regions as those found in the studies on structural effects of aerobic fitness. These findings of association between physical fitness with structural and functional brain imaging suggest that regular aerobic exercise decisively contributes to maintain brain health in older adults. Collectively, these results suggest a complex interplay between physical fitness, motor performance and cognition both at the behavioral and neural levels, which supposedly underlies the diminished risk of cognitive decline [32] and dementia [33] in physically fit older individuals.

Interdimensional associations have also been found among cognition, muscular strength, and motor performance. Analysis of association between cognitive functions and gait in older adults showed that performance on speed/executive attention and memory tests can predict gait velocity [34]. Based on data from a large number of participants in the Spanish Barcelona Brain Health Initiative, Zhou and colleagues [35] found that low cognitive functioning is correlated with increased dual-task costs in different kinematic parameters of walking performance. Evaluating longitudinal aging cohorts, Clouston and colleagues [36] found that grip strength was correlated with a mental state score, while walking speed had a stronger correlation with fluid cognition. Leg strength has been shown to be a good predictor of body balance in older adults [37]. As an additional example of association between distinct behavioral dimensions, in an 8-year prospective study, Anstey and colleagues [38] presented evidence that cognitive performance is associated with chance of falling in very old adults, suggesting an association of body balance with mental functions.

In summary, the dimensions of aerobic fitness, cognition, muscular resistance, and motor performance exhibit interconnectedness at both the behavioral and neural levels. These interdimensional relationships underscore the importance of considering multiple aspects of organismic functioning in research and in the promotion of health and well-being in older adults.

Aerobic, Resistance, and Coordination Training Enhance Cognitive Functioning

One of the main tenets of motor, physical and cognitive training is that a systematic practice of a given skill or physical capacity is expected to lead to improved performance on the specifically trained factor. This is known as the *specificity of practice principle*. Specificity of practice effects were documented in older athletes by comparing runners and tennis players with at least 10 years of training against age-matched and young exercisers [39]. They were tested on six motor tasks requiring different skills, like coincident timing, finger dexterity, fast finger tapping, limit of balance stability and choice reaction time. Results showed that the older tennis players were the single group to achieve distinguished performance on some of the motor tests, with lower simple reaction time and decreased temporal errors in coincident timing than the other two aged groups. Remarkably, performance of the older tennis players was equivalent to that shown by the young participants in the coincident timing task. Considering that fast reactions and accurate coincident timing in striking fast moving balls are mandatory for playing tennis, these data suggest that older tennis players selectively prevented performance decline only in the systematically trained motor functions. Similar specificity of practice effect can be thought to apply to motor [40], muscular resistance [41], and cognitive [42] training.

In dissonance to the specificity of practice principle, several studies have demonstrated that physical training can also lead to cognitive benefits. Systematic reviews and meta-analyses have shown that aerobic training improves cognitive performance in healthy older individuals, slowing down the rate of cognitive decline associated with sedentary lifestyles [9, 43–46]. Furthermore, aerobic training has been linked to a reduced risk of mental diseases such as Alzheimer and dementia [47]. Older individuals engaged in aerobic training have shown improved executive functioning [48, 49], processing speed [50], visuospatial memory [51], attentional flexibility, and time-sharing abilities [52] compared to non-trained controls. Gains in cognitive functions as a result of aerobic training can be thought to result from functional and structural changes in the aging brain. Compared to sedentary controls, highly fit or aerobically trained older participants were shown to have increased task-related activation of the prefrontal and parietal cortices [53]. These cortical regions are conceived to be related to the processing of spatial attention and inhibitory control. An additional effect was seen in the activation of the anterior cingulate cortex, a neural structure conceived to underlie adaptation in the attentional network. Experimental investigation at the structural level has revealed that aerobic training leads to increased cortical thickness in the left frontal region [48] and in the volume of the prefrontal and temporal cortices [54]. Additional research showed that participation in a walking program during 1 year induced enlargement of the anterior hippocampal volume in parallel with memory improvement [55].

Expanding beyond aerobic training, Northey and colleagues [45] and Herold and colleagues [56] reviewed results from studies evaluating the effects of muscular resistance training on cognitive performance. The results supported the conclusion that not only aerobic capacity training but also muscular resistance exercising improves cognitive processing in middle-aged and older individuals, regardless of their cognitive status. As representative experimental evidence, Cassilhas and colleagues [57] compared the effects of moderate- and high-intensity resistance training on cognitive functions in older adults. Results indicated that both experimental groups performed better than age-matched controls on different cognitive tests for evaluation of working memory and attention control. In a 1-year long randomized controlled trial, Liu-Ambrose and colleagues [58] compared the effects of one versus two resistance training sessions per week on cognitive functioning in older women, taking as reference age-matched controls receiving twice-weekly balance and tone training. Results showed that both once- and twice-weekly resistance training groups achieved higher performance when tested for selective attention and inhibitory control at the end of the training program, while balance/tone training failed to lead to gains in the cognitive assessment. In an ensuing randomized controlled trial, Liu-Ambrose et al. [59] tested the effect of resistance training on cortical plasticity in community-dwelling senior women. Results showed that resistance training induced functional changes in the anterior portion of the left middle temporal gyrus and in the left anterior insula, with this cortical plasticity associated with increased response inhibition.

Further empirical evidence has shown that training motor coordination can also lead to improvement of cognitive functions in older adults. Differently from aerobic and muscular resistance training, motor coordination training usually does not require large metabolic resources. Rather, it requires perceptuomotor processes, being oriented to improvement of performance on tasks requiring fine or global motor actions, body balance control, coordination between body segments, or activity-dependent interaction with other people or objects. Voelcker-Rehage and colleagues [49] performed a 1-year longitudinal study in older adults to assess the effects of aerobic versus coordination training (taking as reference a control group practicing relaxation and stretching exercises) on performance of cognitive tests requiring executive control and perceptual speed. Beyond training-related behavioral gains, changes in brain activation patterns after training was evaluated through functional magnetic resonance imaging. Analysis of behavioral data revealed that both experimental groups improved performance on perceptual speed, achieving specific gains on speed and accuracy components as a result of aerobic or motor coordination training. In comparison with controls, functional brain imaging indicated that both the coordination and aerobic training groups presented decreased activation in prefrontal areas during the evaluation of executive functions. This finding can be interpreted as a more efficient task-related information processing induced by either modality of training. Further analysis showed modality-specific training effects in activation of cortical regions. While aerobic training induced higher activation of cortical areas related to sensorimotor processing, coordination training led to higher activation of the visuospatial network. In a further test of the effects of motor coordination training on gains of cognitive functions, Hötting and colleagues [60] compared middle-aged groups receiving coordination (combined with stretching) or aerobic (cycling) training during a 6-month program on psychometric tests for cognitive assessment. Analysis indicated that both the coordination and aerobic training induced gains in episodic memory, while specific gains in selective attention were observed in the coordination compared to the aerobic training group. These findings suggest that motor coordination training leads to specific cognitive gains and strengthening of neurocognitive networks subserving skillful motor performance. Motor complexity in coordination training can be conceived to underlie behavioral and respective neuroplastic changes [61]. Literature reviews have indicated higher cognitive functioning following coordination training than other kinds of exercise [62, 63].

Physiological explanations for the cognitive benefits observed in aerobic, resistance, and coordination training involve distinct mechanisms. Regular aerobic training has been associated with increased neurogenesis and cerebral blood volume in the dentate gyrus of the human hippocampus [64]. Substantiating the association between physiological changes in the brain and cognitive functions, the analysis also showed that higher cerebral blood volume correlated with improved performance on verbal recall. Further investigation on the neurocognitive effects of aerobic training in older individuals showed that higher cerebral blood volume at the end of a training program led also to improved performance on recognition and spatial memory tests [65]. These results suggest that increased cerebral blood flow due to aerobic training provides higher oxygen supply to the brain, favoring neurogenesis and cerebral functioning. Based on a literature review on this topic, Marmeleira [66] discussed evidence that aerobic fitness is associated with changes in mechanisms related with higher cerebral blood flow, neurotrophic factors, neurotransmitters, and reconfiguration of the neural architecture, corresponding to neural changes that have been shown to underlie gains in cognitive performance. Regarding coordination training, Marmeleira suggests that regular practice of motor skills leads to systematic exercising of task-specific executive functions that might benefit performance on pure cognitive tasks loading on the same functions. Stimpson and colleagues [67] have proposed the following sequence of neural events to explain cognitive gains from aerobic training: (a) aerobic fitness leads to cerebral angiogenesis, having as a consequence (b) improved oxygen supply to the brain, causing (c) augmented neurotrophin delivery and (d) associated neurogenesis, followed by (e) connection of the new neurons into functional networks through motor/cognitive task-specific training, (f) having as outcome improved brain functioning. From this proposition, a possible explanation for cognitive gains from physical and motor training is that synapses are randomly generated at diffuse sites in the nervous system as a result of aerobic and resistance training, while their stabilization and functional integration depends on their recruitment to participate of a given neural network to produce the desired response during a motor coordination or cognitive training [68]. In other words, it can be conceived that aerobic training induces higher angiogenesis (and respective oxygen supply) and neurogenesis, while motor/cognitive-related training guides the connectome leading to plastic changes in the brain reflected into functional and structural adaptive gains [69]. This knowledge is of particular relevance for older people in the attempt to attenuate or even revert losses in the gray matter and physical-motor-cognitive functions observed over years in the regular sedentary aging (cf. [18, 19]). See Kempermann and colleagues [70] and Herold and colleagues [56] for reviews on this topic.

Overall, the substantial evidence supporting the positive effects of aerobic, resistance, and coordination training on cognitive functioning, along with the associated physiological adaptations in the brain, emphasizes the importance of physical activity and motor training to mitigate age-related declines in both gray matter and physical-motor-cognitive functions commonly observed in sedentary aging populations.

Sequential Versus Simultaneous Multicomponent Training

In the preceding sections we reviewed major findings on the declines of cognitive, physical, and motor dimensions associated with regular aging, the relationships among these dimensions, and the beneficial effects of aerobic, resistance, and motor training on cognitive functioning in older adults. While the focus in the previous section was on the effects of nonspecific (non-cognitive targeted) training for improving cognitive functioning, it is also conceivable that between-dimension training-related gains can occur in other behavioral dimensions. Cognitive functioning, for example, has been shown to have predictive power for the risk of falls in older adults [38]. Although we have limited empirical evidence, it is plausible that improving cognitive functions through specific cognitive training or indirectly through physical/coordination training could potentially reduce the chances of falling in older people. By enhancing anticipatory and attentional cognitive functions, for example, older individuals might improve the ability to avoid situations that increase the risk of falls, such as monitoring the near space and negotiating obstacles during walking. In another instance that one can devise reciprocal gains between behavioral dimensions, leg muscular resistance has been identified as one of the major predictors of critical balance loss leading to falls in older adults [6]. This relationship between leg strength and body balance is straightforward, as unexpected stance or gait perturbations require vigorous and fast muscular responses in the lower limbs for timely balance recovery [71, 72]. Therefore, training for improvement of fast legs' muscular contractions can be assumed to be an important factor for enhancement of reactive balance responses through a diversity of vigorous and fast compensatory leg movements to sudden extrinsic perturbations (cf. [73]), reducing as a consequence the risk of falls. In the opposite direction, a study evaluating the benefits of a training program aiming at improving dynamic balance in healthy sedentary older adults revealed that one of the major gains was in leg muscular resistance [74]. This finding suggests that regular practice of body balance tasks imposes sufficient muscular demand on the legs to induce muscular resistance gains in older adults. Importantly, this study demonstrated that the resistance gains were achieved through functional tasks, which are more applicable to daily living situations compared to strength training using machines targeting at resistance increment of single-joint muscle groups.

Based on the reviewed findings that the regular aging process is associated with declines in the aerobic, cognitive, muscular resistance, and motor (coordination/balance) dimensions, it is evident that training programs should aim at improving all of these dimensions to achieve comprehensive effectiveness in enhancing the quality of life of older adults. Developing a multicomponent training program for older adults can be approached in two ways: (a) Sequential isolated exercises or tasks targeting specific behavioral dimensions, with minimal overlap in demands across different dimensions. In this strategy, the training session is divided into distinct parts dedicated to exercising separately cognitive functions, aerobic capacity, muscular resistance, or motor skills (coordination and balance). (b) Activities aiming at simultaneously exercising two or more behavioral dimensions during the training session. This approach requires the integration of cognitive and neuromuscular resources to meet the demands of different task components. In the following sections are reviewed the gains achieved from each approach for a holistic multidimensional training of older adults.

In testing the effects of a program based on sequential activities for acquiring motor skills in healthy young individuals, it was shown that providing a single bout of different intensities of aerobic exercise after 20 minutes of practice of a manual motor task favored the learning process compared to motor practice alone [75]. Interestingly, a group that received aerobic exercise at a higher intensity (90% VO_2 maximum) demonstrated higher retention results after 7 days of rest than a group exercising at a lower intensity (45% VO_2 maximum). This strategy of combining motor skill learning with an ensuing bout of aerobic exercise was also successful in individuals with Parkinson's disease, with data showing that providing moderate-intensity cycling after practicing a task of balancing on an unstable platform led to superior 7-day retention of performance gains [76].

Van Het Reve and de Bruin [77] provided healthy older adults with twice-weekly activities aimed at exercising body balance and muscular resistance during the training sessions. In addition to the physical-motor training, one group received additional cognitive training through a computer-based software in separate sessions. Results indicated that the balance-strength training associated with cognitive activities led to higher gains on different tests, including walking dual-task costs, gait initiation, and divided attention [78]. Combined sequential balance-cognitive training for cognitively impaired older adults induced higher gains in static and dynamic balance [79] as well as cognitive functioning [80, 81] compared to dynamic balance training alone. Of particular applied relevance, two studies conducted by Hagovska [79, 80] revealed that training-related gains transferred to daily living activities, leading to self-reports of improved quality of life. Systematic reviews have substantiated the conclusion that sequential physical and cognitive training can lead to higher gains than single training activities [82, 83]. Additionally, a review by Cadore and colleagues [84] concluded that a sequential multicomponent training approach, composed of exercises aiming to develop body balance, muscular resistance, and aerobic capacity, was effective in improving gait performance, body balance, muscular resistance, and reducing the risk of falls in physically frail older adults.

Although the sequential training approach has been shown to concurrently develop the physical, motor, and cognitive dimensions relevant to attenuating age-related declines, further examination of the literature indicates that simultaneously combined physical-cognitive training can lead to greater functional gains. Based on an extensive literature review, Tait and colleagues [85] found inconsistent evidence of cognitive gains from sequential training, with only six out of ten studies showing additional beneficial effects compared to individual cognitive or exercise training. In contrast, combined simultaneous physical/motor-cognitive training consistently demonstrated performance improvements in different behavioral components, with 17 out of 19 studies reporting more pronounced gains in cognitive assessments compared to non-combined training. A more recent systematic review and meta-analysis by Rieker and colleagues [86] confirmed these findings, showing more consistent results indicating that physical exercise combined with simultaneous cognitive tasks leads to higher performance gains in executive functions, global cognition, as well as physical and motor performance. The review also highlighted that multicomponent training, including physical, motor, and cognitive elements, promoted through exergames, resulted in notable performance gains, particularly in the motor and cognitive dimensions. Similar conclusions regarding the increased benefits of combined training were reached in other studies conducted with healthy older adults [87] as well as older individuals suffering from cognitive impairment [88, 89].

Specifically regarding the simultaneous combination of motor and cognitive tasks, Herold and colleagues [90] proposed a distinction between added cognition and natural cognitive-motor tasks. Added cognition refers to contexts in which a cognitive task is performed simultaneously with a motor task, but the two task components are not inherently interconnected. Namely, good performance on the cognitive task is not required for successful completion of the motor component. Examples of this category include dual-tasks like chatting while walking or driving. On the other hand, natural cognitive-motor tasks involve cognitive subcomponents that are integral to the task's overall objective. Activities such as sports, dance, and exergames require associated motor and cognitive functions. For instance, in dance, the performer must perceive the musical rhythm, remember a specific sequence of multilimb movements, synchronize the sequence of movements with the musical rhythm, and maintain dynamic balance while dancing. Sport-related and exergames demand selective attention to those critical events for successful performance, spatial and temporal anticipation, mental flexibility to deal with the changing game demands, and fast decision-making in complex settings, alongside controlled voluntary movements, to achieve the activity's goals. In line with the literature reviewed here, Herold and colleagues [90] hypothesized that the simultaneous combination of motor and cognitive tasks is the most promising approach to effectively enhance the cognitive reserve in older adults.

Training Programs Based on Dual-Tasking

To understand the potential benefits of dual-tasking as a training activity for older adults, it is important to consider the interference between cognitive and motor tasks. Coelho and colleagues [91] conducted a study with healthy young participants and found that performing a cognitive task while responding to a mechanical balance perturbation resulted in increased body sway, wider hip and trunk displacement, and weaker leg muscular activation compared to performing the reactive responses without a concurrent cognitive task. Barra and colleagues [92] observed reciprocal interference between cognitive and balance tasks, with increased balance challenge leading to greater task errors in a cognitive task, while the cognitive task led to higher incidence of falls when standing on a narrow surface. These results are consistent with the expected between-task interference due to competition between the cognitive and motor task components for the available attentional resources (see [93, 94]). Interference between cognitive and balance tasks has also been observed in older individuals [95–98]. Stojan and colleagues [98] investigated the performance of older participants during dual-tasking involving walking on a treadmill associated with either the cognitive Stroop (for inhibitory control) test or a backward counting task. They found that dual-tasking led to increased cortical activation in the prefrontal and parietal cortical regions compared to single-tasking. The degree of cortical activation correlated with a decline in walking performance during dual-tasking, suggesting neural inefficiency in the aging brain.

Interestingly, the interference between motor and cognitive tasks has shown positive effects on performance gains in older individuals. Considering that dual taking is specially challenging for older adults either for cognitive or physical/motor performance, it has been tested as a potential tool for motor-cognitive training for older adults. Donnezan et al. [99] conducted a study with older adults with mild cognitive impairment and assigned them to four groups: simultaneous cognitive and physical training (dual-task), physical training only, cognitive training only, or a no-intervention control group. Results from an extensive battery of neuropsychological and motor tests revealed a clear advantage favoring the dual-task training, with performance gains in 8 out of 11 measurements, including improvements in both the cognitive and motor dimensions. Additionally, only the dual-task training group showed enduring effects for cognition and dynamic balance gains. Single-task training groups showed limited effects, with cognitive training leading to gains in two cognitive variables and physical training leading to gains in one cognitive and one motor task compared to the control group.

To assess effects of dual-task training on different dimensions, Jardim and colleagues [100] provided healthy older adults with a program combining physical exercises/dance and simultaneous cognitive tasks. The effects of the training program were assessed using a battery of tests for cognitive, physical, and functional abilities. The dual-task training group exhibited improvements in cognitive tests for episodic and recognition memory, physical tests for aerobic capacity and lower limb strength, and functional tests for dual-task walking speed and timed up and go. However, this study lacked an active control group under a single-task training scheme, which would have provided a better understanding of the specific benefits of dual-task training. Further investigations comparing dual-task and single-task training have demonstrated greater cognitive gains when combining aerobic and resistance exercises with simultaneous cognitive tasks [101, 102] as well as when combining strength and balance training with cognitive tasks [103, 104].

To examine the effects of motor-cognitive dual-task training, de Lima and colleagues [105] provided healthy older adults with a training program on a task requiring balance and agility in climbing a ladder. One group practiced the motor task alone (single-task regime), while another group practiced the motor task simultaneously with a cognitive task requiring verbal fluency. Analysis of the training effects revealed that both the single-task and dual-task groups achieved gains in muscular resistance, agility, body balance, and short-term memory. Remarkably, the dual-task training group showed exclusive gains in verbal fluency, dual-task timed up and go, and attention/mental flexibility tests. These results suggest that motor-cognitive dual-task training leads to greater improvements, particularly in the cognitive dimension. Additionally, Silsupadol and colleagues [106] investigated the benefits of a motor-cognitive dual-task training program in older adults with balance impairments. They compared a group that practiced multiple motor tasks for balance in a single-task regime with two dual-task training groups. The dual-task groups performed balance exercises concurrently with cognitive tasks and were instructed to either share attention between the cognitive and balance tasks or prioritize one of them. The results indicated that all three groups achieved gains in body balance and walking speed. Remarkably, only the dual-task training groups showed performance gains when walking was associated with a cognitive task, with more enduring effects observed when participants prioritized one of the tasks during the training sessions.

Systematic literature reviews have further supported the effectiveness of motor-cognitive dual-task training in enhancing motor functions such as body balance, mobility, and upper/lower limb motor skills [107, 108], as well as executive functions like set-shifting, working memory, and inhibitory control [109]. Therefore, experimental evidence indicates that motor-cognitive dual-task training is more effective than training in a single-task regime for counteracting motor and cognitive declines associated with aging.

Training Programs Based on Exergames

Playing exergames corresponds to a particular kind of multicomponent training requiring the integration of cognition, motor control, and physical fitness in a virtual reality environment. According to Herold and colleagues [90], exergames can be seen as natural cognitive-motor tasks, in which the cognitive component is inseparable from the overall task demands. For example, in a virtual tennis game, players must engage various cognitive functions such as recognizing the direction and speed of the ball on the screen, in addition to anticipating the appropriate time and space to hit the virtual ball. As further cognitive functions, the player has to select and plan appropriate movements for the intended response, taking into account the position of the virtual opponent on the court through appropriate use of selective attention. To perform the selected response in terms of the desired ball direction (parallel x crossed), velocity (slow x fast) and spin (no spin x topspin x backspin), the manual movements of the hitting arm have to be precisely controlled in space and time to perform the selected response. Fast strikes, in particular, require vigorous muscular activation not only of the hitting arm but also of the whole body in a coordinated way, while dynamically maintaining body balance. Additionally, if the virtual match is sufficiently long, aerobic capacity will be required as well. Therefore, exergames inherently intertwine cognitive, motor, and physical dimensions during their practice.

Research on the potential benefits of exergames for older adults has confirmed their effectiveness in enhancing sensorimotor and cognitive functions. In a randomized controlled trial comparing exergame training with other forms of training, cognitively healthy older adults were assigned to one of three groups: exergame-based dancing using virtual reality, treadmill walking combined with simultaneous verbal memory training (dual-task), or treadmill walking alone [110]. While all three training programs led to performance gains, like improvements in gait, functional fitness, and a reduction in fall frequency, there were specific gains to each group. The dancing exergame group demonstrated reduced step time during fast walking, whereas the walking-memory dual-task group showed reduced gait variability during a walking-cognition dual-task and decreased dual-task costs at the preferred walking speed.

Schättin and colleagues [111] compared the effects of training programs based either on exergame playing or body balance in healthy older adults, assessing both the behavioral and neural dimensions. Participants in the exergame group engaged in interactive whole body movements driven by a video game while standing on a force plate. The games aimed to develop executive functions and provided online feedback on positioning and timing to promote interaction with the virtual environment. The balance group trained on various quiet and dynamic balance tasks. Analysis of the training-related gains revealed that the exergame group improved mainly spatiotemporal parameters (speed, cadence, and stride length) during dual-task walking, while the balance group achieved gains only in single-task walking. Assessment of executive functions showed that the exergame group achieved improvements in working memory, divided attention, and set-shifting, whereas the balance group showed improved performance in set-shifting only. Evaluation of cerebral cortex activation showed a training-related decrease in theta relative power over the prefrontal cortex in the exergame group compared to the balance group. This neural effect from exergame training contrasts with the expected increase of prefrontal activation associated with aging (see also [112, 113]). Conclusions from systematic literature reviews on the effects of exergames on the motor, cognitive, and neural dimensions have indicated that exergame-based training programs for healthy older adults tend to yield comparable or slightly superior results compared to conventional physical or motor exercise-based training programs [114, 115].

Training Programs Based on Dancing

Dancing is another form of natural cognitive-motor task that combines dynamic body balance, interlimb coordination, cognitive functions, and aerobic fitness [90]. When following a predetermined sequence of steps harmonized with music, dancers need to remember the movements, perceive the rhythm, and integrate their actions with the music's timing. Learning new stepping sequences in dancing also exercises episodic and working memory functions. As dancing requires also a frequent change of the support base, often supporting the body on a single leg, this represents a challenging dynamic balance task for older adults. Moreover, the continuous and rhythmic nature of dancing may incorporate aerobic fitness training into various motor and cognitive functions. Empirical studies have confirmed the multidimensional benefits of regular dancing on motor and cognitive functions in older adults.

To evaluate the effects of long-term dancing on motor and cognitive functions, Kattenstroth and colleagues [116] compared older adults who had been practicing dance for an average of 16.5 years against age-, education-, and gender-matched controls. Results from a comprehensive test battery indicated that the dancers reached better performance in most tests, including quiet and dynamic balance, reaction time, manual dexterity, manual accuracy, and cognitive functions. Long-term dancing was also associated with higher independence in daily activities and mobility. Further research has shown that much shorter periods of dance training can lead to multidimensional gains in older adults. A 6-month dance program for a group of healthy older adults resulted in improved balance, reaction time, cognitive function, and motor performance in different tests. In contrast, the age-matched passive control group showed no positive changes and even impoverished performance compared to the baseline assessment [117].

The behavioral gains observed in older adults participating in dance programs have been shown to be associated with adaptive changes in the brain. A study comparing dance-based training with conventional fitness activities revealed that dance led to cognitive gains along with structural changes in the aging brain [118]. Both the dance and fitness groups showed improvements in attention after 6 months of training, and in working memory after 18 months of training. Magnetic resonance imaging analysis revealed increased gray matter volume in the left precentral gyrus after 6 months and in the parahippocampal gyrus after 18 months of dance training compared to the fitness training group. These structural changes are likely a result of the demands associated with learning complex dance movements and engaging working and episodic memory during dance training. Another study comparing dance and physical fitness training programs for older adults showed that both groups achieved increases in hippocampal volume [119]. However, dancers exhibited greater volume increases in specific hippocampal regions associated with early memory retrieval, recognition, and memory consolidation. At the behavioral level, only the dance group showed improved performance after the training program. A recent systematic review by Muiños and Ballesteros [120] compiled consistent evidence indicating that regular participation in dance activities by middle-aged and older adults induces neuroplasticity, counteracting age-related declines in cognition, motor control, and brain structure. Based on the reviewed findings, dance can be considered an effective activity for attenuating, stabilizing, or even reversing age-related declines across multiple dimensions.

Proposed Approach for Training Older Adults

Based on the reviewed evidence, the most effective approach for training older adults involves combining aerobic or resistance training with simultaneous motor and cognitive tasks. This approach takes advantage of the synergistic effect between these dimensions, leading to higher functional gains compared to training each component separately. A fundamental point to be considered is that in every imaginable action all organismic dimensions are involved, varying between very low and very high demands. When selecting/elaborating a training task we can set individually the physical, motor and cognitive demands. To illustrate this point, let us start from a simple task and understand how it could be made more complex by combining simultaneous requirements in different dimensions. As the initial task, consider the context of reproducing observed cyclic movements of oscillating the two arms in a given pattern, like alternating lateral up and down in-phase movements, while stably standing supported on the two legs. In this case, not only the aerobic and resistance demands are low, but also the demands of body balance, coordination and cognitive functions are minimally challenged even for a sedentary older participant. How could this task be modified to achieve higher multidimensional gains? Moving forward the control switch to increase motor complexity, the same arm movements might be made while supported on a single leg, noticeably reducing the support base area. With this task demand upgrade, the requirements of body balance would be considerably increased, and so the potential balance improvements as a result of training [121]. To further increase the gains in the motor dimension, the task could be changed into one requiring coordinated movements between the two arms and the free non-supporting leg. This new version of the task would impose a complex multilimb coordination associated with a challenging balance component. At the mental level, the challenge would be to share attentional resources between the production of the desired coordination pattern and dynamic balance control. In addition, the mind would face the high processing demand of anticipating the consequences of the self-produced movements on body balance in the attempt to achieve the aim of maintaining body balance while supported on a single leg. As in this kind of dynamic balance task, participants produce self-perturbation movements, they frequently suffer body disequilibrium requiring compensatory arm and leg movements for balance recovery. Thus, this task can be assumed to bring also beneficial effects from a perturbation-based balance training [122, 123].

Evaluating the situation of repeating the movements presented by an instructor, the task can be rated as one demanding very low from cognitive functions. While maintaining the upgraded version of the example task, a higher involvement of cognitive functions might be achieved through different procedures. To exercise *working memory*, the task could be changed from the cyclic between-limb coordination performed in unipedal stance into a serial task. More specifically, three or four variations of the multilimb coordination pattern could be sequenced to compose a serial task for practicing. The movement sequence should be presented some times for memorization by the exercisers, and then they should try to reproduce the specified movement sequence in the absence of the online instructor's demonstration. The length of serial movements can be increased over time, progressively recurring to the memory capacity to keep in mind the sequence of movements to be performed. By changing the multilimb movement coordination every cycle, instead of making repetitive movements over time, the exerciser will also need to inhibit the tendency to repeat the coordination mode produced in the previous movement cycle. In this case, the executive function *inhibitory control* would be required to achieve the task aim, while favoring the motor skill learning due the high contextual interference effect (cf. [124]). To further increase the demand of cognitive functions, *divided attention* could be required by adopting a special counting of the performed movement cycles. This strategy can be implemented by asking the exercisers to add/subtract n digits every movement cycle completed. Thus, if the counting rule is summing up 3 digits every movement cycle, rather than counting 1–2-3 …n, participants would count the cycles as 3–6-9 …$n + 3$. In the new version of our task, then, the attention capacity would have to be shared among the multilimb coordination, balance, and cognitive task demands for the due sequence of coordinated movements and counting operations. To exercise *cognitive flexibility*, the counting rule could be frequently changed over the training session. For instance, in the first sequence of movements the counting rule might be adding n digits, in the second sequence subtracting n digits from a given number, in the third using an alphanumeric counting by alternating numbers and letters (1-A-2-B-3-C ...), alternating between different languages (English-Spanish: one, *dos*, three, *cuatro* ...), presetting a rule change when a given number is reached in the counting, and so on. The same principle could be applied to the multilimb coordination component of the task by changing the movement sequence after a number of repetitions (see Fig. 25.1 for a representation).

The explored example shows an illustration of how the demands of a global motor task could be upscaled in the motor and cognitive dimensions. As functional improvement by training can be expected to be also task-specific, it would be desirable to plan the training activities to encompass the different motor (e.g., balance, interlimb coordination) and cognitive function (e.g., attention, memory) demands. Based on the findings reviewed in this chapter, one could expect reciprocal gains between the motor and cognitive task components when they are integrated into a single combined task. To induce the largest training-related benefits in older exercisers, the planned activities should also induce gains of aerobic capacity and muscular resistance. Continuing with our example task, aerobic capacity could be developed in parallel with the motor-cognitive tasks by requesting the participants to perform the training activities in the due rhythm and intensity for maintaining the heart rate at the appropriate level to improve aerobic fitness. Increment of muscular resistance can be achieved by performing a sufficient number of repetitions, using body weight or extra loads, to induce physiological and functional gains. By simultaneously combining aerobic, resistance, motor and cognitive demands in a training

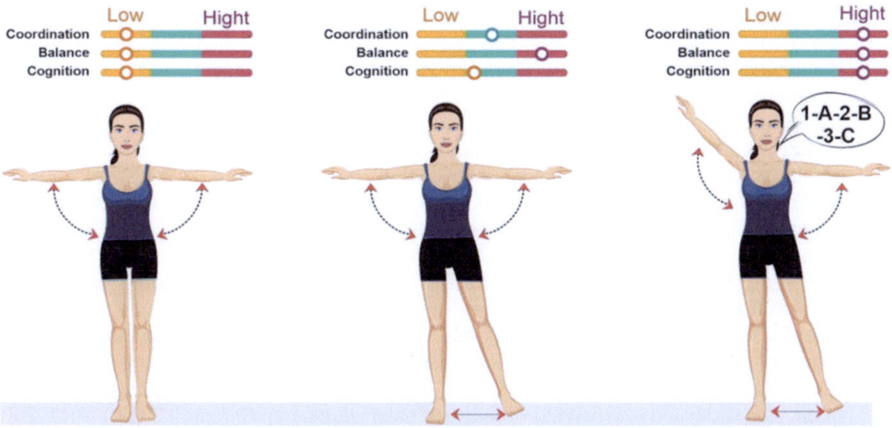

Fig. 25.1 Demands of coordination, body balance, and cognition for each variation of a global motor task. The left-sided image indicates the simplest version, requiring cyclically moving the two arms up and down while standing. The central image represents inclusion of one leg sway in the task, leading to increments in the three dimensions, more noticeably in the balance demand. The right-sided image represents variations in the sequence of multilimb coordination over repetitions associated with alphanumeric counting of the movement cycles, leading to high processing demands in the three behavioral dimensions

program for older adults one could expect to achieve distinctive functional gains contributing decisively to achievement of successful aging.

Acknowledgments I am grateful to Carla Rinaldin for the artwork of Fig. 25.1, and to Pedro Monteiro for technical assistance to format the references.

Funding This work was supported by the Brazilian Council of Science and Technology (CNPq) under the grant number 302798/2022–6.

References

1. Atchley RC, Barusch AS. The demography of aging. In: Atchley RC, Barusch AS, editors. Social forces and aging: an introduction to social gerontology. Belmont, CA: Wadsworth/Thomson Learning; 2004.
2. Fleg JL, Morrell CH, Bos AG, et al. Accelerated longitudinal decline of aerobic capacity in healthy older adults. Circulation. 2005;112:674–82.
3. Dodds RM, Syddall HE, Cooper R, et al. Grip strength across the life course: normative data from twelve British studies. PLoS One. 2014;9:1–15.
4. Mayhew AJ, So HY, Ma J, et al. Normative values for grip strength, gait speed, timed up and go, single leg balance, and chair rise derived from the Canadian longitudinal study on ageing. Age Ageing. 2023;52(4):afad0542023.
5. Daly RM, Rosengren BE, Alwis G, et al. Gender specific age-related changes in bone density, muscle strength and functional performance in the elderly: A-10 year prospective population-based study. BMC Geriatr. 2013;13:1471–2318.
6. Lusardi MM, Fritz S, Middleton A, et al. Determining risk of falls in community dwelling older adults: a systematic review and meta-analysis using posttest probability. J Geriatr Phys Ther. 2017;40:1–36.
7. Den Ouden MEM, Schuurmans MJ, Arts IEMA, et al. Physical performance characteristics related to disability in older persons: a systematic review. Maturitas. 2011;69:208–19.
8. Diamond A. Executive functions. Annu Rev Psychol. 2013;64:135–68.
9. Colcombe S, Kramer AF. Fitness effects on the cognitive function of older adults: a meta-analytic study—revisited. Psychol Sci. 2003;14:125–30.
10. Lopez OL, Kuller LH, Fitzpatrick A, et al. Evaluation of dementia in the cardiovascular health cognition study. Neuroepidemiology. 2003;22:1–12.
11. Buckner RL. Memory and executive function in aging and AD: multiple factors that cause decline and reserve factors that compensate. Neuron. 2004;44:195–208.
12. Grady C. The cognitive neuroscience of ageing. Nat Rev Neurosci. 2012;13:491–505.
13. Ferguson HJ, Brunsdon VEA, Bradford EEF. The developmental trajectories of executive function from adolescence to old age. Sci Rep. 2021;11:1–17.
14. Kim K, Deller L, Vinent M, et al. Age-related effects of repeated task switching in a novel voluntary gait adaptability task. Exp Brain Res. 2023;241:1533–42.
15. Hennah C, Doumas M. Dual-task walking on real-world surfaces: adaptive changes in walking speed, step width and step height in young and older adults. Exp Gerontol. 2023;177:112200.
16. Raz N, Gunning-Dixon F, Head D, et al. Aging, sexual dimorphism, and hemispheric asymmetry of the cerebral cortex: replicability of regional differences in volume. Neurobiol Aging. 2004;25:377–96.
17. Driscoll I, Hamilton DA, Petropoulos H, et al. The aging hippocampus: cognitive, biochemical and structural findings. Cereb Cortex. 2003;13:1344–51.
18. Raz N, Lindenberger U, Rodrigue KM, et al. Regional brain changes in aging healthy adults: general trends, individual differences and modifiers. Cereb Cortex. 2005;15:1676–89.

19. Jack CR, Wiste HJ, Vemuri P, et al. Brain beta-amyloid measures and magnetic resonance imaging atrophy both predict time-to-progression from mild cognitive impairment to Alzheimer's disease. Brain. 2010;133:3336–48.
20. Spirduso WW. Reaction and movement time as a function of age and physical activity level. J Gerontol. 1975;30:435–40.
21. Spirduso WW, MacRae HH, MacRae PG, et al. Exercise effects on aged motor function. Ann N Y Acad Sci. 1988;515:363–75.
22. McGregor KM, Nocera JR, Sudhyadhom A, et al. Effects of aerobic fitness on aging-related changes of interhemispheric inhibition and motor performance. Front Aging Neurosci. 2013;5:1–14.
23. Barnes DE, Yaffe K, Satariano WA, et al. A longitudinal study of cardiorespiratory fitness and cognitive function in healthy older adults. J Am Geriatr Soc. 2003;51:459–65.
24. Middleton LE, Barnes DE, Lui LY, et al. Physical activity over the life course and its association with cognitive performance and impairment in old age. J Am Geriatr Soc. 2010;58:1322–6.
25. Gouveia ÉR, Gouveia BR, Ihle A, et al. Balance and mobility relationships in older adults: a representative population-based cross-sectional study in Madeira, Portugal. Arch Gerontol Geriatr. 2019;80:65–9.
26. Gordon BA, Rykhlevskaia EI, Brumback CR, et al. Neuroanatomical correlates of aging, cardiopulmonary fitness level, and education. Physiology. 2008;45:825–38.
27. Van Gelder BM, Tijhuis MAR, Kalmijn S, et al. Physical activity in relation to cognitive decline in elderly men: the FINE study. Neurology. 2004;63:2316–21.
28. Biasin F, Ceolin C, Celli S, et al. Interrelation between functional decline and dementia: the potential role of balance assessment. Hum Mov Sci. 2023;89:103095.
29. Voelcker-Rehage C, Godde B, Staudinger UM. Physical and motor fitness are both related to cognition in old age. Eur J Neurosci. 2010;31:167–76.
30. Erickson KI, Raji CA, Lopez OL, et al. Physical activity predicts gray matter volume in late adulthood: the cardiovascular health study. Neurology. 2010;75:1415–22.
31. Hayes SM, Hayes JP, Cadden M, et al. A review of cardiorespiratory fitness-related neuroplasticity in the aging brain. Front Aging Neurosci. 2013;5:1–16.
32. Sofi F, Valecchi D, Bacci D, et al. Physical activity and risk of cognitive decline: a meta-analysis of prospective studies. J Intern Med. 2011;269:107–17.
33. Hamer M, Chida Y. Physical activity and risk of neurodegenerative disease: a systematic review of prospective evidence. Psychol Med. 2008;39:3–11.
34. Holtzer R, Verghese J, Xue X, et al. Cognitive processes related to gait velocity: results from the Einstein aging study. Neuropsychology. 2006;20:215–23.
35. Zhou J, Cattaneo G, Yu W, et al. The age-related contribution of cognitive function to dual-task gait in middle-aged adults in Spain: observations from a population-based study. Lancet Heal Longev. 2023;4:e98–e106.
36. Clouston SAP, Brewster P, Kuh D, et al. The dynamic relationship between physical function and cognition in longitudinal aging cohorts. Epidemiol Rev. 2013;35:33–50.
37. Lapszo J, Giovanis V, Prusik K, et al. Balance control contributors—the relationships between leg strength and balance control ability in seniors. Acta Bioeng Biomech. 2012;14:3–8.
38. Anstey KJ, Von Sanden C, Luszcz MA. An 8-year prospective study of the relationship between cognitive performance and falling in very old adults. J Am Geriatr Soc. 2006;54:1169–76.
39. Dascal JB, Teixeira LA. Selective maintenance of motor performance in older adults from long-lasting sport practice. Res Q Exerc Sport. 2016;87:262–70.
40. Proteau L, Marteniuk RG, Lévesque L. A sensorimotor basis for motor learning:evidence indicating specificity of practice. Q J Exp Psychol. 1992;44:557–75.
41. Behm DG, Sale DG. Velocity specificity of resistance training. Sports Med. 1993;15:374–88.
42. Giuli C, Papa R, Lattanzio F, et al. The effects of cognitive training for elderly: results from my mind project. Rejuvenation Res. 2016;19:485–94.

43. Angevaren M, Aufdemkampe G, Verhaar HJJ, et al. Physical activity and enhanced fitness to improve cognitive function in older people without known cognitive impairment. Cochrane Database Syst Rev. 2008;2:CD005381. https://doi.org/10.1002/14651858.CD005381.
44. Hötting K, Röder B. Beneficial effects of physical exercise on neuroplasticity and cognition. Neurosci Biobehav Rev. 2013;37:2243–57.
45. Northey JM, Cherbuin N, Pumpa KL, et al. Exercise interventions for cognitive function in adults older than 50: a systematic review with meta-analysis. Br J Sports Med. 2018;52:154–60.
46. Hindin S, Zelinski EM. Extended practice and aerobic exercise interventions benefit untrained cognitive outcomes in older adults: a meta-analysis. J Am Geriatr Soc. 2012;60:136–41.
47. Kennedy G, Hardman RJ, MacPherson H, et al. How does exercise reduce the rate of age-associated cognitive decline? A review of potential mechanisms. J Alzheimers Dis. 2016;55:1–18.
48. Stern Y, Mackay-Brandt A, Lee S, et al. Effect of aerobic exercise on cognition in younger adults: a randomized clinical trial. Neurology. 2019;92:E905–16.
49. Voelcker-Rehage C, Godde B, Staudinger UM. Cardiovascular and coordination training differentially improve cognitive performance and neural processing in older adults. Front Hum Neurosci. 2011;5:1–12.
50. Moul JL, Goldman B, Warren B. Physical activity and cognitive performance in the older population. J Aging Phys Act. 1995;3:135–45.
51. Stroth S, Hille K, Spitzer M, et al. Aerobic endurance exercise benefits memory and affect in young adults. Neuropsychol Rehabil. 2009;19:223–43.
52. Hawkins HL, Kramer AF, Capaldi D. Aging, exercise, and attention. Psychol Aging. 1992;7:643–53.
53. Colcombe SJ, Kramer AF, Erickson KI, et al. Cardiovascular fitness, cortical plasticity, and aging. Proc Natl Acad Sci. 2004;101:3316–21.
54. Colcombe SJ, Erickson KI, Scalf PE, et al. Aerobic exercise training increases brain volume in aging humans. J Gerontol—Ser A Biol Sci Med Sci. 2006;61:1166–70.
55. Erickson KI, Voss MW, Shaurya R, et al. Exercise training increases size of hippocampus and improves memory. Proc Natl Acad Sci. 2011;108:3017–22.
56. Herold F, Törpel A, Schega L, et al. Functional and/or structural brain changes in response to resistance exercises and resistance training lead to cognitive improvements—a systematic review. Eur Rev Aging Phys Act. 2019;16:1–33.
57. Cassilhas RC, Viana VAR, Grassmann V, et al. The impact of resistance exercise on the cognitive function of the elderly. Med Sci Sports Exerc. 2007;39:1401–7.
58. Liu-Ambrose T, Nagamatsu LS, Graf P, et al. Resistance training and executive functions: a 12-month randomized controlled trial. Arch Intern Med. 2010;170:170–8.
59. Liu-Ambrose T, Nagamatsu LS, Voss MW, et al. Resistance training and functional plasticity of the aging brain: a 12-month randomized controlled trial. Neurobiol Aging. 2012;33:1690–8.
60. Hötting K, Reich B, Holzschneider K, et al. Differential cognitive effects of cycling versus stretching/coordination training in middle-aged adults. Health Psychol. 2012;31:145–55.
61. Carey JR, Bhatt E, Nagpal A. Neuroplasticity promoted by task complexity. Exerc Sport Sci Rev. 2005;33:24–31.
62. Ludyga S, Gerber M, Pühse U, et al. Systematic review and meta-analysis investigating moderators of long-term effects of exercise on cognition in healthy individuals. Nat Hum Behav. 2020;4:603–12.
63. Voelcker-Rehage C, Niemann C. Structural and functional brain changes related to different types of physical activity across the life span. Neurosci Biobehav Rev. 2013;37:2268–95.
64. Pereira AC, Huddleston DE, Brickman A, et al. An in vivo correlate of exercise-induced neurogenesis in the adult dentate gyrus. Proc Natl Acad Sci USA. 2007;104:5638–43.
65. Maass A, Düzel S, Goerke M, et al. Vascular hippocampal plasticity after aerobic exercise in older adults. Mol Psychiatry. 2015;20:585–93.

66. Marmeleira J. An examination of the mechanisms underlying the effects of physical activity on brain and cognition: a review with implications for research. Eur Rev Aging Phys Act. 2013;10:83–94.
67. Stimpson NJ, Davison G, Javadi AH. Joggin' the noggin: towards a physiological understanding of exercise-induced cognitive benefits. Neurosci Biobehav Rev. 2018;88:177–86.
68. Bamidis PD, Vivas AB, Styliadis C, et al. A review of physical and cognitive interventions in aging. Neurosci Biobehav Rev. 2014;44:206–20.
69. Fissler P, Küster O, Schlee W, et al. Novelty interventions to enhance broad cognitive abilities and prevent dementia: synergistic approaches for the facilitation of positive plastic change. Progr Brain Res. 2013;207:403–34.
70. Kempermann G, Fabel K, Ehninger D, et al. Why and how physical activity promotes experience-induced brain plasticity. Front Neurosci. 2010;4:1–9.
71. Coelho DB, Silva MB, de Lima-Pardini AC, et al. Young and older adults adapt automatic postural responses equivalently to repetitive perturbations but are unable to use predictive cueing to optimize recovery of balance stability. Neurosci Lett. 2018;685:167–72.
72. Teixeira LA, Maia Azzi N, de Oliveira JA, et al. Automatic postural responses are scaled from the association between online feedback and feedforward control. Eur J Neurosci. 2020;51:2023–32.
73. de Souza CR, Betelli MT, Takazono PS, et al. Evaluation of balance recovery stability from unpredictable perturbations through the compensatory arm and leg movements (CALM) scale. PLoS One. 2019;14:1–17.
74. Marcori AJ. Single leg balance training: systematic review of the literature and effects in older individuals. Doctoral dissertation. University of São Paulo. 2022.
75. Thomas R, Johnsen LK, Geertsen SS, et al. Acute exercise and motor memory consolidation: the role of exercise intensity. PLoS One. 2016;11:1–16.
76. Wanner P, Winterholler M, Gaßner H, et al. Acute exercise following skill practice promotes motor memory consolidation in Parkinson's disease. Neurobiol Learn Mem. 2021;178:107366.
77. Van Het Reve E, De Bruin ED. Strength-balance supplemented with computerized cognitive training to improve dual task gait and divided attention in older adults: a multicenter randomized-controlled trial. BMC Geriatr. 2014;14:1–15.
78. Sipilä S, Tirkkonen A, Savikangas T, et al. Effects of physical and cognitive training on gait speed and cognition in older adults: a randomized controlled trial. Scand J Med Sci Sport. 2021;31:1518–33.
79. Hagovská M, Olekszyová Z. Impact of the combination of cognitive and balance training on gait, fear and risk of falling and quality of life in seniors with mild cognitive impairment. Geriatr Gerontol Int. 2016;16:1043–50.
80. Hagovska M, Nagyova I. The transfer of skills from cognitive and physical training to activities of daily living: a randomised controlled study. Eur J Ageing. 2017;14:133–42.
81. Shimada H, Makizako H, Doi T, et al. Effects of combined physical and cognitive exercises on cognition and mobility in patients with mild cognitive impairment: a randomized clinical trial. J Am Med Dir Assoc. 2018;19:584–91.
82. Bruderer-Hofstetter M, Rausch-Osthoff AK, Meichtry A, et al. Effective multicomponent interventions in comparison to active control and no interventions on physical capacity, cognitive function and instrumental activities of daily living in elderly people with and without mild impaired cognition—a systematic review. Ageing Res Rev. 2018;45:1–14.
83. Lauenroth A, Ioannidis AE, Teichmann B. Influence of combined physical and cognitive training on cognition: a systematic review. BMC Geriatr. 2016;16:21–3.
84. Cadore EL, Rodríguez-Mañas L, Sinclair A, et al. Effects of different exercise interventions on risk of falls, gait ability, and balance in physically frail older adults: a systematic review. Rejuvenation Res. 2013;16:105–14.
85. Tait JL, Duckham RL, Milte CM, et al. Influence of sequential vs. simultaneous dual-task exercise training on cognitive function in older adults. Front Aging Neurosci. 2017;9:3689.

86. Rieker JA, Reales JM, Muiños M, et al. The effects of combined cognitive-physical interventions on cognitive functioning in healthy older adults: a systematic review and multilevel meta-analysis. Front Hum Neurosci. 2022;16:112.
87. Law LLF, Barnett F, Yau MK, et al. Effects of combined cognitive and exercise interventions on cognition in older adults with and without cognitive impairment: a systematic review. Ageing Res Rev. 2014;15:61–75.
88. Levin O, Netz Y, Ziv G. The beneficial effects of different types of exercise interventions on motor and cognitive functions in older age: a systematic review. Eur Rev Aging Phys Act. 2017;14:1–23.
89. Yang C, Moore A, Mpofu E, et al. Effectiveness of combined cognitive and physical interventions to enhance functioning in older adults with mild cognitive impairment: a systematic review of randomized controlled trial. Gerontologist. 2020;60:E633–42.
90. Herold F, Hamacher D, Schega L, et al. Thinking while moving or moving while thinking—concepts of motor-cognitive training for cognitive performance enhancement. Front Aging Neurosci. 2018;10:1–11.
91. Coelho DB, Bourlinova C, Teixeira LA. Higher order balance control: distinct effects between cognitive task and manual steadiness constraint on automatic postural responses. Hum Mov Sci. 2016;50:62–72.
92. Barra J, Bray A, Sahni V, et al. Increasing cognitive load with increasing balance challenge: recipe for catastrophe. Exp Brain Res. 2006;174:734–45.
93. Kahneman D. Attention and effort. Englewood Cliffs, NJ: Prentice-Hall; 1973.
94. Pashler H, Johnston JC, Ruthruff E. Attention and performance. Annu Rev Psychol. 2001;52:629–51.
95. Brown LA, Shumway-Cook A, Woollacott MH. Attentional demands and postural recovery: the effects of aging. J Gerontol—Ser A Biol Sci Med Sci. 1999;54:165–71.
96. Little CE, Woollacott M. Effect of attentional interference on balance recovery in older adults. Exp Brain Res. 2014;232:2032–49.
97. Rosso AL, Cenciarini M, Sparto PJ, et al. Neuroimaging of an attention demanding dual-task during dynamic postural control. Gait Posture. 2017;57:193–8.
98. Stojan R, Mack M, Bock O, et al. Inefficient frontal and parietal brain activation during dual-task walking in a virtual environment in older adults. NeuroImage. 2023;273:120070.
99. Donnezan LC, Perrot A, Belleville S, et al. Effects of simultaneous aerobic and cognitive training on executive functions, cardiovascular fitness and functional abilities in older adults with mild cognitive impairment. Ment Health Phys Act. 2018;15:78–87.
100. Jardim NYV, Bento-Torres NVO, Costa VO, et al. Dual-task exercise to improve cognition and functional capacity of healthy older adults. Front Aging Neurosci. 2021;13:1–16.
101. Uysal İ, Başar S, Aysel S, et al. Aerobic exercise and dual-task training combination is the best combination for improving cognitive status, mobility and physical performance in older adults with mild cognitive impairment. Aging Clin Exp Res. 2023;35:271–81.
102. Yokoyama H, Okazaki K, Imai D, et al. The effect of cognitive-motor dual-task training on cognitive function and plasma amyloid β peptide 42/40 ratio in healthy elderly persons: a randomized controlled trial. BMC Geriatr. 2015;15:1–10.
103. Hiyamizu M, Morioka S, Shomoto K, et al. Effects of dual task balance training on dual task performance in elderly people: a randomized controlled trial. Clin Rehabil. 2012;26:58–67.
104. Norouzi E, Vaezmosavi M, Gerber M, et al. Dual-task training on cognition and resistance training improved both balance and working memory in older people. Phys Sportsmed. 2019;47:471–8.
105. de Lima VC, Castaño LAA, Sampaio RAC, et al. Effect of agility ladder training with a cognitive task (dual task) on physical and cognitive functions: a randomized study. Front Public Heal. 2023;11:1159343. https://doi.org/10.3389/fpubh.2023.1159343.
106. Silsupadol P, Shumway-cook A, Woollacott M. Effects of single-task versus dual-task training on balance in order adults. Arch Phys Med Rehabil. 2009;90:381–7.
107. Pichierri G, Wolf P, Murer K, et al. Cognitive and cognitive-motor interventions affecting physical functioning: a systematic review. BMC Geriatr. 2011;11:29.

108. Wollesen B, Voelcker-Rehage C. Training effects on motor-cognitive dual-task performance in older adults: a systematic review. Eur Rev Aging Phys Act. 2014;11:5–24.
109. Wollesen B, Wildbredt A, Schooten K, et al. Effects of exercise training interventions on executive function in older adults: a systematic review and meta-analysis. Eur Rev Aging Phys Act. 2020;51:597–8.
110. Eggenberger P, Theill N, Holenstein S, et al. Multicomponent physical exercise with simultaneous cognitive training to enhance dual-task walking of older adults: a secondary analysis of a 6-month randomized controlled trial with I-year follow-up. Clin Interv Aging. 2015;10:1711–32.
111. Schättin A, Arner R, Gennaro F, et al. Adaptations of prefrontal brain activity, executive functions, and gait in healthy elderly following exergame and balance training: a randomized-controlled study. Front Aging Neurosci. 2016;8:278.
112. Adcock M, Fankhauser M, Post J, Lutz K, Zizlsperger L, Luft AR, et al. Effects of an in-home multicomponent exergame training on physical functions, cognition, and brain volume of older adults: a randomized controlled trial. Front Med. 2020;6:321.
113. Eggenberger P, Wolf M, Schumann M, et al. Exergame and balance training modulate prefrontal brain activity during walking and enhance executive function in older adults. Front Aging Neurosci. 2016;8:66.
114. Chen Y, Zhang Y, Guo Z, et al. Comparison between the effects of exergame intervention and traditional physical training on improving balance and fall prevention in healthy older adults: a systematic review and meta-analysis. J Neuroeng Rehabil. 2021;18:1–17.
115. Stojan R, Voelcker-Rehage C. A systematic review on the cognitive benefits and neurophysiological correlates of exergaming in healthy older adults. J Clin Med. 2019;8:2–27.
116. Kattenstroth JC, Kolankowska I, Kalisch T, et al. Superior sensory, motor, and cognitive performance in elderly individuals with multi-year dancing activities. Front Aging Neurosci. 2010;2:1–9.
117. Kattenstroth JC, Kalisch T, Holt S, et al. Six months of dance intervention enhances postural, sensorimotor, and cognitive performance in elderly without affecting cardio-respiratory functions. Front Aging Neurosci. 2013;5:1–16.
118. Müller P, Rehfeld K, Schmicker M, et al. Evolution of neuroplasticity in response to physical activity in old age: the case for dancing. Front Aging Neurosci. 2017;9:1–8.
119. Rehfeld K, Müller P, Aye N, et al. Dancing or fitness sport? The effects of two training programs on hippocampal plasticity and balance abilities in healthy seniors. Front Hum Neurosci. 2017;11:1–9.
120. Muiños M, Ballesteros S. Does dance counteract age-related cognitive and brain declines in middle-aged and older adults? A systematic review. Neurosci Biobehav Rev. 2021;121:259–76.
121. Marcori AJ, Monteiro PHM, Oliveira AJ, et al. Single leg balance training: a systematic review. Percept Mot Skills. 2022;129:232–52.
122. Ribeiro de Souza C, Ávila de Oliveira J, Takazono PS, et al. Perturbation-based balance training leads to improved reactive postural responses in individuals with Parkinson's disease and freezing of gait. Eur J Neurosci. 2023;57:2174–86.
123. Takazono PS, Ribeiro de Souza C, Ávila de Oliveira J, et al. High contextual interference in perturbation-based balance training leads to persistent and generalizable stability gains of compensatory limb movements. Exp Brain Res. 2020;238(5):1249–63.
124. Lage GM, Ugrinowitsch H, Apolinário-Souza T, et al. Repetition and variation in motor practice: a review of neural correlates. Neurosci Biobehav Rev. 2015;57:132–41.

Exercise and Balance in Older Adults with Movement Disorders

26

Madeleine E. Hackney, Trisha Kesar, Joe R. Nocera, Tricia Creel, and Doherty Riebesell

Abstract

This chapter concerns balance, gait function, exercise, and current rehabilitation options for older adults with Parkinson's disease (PD) and stroke, within the context of aging in the absence of neurodegenerative disease or neuroinsult. We outline the primary balance and gait deficits and their impact on falls' rates for PD and stroke, with discussion regarding impairment in dual tasking and cognitive disturbances. We consider current options in physical therapy and exercise-based therapy for PD and stroke, particularly for interlimb coordination and gait function. Crossover approaches in rehabilitative techniques from PD/stroke to normal aging motor impairments often go under-utilized in the clinic. Therefore, implications for older adults without movement disorders, who often have purely aging-related symptoms similar to those of PD are discussed. Currently, research is especially engaged in investigating novel approaches to multimodal exercise, which have

M. E. Hackney (✉)
Department of Medicine, Emory University School of Medicine, Atlanta, GA, USA
e-mail: mehackn@emory.edu

T. Kesar
Department of Rehabilitation Medicine, Emory University School of Medicine, Atlanta, GA, USA
e-mail: tkesar@emory.edu

J. R. Nocera
Departments of Neurology and Rehabilitation Medicine, Emory University School of Medicine, Atlanta, GA, USA
e-mail: jnocera@emory.edu

T. Creel
Division of Physical Therapy, Washington University, St. Louis, MO, USA

D. Riebesell
North Carolina, USA

F. A. Barbieri et al. (eds.), *Locomotion and Posture in Older Adults*,
https://doi.org/10.1007/978-3-031-74123-4_26

emerged as promising therapies for balance impairments including aerobic exercise, tai chi, and dance. Efficacy of such interventions is presented with respect to new research showing cognitive effects. We conclude this chapter by discussing hypotheses regarding mechanisms underlying deficit and recovery in these populations. Understanding the mechanisms for rehabilitative gains is crucial for developing targeted and efficient therapy for PD and stroke populations.

Primary Balance and Gait Deficits in Aging and Neurodegenerative Disease

Aging in the absence of disease encompasses alterations in sensorimotor processing that lead to deterioration of motor performance, including coordination impairments, increased variability of movement, slowing of movement, and gait and balance impairments [1, 2]. These impairments are thought to result from cumulative changes in central and peripheral nervous systems, the neuromuscular system, and the peripheral vestibular system [3–5]. In the peripheral nervous systems, older adults have decreased number and density of both articular and cutaneous mechanoreceptors, and alterations in muscle spindles [6, 7]. In the central nervous systems, older adults have delayed impulse conduction, decreased impulse velocity, delayed synaptic transmission, declining prevalence of all neurotransmitters, and a loss of large, myelinated fibers that decreases axonal ability to transmit impulses [8]. Cell loss from aging is most notable in the cerebral cortex lobes, cerebellar area, and frontal lobe gray matter. Thus, there is a direct impact on memory, attention, awareness, motor control, coordination, and the ability to perform executive function tasks. The culmination of this overall central decline results in decreased automaticity of movement and increased reliance on workaround strategies along with a slower processing speed and deficit in the ability to handle multiple processes simultaneously.

Individuals with movement disorders resulting from disease or neurological insult must cope with impairments that go above and beyond those experienced from normal aging. This chapter will cover these impairments for the common disorders, Parkinson's disease (PD) and stroke. Potentially, to address impairment stemming from normal aging, one can apply knowledge gained from research into rehabilitative approaches developed for PD and stroke.

Parkinson's Disease—Impact on Falls' Risk and Balance

PD is a neurological disorder characterized by rigidity, bradykinesia, postural abnormalities, resting tremor, and changes in gait [9, 10]. Over 70% of persons with PD fall during the course of their disease [11, 12], often resulting in decreased mobility, loss of independence, and injuries [13–18]. Lower extremity impairments contributing to gait dysfunction and postural instability also have powerful effects on self-reported motor and psychological quality of life [19–22].

Impairments in the motor and cognitive domains intersect for people with PD during the performance of a secondary, goal-oriented task, often referred to as dual tasking. Unfortunately, gait disturbance increases in individuals with PD during performance of a secondary task (both non-motor and motor) [23]. Camicioli et al. reported dual-task performance (verbal recitation of numbers) in people with PD led to decreased step size and gait speed [24, 25]. Gait speed and stride length reduce significantly in PD patients while carrying a tray of glasses filled with water compared to free walking [26]. O'Shea evaluated the gait of PD participants while performing coin transference or digit subtraction. Persons with PD demonstrated a greater decrease in stride length, walking speed, and cadence during the dual-task conditions than did the matched comparison groups [27]. The effect of a dual task on motor performance can be described as "cognitive-motor" interference and appears to negatively affect walking speed regardless of the type of dual task [28]. One of the reasons for the strong association between deterioration of gait with dual-task performance in patients with PD is the underlying decrease in automaticity of motor tasks commonly found in PD. Automaticity is defined as "performance of task without attention directed to task execution" and is frequently impaired in PD, worse among those who experience freezing of gait (FOG). Automaticity has also been found to be impaired among individuals with cognitive impairment resulting from other pathologies, including Alzheimer's disease.

Surprisingly, Longhurst et al. 2022 found little association between dual-task performance and falls in people with PD but did find an association in the healthy older adult population [29]. The study authors hypothesize that impaired dual-task performance is related to falls, but that patients with PD recognize this and avoid participation in activities that put them at higher risk for falls, thereby reducing their fall rate. This may indicate a potential avenue for rehabilitation intervention in the healthy older adult population. Additionally, for patients with PD who experience freezing of gait, simple avoidance of risky activities involving dual tasking may not be enough to prevent falls. A study on falls in PD by Pelicioni et al. in 2019 found that of 2043 reported falls, 1249 were freezing of gait related. These falls were also more likely to occur at home, perhaps reflecting difficulty walking in more confined spaces and that people who experience (FOG) spend less time participating in community activities [30].

In addition to FOG, people with PD can fall due to a host of other factors, including impaired anticipatory and reactive postural control, decreased lower extremity muscle strength, impaired proprioception, decreased gait speed, increased gait variability. In addition to the motor symptoms, impaired cognition has also shown significant association with falling. However, the strongest predictor of falling is having had a previous fall [31].This overlaps with the major risk factors for falls in older adults, including impaired balance and gait, polypharmacy, visual impairments, cognitive decline—especially attention and executive dysfunction, and history of previous falls [32]. A better understanding of the intersection between gait and cognition in both PD and in older adults can lead to improved interventions in both populations to manage fall risk and improve quality of life.

Gandolfi et al. discovered that patients with PD experienced poorer gait performance when performing dual tasks, as both stride length and gait speed decreased significantly [33]. The impact of performing two tasks simultaneously on gait impairment may uncover non-motor symptoms linked to PD. [34]. Gait disturbances associated with PD typically include slowed walking as well as increased gait variability. Hausdorff reported that dual-task performance markedly heightens gait variability and had less effect on bradykinetic manifestations such as stride time [35].

Dual tasking can significantly impact cognitive function, leading to a decrease in the ability to switch between tasks. In addition, it can hinder walking ability by affecting various factors such as speed, stride length, and frequency. Salazar's research findings show that this phenomenon is noticeable in both healthy individuals and those who have PD. However, individuals with PD tend to experience a more pronounced effect on their walking speed and stride frequency compared to their healthy counterparts [36].

This finding is troubling because of the strong relationship between increased gait variability and fall risk in older populations [37]. In the study conducted by Callisaya et al., it was found that older people with poorer gait are at a higher risk of experiencing multiple falls. The research indicates that specific measurements of gait and gait variability are the main factors that contribute to the increased risk of multiple falls in older adults. The study also revealed that an increase in step length variability has a linear correlation with an increased risk of multiple falls, while gait speed, cadence, and step time variability have non-linear relationships with fall risk in older adults [38].

Both cognitively healthy and cognitively impaired older adults exhibit abnormal gait variability that is correlated with functional and morphological changes in cortical and subcortical brain areas. These changes are also associated with an increased risk of falling [39].

Rochester and colleagues evaluated the interference effects on walking performance by dual-motor tasks, dual cognitive tasks, and a combination motor-cognitive task (talking and carrying a tray while walking) in individuals with PD as well as the influence of cognition, depression, fatigue, and balance. Walking speed and step length decreased significantly in the dual cognitive and multi-task trials. Furthermore, cognitive function, depression, physical fatigue, and balance were significantly related to walking speed and both cognitive function and fatigue affected dual-task performance [40]. Fatigue's contribution to aspects of gait quality related to falls [41], mobility and walking capacity [42] in patients with PD is well known. Besides, individuals in the later stages of PD may be particularly affected by muscle fatigue and this can impact the spatiotemporal gait parameters [43].

Cognitive status was linked to dual-task costs on gait and cognition [44]. Non-motor experiences of daily living and TUG-cog were associated with dual-task costs on cognition and gait, respectively. PD MCI showed higher dual-task costs on gait than PD non-MCI [45].

Combined, these studies identify a dual-task interference with steady state walking in patients with PD. Apparently, a critical level of task complexity exists after which gait deteriorates significantly.

Stroke—Impact on Falls' Risk and Balance

Stroke is a leading cause of death and disability worldwide, with about 15 million people suffering from stroke every year. Stroke is the second-leading cause of death and the third-leading cause of death and disability combined worldwide, with a global cost of over US$721 billion [46]. At the global level in 2019, the number of DALYs due to stroke was higher in males (77.0 million) than in females (66.0 million) [47].

The symptoms and prognosis of stroke, caused by a loss of blood supply to neural tissue, vary widely depending on the site and size of the lesion [48, 49]. Motor disabilities are often a consequence and can affect speech [50], grasp, balance [51], gait, significantly impacting activities of daily living and quality of life [52]. Impairments such as muscle weakness, spasticity, decreased intra- and interlimb coordination contribute to deficits in balance and gait function [53]. Even after discharge from rehabilitation, a majority of stroke survivors have balance dysfunction, leading to increased risk of falls [54, 55]. The majority of falls occur within the first few months following discharge from rehabilitation [56–60]. Stroke survivors who experience a fall are less likely to be socially active in the community and more likely to have symptoms of depression [61] [56]. Furthermore, post-stroke hemiparesis is accompanied by a myriad of gait deficits that further add to the risk for falls. For example, reduced flexion of the hip, knee, and ankle during paretic swing phase may prevent the paretic foot from clearing the ground during swing, which may contribute to falls [62].

Considerable evidence exists about the impairments in balance observed in individuals with post-stroke hemiparesis [63]. During standing, stroke survivors demonstrate increased postural sway, with a shift in center of body sway toward the non-paretic limb, with an asymmetric distribution of body weight [64, 65]. Interestingly, related to the increased postural sway during quiet standing, compared to able-bodied individuals, stroke participants show less between-limb synchronization, i.e., correlation between the antero-posterior and medio-lateral center of pressure sway [66, 67]. As can be expected, stroke survivors also present with deficits in dynamic balance, and lower scores on clinical function tests such as the Timed Up and Go or the Berg Balance Scale [68]. Studies have shown that in response to a balance perturbation, stroke survivors demonstrate impairments in reactive stepping characterized by the need for assistance, inability to step with either leg, or the need for multiple-step responses [69]. Impaired stepping responses can increase the risk of falls when faced with challenges and obstacles during community ambulation [70]. Asymmetry in weight-distribution during standing is commonly observed in individuals post-stroke, with greater weight shifted toward the non-paretic limb [71]. Interestingly, asymmetric weight-bearing during standing has been shown to correlate with asymmetry during gait [72–75], suggesting that some common mechanisms might underlie deficits in balance and gait. Emerging literature results show that cortical activity (e.g., Beta power and coherence in the motor cortex measured using electroencephalography, connectivity between prefrontal-motor cortical networks) may have promise as a biomarker for individualizing balance challenge, providing a neural target for precision-medicine efforts aimed at fall prevention with aging [76, 77]. A better understanding of the impairments in balance and gait that contribute to falls is warranted for the development of more effective post-stroke fall prevention programs.

Motor-Cognitive Interaction and Falls: Dual Tasking and Cognitive Disturbances

In the past, movement and cognition were thought to be controlled by isolated, proprietary, cortical regions. However, functional neuroimaging techniques have graphically demonstrated considerable overlap in brain regions for many disparate behaviors. Overlapping neural systems likely serve both cognitive and motor function [78, 79]. Two primary regions have been identified that are activated by both cognitive and motor tasks: sensorimotor cortex and the dorso-lateral prefrontal cortex (dlPFC) [80]. While it is axiomatic that motor tasks will activate sensorimotor cortices and their association cortices, action words, both verbs and nouns, can activate somatotopically appropriate locations within sensorimotor cortices [81, 82] and supplementary motor cortex [83, 84]. The cortical representation of action word meaning includes cortex used for *enacting* a particular verb (e.g., writing, painting) or *using* an action-related noun (e.g., pencil, paintbrush) [85, 86]. From a behavioral standpoint, processing hand action-related words can impact finger and hand movements but not foot movement. Conversely, hand and arm movements also impact processing of hand-related words [87] [88]. However, both facilitation and inhibition of movement are possible following action word processing [89, 90].

The dlPFC is a region receiving input from multiple sensory and multimodal areas with projections to and from occipital, temporal and parietal lobes, as well as sensorimotor cortices. The dlPFC may provide "processing resources" (i.e., computational resources for calculating complex behaviors) for resource-demanding tasks, including non-automatic movement, executive function, working memory, and language [91]. The dlPFC is vulnerable to age-related declines in function due to loss of synapses [92, 93]. Because the dlPFC supports processing in multiple domains [94], there is often competition for processing resources during concurrent tasks [95]. More study is necessary to determine the involvement of various cortical and subcortical areas that underlie healthy motor-cognitive integration.

Parkinson's Disease

In PD, declines in dlPFC functional connectivity are more pronounced than in age-matched peers [96, 97], resulting in fewer resources available for calculating complex behaviors [98–100]; therefore, people with PD often experience exaggerated dual-task impairments relative to their age-matched peers [101] [27]. The magnitude of dual-task effects, or decrement in performance during concurrent tasks, is highly dependent on the task difficulty: as the secondary cognitive task increases in difficulty, so does the impairment in the primary motor task [102]. To effectively assess and treat dual-task gait decline in older adults, it is crucial to consider the type and difficulty level of the secondary cognitive task. Goh's research has demonstrated that both factors significantly influence older adults' susceptibility to dual-task interference [103].

When considering the disease process and manifestation of PD, the link between motor and cognitive function is especially clear. Motor learning is slower and likely uses more brain activity in individuals with PD than those without [104, 105]. It has been indicated that the basal ganglia and striatum play an important role in movement and skill acquisition in PD. PD patients have difficulty learning new motor skills or multitasking, even if they have already mastered these tasks. Increased bradykinesia—a reliable clinical measure of the nigrostriatal lesion in PD—is associated with the presence of [106, 107]. With careful concentration on critical movement aspects, those with PD can achieve close to normal movement amplitudes [108, 109]. During externally cued movements, people with PD might be able to bypass the malfunctioning basal ganglia [110] and activate the Cerebellar-Thalamo-Cortical (CTC) neural network, in a manner similar to that noted in age-matched controls. It is well known that external cues can often alleviate FOG [111]. Cueing, particularly rhythmic auditory cueing, is recognized as a valuable component of locomotor therapy for individuals with PD facing gait challenges. Auditory cueing primarily impacts temporal gait parameters. On the other hand, visual cueing is effective in enhancing spatial aspects such as step/stride length and reducing variability and asymmetry. However, the effectiveness of cueing in PD rehabilitation may vary based on disease stage and predominant symptoms. Researchers believe external cueing affects movement control by modulating neural circuits to bypass hypoactive basal ganglia-supplementary motor cortex (SMA) circuits [112, 113].

The rationale for "dual-task interference" is that performing multiple tasks requires more executive resources, which, in aging [114, 115] and more so in PD, are often limited [98]. The performance decrement during the dual task, termed the dual-task cost, depends on the type of task being performed and, more importantly, the population being tested. Activities of daily living are typically performed under modestly complex conditions and require the simultaneous performance of cognitive and motor tasks [116]. Due to the additional cognitive load in the dual-task situation, older adults' task performance exhibits deficits in the situation of high cognitive load. Dual-task interference in older adults is strongly influenced by task prioritization [117]. The cognitive effects of dual tasking while walking are affected by factors such as task complexity, task prioritization, cross-talk interaction, and learning processes [118]. Dual task (DT) presents greater difficulties for people with PD compared to healthy older adults [45].

Therefore, even slight, or subtle declines in cognitive function for people with PD may impact performance of routine activities such as dressing, grooming, cooking, walking, and driving. Even in healthy older adults, evidence suggests that the dual-task cost on cognitive and motor performance increases with age [119]. Pass Oliveros et al., suggests that aging is associated with increased confusion in response selection and decreased efficiency in flexibly sharing processing capacity during dual-task situations [120].

When two tasks are performed simultaneously, the more familiar task may be more reliant on basal ganglia control and processing; while the less familiar or attention-demanding task is modulated by the frontal cortex [27, 121–123]. Therefore, impaired functioning of the basal ganglia would be hypothesized to result in automatic tasks becoming slow, reduced in amplitude or ceasing altogether. This is consistent with the lack of spontaneous movements, development of bradykinesia and FOG) seen in patients with PD. Dalrymple-Alford and colleagues examined the effects of adding a cognitive task during an upper extremity tracking task with controls and individuals with PD [124]. Dual tasking inhibits cognition and gait development of individuals with PD due to their inability to manage the complex cognitive and motor demands of locomotion [125]. Those with PD showed an increase in tracking errors when asked to recall a series of digits. These data support the hypothesis that executive function deficits can be caused by disruptions of the basal ganglia circuits and contribute to increased motor performance variability under dual-task conditions. Dual-task walking issues in PD impact both motor and cognitive functions. The severity varies based on individual, task, and environment, with notable implications for gait impairments [126].

Stroke

There was a significant correlation between motor and cognitive functioning among stroke patients, regardless of the severity of the stroke [127]. The impact of stroke on the interaction between cognitive functions and motor tasks such as walking has been the focus of investigation in recent studies [127, 128]. In stroke survivors, postural sway reduces during standing balance tasks performed concurrently with a cognitive task [129, 130]. In another study, comparison of cognitive-motor dual tasking during reactive versus intentional balance task showed that cognitive performance only decreased during the reactive balance task, suggesting the nervous system's prioritization of reactive over intentional balance post-stroke [131]. During dual-task walking, cognitive cost during a serial subtraction task performed while walking was greater for stroke survivors versus young, able-bodied individuals [132, 133]. Another recent study tracked cognitive decline, the Timed Up and Go test, the Berg Balance Scale, dual-task performance, as well as gait speed in stroke survivors over a 20-year period, and suggested that gait and balance measures may be useful as predictors of future cognitive decline following stroke [134]. Tsang et al., showed that dual-task interference, particularly during walking, can significantly affect stroke survivors. The tasks involving manual and mental tracking impose the most interference on gait speed. The study also notes that the nature of the concurrent task affects interference, while the time since the stroke does not [135]. Further study of the inter-relationships between cognitive-motor performance post-stroke is greatly needed.

Dual Tasking: Effects on Gait and Balance

The capacity to perform a second task during locomotion is highly advantageous. Many activities of daily living require multitasking, e.g., carrying objects or thinking while walking in a crowded environment, thus increasing older individuals' risk for falling [136, 137]. Dual-task walking is crucial for daily activities, often involving concurrent cognitive tasks. Successful performance requires adjusting gait, efficient cognitive processing, and appropriate visual scanning. Age-related declines in coordination and cognitive function can make dual tasking common and increase the risk of falls. These declines impact gait adjustment, cognitive speed, selective attention, and spatial working memory, contributing to dual-tasking challenges [138].

In fact, most falls in community-living older adults occur during routine, nonathletic activities of daily life [139]. Nagarkar's study (2017–18) on 31,477 older adults in India showed a clear connection between daily activities, difficulty in performing them, and an increased risk of falls. The study explored the relationship between daily living activities and falls [140], and in proportion to the disruption of daily activities, the risk of falling increases [141]

Using the dual-task paradigm, researchers have demonstrated that maintaining balance requires attentional resources and demands on those resources increase with impaired balance [142]. It was found that children exhibited a relationship between attention needs and balance while performing dual tasking [143]. Small et al. found that young adults have decreased balance control during dual-task treadmill walking as cognitive loads increase [144]. Shumway-Cook and Woollacott demonstrated that older adults with impaired balance could maintain standing balance under a single-task condition, but fell under dual-task conditions [145]. Gait assessment under dual-task conditions may be sensitive for fall risk identification in older adults [103, 146–148]. Based on the findings, there was a notable correlation between the frequency of falls and the mean results of the single and dual Timed Up and Go (TUG) assessments. Nonetheless, the outcome of the single TUG examination was not conclusive in identifying whether the subjects were prone to falls or not [149]. However, a review suggests that only some fallers are identified by dual-task conditions [150]. Recent systematic literature review has shown that cognitive-motor DT can be a helpful indicator of fall risk in healthy older adults [151]. However, it remains unclear whether DT is more valuable than ST. Additionally, the overall motor capacity of the subject has also been identified as a strong predictor of falls and a potential marker of cognitive decline in older adults. At present, there is insufficient evidence to determine the predictive power of cognitive-motor DT for GI or postural control during motor tasks. While cognitive-walking DT tests are frequently used, there are various DT paradigms, and only about half of the studies have demonstrated that DT is more effective than ST in predicting future falls [151]. Thus it is unclear if they are more effective than single-task assessments. Also, Abou's research suggests that dual-task testing may not be a reliable predictor of future falls in PwMS. More complex tasks and longer monitoring periods are needed to establish its dependability [152]. Diverse cognitive and manual tasks have been used to assess the ability to divide attention while walking and to identify fall risk.

Research shows cognitive-walking DT tests are more common than those involving GI or postural control. This diversity can make comparing findings across studies challenging [150, 151].

Parkinson's Disease—Impact on Gait and Cognitive-Motor Dual Tasking

Many individuals with PD use attentional strategies to maintain stability and reduce their fall risk [153–155]. However, balance-enhancing strategies are often ineffective when presented with attention dividing challenges. The introduction of a concurrent verbal cognitive task led to deterioration in postural stability especially in demanding balance conditions and that this deterioration placed people with PD at a high risk of falling [153]. Similarly, greater postural sway was observed in PD fallers while completing an attention distracting cognitive task [156]. PD impairs standing stability and requires extra attention to postural balance. This makes it difficult for individuals with PD to perform well when multitasking, affecting their cognitive performance [157]. The addition of a cognitive task to the TUG enhanced the identification of fall risk in people with PD. This finding underscores the importance of assessing cognitive function in individuals with PD, as it has been shown to be a crucial factor contributing to fall risk [158]. There is also evidence that motor dual-tasking impairments contribute to falls among people with PD, which may be prevented by avoiding dual-task situations and practicing motor dual tasking [24].

Recently researchers have explored how the scaling and coordination aspects of motor control are affected by the disorder. Basal ganglia dysfunction causes deficits in the temporal and spatial coordination of multi-segment movements. Increased bradykinesia and rigidity have also been associated with decreased motor adaptive ability in movement coordination [159, 160]. Although dopamine replacement is the most common pharmacological treatment of motor symptoms in PD, its effects on motor coordination are not completely understood.

A recent study revealed that patients with PD presented with varying degrees of movement deficit, including intensive (scaling) and coordinated deficits [161]. This implies that the basal ganglia-thalamocortical circuits might have a crucial role in these aspects of movement. However, when these patients were administered dopaminergic therapy, which boosts the level of tonic dopamine, their intensive movements showed significant improvement. The reason behind this is that the dorsal striatum's tonic dopamine levels encode the energetic cost of a movement. Despite this, their coordinative movements did not improve, suggesting that merely increasing the tonic levels of dopamine is insufficient to restore the precise and differentiated activity of corticostriatal circuits necessary for finely coordinated movement [160].

Interlimb coordination is important for dynamic stability during gait and contributes to the ability to achieve a normal gait speed. However, studies show that both ipsilateral and contralateral interlimb coordination is reduced in persons with PD compared to the healthy older adults. The normal close coupling of arm and leg movements during gait is disrupted in PD, although the mechanism for this is unclear. This occurs even when the disease progression is mild [162]. In addition, an increased cognitive load (e.g., under dual-tasking conditions) is significantly correlated with increased gait variability. In people with PD, higher cognitive demands are imposed on the patient to maintain a consistent and accurate alternate stepping pattern [163]. It has been established that dual tasks have a substantial negative impact on the walking performance of individuals with PD. It has been noted that the execution of multiple tasks simultaneously has an adverse effect on gait performance, irrespective of the level of single-task gait speed. Additionally, the type of dual task performed does not influence the significant negative effect of performing dual tasks on dual-task walking speed. These findings confirm that individuals with PD have significant difficulty walking when they are performing dual tasks [28, 164].

One manifestation of dyscoordination in PD is the occurrence of motor blocks, the inability to initiate or the sudden discontinuation in voluntary movements. This can manifest as FOG in the lower limbs. FOG occurs when a person with PD is temporarily unable to initiate or continue effective stepping, usually for only a few seconds. FOG is a common issue experienced by more than half of individuals with advanced PD. FOG is a debilitating symptom characterized by brief episodes of inability to step or extremely short steps that usually occur while initiating gait or turning while walking. This symptom is often responsible for falls in PD and is highly associated with recurrent falls, which may be caused by multilevel network failure [165] but can then overcome and continue walking at their normal cadence [166]. Although the mechanisms underlying FOG) are poorly understood, FOG is associated with decreased gait rhythmicity and asymmetry, and bilateral dyscoordination of left-right stepping [163, 165]. FOG also tends to manifest in functional situations requiring increased interlimb coordination, such as turning [166]. Three hundred sixty degree turning in combination with dual tasking has been shown to be a significant trigger for FOG. People who freeze tend to increase their cadence and adopt a posture second strategy in contrast to non-freezers when presented with a dual-task situation. Freezers take significantly more steps to turn and are slower than people without FOG. Activities of daily living are significantly impacted given that functional mobility in the home tends to involve frequent turns [167].

People with FOG have less automatic gait and impaired cognition, balance, and postural transitions compared to those without FOG in PD [168]. Concurrent engagement in multiple activities, such as tracking days and walking, may adversely affect the gait of individuals with PD. This is likely due to the heightened demands of both tasks, which can overwhelm the individual's ability to concentrate, further compromised in PD [169]. Or people with PD and FOG may experience unilateral motor impairments leading to difficulty during postural transitions, such as turning during daily activities. Increased FOG severity may be indicated by lower turning performance, with a high explanatory power of 50.1%, such as the associations between NFOGQ scores and turning characteristics [170]. FOG symptoms not only affect the daily life and movements of people with PD but are also related to an increased risk of falls [171, 172].

Motor blocks can also occur with upper extremity use. A recent study by Brown et al. also showed motor blocks during rhythmic bimanual coordination when switching between phase patterns (e.g. between in-phase and anti-phase). The study concluded that upper limb motor blocks occurred in PD participants both without ("off") and with ("on") dopamine replacement. Specifically, the motor blocks may be caused by difficulty shifting attention under increased cognitive demand, implicating hypoactivation in motor and prefrontal areas [173]. Cognition affects and is constrained by intrinsic coordination dynamics. Switching from less stable to more stable patterns incur a higher cognitive load when going from AP to IP. Switching patterns between groups is difficult in both directions. Older participants take longer to switch from AP to IP patterns [174].

Studies have also shown that the rapid alternating task category in the United Parkinson's Disease Rating Scale (UPDRS) is an independent predictor of falls, suggesting a correlation between impaired intersegmental coordination and fall risk [175].

Turning is a multifaceted movement. The coordination between different body segments, especially during ambulation, is a frequent component of daily activities. A decline in this turning coordination heightens the risk of falls. Simultaneously engaging in cognitive tasks while turning can strain neural processing, potentially leading to hazardous turning maneuvers. This risk is particularly amplified in individuals diagnosed with PD [176].

Stroke—Impact on Gait and Cognitive-Motor Dual Tasking

Gait impairments in people post-stroke span multiple lower extremity joints and all phases of the gait cycle. In addition to the multitude of deficits in kinematics and kinetics in post-stroke gait, asymmetry of temporal and spatial gait parameters is common post-stroke [177]. In healthy individuals, gait tends to be symmetric both spatially (between left and right joint angles, step and stride lengths) and temporally (between right and left swing, stance, step and stride times). The unilateral deficits in the paretic limb affected by the stroke result in asymmetry, usually visibly observable as a "limp" during walking. Spatial asymmetry is manifested as a difference in step length, with the paretic leg being either longer or shorter steps compared to the non-paretic. Temporal asymmetry is reflected in reduced double support and single-leg stance duration on the paretic leg [178]. Post-stroke gait asymmetry may have important implications for gait speed, energy expenditure during gait, musculoskeletal overuse and loading on the non-paretic leg, and the incidence of falls.

Further adding to the complexity of balance and gait dysfunction observed post-stroke, deficits in adaptation and response to perturbations have been observed during dynamic balance tasks post-stroke. Post-stroke individuals with foot drop using an ankle-foot orthosis had reduced gait adaptability, as shown by reduced success with avoiding obstacles and reduced capacity to restore gait after crossing the obstacle [179]. Difficulty with safely navigating obstacles and incorporating step modifications during community ambulation would predispose stroke survivors to falls and injuries. Post-stroke persons may also show normal obstacle-avoidance strategies but have delayed and reduced electromyography responses, smaller joint angle deviations from unperturbed walking, and smaller horizontal margins from the foot to the obstacle, suggesting possible mechanisms that could be targeted with rehabilitation [180].

Dual-task training has also received attention in stroke rehabilitation research. Interventions designed to train cognitive-motor dual tasking, and incorporating visual or auditory cues, may show superior effects on post-stroke motor function compared to interventions not including dual-task practice [181, 182]. Although evidence supporting the incorporation of cognitive-motor interference tasks into stroke rehabilitation is still inconclusive, the use of dual-task training paradigms for improving community ambulation and reducing falls in post-stroke individuals merits systematic investigation [183].

Options in Physical Therapy and Exercise-Based Therapies

Assessment

The previous sections have highlighted the fact that a reduced capacity for dual-task walking and/or limited ability to adapt to changes in environmental context may substantially restrict the degree to which a person is able to participate in life roles. Conventional rehabilitation does not always adequately address the interaction of these two impairments, which can contribute to lower levels of participation and physical activity. As a result, the physical therapy assessment of older adults with and without neurological insult or disease should encompass a careful analysis of both coordination and dual-task ability and their impact on the patient's functional mobility.

Assessment of dual-task ability can include the Timed Up and Go Cognitive and the Timed Up and Go Manual. These tests are quick, dynamic measures for identifying individuals who are at risk for falls. Cut off scores are available for both community dwelling elderly [184] and for people with PD [185]. A 2012 study by Plummer-D'Amato et al. showed dual-task ability for community dwelling older adults could be assessed by timing participants completing a 6-m obstacle course under single-task and three different dual-task conditions (spontaneous speech, alphabet recitation and coin transfer) [186]. The therapist should be aware of the different types of cognitive interference tasks and evaluate several if necessary to determine the impairments most requiring intervention. The therapist's assessment may also include looking at spatiotemporal gait parameters under single and dual-task conditions, such as time to complete, stride length and number of steps taken on a 10-m Walk Test.

A careful assessment of coordination will include detailed observation of the patient's movements during sequential tasks under various conditions. An examination of upper extremity coordination in sitting might include rapid alternating movements, finger to nose, and rapid tapping of the first finger on the crease of the thumb.

Lower extremity coordination testing could include heel to shin testing and timed tapping of the patient's foot into the examiner's hand. The Perdue Pegboard Test is a test of upper extremity dexterity and coordination recommended by the American Physical Therapy Association's Parkinson EDGE Task Force (PDEDGE) and takes less than 5 minutes to administer.

Work by Gammon Earhart concludes that while much insight can be gained through assessing isolated coordination of movement, there is increasing recognition that consistency of step-to-step performance across longer periods of gait provides important information about dynamic postural control. Consequently, gait analysis should play an important role in the assessment of coordination in both normal aging and in people with PD. The phase coordination index examines temporal coordination of interlimb phasing and variability of this phasing across strides. Decreased and less consistent phase coordination index is shown with aging, PD, and FOG. Earhart also points out that performance of more challenging gait tasks such as backward walking and turning are associated with reduced coordination as measured by phase coordination index. These tasks show that older adults are more affected then younger, those with PD are more affected than age-matched controls, and those with PD and history of freezing are more affected than those with PD but no history of freezing. Assessment of coordination and consistency over a longer duration, including when faced with dual-task challenges, is key to a comprehensive evaluation of dynamic postural control in both older adults and those with PD [187].

Gait analysis is important. Gait speed has been suggested to be "almost the perfect measure" as it correlates well with functional ability and balance confidence and has the ability to predict future health status and functional decline [188]. Self-selected walking speed has also been found to be reliable, valid, sensitive, and specific. Both age and sex gait speed norms have been derived, along with correlations for functional mobility that range from "household ambulator" to "crosswalk and community ambulatory." Gait speed can also be used to determine amount of assistance needed [188]. Horak et al., suggest use of the Balance Evaluation Systems Test (BESTest) as a reliable and valid means to determine balance problems for patients and appropriately direct treatment [189]. The test is designed to identify underlying postural control mechanisms that may be responsible for poor functional balance.

Novel Approaches to Multimodal Exercise

In 2009, King and Horak introduced a novel framework of progressive sensorimotor agility exercises to delay mobility disability in people with PD [190]. Their framework has a strong evidence-based foundation, and includes challenges to coordination and cognitive interference. These principles can be incorporated into an ongoing exercise program for both people with PD and those with mobility impairments as a result a stroke or from the normal aging process. The exercises should:

- Be complex, multi-segmental, whole-body and require quick selection and sequencing of motor programs
- Address axial rigidity
- Be task and environment specific
- Teach patients to increase speed, amplitude and temporal pacing of self-initiated and reactive movements
- Involve complex gait training, and in environments where freezing typically occurs
- Facilitate increased use of proprioceptive information and decreased visual reliance
- Introduce cognitive constraints to progress an agility or mobility task

Preliminary evidence shows the effectiveness of coordination and dual-task training for older adults and people with PD. A 2012 pilot randomized controlled trial found that once weekly group circuit training, with or without simultaneous cognitive tasks, resulted in significantly improved walking speed among older adults. However, group-format dual-task training once per week did not improve walking time or dual-task cost on an obstacle negotiation task [186]. Small studies and pilot studies suggest that divided attention training can lead to larger steps, increased speed and decreased gait variability during gait under dual-task conditions in people with PD [191, 192]. A more recent randomized, controlled pilot study confirmed the efficacy of specific physical therapy intervention focused on asymmetry of motor control during gait [193].

More research has been completed on physical therapy interventions for FOG. Although the neural mechanism underlying FOG in PD is poorly understood, prolonged initial step duration is a physical predictor of FOG in PD. Therapists can easily incorporate specific interventions designed to decrease this step duration into a fall prevention training program for PD [194]. Other studies have shown that an individualized program of auditory cueing (using metronomes or similar devices) is easy and inexpensive to implement and has an immediate effect on gait. Improvements are seen in walking speed, stride length and freezing [195–197]. Auditory and visual cues in combination with treadmill training have been shown to be effective in improving functional indicators for people with PD + FOG. The treadmill likely acts as a supplementary external cue and works to decrease asymmetry in gait [198, 199]. Another intervention target for decreasing FOG is improvement of motor set switching. For example, people with PD could repeatedly practice changing step direction from one trial to the next [200]. Because FOG is one of the most disabling symptoms of PD and tends to occur more often in the advanced disease state, therapists should also consider incorporating compensatory techniques, modification of the patient's home environment and care partner/giver training into the treatment plan.

Similar to the beneficial effects of aerobic exercise shown in older adults and PD, several studies have demonstrated the benefits of treadmill-based walking exercise interventions in individuals with chronic stroke. Macko and colleagues showed that participation in a 6-month treadmill-based aerobic exercise program resulted in greater increases in cardiovascular fitness and walking function in individuals with chronic post-stroke hemiparesis [201, 202]. Considerable evidence supports the incorporation of cardiorespiratory and aerobic exercise training within post-stroke rehabilitation programs to improve post-stroke gait and balance function [203, 204]. Single-session as well as long-term training studies in stroke survivors have shown that in addition to cardiovascular benefits obtained by aerobic exercise such as fast treadmill walking, gait training at a faster than self-selected speed also imparts beneficial effects on biomechanical gait impairments, gait asymmetry, and muscle activation post-stroke [205–207].

Consistent with the beneficial effects of exercise on neuroplasticity and cognition in older adults, evidence in stroke also suggests that exercise promotes neuroplasticity by increasing brain-derived neurotrophic factor (BDNF) production, and can facilitate motor learning during post-stroke rehabilitation [208, 209].

Ongoing studies are evaluating if physical exercise programs can prevent cognitive decline in individuals after a minor ischemic stroke [210]. Also, similar to PD and older adults, community-based and group exercise programs have potential for maintaining or improving post-stroke motor function [211]. Over the past decade, interest in stroke rehabilitation research has grown toward development of novel exercise interventions that capitalize on combined approaches such as treadmill training plus functional electrical stimulation [212, 213], task-specific exercises and non-invasive brain stimulation [214], etc. and toward treatments that maximally harness neuroplasticity.

While it is clear that exercise addresses mobility issues in older adults and those with PD, investigation into the cognitive effects of exercise have come to the fore. A review of six pre-clinical studies in rodent models of PD revealed positive effects of exercise on cognition in rodents, improving long-term memory, motor learning, and short-term social memory [215]. Along with these behavioral changes were neurobiological changes including upregulation of the neurotrophic factors, brain-derived neurotrophic factor (BDNF), and GDNF in striatum and increased dopamine in the striatum. These findings are in line with three proposed mechanisms of improved cognition via exercise specifically for individuals with PD: enhanced availability of dopamine (DA) projections to the dorsal and/or ventral striatum; increased neurotrophic factor availability; and/or decreased neuroinflammation in the basal ganglia. The same review also covered recent human studies and found eight studies that demonstrated improved cognitive function as a result of exercise [215].

Other researchers have demonstrated both motor and cognitive effects of dance exercise. Tango instruction has led to improvement in PD mobility and QOL versus other partnered dances [216], non-partnered dance [217] and generalized exercise [218]. McKee and Hackney demonstrated that, in addition to expected motor improvements, 30 hours of adapted tango over 12 weeks improved disease severity and spatial cognition (as measured with the mental imagery, Brooks task) in individuals with mild-moderate PD [219]. Importantly, the exercise dose in this study—30 hours over 10–12 weeks— exceeds weekly exercise dosage recommendations for deconditioned older adults with chronic illness [220], which may have contributed to cognitive and motor improvements. Tango could be considered light-moderate exercise. Participants are stepping at 60–120 beats/minute (tempi of tango music) and expending at least three Metabolic Equivalent of Tasks (METs) per minute [221]. Thus, cognitive gains noted in the adapted tango group could have occurred because aerobic exercise has beneficial effects upon cognition [222, 223]. Notably, the researchers in this study ruled out partnered/social learning and interaction as being responsible for gains. Thus, adapted tango elements, including structured motor components that engage memory of steps and directions while encouraging keen awareness of spatial relationships, could have contributed to cognitive gains.

Several other small studies have examined the benefits of exercise for those with PD on various aspects of cognition. Six months of generalized moderate-intensity, multimodal physical training (consisting of aerobic, resistance, coordination and balance elements) led to improvements in the capacity for abstraction and mental flexibility as measured by the Wisconsin Card Sorting Task in 10 older individuals with PD in comparison to a non-exercising control group [224]. Fifteen individuals with PD who participated in programs of anabolic and aerobic exercise two times weekly for 12 weeks showed improvements in verbal fluency [225]. Low intensity passive cycling on a tandem bike, in a "forced exercise" situation one time per week over 4 weeks has led to improvements by 19 people with PD on the Trails Making Test A&B, an EF measure [226]. Dos Santos Mendes et al. assigned 16 individuals with early PD to Wii Fit training, to evaluate the motor and cognitive demands of the games on people with PD, in comparison to 11 healthy older adults. Compared to healthy controls, those with PD had no deficit in motor learning or retention on seven of the ten games but had marked learning deficits on three games. However, the PD cohort was able to transfer motor ability gained from the games to a similar, but untrained task [227]. Muller and Muhlack investigated the effects of a single bout (rather than an intervention) of high-intensity endurance aerobic exercise (heart rate-targeted cycling) or rest following L-dopa administration on reaction time, and complex movement sequence ability in 22 individuals with PD in a cross-over design. Participants improved on reaction time, tapping rate and peg insertion interval time after exercise, whereas they gave fewer correct answers after rest, and reaction time increased after rest [228].

These recent studies are encouraging and provide preliminary evidence that supports the effects of exercise on aspects of cognition in addition to motor gains, for those with PD. The findings by Uc et al. are encouraging because they agree with research supporting the beneficial effects of aerobic exercise on cognition in older adults; but these findings must be replicated in Phase III clinical trials. Furthermore, all of these studies employed a range of cognitive outcome tasks, and improvements were limited to one or two executive function measures. The exception is the improvement noted by McKee & Hackney, which provides novel evidence that supports further study into application of complex exercise programs, like adapted tango, for improving cognition. Such study is warranted and definitely needed [229] given the prevalence of MCI in PD, which affects the spectrum of mental function, and has deleterious effects on mobility because of a motor-cognitive interaction.

Hypotheses for Mechanisms Underlying Deficit and Recovery in Stroke and PD

Neuroplasticity is the phenomenon of changes or adaptations in structure or function of the nervous system on the basis of experience and practice. Plastic changes can occur on anatomical, molecular, genetic, structural, and functional levels within the nervous system. A possible neurobiological mechanism underlying the positive effects of exercise is the increased synthesis and release of neurotransmitters and neurotrophins, which could enhance neurogenesis, angiogenesis and thus neuroplasticity [230]. Additionally, reorganization of cortical representations, synaptogenesis, and synaptic potentiation play a role.

Typically, increased usage of or skill acquisition by one body part is followed by increase spread in the cortical map for that body part. Some changes have been attributed to competitive plasticity, referring to competition between body parts for limited cortical space, while others attribute the changes to the unmasking of previously silent or inactive neural connections. Changes in the horizontal spread of cortical representations of a particular body segment or movement in response to a change in stimulus leads to reorganization of cortical maps. Changes in map representations with training and experience have been demonstrated in both animal and human models of injury [231, 232].

Significant progress has been made in understanding how neuroplasticity mechanisms primed through physical activity exert an effect on the brain. Exercise effects on hippocampal neuronal regeneration are especially well documented in populations including stroke, PD and normal aging [233–236]. Erickson and colleagues longitudinally demonstrated 1–2% increases in hippocampal volume following a year- long aerobic exercise intervention in older adults. Significantly, a non-aerobic exercise control group experienced a 1–2% degradation of hippocampal volume over that same time course [237]. Furthermore, researchers have examined associations between cardiovascular fitness levels and the density of gray and white matter in adults ages 55–79. Older adults with greater levels of cardiovascular fitness had significantly less atrophy of gray matter in the frontal cortex as well as significantly less tissue loss in both the anterior and posterior white matter tracts [238].

Alterations in structure may correlate to improved behavioral and functional outcomes. Neuronal regeneration in the hippocampus is critical because of its vital role in memory formation and spatial navigation. In the Erickson study, the increase in hippocampal volume following exercise was associated with more accurate performance on a spatial memory task. However, Ten Brinke and colleagues demonstrated that increased left hippocampal volume was significantly associated with greater loss in word recollection after interference. In the same sample, aerobic training significantly improved word recall after a delay as measured by The Rey Auditory Verbal Learning Test [239]. Other factors, such as white matter degeneration, may significantly moderate the association between brain volume and cognitive performance. For example, the connectivity between the hippocampus and other brain areas may be greatly disrupted by white matter abnormalities, which is likely the case in MCI [240]. Thus, increasing hippocampal volume alone, through aerobic, other exercise, or other means, in older populations may not always result in improved memory performance.

Similarly, demonstrated enhancement in frontal connectivity associated with aerobic fitness is correlated with improvements in frontally mediated EFs. For example, aerobic exercise is associated with improvements in attention and processing speed, EF, and memory in healthy and impaired individuals, including aged individuals [241]. Seminal work demonstrated that 124 older adults randomly assigned to receive aerobic training experienced substantial improvement in performance of tasks dependent on executive control processes and the integrity of the prefrontal and frontal cortex [242]. A study assigned older individuals (65 years and over) to ride stationary bicycles for three "spin" sessions per week for 12 weeks in comparison to a control group. The exercise group demonstrated significantly higher category verbal fluency after the intervention. Furthermore, follow-up analysis demonstrated significant correlations between increase in cardiovascular fitness correlated with improvements in verbal fluency [243]. Most notably, these results report that the effects of aerobic training on executive cognitive functions may be selective. The mechanism for these changes comes from cross-sectional studies, which indicate that exercise may mitigate decreases in vital cortical inhibitory mechanisms in older adults [244, 245].

Not all of the effects of exercise are mediated by neurogenesis in the neocortex. Exercise has effects in other central nervous systems structures particularly implicated in PD including substantia nigra and basal ganglia [246–248], corticostriatal synapses [249], and the cerebellum [250].

In individuals with PD, neuroprotective mechanisms of exercise may be related to engagement in ongoing, vigorous exercise that increases heart rate and oxygen uptake [251]. A mechanism through which aerobic activity engenders improvement, may be plasticity-related changes in synaptogenesis, angiogenesis and neurogenesis [252]. "Forced exercise" has been shown to be an interesting potential mechanism of rehabilitation in the case of tandem biking [253]. The complex movement patterns experienced in adapted tango for people with PD may cause beneficial neural plasticity in neural pathways for movement. Multiple studies demonstrate that improvements in mobility, balance, spatial cognition, and disease severity may be retained for up to 3 months after adapted tango in individuals with mild-moderate PD [216–219, 254]. A link between activity, mental engagement and neural pathways may be primed by dancing, which involves complex, unfamiliar tasks like walking backward, problem solving and movement improvisation.

Going forward, uncovering mechanisms may be the most important area of discovery for enhancing non-pharmacological interventions that address mobility and motor-cognitive issues in older adults with and without movement disorders. The knowledge and principles gained could impact not only exercise disciplines but also pharmacological, surgical, physical, and occupational therapy for older adults with and without neurological disorders. Future work related to neurobiological mechanisms will be crucial to informing rehabilitative interventions as well as pharmacological and surgical treatments. Imaging with positron emission tomography (PET) and functional magnetic resonance imaging (fMRI) hold promise as well, given that lower limb neural pathways, implicated in exercise, are virtually unexplored in connection with rehabilitative efforts in PD.

Neuroplasticity mechanisms underlying recovery of sensorimotor function following stroke have been extensively investigated. During days and weeks following a stroke, changes in synaptic efficacy of cortical neurons begin to emerge in and immediately around the lesioned cortex, in distant parts of the side affected by the stroke, as well as in the contra-lesional cortex. Assessment of corticomotor excitability using transcranial magnetic stimulation (TMS) reveal depressed cortical excitability in the lesioned motor cortex early after stroke, and a slow increase in corticomotor excitability over the course of recovery of post-stroke function [255]. Studies using TMS-derived measures also suggest that an abnormal imbalance of inter-hemispheric inhibition, i.e., increased inhibition of the lesioned hemisphere by the non-lesioned hemisphere, may be an important neural correlate underlying post-stroke motor impairment, as well as a potential target for post-stroke rehabilitation. Imaging studies reveal marked changes in brain activation during movements of the paretic limb post-stroke. Interestingly, fMRI evidence of bilateral activation during unilateral movements is also observed in older adults as well as in young individuals during performance of complex motor tasks, suggesting that overlapping neural mechanisms may be at play in aging and movement disorders such as stroke.

Plausibly, greater activity in the unaffected hemisphere and secondary motor areas is a mechanism through which activity in residual neural networks compensates for the functions lost by the cortical tissue damaged due to the stroke (also referred to as the vicariation model of stroke recovery) [255]. In contrast, the inter-hemispheric competition model of stroke recovery posits that lesion to one hemisphere due to stroke disrupts the balance of inter-hemispheric interactions, and excess activity in the non-lesioned hemisphere can be detrimental to function. Post-stroke cortical reorganization is complex with high inter-individual variability, and its mechanisms and causal factors are still incompletely understood. A better understanding of the neuroplasticity mechanisms underlying post-stroke recovery can help develop new treatments and clinical decision-making protocols for maximizing sensorimotor function and QOL post-stroke.

Conclusion

Rehabilitation to restore and/or improve motor-cognitive function in older adults with neurological insult must be efficient and effective, because adherence to an exercise regimen is critical. Thus, identifying aspects of exercise and rehabilitative therapy, which are most responsible for benefits to mobility- and cognitive-mediating symptoms, i.e., axial impairment and depression, will impact adherence to exercise. Understanding these crucial aspects will help determine foundational principles of exercise training to evince motor and cognitive maintenance and/or gains. With improved and/or maintained independence via enhanced mobility, and targeted application of neuroplasticity principles, the overall goal of improving mobility and motor-cognitive function in older adults with and without neurological disorder can be reached.

References

1. Campos JL, Marusic U, Mahoney JR. The intersection of cognitive, motor, and sensory processing in aging: links to functional outcomes, Volume I. Front Aging Neurosci. 2022;30(14):1009532.
2. Vieweg J, Panzer S, Schaefer S. Effects of age simulation and age on motor sequence learning: interaction of age-related cognitive and motor decline. Human Move Sci. 2023;1(87):103025.
3. Nnodim JO, Yung RL. Balance and its clinical assessment in older adults–a review. J Geriatr Med Gerontol. 2015;1(1):3.
4. Xing L, Bao Y, Wang B, Shi M, Wei Y, Huang X, Dai Y, Shi H, Gai X, Luo Q, Yin Y. Falls caused by balance disorders in the elderly with multiple systems involved: pathogenic mechanisms and treatment strategies. Front Neurol. 2023;23(14):1128092.
5. CIFU DX. Central nervous system disorders affecting mobility in older adults. Geriatric Rehab. 2018;20:57.
6. Landelle C, El Ahmadi A, Kavounoudias A. Age-related impairment of hand movement perception based on muscle proprioception and touch. Neuroscience. 2018;15(381):91–104.
7. Shaffer SW, Harrison AL. Aging of the somatosensory system: a translational perspective. Phys Therap. 2007;87(2):193–207.
8. Lee J, Kim HJ. Normal aging induces changes in the brain and neurodegeneration progress: review of the structural, biochemical, metabolic, cellular, and molecular changes. Front Aging Neurosci. 2022;30(14):931536.
9. Balestrino R, Schapira A. Parkinson disease. Eur J Neurol. 2020;27(1):27–42.
10. Raza C, Anjum R. Parkinson's disease: mechanisms, translational models and management strategies. Life Sci. 2019;226:77–90.
11. Hoffman GJ, Malani PN, Solway E, Kirch M, Singer DC, Kullgren JT. Changes in activity levels, physical functioning, and fall risk during the COVID-19 pandemic. J Am Geriatr Soc. 2022;70(1):49–59.
12. Silva de Lima AL, Smits T, Darweesh SK, Valenti G, Milosevic M, Pijl M, et al. Home-based monitoring of falls using wearable sensors in Parkinson's disease. Mov Disord. 2020;35(1):109–15.
13. Melton LJ, Leibson CL, Achenbach SJ, Bower JH, Maraganore DM, Oberg AL, et al. Fracture risk after the diagnosis of Parkinson's disease: influence of concomitant dementia. Mov Disord. 2006;21(9):1361–7.
14. Johnell O, Melton LJ 3rd, Atkinson EJ, O'Fallon WM, Kurland LT. Fracture risk in patients with parkinsonism: a population-based study in Olmsted County, Minnesota. Age Ageing. 1992;21(1):32–8.
15. Hely MA, Reid WGJ, Adena MA, Halliday GM, Morris JGL. The Sydney multicenter study of Parkinson's disease: the inevitability of dementia at 20 years. Mov Disord. 2008;23(6):837–44.
16. Bloem BR, Hausdorff JM, Visser JE, Giladi N. Falls and freezing of gait in Parkinson's disease: a review of two interconnected, episodic phenomena. Mov Disord. 2004;19(8):871–84.
17. Mei S, Li J, Middlebrooks EH, Almeida L, Hu W, Zhang Y, et al. New onset on-medication freezing of gait after STN-DBS in Parkinson's disease. Front Neurol. 2019;10:659.
18. Mühlenfeld N, Söhling N, Marzi I, Pieper M, Paule E, Reif PS, et al. Fractures in Parkinson's disease: injury patterns, hospitalization, and therapeutic aspects. Eur J Trauma Emerg Surg. 2021;47:573–80.
19. Stewart KC, Fernandez HH, Okun MS, Jacobson CE, Hass CJ. Distribution of motor impairment influences quality of life in Parkinson's disease. Mov Disord. 2008;23(10):1466–8.

20. Chen J, Devine A, Dick IM, Dhaliwal SS, Prince RL. Prevalence of lower extremity pain and its association with functionality and quality of life in elderly women in Australia. J Rheumatol. 2003;30(12):2689–93.
21. Wu Y, Guo XY, Wei QQ, Ou RW, Song W, Cao B, et al. Non-motor symptoms and quality of life in tremor dominant vs postural instability gait disorder Parkinson′ s disease patients. Acta Neurol Scand. 2016;133(5):330–7.
22. Oliveira RCCD, Labanca L, Meireles PGZ, Diniz ML, Pires APBÀ, Barroso JC, et al. Galvanic vestibular stimulation to improve postural instability, voluntary attention, and quality of life in Parkinson's disease patients. Revista CEFAC. 2023;25:e0423.
23. Li Z, Wang T, Liu H, Jiang Y, Wang Z, Zhuang J. Dual-task training on gait, motor symptoms, and balance in patients with Parkinson's disease: a systematic review and meta-analysis. Clin Rehabil. 2020;34(11):1355–67.
24. Heinzel S, Maechtel M, Hasmann SE, Hobert MA, Heger T, Berg D, et al. Motor dual-tasking deficits predict falls in Parkinson's disease: a prospective study. Parkinsonism Relat Disord. 2016;26:73–7.
25. Camicioli R, Oken BS, Sexton G, Kaye JA, Nutt JG. Verbal fluency task affects gait in Parkinson's disease with motor freezing. J Geriatr Psychiatry Neurol. 1998;11(4):181–5.
26. Bond JM, Morris M. Goal-directed secondary motor tasks: their effects on gait in subjects with Parkinson disease. Arch Phys Med Rehabil. 2000;81(1):110–6.
27. O'Shea S, Morris ME, Iansek R. Dual task interference during gait in people with Parkinson disease: effects of motor versus cognitive secondary tasks. Phys Ther. 2002;82(9):888–97.
28. Raffegeau TE, Krehbiel LM, Kang N, Thijs FJ, Altmann LJ, Cauraugh JH, et al. A meta-analysis: Parkinson's disease and dual-task walking. Parkinsonism Relat Disord. 2019;62:28–35.
29. Longhurst JK, Rider JV, Cummings JL, John SE, Poston B, Held Bradford EC, et al. A novel way of measuring dual-task interference: the reliability and construct validity of the dual-task effect battery in neurodegenerative disease. Neurorehabil Neural Repair. 2022;36(6):346–59.
30. Pelicioni PH, Menant JC, Latt MD, Lord SR. Falls in Parkinson's disease subtypes: risk factors, locations and circumstances. Int J Environ Res Public Health. 2019;16(12):2216.
31. Ashburn A, Pickering R, McIntosh E, Hulbert S, Rochester L, Roberts HC, et al. Exercise- and strategy-based physiotherapy-delivered intervention for preventing repeat falls in people with Parkinson's: the PDSAFE RCT. Health Technol Assess. 2019;23(36):1.
32. Ambrose AF, Paul G, Hausdorff JM. Risk factors for falls among older adults: a review of the literature. Maturitas. 2013;75(1):51–61.
33. Gandolfi M, Fiorio M, Geroin C, Torneri P, Menaspà Z, Smania N, et al. Dual tasking affects gait performance but not automaticity in functional gait disorders: a new diagnostic biomarker. Parkinsonism Relat Disord. 2023;108:105291.
34. Zhang M, Gan Y, Wang X, Wang Z, Feng T, Zhang Y. Gait performance and non-motor symptoms burden during dual-task condition in Parkinson's disease. Neurol Sci. 2023;44(1):181–90.
35. Hausdorff JM, Balash J, Giladi N. Effects of cognitive challenge on gait variability in patients with Parkinson's disease. J Geriatr Psychiatry Neurol. 2003;16(1):53–8.
36. Salazar RD, Ren X, Ellis TD, Toraif N, Barthelemy OJ, Neargarder S, et al. Dual tasking in Parkinson's disease: cognitive consequences while walking. Neuropsychology. 2017;31(6):613.
37. Maki BE. Gait changes in older adults: predictors of falls or indicators of fear. J Am Geriatr Soc. 1997;45(3):313–20.
38. Callisaya ML, Blizzard L, Schmidt MD, Martin KL, McGinley JL, Sanders LM, et al. Gait, gait variability and the risk of multiple incident falls in older people: a population-based study. Age Ageing. 2011;40(4):481–7.
39. Pieruccini-Faria F, Montero-Odasso M, Hausdorff JM. Gait variability and fall risk in older adults: the role of cognitive function. In: Montero-Odasso M, Camicioli R, editors. Falls and cognition in older persons: fundamentals, assessment and therapeutic options. Springer Nature Switzerland AG; 2020. p. 107–38. https://doi.org/10.1007/978-3-030-24233-6_7.

40. Rochester L, Hetherington V, Jones D, Nieuwboer A, Willems AM, Kwakkel G, et al. Attending to the task: interference effects of functional tasks on walking in Parkinson's disease and the roles of cognition, depression, fatigue, and balance. Arch Phys Med Rehabil. 2004;85(10):1578–85.
41. Huang Y-Z, Chang F-Y, Liu W-C, Chuang Y-F, Chuang L-L, Chang Y-J. Fatigue and muscle strength involving walking speed in Parkinson's disease: insights for developing rehabilitation strategy for PD. Neural Plast. 2017;2017:1941980. https://doi.org/10.1155/2017/1941980.
42. Carvalho DV, Santos RMS, Magalhães HC, Souza MS, Christo PP, Almeida-Leite CM, et al. Can fatigue predict walking capacity of patients with Parkinson's disease? Arq Neuropsiquiatr. 2020;78:70–5.
43. Abd Ghani H, Alghwiri AA, Hisham H, Manaf H. Lower limb muscle fatigue alters spatiotemporal gait parameters and turning difficulty characteristics in Parkinson's disease. Ann Rehabil Med. 2023;47(4):282–90.
44. Stegemöller EL, Wilson JP, Hazamy A, Shelley MC, Okun MS, Altmann LJ, et al. Associations between cognitive and gait performance during single-and dual-task walking in people with Parkinson disease. Phys Ther. 2014;94(6):757–66.
45. Johansson H, Ekman U, Rennie L, Peterson DS, Leavy B, Franzén E. Dual-task effects during a motor-cognitive task in Parkinson's disease: patterns of prioritization and the influence of cognitive status. Neurorehabil Neural Repair. 2021;35(4):356–66.
46. Feigin VL, Brainin M, Norrving B, Martins S, Sacco RL, Hacke W, et al. World stroke organization (WSO): global stroke fact sheet 2022. Int J Stroke. 2022;17(1):18–29.
47. Feigin VL, Stark BA, Johnson CO, Roth GA, Bisignano C, Abady GG, et al. Global, regional, and national burden of stroke and its risk factors, 1990–2019: a systematic analysis for the global burden of disease study 2019. The Lancet Neurology. 2021;20(10):795–820.
48. Thye M, Mirman D. Relative contributions of lesion location and lesion size to predictions of varied language deficits in post-stroke aphasia. NeuroImage: Clinical. 2018;20:1129–38.
49. Cheng B, Forkert ND, Zavaglia M, Hilgetag CC, Golsari A, Siemonsen S, et al. Influence of stroke infarct location on functional outcome measured by the modified Rankin scale. Stroke. 2014;45(6):1695–702.
50. Sherman V, Martino R, Bhathal I, DeVeber G, Dlamini N, MacGregor D, et al. Swallowing, oral motor, motor speech, and language impairments following acute pediatric ischemic stroke. Stroke. 2021;52(4):1309–18.
51. Lin Q, Zheng Y, Lian P, Guo Y, Huang H, Luo Z, et al. Quantitative static and dynamic assessment of balance control in stroke patients. JoVE. 2020;159:e60884.
52. Chen Q, Cao C, Gong L, Zhang Y. Health related quality of life in stroke patients and risk factors associated with patients for return to work. Medicine. 2019;98(16):e15130. https://doi.org/10.1097/MD.0000000000015130.
53. Darak V, Karthikbabu S. Lower limb motor function and hip muscle weakness in stroke survivors and their relationship with pelvic tilt, weight-bearing asymmetry, and gait speed: a cross-sectional study. Current Journal of Neurology. 2020;19(1):1.
54. Đurović O, Radovanović S, Đonović N, Simić-Vukomanović I, Gajović G, Radević S. Risk factors and characteristics of falls among hospitalized stroke patients. Serb J Exp Clin Res. 2021;22(4):301–7.
55. Xu T, Clemson L, O'Loughlin K, Lannin NA, Dean C, Koh G. Risk factors for falls in community stroke survivors: a systematic review and meta-analysis. Arch Phys Med Rehabil. 2018;99(3):563–73. e5.
56. Forster A, Young J. Incidence and consequences of falls due to stroke: a systematic inquiry. BMJ. 1995;311(6997):83–6.
57. Andersson AG, Kamwendo K, Appelros P. Fear of falling in stroke patients: relationship with previous falls and functional characteristics. Int J Rehabil Res. 2008;31(3):261–4.
58. Mackintosh SF, Goldie P, Hill K. Falls incidence and factors associated with falling in older, community-dwelling, chronic stroke survivors (> 1 year after stroke) and matched controls. Aging Clin Exp Res. 2005;17(2):74–81.

59. Mackintosh SF, Hill K, Dodd KJ, Goldie P, Culham E. Falls and injury prevention should be part of every stroke rehabilitation plan. Clin Rehabil. 2005;19(4):441–51.
60. Jalayondeja C, Sullivan PE, Pichaiyongwongdee S. Six-month prospective study of fall risk factors identification in patients post-stroke. Geriatr Gerontol Int. 2014;14(4):778–85.
61. Alghwiri AA. The correlation between depression, balance, and physical functioning post stroke. J Stroke Cerebrovasc Dis. 2016;25(2):475–9.
62. Wei T-S, Liu P-T, Chang L-W, Liu S-Y. Gait asymmetry, ankle spasticity, and depression as independent predictors of falls in ambulatory stroke patients. PLoS One. 2017;12(5):e0177136.
63. Vistamehr A, Kautz SA, Bowden MG, Neptune RR. Correlations between measures of dynamic balance in individuals with post-stroke hemiparesis. J Biomech. 2016;49(3):396–400.
64. Kiyota Y, Hase K, Nagashima H, Obara T, Liu M. Adaptation process for standing postural control in individuals with hemiparesis. Disabil Rehabil. 2011;33(25–26):2567–73.
65. Oliveira FA, Martins CP, de Oliveira LA, Rodrigues EC, Ferreira AS, Lemos T. Poststroke consequences upon optimization properties of postural sway during upright stance: a cross-sectional study. Top Stroke Rehabil. 2023;30(7):663–71.
66. Mansfield A, Danells CJ, Inness E, Mochizuki G, McIlroy WE. Between-limb synchronization for control of standing balance in individuals with stroke. Clin Biomech (Bristol, Avon). 2011;26(3):312–7.
67. Jagroop D, Aryan R, Schinkel-Ivy A, Mansfield A. Reliability of unconventional Centre of pressure measures of quiet standing balance in people with chronic stroke. Gait Posture. 2023;102:159–63.
68. Alghadir AH, Al-Eisa ES, Anwer S, Sarkar B. Reliability, validity, and responsiveness of three scales for measuring balance in patients with chronic stroke. BMC Neurol. 2018;18(1):1–7.
69. Inness EL, Mansfield A, Lakhani B, Bayley M, McIlroy WE. Impaired reactive stepping among patients ready for discharge from inpatient stroke rehabilitation. Phys Ther. 2014;94(12):1755–64.
70. Salot P, Patel P, Bhatt T. Reactive balance in individuals with chronic stroke: biomechanical factors related to perturbation-induced backward falling. Phys Ther. 2016;96(3):338–47.
71. de Kam D, Kamphuis JF, Weerdesteyn V, Geurts AC. The effect of weight-bearing asymmetry on dynamic postural stability in people with chronic stroke. Gait Posture. 2017;53:5–10.
72. Hendrickson J, Patterson KK, Inness EL, McIlroy WE, Mansfield A. Relationship between asymmetry of quiet standing balance control and walking post-stroke. Gait Posture. 2014;39(1):177–81.
73. Adegoke BO, Olaniyi O, Akosile CO. Weight bearing asymmetry and functional ambulation performance in stroke survivors. Global J Health Sci. 2012;4(2):87–94.
74. Szopa A, Domagalska-Szopa M, Lasek-Bal A, Żak A. The link between weight shift asymmetry and gait disturbances in chronic hemiparetic stroke patients. Clin Interv Aging. 2017;12:2055–62.
75. Ravichandran H, Shetty KS, Janakiraman B. Effect of gait-specific weight-bearing interventions on physical performance among subjects with stroke: a systematic review and meta-analysis. Journal of Stroke Medicine. 2022;5(2):107–18.
76. Palmer JA, Payne AM, Ting LH, Borich MR. Cortical engagement metrics during reactive balance are associated with distinct aspects of balance behavior in older adults. Front Aging Neurosci. 2021;13:684743.
77. Ghosn NJ, Palmer JA, Borich MR, Ting LH, Payne AM. Cortical beta oscillatory activity evoked during reactive balance recovery scales with perturbation difficulty and individual balance ability. Brain Sci. 2020;10(11):860. https://doi.org/10.3390/brainsci10110860. PMID: 33207570; PMCID: PMC7697848.
78. Domellof ME, Elgh E, Forsgren L. The relation between cognition and motor dysfunction in drug-naive newly diagnosed patients with Parkinson's disease. Mov Disord. 2011;26(12):2183–9.
79. Patel R, Spreng RN, Turner GR. Functional brain changes following cognitive and motor skills training: a quantitative meta-analysis. Neurorehabil Neural Repair. 2013;27(3):187–99.

80. Lee J, Dong S, Jeong J, Yoon B. Effects of transcranial direct current stimulation over the dorsolateral prefrontal cortex (PFC) on cognitive-motor dual control skills. Percept Mot Skills. 2020;127(5):803–22.
81. Pulvermuller F. Brain reflections of words and their meaning. Trends Cogn Sci. 2001;5(12):517–24.
82. Popp M, Trumpp NM, Sim E-J, Kiefer M. Brain activation during conceptual processing of action and sound verbs. Adv Cogn Psychol. 2019;15(4):236.
83. Kemmerer D, Castillo JG, Talavage T, Patterson S, Wiley C. Neuroanatomical distribution of five semantic components of verbs: evidence from fMRI. Brain Lang. 2008;107(1):16–43.
84. Raposo A, Moss HE, Stamatakis EA, Tyler LK. Modulation of motor and premotor cortices by actions, action words and action sentences. Neuropsychologia. 2009;47(2):388–96.
85. Grossi JA, Maitra KK, Rice MS. Semantic priming of motor task performance in young adults: implications for occupational therapy. Am J Occup Ther. 2007;61(3):311–20.
86. Shebani Z, Carota F, Hauk O, Rowe JB, Barsalou LW, Tomasello R, et al. Brain correlates of action word memory revealed by fMRI. Sci Rep. 2022;12(1):16053.
87. Togato G, Andras F, Miralles E, Macizo P. Motor processing modulates word comprehension. Br J Psychol. 2021;112(4):1028–52.
88. Rodriguez AD. Semantic-motor representations: effects on language and motor production. Ann Arbor, MI: ProQuest Information & Learning; 2010.
89. Dalla Volta R, Gianelli C, Campione GC, Gentilucci M. Action word understanding and overt motor behavior. Exp Brain Res. 2009;196(3):403–12.
90. Borelli E, Butera C, Katirai A, Adams TC, Aziz-Zadeh L. Impact of motor stroke on novel and conventional action metaphor comprehension. Brain Lang. 2022;226:105081.
91. Friedman NP, Robbins TW. The role of prefrontal cortex in cognitive control and executive function. Neuropsychopharmacology. 2022;47(1):72–89.
92. Ibañez S, Luebke JI, Chang W, Draguljić D, Weaver CM. Network models predict that pyramidal neuron hyperexcitability and synapse loss in the dlPFC lead to age-related spatial working memory impairment in rhesus monkeys. Front Comput Neurosci. 2020;13:89.
93. Raz N. Aging of the brain and its impact on cognitive performance: integration of structural and functional findings. In: Craik FIM, Salthouse TA, editors. The handbook of aging and cognition. 2nd ed. Mahwah, NJ: Lawrence Erlbaum; 2000. p. 1–90.
94. Cabeza R. Functional neuroimaging of cognitive aging. In: Cabeza R, Kingstone A, editors. Handbook of functional neuroimaging of cognition. Cambridge, MA: MIT Press; 2001. p. 331–77.
95. Fiske A, Holmboe K. Neural substrates of early executive function development. Dev Rev. 2019;52:42–62.
96. Rowe J, Stephan KE, Friston K, Frackowiak R, Lees A, Passingham R. Attention to action in Parkinson's disease: impaired effective connectivity among frontal cortical regions. Brain. 2002;125(2):276–89.
97. White LK, Makhoul W, Teferi M, Sheline YI, Balderston NL. The role of dlPFC laterality in the expression and regulation of anxiety. Neuropharmacology. 2022;224:109355.
98. Orcioli-Silva D, Vitório R, Nóbrega-Sousa P, da Conceição NR, Beretta VS, Lirani-Silva E, et al. Levodopa facilitates prefrontal cortex activation during dual task walking in Parkinson disease. Neurorehabil Neural Repair. 2020;34(7):589–99.
99. Orcioli-Silva D, Vitório R, Nóbrega-Sousa P, Beretta VS, Conceição NR, Oliveira AS, et al. Cortical activity underlying gait improvements achieved with dopaminergic medication during usual walking and obstacle avoidance in Parkinson disease. Neurorehabil Neural Repair. 2021;35(5):406–18.
100. Vitório R, Lirani-Silva E, Orcioli-Silva D, Beretta VS, Oliveira AS, Gobbi LTB. Electrocortical dynamics of usual walking and the planning to step over obstacles in Parkinson's disease. Sensors. 2023;23(10):4866.
101. Roeder L, Boonstra TW, Kerr GK. Corticomuscular control of walking in older people and people with Parkinson's disease. Sci Rep. 2020;10(1):2980.

102. Al-Yahya E, Dawes H, Smith L, Dennis A, Howells K, Cockburn J. Cognitive motor interference while walking: a systematic review and meta-analysis. Neurosci Biobehav Rev. 2011;35(3):715–28.
103. Goh H-T, Pearce M, Vas A. Task matters: an investigation on the effect of different secondary tasks on dual-task gait in older adults. BMC Geriatr. 2021;21(1):1–12.
104. Nieuwboer A, Rochester L, Muncks L, Swinnen SP. Motor learning in Parkinson's disease: limitations and potential for rehabilitation. Parkinsonism Relat Disord. 2009;15(Suppl 3):S53–8.
105. Olson M, Lockhart TE, Lieberman A. Motor learning deficits in Parkinson's disease (PD) and their effect on training response in gait and balance: a narrative review. Front Neurol. 2019;10:62.
106. Fang C, Lv L, Mao S, Dong H, Liu B. Cognition deficits in Parkinson's disease: mechanisms and treatment. Parkinson's Disease. 2020;2020:2076942. https://doi.org/10.1155/2020/2076942.
107. Poletti M, Frosini D, Pagni C, Baldacci F, Nicoletti V, Tognoni G, et al. Mild cognitive impairment and cognitive-motor relationships in newly diagnosed drug-naive patients with Parkinson's disease. J Neurol Neurosurg Psychiatry. 2012;83(6):601–6.
108. Baker K, Rochester L, Nieuwboer A. The immediate effect of attentional, auditory, and a combined cue strategy on gait during single and dual tasks in Parkinson's disease. Arch Phys Med Rehabil. 2007;88(12):1593–600.
109. Morris ME, Huxham FE, McGinley J, Iansek R. Gait disorders and gait rehabilitation in Parkinson's disease. Adv Neurol. 2001;87:347–61.
110. Freedland RL, Festa C, Sealy M, McBean A, Elghazaly P, Capan A, et al. The effects of pulsed auditory stimulation on various gait measurements in persons with Parkinson's disease. NeuroRehabilitation. 2002;17(1):81–7.
111. Jiang Y, Norman KE. Effects of visual and auditory cues on gait initiation in people with Parkinson's disease. Clin Rehabil. 2006;20(1):36–45.
112. Muthukrishnan N, Abbas JJ, Shill HA, Krishnamurthi N. Cueing paradigms to improve gait and posture in Parkinson's disease: a narrative review. Sensors. 2019;19(24):5468.
113. Sweeney D, Quinlan LR, Browne P, Richardson M, Meskell P, ÓLaighin G. A technological review of wearable cueing devices addressing freezing of gait in Parkinson's disease. Sensors. 2019;19(6):1277.
114. Stuart S, Alcock L, Rochester L, Vitorio R, Pantall A. Monitoring multiple cortical regions during walking in young and older adults: dual-task response and comparison challenges. Int J Psychophysiol. 2019;135:63–72.
115. Nóbrega-Sousa P, Gobbi LTB, Orcioli-Silva D, Conceição NR, Beretta VS, Vitório R. Prefrontal cortex activity during walking: effects of aging and associations with gait and executive function. Neurorehabil Neural Repair. 2020;34(10):915–24.
116. Cahn-Weiner DA, Boyle PA, Malloy PF. Tests of executive function predict instrumental activities of daily living in community-dwelling older individuals. Appl Neuropsychol. 2002;9(3):187–91.
117. Fallahtafti F, Boron JB, Venema DM, Kim HJ, Yentes JM. Task specificity impacts dual-task interference in older adults. Aging Clin Exp Res. 2021;33:581–7.
118. Bianchini E, Warmerdam E, Romijnders R, Hansen C, Pontieri FE, Maetzler W. Cognitive dual-task cost depends on the complexity of the cognitive task, but not on age and disease. Front Neurol. 2022;13:964207.
119. Li KZH, Lindenberger U, Freund AM, Baltes PB. Walking while memorizing: age-related differences in compensatory behavior. Psychol Sci. 2001;12(3):230–7.
120. Paas Oliveros LK, Pieczykolan A, Pläschke RN, Eickhoff SB, Langner R. Response-code conflict in dual-task interference and its modulation by age. Psychol Res. 2023;87(1):260–80.
121. Iansek R, Bradshaw J, Phillips J, Morris ME, Cunnington R. The functions of the basal ganglia and the paradox of stereotaxic surgery in Parkinson's disease. Brain. 1995;118(Part 6):1613–5.
122. Temel Y, Blokland A, Steinbusch HW, Visser-Vandewalle V. The functional role of the subthalamic nucleus in cognitive and limbic circuits. Prog Neurobiol. 2005;76(6):393–413.

123. Desrochers TM, Burk DC, Badre D, Sheinberg DL. The monitoring and control of task sequences in human and non-human primates. Front Syst Neurosci. 2016;9:185.
124. Dalrymple-Alford J, Kalders A, Jones R, Watson R. A central executive deficit in patients with Parkinson's disease. J Neurol Neurosurg Psychiatry. 1994;57:360–7.
125. Xiao Y, Yang T, Shang H. The impact of motor-cognitive dual-task training on physical and cognitive functions in Parkinson's disease. Brain Sci. 2023;13(3):437.
126. Kelly VE, Eusterbrock AJ, Shumway-Cook A. A review of dual-task walking deficits in people with Parkinson's disease: motor and cognitive contributions, mechanisms, and clinical implications. Parkinson's disease. 2012;2012:918719. https://doi.org/10.1155/2012/918719.
127. Verstraeten S, Mark RE, Dieleman J, van Rijsbergen M, de Kort P, Sitskoorn MM. Motor impairment three months post stroke implies a corresponding cognitive deficit. J Stroke Cerebrovasc Dis. 2020;29(10):105119.
128. Plummer P, Eskes G, Wallace S, Giuffrida C, Fraas M, Campbell G, et al. Cognitive-motor interference during functional mobility after stroke: state of the science and implications for future research. Arch Phys Med Rehabil. 2013;94(12):2565–74 e6.
129. Hyndman D, Pickering RM, Ashburn A. Reduced sway during dual task balance performance among people with stroke at 6 and 12 months after discharge from hospital. Neurorehabil Neural Repair. 2009;23(8):847–54.
130. Bohlke K, Zhu X, Sparto PJ, Redfern MS, Rosano C, Sejdic E, et al. The effect of a verbal cognitive task on postural sway does not persist when the task is over. Sensors. 2021;21(24):8428.
131. Subramaniam S, Hui-Chan CW, Bhatt T. Effect of dual tasking on intentional vs. reactive balance control in people with hemiparetic stroke. J Neurophysiol. 2014;112(5):1152–8.
132. Patel P, Bhatt T. Task matters: influence of different cognitive tasks on cognitive-motor interference during dual-task walking in chronic stroke survivors. Top Stroke Rehabil. 2014;21(4):347–57.
133. Timmermans C, Roerdink M, Janssen TW, Meskers CG, Beek PJ. Dual-task walking in challenging environments in people with stroke: cognitive-motor interference and task prioritization. Stroke research and treatment. 2018;2018:7928597. https://doi.org/10.1155/2018/7928597.
134. Assayag EB, Shenhar-Tsarfaty S, Korczyn AD, Kliper E, Hallevi H, Shopin L, et al. Gait measures as predictors of Poststroke cognitive function: evidence from the TABASCO study. Stroke. 2015;46(4):1077–83. https://doi.org/10.1161/STROKEAHA.114.007346.
135. Tsang CS-L, Wang S, Miller T, Pang MY-C. Degree and pattern of dual-task interference during walking vary with component tasks in people after stroke: a systematic review. J Physiother. 2022;68(1):26–36.
136. Hollman JH, Kovash FM, Kubik JJ, Linbo RA. Age-related differences in spatiotemporal markers of gait stability during dual task walking. Gait Posture. 2007;26(1):113–9.
137. Faulkner KA, Redfern MS, Cauley JA, Landsittel DP, Studenski SA, Rosano C, et al. Multitasking: association between poorer performance and a history of recurrent falls. J Am Geriatr Soc. 2007;55(4):570–6.
138. Zukowski LA, Tennant JE, Iyigun G, Giuliani CA, Plummer P. Dual-tasking impacts gait, cognitive performance, and gaze behavior during walking in a real-world environment in older adult fallers and non-fallers. Exp Gerontol. 2021;150:111342.
139. Soriano TA, DeCherrie LV, Thomas DC. Falls in the community-dwelling older adult: a review for primary-care providers. Clin Interv Aging. 2007;2(4):545–54.
140. Nagarkar A, Kulkarni S. Association between daily activities and fall in older adults: an analysis of longitudinal ageing study in India (2017–18). BMC Geriatr. 2022;22(1):1–7.
141. Giovannini S, Brau F, Galluzzo V, Santagada DA, Loreti C, Biscotti L, et al. Falls among older adults: screening, identification, rehabilitation, and management. Appl Sci. 2022;12(15):7934.
142. Kerr B, Condon SM, McDonald LA. Cognitive spatial processing and the regulation of posture. J Exp Psychol Hum Percept Perf. 1985;11(5):617–22.
143. Abuin-Porras V, Villafañe JH, Jiménez-Antona C, Palacios A, Martínez-Pascual B, Rodríguez-Costa I. Relationship between attention and balance: a dual-task condition study in children. J Exer Rehab. 2018;14(3):349.

144. Small GH, Brough LG, Neptune RR. The influence of cognitive load on balance control during steady-state walking. J Biomech. 2021;122:110466.
145. Shumway-Cook A, Woollacott MH. Attentional demands and postural control: the effect of sensory context. J Gerontol Med Sci. 2000;55A(1):M10–M6.
146. Melzer I, Oddsson LI. The effect of a cognitive task on voluntary step execution in healthy elderly and young individuals. J Am Geriatr Soc. 2004;52(8):1255–62.
147. Verghese J, Buschke H, Viola L, Katz M, Hall C, Kuslansky G, et al. Validity of divided attention tasks in predicting falls in older individuals: a preliminary study. J Am Geriatr Soc. 2002;50(9):1572–6.
148. Yogev-Seligmann G, Hausdorff JM, Giladi N. The role of executive function and attention in gait. Mov Disord. 2008;23(3):329–42; quiz 472.
149. Tomas-Carus P, Biehl-Printes C, Pereira C, Veiga G, Costa A, Collado-Mateo D. Dual task performance and history of falls in community-dwelling older adults. Exp Gerontol. 2019;120:35–9.
150. Zijlstra A, Ufkes T, Skelton DA, Lundin-Olsson L, Zijlstra W. Do dual tasks have an added value over single tasks for balance assessment in fall prevention programs? A mini-review. Gerontology. 2008;54(1):40–9.
151. Bayot M, Dujardin K, Dissaux L, Tard C, Defebvre L, Bonnet CT, et al. Can dual-task paradigms predict falls better than single task?–a systematic literature review. Neurophysiol Clin. 2020;50(6):401–40.
152. Abou L, Peters J, Fritz NE, Sosnoff JJ, Kratz AL. Motor cognitive dual-task testing to predict future falls in multiple sclerosis: a systematic review. Neurorehabil Neural Repair. 2022;36(12):757–69.
153. Morris M, Iansek R, Smithson F, Huxham F. Postural instability in Parkinson's disease: a comparison with and without a concurrent task. Gait Posture. 2000;12(3):205–16.
154. Smithson F, Morris ME, Iansek R. Performance on clinical tests of balance in Parkinson's disease. Phys Ther. 1998;78(6):577–92.
155. Fok P, Farrell M, McMeeken J. The effect of dividing attention between walking and auxiliary tasks in people with Parkinson's disease. Hum Mov Sci. 2012;31(1):236–46.
156. Ashburn A, Stack E, Pickering RM, CD. W. Predicting fallers in a community-based sample of people with Parkinson's disease. Gerontology. 2001;47(5):277–81.
157. Morenilla L, Márquez G, Sánchez JA, Bello O, López-Alonso V, Fernández-Lago H, et al. Postural stability and cognitive performance of subjects with Parkinson's disease during a dual-task in an upright stance. Front Psychol. 2020;11:1256.
158. Vance RC, Healy DG, Galvin R, French HP. Dual tasking with the timed "up & go" test improves detection of risk of falls in people with Parkinson disease. Phys Ther. 2015;95(1):95–102.
159. Winogrodzka A, Wagenaar RC, Booij J, Wolters EC. Rigidity and bradykinesia reduce interlimb coordination in parkinsonian gait. Arch Phys Med Rehabil. 2005;86(2):183–9.
160. Snider J, Lee D, Harrington DL, Poizner H. Scaling and coordination deficits during dynamic object manipulation in Parkinson's disease. J Neurophysiol. 2014;112(2):300–15.
161. Vervoort G, Bengevoord A, Nackaerts E, Heremans E, Vandenberghe W, Nieuwboer A. Distal motor deficit contributions to postural instability and gait disorder in Parkinson's disease. Behav Brain Res. 2015;287:1–7.
162. Roemmich RT, Field AM, Elrod JM, Stegemoller EL, Okun MS, Hass CJ. Interlimb coordination is impaired during walking in persons with Parkinson's disease. Clin Biomech (Bristol, Avon). 2013;28(1):93–7.
163. Plotnik M, Giladi N, Hausdorff JM. Bilateral coordination of gait and Parkinson's disease: the effects of dual tasking. J Neurol Neurosurg Psychiatry. 2009;80(3):347–50.
164. Strouwen C, Molenaar EA, Keus SH, Münks L, Heremans E, Vandenberghe W, et al. Are factors related to dual-task performance in people with Parkinson's disease dependent on the type of dual task? Parkinsonism Relat Disord. 2016;23:23–30.

165. Marquez JS, Hasan SS, Siddiquee MR, Luca CC, Mishra VR, Mari Z, et al. Neural correlates of freezing of gait in Parkinson's disease: an electrophysiology mini-review. Front Neurol. 2020;11:571086.
166. Tanahashi T, Yamamoto T, Endo T, Fujimura H, Yokoe M, Mochizuki H, et al. Noisy inter-limb coordination can be a main cause of freezing of gait in patients with little to no parkinsonism. PLoS One. 2013;8(12):e84423.
167. Spildooren J, Vercruysse S, Desloovere K, Vandenberghe W, Kerckhofs E, Nieuwboer A. Freezing of gait in Parkinson's disease: the impact of dual-tasking and turning. Mov Disord. 2010;25(15):2563–70.
168. de Souza Fortaleza AC, Mancini M, Carlson-Kuhta P, King LA, Nutt JG, Chagas EF, et al. Dual task interference on postural sway, postural transitions and gait in people with Parkinson's disease and freezing of gait. Gait Posture. 2017;56:76–81.
169. Onder H, Ozyurek O. The impact of distinct cognitive dual-tasks on gait in Parkinson's disease and the associations with the clinical features of Parkinson's disease. Neurol Sci. 2021;42:2775–83.
170. Choi H, Youm C, Park H, Kim B, Cheon S-M, Lee M. Association between severity of freezing of gait and turning characteristics in people with Parkinson's disease. Int J Environ Res Public Health. 2022;19(19):12131.
171. Mancini M, Shah VV, Stuart S, Curtze C, Horak FB, Safarpour D, et al. Measuring freezing of gait during daily-life: an open-source, wearable sensors approach. J Neuroeng Rehabil. 2021;18:1–13.
172. Steinbach MJ, Campbell RW, DeVore BB, Harrison DW. Laterality in Parkinson's disease: a neuropsychological review. Appl Neuropsychol Adult. 2023;30(1):126–40.
173. Brown MJ, Almeida QJ, Rahimi F. The dopaminergic system in upper limb motor blocks (ULMB) investigated during bimanual coordination in Parkinson's disease (PD). J Neurol. 2015;262(1):41–53.
174. Temprado J-J, Torre MM, Langeard A, Julien-Vintrou M, Devillers-Réolon L, Sleimen-Malkoun R, et al. Intentional switching between bimanual coordination patterns in older adults: is it mediated by inhibition processes? Front Aging Neurosci. 2020;12:29.
175. Kerr GK, Worringham CJ, Cole MH, Lacherez PF, Wood JM, Silburn PA. Predictors of future falls in Parkinson disease. Neurology. 2010;75(2):116–24.
176. Bianchini E, Warmerdam E, Romijnders R, Stürner KH, Baron R, Heinzel S, et al. Turning when using smartphone in persons with and those without neurologic conditions: observational study. J Med Internet Res. 2023;25:e41082.
177. Awad LN, Palmer JA, Pohlig RT, Binder-Macleod SA, Reisman DS. Walking speed and step length asymmetry modify the energy cost of walking after stroke. Neurorehabil Neural Repair. 2015;29(5):416–23. https://doi.org/10.1177/1545968314552528.
178. Patterson KK, Parafianowicz I, Danells CJ, Closson V, Verrier MC, Staines WR, et al. Gait asymmetry in community-ambulating stroke survivors. Arch Phys Med Rehabil. 2008;89(2):304–10.
179. van Swigchem R, Roerdink M, Weerdesteyn V, Geurts AC, Daffertshofer A. The capacity to restore steady gait after a step modification is reduced in people with poststroke foot drop using an ankle-foot orthosis. Phys Ther. 2014;94(5):654–63.
180. van Swigchem R, van Duijnhoven HJ, den Boer J, Geurts AC, Weerdesteyn V. Deficits in motor response to avoid sudden obstacles during gait in functional walkers poststroke. Neurorehabil Neural Repair. 2013;27(3):230–9.
181. Choi W, Lee G, Lee S. Effect of the cognitive-motor dual-task using auditory cue on balance of surviviors with chronic stroke: a pilot study. Clin Rehabil. 2014;29(8):763–70. https://doi.org/10.1177/0269215514556093.
182. Choi JH, Kim BR, Han EY, Kim SM. The effect of dual-task training on balance and cognition in patients with subacute post-stroke. Ann Rehabil Med. 2015;39(1):81–90.
183. Wang XQ, Pi YL, Chen BL, Chen PJ, Liu Y, Wang R, et al. Cognitive motor interference for gait and balance in stroke: a systematic review and meta-analysis. Eur J Neurol. 2015;22(3):555–e37.

184. Shumway-Cook A, Brauer S, Woollacott M. Predicting the probability for falls in community-dwelling older adults using the timed up & go test. Phys Ther. 2000;80(9):896–903.
185. Maranhao-Filho PA, Maranhao ET, Lima MA, Silva MM. Rethinking the neurological examination II: dynamic balance assessment. Arq Neuropsiquiatr. 2011;69(6):959–63.
186. Plummer-D'Amato P, Cohen Z, Daee NA, Lawson SE, Lizotte MR, Padilla A. Effects of once weekly dual-task training in older adults: a pilot randomized controlled trial. Geriatr Gerontol Int. 2012;12(4):622–9.
187. Earhart GM. Dynamic control of posture across locomotor tasks. Mov Disord. 2013;28(11):1501–8.
188. Fritz S, Lusardi M. White paper: "walking speed: the sixth vital sign". J Geriatr Phys Ther. 2009;32(2):46–9.
189. Horak FB, Wrisley DM, Frank J. The balance evaluation systems test (BESTest) to differentiate balance deficits. Phys Ther. 2009;89(5):484–98.
190. King LA, Horak FB. Delaying mobility disability in people with Parkinson disease using a sensorimotor agility exercise program. Phys Ther. 2009;89(4):384–93.
191. Brauer SG, Morris ME. Can people with Parkinson's disease improve dual tasking when walking? Gait Posture. 2010;31(2):229–33.
192. Yogev-Seligmann G, Giladi N, Brozgol M, Hausdorff JM. A training program to improve gait while dual tasking in patients with Parkinson's disease: a pilot study. Arch Phys Med Rehabil. 2012;93(1):176–81.
193. Ricciardi L, Ricciardi D, Lena F, Plotnik M, Petracca M, Barricella S, et al. Working on asymmetry in Parkinson's disease: randomized, controlled pilot study. Neurol Sci. 2015;36(8):1337–43. https://doi.org/10.1007/s10072-015-2082-8.
194. Chong RK, Lee KH, Morgan J, Wakade C. Duration of step initiation predicts freezing in Parkinson's disease. Acta Neurol Scand. 2015;132(2):105–10. https://doi.org/10.1111/ane.12361.
195. Ledger S, Galvin R, Lynch D, Stokes EK. A randomised controlled trial evaluating the effect of an individual auditory cueing device on freezing and gait speed in people with Parkinson's disease. BMC Neurol. 2008;8:46.
196. Lim I, van Wegen E, de Goede C, Deutekom M, Nieuwboer A, Willems A, et al. Effects of external rhythmical cueing on gait in patients with Parkinson's disease: a systematic review. Clin Rehabil. 2005;19(7):695–713.
197. Ellis T, de Goede CJ, Feldman RG, Wolters EC, Kwakkel G, Wagenaar RC. Efficacy of a physical therapy program in patients with Parkinson's disease: a randomized controlled trial. Arch Phys Med Rehabil. 2005;86(4):626–32.
198. Frazzitta G, Maestri R, Uccellini D, Bertotti G, Abelli P. Rehabilitation treatment of gait in patients with Parkinson's disease with freezing: a comparison between two physical therapy protocols using visual and auditory cues with or without treadmill training. Mov Disord. 2009;24(8):1139–43.
199. Frazzitta G, Pezzoli G, Bertotti G, Maestri R. Asymmetry and freezing of gait in parkinsonian patients. J Neurol. 2013;260(1):71–6.
200. Smulders K, Esselink RA, Bloem BR, Cools R. Freezing of gait in Parkinson's disease is related to impaired motor switching during stepping. Mov Disord. 2015;30(8):1090–7. https://doi.org/10.1002/mds.26133.
201. Macko RF, Ivey FM, Forrester LW, Hanley D, Sorkin JD, Katzel LI, et al. Treadmill exercise rehabilitation improves ambulatory function and cardiovascular fitness in patients with chronic stroke: a randomized, controlled trial. Stroke. 2005;36(10):2206–11.
202. Silver KH, Macko RF, Forrester LW, Goldberg AP, Smith GV. Effects of aerobic treadmill training on gait velocity, cadence, and gait symmetry in chronic hemiparetic stroke: a preliminary report. Neurorehabil Neural Repair. 2000;14(1):65–71.
203. Saunders DH, Sanderson M, Brazzelli M, Greig CA, Mead GE. Physical fitness training for stroke patients. Cochrane Database Syst Rev. 2013;10:CD003316.
204. Brazzelli M, Saunders DH, Greig CA, Mead GE. Physical fitness training for patients with stroke: updated review. Stroke. 2012;43(4):e39–40.

205. Lamontagne A, Fung J. Faster is better: implications for speed-intensive gait training after stroke. Stroke. 2004;35(11):2543–8.
206. Pohl M, Mehrholz J, Ritschel C, Ruckriem S. Speed-dependent treadmill training in ambulatory hemiparetic stroke patients: a randomized controlled trial. Stroke. 2002;33(2):553–8.
207. Tyrell CM, Roos MA, Rudolph KS, Reisman DS. Influence of systematic increases in treadmill walking speed on gait kinematics after stroke. Phys Ther. 2011;91(3):392–403.
208. Mang CS, Campbell KL, Ross CJ, Boyd LA. Promoting neuroplasticity for motor rehabilitation after stroke: considering the effects of aerobic exercise and genetic variation on brain-derived neurotrophic factor. Phys Ther. 2013;93(12):1707–16.
209. Dimyan MA, Cohen LG. Neuroplasticity in the context of motor rehabilitation after stroke. Nat Rev Neurol. 2011;7(2):76–85.
210. Boss HM, Van Schaik SM, Deijle IA, de Melker EC, van den Berg BT, Scherder EJ, et al. A randomised controlled trial of aerobic exercise after transient ischaemic attack or minor stroke to prevent cognitive decline: the MoveIT study protocol. BMJ Open. 2014;4(12):e007065.
211. Moore SA, Hallsworth K, Jakovljevic DG, Blamire AM, He J, Ford GA, et al. Effects of community exercise therapy on metabolic, brain, physical, and cognitive function following stroke: a randomized controlled pilot trial. Neurorehabil Neural Repair. 2014;29(7):623–35. https://doi.org/10.1177/1545968314562116.
212. Kesar TM, Reisman DS, Perumal R, Jancosko AM, Higginson JS, Rudolph KS, et al. Combined effects of fast treadmill walking and functional electrical stimulation on post-stroke gait. Gait Posture. 2011;33(2):309–13.
213. Awad LN, Reisman DS, Kesar TM, Binder-Macleod SA. Targeting paretic propulsion to improve poststroke walking function: a preliminary study. Arch Phys Med Rehabil. 2014;95(5):840–8.
214. Madhavan S, Shah B. Enhancing motor skill learning with transcranial direct current stimulation - a concise review with applications to stroke. Front Psych. 2012;3:66.
215. Murray DK, Sacheli MA, Eng JJ, Stoessl AJ. The effects of exercise on cognition in Parkinson's disease: a systematic review. Transl Neurodegener. 2014;3(1):5.
216. Hackney ME, Earhart GM. Effects of dance on movement control in Parkinson's disease: a comparison of Argentine tango and American ballroom. J Rehab Med. 2009;41(6):475–81.
217. Hackney ME, Earhart GM. Effects of dance on gait and balance in Parkinson's disease: a comparison of partnered and nonpartnered dance movement. Neurorehabil Neural Repair. 2010;24(4):384–92.
218. Hackney ME, Kantorovich S, Levin R, Earhart GM. Effects of tango on functional mobility in Parkinson's disease: a preliminary study. J Neurol Phys Therapy. 2007;31(4):173–9.
219. McKee KE, Hackney ME. The effects of adapted tango on spatial cognition and disease severity in Parkinson's disease. J Mot Behav. 2013;45(6):519–29.
220. Chodzko-Zajko WJ, Proctor DN, Fiatarone Singh MA, Minson CT, Nigg CR, Salem GJ, et al. American College of Sports Medicine position stand. Exercise and physical activity for older adults. Med Sci Sports Exerc. 2009;41(7):1510–30.
221. Heyward VH. Advanced fitness assessment and exercise prescription. 6th ed. Champaign, IL: Human Kinetics; 2010.
222. Kraft E. Cognitive function, physical activity, and aging: possible biological links and implications for multimodal interventions. Neuropsychol Dev Cogn B Aging Neuropsychol Cogn. 2012;19(1–2):248–63.
223. Ratey JJ, Loehr JE. The positive impact of physical activity on cognition during adulthood: a review of underlying mechanisms, evidence and recommendations. Rev Neurosci. 2011;22(2):171–85.
224. Tanaka K, Quadros AC Jr, Santos RF, Stella F, Gobbi LT, Gobbi S. Benefits of physical exercise on executive functions in older people with Parkinson's disease. Brain Cogn. 2009;69(2):435–41.
225. Cruise KE, Bucks RS, Loftus AM, Newton RU, Pegoraro R, Thomas MG. Exercise and Parkinson's: benefits for cognition and quality of life. Acta Neurol Scand. 2011;123(1):13–9.

226. Ridgel AL, Kim CH, Fickes EJ, Muller MD, Alberts JL. Changes in executive function after acute bouts of passive cycling in Parkinson's disease. J Aging Phys Act. 2011;19(2):87–98.
227. dos Santos Mendes FA, Pompeu JE, Modenesi Lobo A, Guedes da Silva K, Oliveira Tde P, Peterson Zomignani A, et al. Motor learning, retention and transfer after virtual-reality-based training in Parkinson's disease—effect of motor and cognitive demands of games: a longitudinal, controlled clinical study. Physiotherapy. 2012;98(3):217–23.
228. Muller T, Muhlack S. Effect of exercise on reactivity and motor behaviour in patients with Parkinson's disease. J Neurol Neurosurg Psychiatry. 2010;81(7):747–53.
229. Hindle JV, Petrelli A, Clare L, Kalbe E. Nonpharmacological enhancement of cognitive function in Parkinson's disease: a systematic review. Mov Disord. 2013;28(8):1034–49. https://doi.org/10.1002/mds.25377.
230. Voss MW, Erickson KI, Prakash RS, Chaddock L, Kim JS, Alves H, et al. Neurobiological markers of exercise-related brain plasticity in older adults. Brain Behav Immun. 2013;28:90–9.
231. Merzenich MM, Nelson RJ, Stryker MP, Cynader MS, Schoppmann A, Zook JM. Somatosensory cortical map changes following digit amputation in adult monkeys. J Comp Neurol. 1984;224(4):591–605.
232. Buonomano DV, Merzenich MM. Cortical plasticity: from synapses to maps. Annu Rev Neurosci. 1998;21:149–86.
233. McCrate ME, Kaspar BK. Physical activity and neuroprotection in amyotrophic lateral sclerosis. NeuroMolecular Med. 2008;10(2):108–17.
234. Klaus F, Amrein I. Running in laboratory and wild rodents: differences in context sensitivity and plasticity of hippocampal neurogenesis. Behav Brain Res. 2012;227(2):363–70. https://doi.org/10.1016/j.bbr.2011.04.027.
235. Sahay A, Scobie KN, Hill AS, O'Carroll CM, Kheirbek MA, Burghardt NS, et al. Increasing adult hippocampal neurogenesis is sufficient to improve pattern separation. Nature. 2011;472(7344):466–70.
236. Lau YS, Patki G, Das-Panja K, Le WD, Ahmad SO. Neuroprotective effects and mechanisms of exercise in a chronic mouse model of Parkinson's disease with moderate neurodegeneration. Eur J Neurosci. 2011;33(7):1264–74.
237. Erickson KI, Voss MW, Prakash RS, Basak C, Szabo A, Chaddock L, et al. Exercise training increases size of hippocampus and improves memory. Proc Natl Acad Sci USA. 2011;108(7):3017–22.
238. Colcombe SJ, Erickson KI, Raz N, Webb AG, Cohen NJ, McAuley E, et al. Aerobic fitness reduces brain tissue loss in aging humans. J Gerontol A Biol Sci Med Sci. 2003;58(2):176–80.
239. Ten Brinke LF, Bolandzadeh N, Nagamatsu LS, Hsu CL, Davis JC, Miran-Khan K, et al. Aerobic exercise increases hippocampal volume in older women with probable mild cognitive impairment: a 6-month randomised controlled trial. Br J Sports Med. 2015;49(4):248–54. https://doi.org/10.1136/bjsports-2013-093184.
240. Rowley J, Fonov V, Wu O, Eskildsen SF, Schoemaker D, Wu L, et al. White matter abnormalities and structural hippocampal disconnections in amnestic mild cognitive impairment and Alzheimer's disease. PLoS One. 2013;8(9):e74776.
241. Voss MW, Heo S, Prakash RS, Erickson KI, Alves H, Chaddock L, et al. The influence of aerobic fitness on cerebral white matter integrity and cognitive function in older adults: results of a one-year exercise intervention. Hum Brain Mapp. 2013;34(11):2972–85.
242. Kramer AF, Hahn S, Cohen NJ, Banich MT, McAuley E, Harrison CR, et al. Ageing, fitness and neurocognitive function. Nature. 1999;400(6743):418–9.
243. Nocera J, McGregor KM, Hass C, Crosson B. Spin exercise improves semantic fluency in previously sedentary older adults. J Aging Phys Act. 2015;23(1):90–4. https://doi.org/10.1123/japa.2013-0107.
244. McGregor KM, Heilman KM, Nocera JR, Patten C, Manini TM, Crosson B, et al. Aging, aerobic activity and interhemispheric communication. Brain Sci. 2012;2(4):634–48.
245. McGregor KM, Nocera JR, Sudhyadhom A, Patten C, Manini TM, Kleim JA, et al. Effects of aerobic fitness on aging-related changes of interhemispheric inhibition and motor performance. Front Aging Neurosci. 2013;5:66.

246. Smith BA, Goldberg NR, Meshul CK. Effects of treadmill exercise on behavioral recovery and neural changes in the substantia nigra and striatum of the 1-methyl-4-phenyl-1,2,3,6-tetrahydropyridine-lesioned mouse. Brain Res. 2011;1386:70–80.
247. Wu SY, Wang TF, Yu L, Jen CJ, Chuang JI, Wu FS, et al. Running exercise protects the substantia nigra dopaminergic neurons against inflammation-induced degeneration via the activation of BDNF signaling pathway. Brain Behav Immun. 2011;25(1):135–46.
248. Vucckovic MG, Li Q, Fisher B, Nacca A, Leahy RM, Walsh JP, et al. Exercise elevates dopamine D2 receptor in a mouse model of Parkinson's disease: in vivo imaging with [(1)F]fallypride. Mov Disord. 2010;25(16):2777–84.
249. Cepeda C, Cummings DM, Hickey MA, Kleiman-Weiner M, Chen JY, Watson JB, et al. Rescuing the Corticostriatal synaptic disconnection in the R6/2 mouse model of Huntington's disease: exercise, adenosine receptors and Ampakines. PLoS Curr. 2010;2:RRN1182. https://doi.org/10.1371/currents.RRN1182.
250. Ben-Ari S, Ofek K, Barbash S, Meiri H, Kovalev E, Greenberg DS, et al. Similar cation channels mediate protection from cerebellar exitotoxicity by exercise and inheritance. J Cell Mol Med. 2012;16(3):555–68. https://doi.org/10.1111/j.1582-4934.2011.01331.x.
251. Ahlskog JE. Does vigorous exercise have a neuroprotective effect in Parkinson disease? Neurology. 2011;77(3):288–94.
252. Hirsch MA, Farley BG. Exercise and neuroplasticity in persons living with Parkinson's disease. Eur J Phys Rehabil Med. 2009;45(2):215–29.
253. Alberts JL, Linder SM, Penko AL, Lowe MJ, Phillips M. It is not about the bike, it is about the pedaling: forced exercise and Parkinson's disease. Exerc Sport Sci Rev. 2011;39(4):177–86.
254. Hackney ME, Earhart GM. Health-related quality of life and alternative forms of exercise in Parkinson disease. Parkinsonism Relat Disord. 2009;15(9):644–8.
255. Di Pino G, Pellegrino G, Assenza G, Capone F, Ferreri F, Formica D, et al. Modulation of brain plasticity in stroke: a novel model for neurorehabilitation. Nat Rev Neurol. 2014;10(10):597–608.

Contribution of Virtual Reality (Nintendo Wii) for Exercise Training and Rehabilitation

27

Cynthia Y. Hiraga, Maria G. M. Tonello, Marcela C. Ferracioli-Gama, and Ana M. Pellegrini

Abstract

This chapter discusses using a commercially available video game console for motor intervention and rehabilitation. This chapter presents four main topics. The first one focuses on technology and the basic principles and concepts of Nintendo Wii. The technology behind the Wii gaming system emphasizes the relevance of such technology to motor behavior. The second topic describes the effect of the Wii gaming system on older adults without movement disorders. Exercise training based on Wii gaming may positively impact metabolic parameters and functional capacity, such as balance, as a result of the aging process. The third topic describes the effect of Wii gaming on the rehabilitation of individuals post-stroke and with Parkinson's disease. Wii gaming for these individuals may bring some positive outcomes for motor recovery. Finally, the fourth topic discusses some of the relevant underlying mechanisms of motor learning related to using the Wii gaming system for health exercise and rehabilitation.

Abbreviations

VR Virtual reality
WBB Wii Balance Board.

C. Y. Hiraga (✉) · A. M. Pellegrini
Biosciences Institute, São Paulo State University, Rio Claro, SP, Brazil
e-mail: cynthia.hiraga@unesp.br; anapell@rc.unesp.br

M. G. M. Tonello
Association of Parents and Friends of Exceptional Individuals, Franca, SP, Brazil
e-mail: gina@ginatonello.com.br

M. C. Ferracioli-Gama
Institute of Physical Education and Sports, Federal University of Ceará, Fortaleza, CE, Brazil
e-mail: marcelaferracioli@ufc.br

F. A. Barbieri et al. (eds.), *Locomotion and Posture in Older Adults*,
https://doi.org/10.1007/978-3-031-74123-4_27

COP	Center of pressure
MET	Metabolic equivalent of task
PD	Parkinson's disease
TUG	Timed Up and Go test
BBS	Berg Balance Scale
FES	Functional Electrical Stimulation
CIMT	Constraint-induced movement therapy
KR	Knowledge of results
KP	Knowledge of performance

Virtual Reality: Focus on Nintendo Wii

Virtual reality (VR) is the term mainly used to describe technologies involving the interaction between a person and a computer-generated environment. The concept of virtual reality resides in the idea of presence [1]. According to Steuer, "*virtual reality is defined as a real or simulated environment in which a perceiver experiences telepresence*" [p. 76–77]. In this context, the user becomes part of this virtual environment. A person may perform various actions and have sensory experiences through a combination of devices. Products designed for educational, medical, industrial, military, and entertainment purposes, such as head-mounted displays, motion-sensing gloves, and stereoscopic 3D displays, are available to customers to explore the virtual world [1]. Sensory experiences by virtual reality systems provide advantages according to their applications (e.g., [1, 2]). An environment with virtual hands involving motion-sensing gloves provides an application for risk prevention and training workers in tasks to increase their skill and safety [2].

The sense of existence from the user distinguishes two main types of VR: immersive and nonimmersive [3]. According to Man [3], immersive VR systems project the user into a 3-D environment produced by a sophisticated system. Immersive VR systems combine devices such as head-mounted displays or motion-sensor gloves (e.g., PneuGlove) into an integrated system with a computer and customized software. It permits the user to interact directly with the simulated world (e.g., [4]). Recent generation devices for immersive VR maximize the user's experience. A stereoscopic 3D view moves relative to the user with such realism that he/she perceives himself/herself in a real world that may be miles away from his/her actual location [5]. The idea of immersion in the artificial environment, therefore, is for complete interaction that allows the person to explore that environment fully.

A current type of immersive virtual environment trend is the "metaverse." The metaverse concept appeared for the first time in the science fiction book "Snow Crash" by Neal Stephenson in 1992. The idea of a metaverse is an internet-based network of virtual worlds that tries to replicate reality. It is a three-dimensional experience in a virtual world where people do daily activities using avatars representing them [6]. Avatars are "*general graphic representations that are personified using computer technology*" [7], p. 20. Avatars is a digital profile representing a person in a scenario. Metaverse blends "beyond" and "universe" words referring to a virtual reality existing beyond reality. Nuñes and colleagues [8] resume that the metaverse is an alternative life where avatars engage in various social, cultural, academic, and leisure activities. The emergence of the metaverse creates new challenges and opportunities in multiple areas: education, health care, entertainment, etc.

The metaverse, a significant immersive virtual reality, is already drawing attention to clinical applications. The metaverse can benefit the rehabilitation of patients with neurological disorders, such as individuals with Alzheimer's and Parkinson's or post-stroke [9]. The metaverse would allow them to move and interact with others in the virtual world, an experience they would not have in the real world. Neurological patients can use the metaverse to practice physical activities or perform cognitive training in a controlled environment. According to Moon and colleagues [9], the benefits could be on sensory motor, social, and cognitive functions. The metaverse can potentially improve interaction and communication between patients and health professionals. Patients can use the metaverse to see doctors and receive treatments. Moreover, the metaverse may be helpful to have fun and connect with others to reduce stress, anxiety, and depression symptoms.

Nonimmersive VR systems implement a simulated world using a high-resolution monitor. The user is not fully immersed in the artificial environment, but he/she interacts with simple devices such as a computer mouse [10]. Furthermore, the interaction may be enhanced using input devices such as motion tracker or sensor glove, which the user may act more naturally [11, 12]. Both systems are widely used in various applications, but immersive VR systems provide a closer experience of a real situation than nonimmersive VR systems. An immersive VR system is expensive and demands sophisticated technology. In contrast, a nonimmersive VR system is a low-cost solution for easy access and is still effective for many applications. The gaming and entertainment industry has developed various low-cost, nonimmersive VR systems, such as the Wii.

The Wii gaming system, a video game by Nintendo (Kyoto, Japan), was released in 2006 as the fifth company's home console. In his review, Row [13] comments on the mimetic motion-control interface between user and machine, an idea that revolutionized the video game concept. It means the user may control the game using physical gestures and pressing buttons of the controller (i.e., Wii remote or *Wiimote*). For example, in Wii Sports, playing a tennis match, the user performs the gesture of forehand (i.e., the action of striking a ball with a racket held by the hand on the same side of the body), keeping the Wii remote as if he/she had a racquet in the real tennis game. Thus, as part of real and virtual reality, the user interacts with virtual reality, activating perceptual and motor systems to act appropriately in such virtual reality. On the other side, the Wii system can detect responses from the user, and the virtual environment immediately challenges the user to a different scenario.

A relevant feature of the Wii remote is a wireless motion-sensitive controller. It is used either as a handheld pointing device or as an implement serving as a racquet, a paddle, a ball, a steering wheel, and others [14]. As reported by Jones and Thiruvathukal [14], the Wii remote detects changes in direction, speed, and acceleration in three dimensions with high precision due to the built-in accelerometer and gyrosensors. An optical sensor at one end of the Wii remote helps determine where it points [15]. Some games on Wii need a second controller, the Nunchuk, which plugs into the Wii remote and requires two-handed coordination. The Wii remote communicates with a sensor bar at the center and above or below the television. The Wii remote sends via Bluetooth data regarding position, acceleration, and the button's state to the Wii console [16].

Bluetooth technology changed the concept of playing video games. The control of the games is now based on movements generated by the user (holding the Wii remote). Actions from the user holding and manipulating the Wii remote reflect on the TV display through his/her avatar. The avatar in the Wii gaming system is called Mii [14]. The user controls a Mii with his/her actions by holding the Wii remote, giving him/her the perception of being part of such a virtual world. The games in the Wii system (e.g., Wii Sports, Wii Fit, Wii Sports Resort, Wii Play—these are some of the packages of games and exercises collected in a compact disc) show the user visual feedback of his/her performance. Also, the games give the user motivational feedback, positive comments, and progress information. The Wii system shows the potential to contribute to motor and perceptual development, motor skill acquisition, and physical training.

Another wireless device that communicates via Bluetooth with the Wii gaming system is the Wii Balance Board (WBB). Such a device comprises four force transducers placed at each corner of the platform, and then it precisely measures the body weight and motion [17]. Also, the built-in concept of the WBB is similar to that of a laboratory force platform that contains four force transducers that assess force distribution and the resultant movements in the center of pressure (COP). The concept of this rigid platform is that the user uses the body over the WBB to control the game [14]. The user can control the balance games by adjusting the weight on either leg. A Mii displayed on a screen shows the adjustments done by the user over the WBB. COP shown on the screen generally requires displacement on media-lateral and anterior–posterior axes. The most popular games for WBB are the Wii Fit and Wii Fit Plus, which include yoga, strength training, aerobics, and balance games. The Wii Fit focuses on offering users a program that he/she can work toward personal goals to enhance health and motor control and coordination, mainly for balance and posture.

Some of the games featured in the Wii require users to be physically active or exercise with physical effort. This gaming style is known as "active video game" or "exergaming," which means to exercise using video games [18]. Games such as bowling and boxing (Wii Sports) require whole-body movement to participate in virtual games. However, the intensity of exercising in the games is still low compared to real boxing and bowling games. Activities in the Wii Fit, particularly in aerobics or strength training, appear to require more energy expenditure, and therefore, it would be helpful to promote an active lifestyle. Moreover, the need for motivating and enjoyable physical training or motor rehabilitation is one of the reasons for the growing interest in incorporating video game systems into clinical and fitness settings.

The Use of Wii Gaming for Healthy Aging

Regular practice of exercise contributes to a healthy aging process. According to the World Health Organization [19], physical exercises for older adults should include exercises based on aerobic capacity (150–300 min of moderate intensity or 75–150 min of vigorous intensity throughout the week), muscle strengthening and flexibility (that involve major muscle groups on two or more days a week), and functional capacity, (doing a multicomponent physical activity on three or more days a week). The lack of physical activity in older adults leads to obesity, higher body weight conditions, and risks for falls and fall-related injuries (e.g., [20, 21]). Physical activity programs for older adults must be designed to encourage them to maintain an active daily routine, minimizing the effects of a sedentary lifestyle. All alternative ways must be available to adults and older adults to engage in physical activity practices, particularly those who did not have previous physical exercise experiences and do not feel motivated to begin practicing.

Video game consoles like Wii have been mainly incorporated into physical fitness programs. The technology from the entertainment industry is an enjoyable way that has recently been explored to encourage people of all ages to physical exercise. It provides at least an ambiance with fun and an opportunity to discover the level of his/her abilities (throughout his/her avatar) and to experience all sorts of motor skills. A benefit of such one-to-one interaction (i.e., user and machine) is the time available to the user to familiarize with motor skills required for playing and exercising without exposing himself/herself to others. Therefore, Wii gaming may constitute an opportunity to provide extra motivation for physical activity adherence. It would also be an excellent opportunity for those unfamiliar with physical exercises and sports to initiate a fitness program.

Are the exergames, such as the Wii system, enough to activate energy expenditure rates for general health? Graves and colleagues [22] revealed that the physiological cost of exercising—such as heart rate, oxygen consumption, VO2, and energy expenditure—on Wii Fit games was more significant than that of handheld video gaming. However, the cost of exercising with the Wii Fit games was lower than treadmill exercise for older adults, young adults, and adolescents. Guderian and colleagues [23] found similar results showing that a session of Wii Fit games of approximately 25 min in middle-aged and older adults activates physiological and metabolic responses. In both studies [22, 23], the Wii Fit games applied to older people were considered moderate according to the metabolic equivalent of task (MET). MET expresses the energy cost of physical activity. Therefore, exercising with Wii Fit games benefits health and is within the recommendations for improving and maintaining cardiorespiratory fitness.

The Wii Sports and Wii Fit are the most frequently explored games for research. The energy expenditure measure in the games and exercises of the Wii Fit and Wii Sports were classified as light and moderate intensities [24]. Specifically, the mean MET values in yoga and balance exercises in the Wii Fit were 2.1 and 2.0, reflecting light-intensity activity. Resistance and aerobic exercise of Wii Fit and a set of Wii Sports games (golf, bowling, tennis, baseball, and boxing) were, respectively, 3.2,

3.4, and 3.0 METs, classified as moderate intensity. Games and exercises of vigorous intensity were not found on Wii Fit or Wii Sports. These findings are relevant to designing exercise training programs for young and older adults. Wii Fit and Wii Sports games may enhance cardiorespiratory fitness and muscle strength, motor coordination, and balance, which are critical for physiological capacities.

The intervention based on the Wii gaming in healthy older adults positively affects balance. Cho and colleagues [25] showed that Wii Fit training effectively improves the balance of older participants in a program with three sessions per week for 8 weeks. Similarly, Chao and colleagues [26] showed that the Wii Fit exercise group improved in balance and mobility, practicing twice a week for 4 weeks compared with a group that received a health education program. In a well-elaborated research protocol, Toulotte and colleagues [27] showed that Wii Fit games improved static balance in bipedal conditions. In contrast, the adapted physical activities improved dynamic balance after 20 weeks of one oriented session per week lasting 1 h each. Furthermore, the authors showed that adapted physical activities combined with Wii Fit games did not have significant additional benefits. Overall, the Wii Fit games, featuring yoga, balance games, strength training, and aerobics activities, appear to be an alternative for older adults to exercise and improve balance.

Other attempts, however, showed little or no effects of Wii gaming on the motor abilities of older individuals. For example, Franco and colleagues [28] found slight improvements in balance using the Wii Fit training program twice a week for 3 weeks. The improvement was not more significant than that observed for the control group, which received no training intervention. A serious limitation of the previous study is the number of training sessions, which might impact the lack of effect. An intervention protocol comparing exercises based on video games and physical exercise training [29] for 8 weeks of two training sessions per week showed that activities in the Wii Fit are as effective as the Tai Chi program on postural control and balance measures. Therefore, there was no distinction between the results of both virtual and real training programs. Improvements in postural and balance measures with Wii Fit may be due to the activation of neuromuscular mechanisms similar to those of the physical training programs.

If Wii gaming improves mobility and balance control, such improvements may affect fall prevention. Jung and colleagues [30] reported that an 8-week Wii Sports program improved balance and obstacle negotiation in older women. Recently, a systematic review [31] included 12 research trials that compared exergames interventions ([9] with the Wii system) with no intervention for older adults with impaired balance. The results showed significant improvements in balance and mobility based on the COP, Berg Balance Scale (BBS), and Timed Up and Go test (TUG). Evidence of using Wii gaming as an adjunctive method shows great potential to improve physical functions related to balance control in healthy older adults. Active video games offer variations in feedback, improve motor learning and gait, and reduce the risk of falls for older adults.

The underlying motor process of positive effects for balance control with Wii gaming in older people is still under discussion. Exercises with Wii Fit improve muscle strength because this practice demands single-leg balance and body weight resistance workouts [32]. Furthermore, the visual feedback of the center of gravity or altering body postures to meet task requirements, for instance, promotes motor learning [32]. Also, many of the Wii gaming favorable results for posture and balance represent its sensitivity in integrating sensory modalities. For example, Wii Fit activities require static and dynamic balance and demand higher postural adjustments, thus activating sensory-motor pathways [31].

Wii gaming is safe and feasible to engage older adults in exercise training [33]. The previously cited systematic review [31] showed, through qualitative data, that using Wii games had a relevant effect on motivation and physical activity enjoyment for older adults. Based on previous findings, Chao and colleagues [26] described that Wii gaming increases social interaction, alleviates symptoms of depression, improves adherence to exercises, and improves mood. Such positive effects may benefit a long-term effective intervention program. In addition, older adults have reported that Wii gaming was an enjoyable and acceptable method for exercise and that they would continue to practice after the research protocol. The use of Wii seems attractive for the positive results and stimulates settings for therapists and the older population.

The Use of Wii Gaming for Stroke and Parkinson's Disease Rehabilitation

The Wii system serves for motor rehabilitation in patients with movement impairments. This chapter will focus on individuals post-stroke and with Parkinson's disease (PD) to understand the effects of Wii gaming rehabilitation on motor impairments. Stroke is the second major cause of death worldwide and one of the leading causes of disability [34]. Among several factors, the clinical condition following a stroke depends on the affected cerebral region and the extent of the injury. Often, individuals who have stroke experience sensory, motor, and cognitive impairments, impacting their abilities to perform daily activities. The recovery to maintaining an upright posture, walking, reaching, and manipulating objects with the affected arm following a stroke is the objective of any rehabilitation. Various rehabilitation techniques are available; some are more effective than others [35], and no gold standard treatment exists. Research focusing on recent technologies for stroke rehabilitation is an avenue to establish effective protocols that may maximize motor and functional recovery.

The high cost associated with stroke-related healthcare encourages clinicians and researchers to explore the effectiveness of low-cost devices and a broad range of environments for movements. There is a consensus that the Wii gaming after a stroke displays a series of advantages [36]. For instance, the Wii gaming system provides repetitive task-specific training; it offers training in an enriched environment; it simulates real-world activities, giving more ecological validity; it is exciting and enjoyable, encouraging patients to train. The Wii gaming appears to be an alternative to establishing innovative and stimulating rehabilitation in clinical settings and at home. A further aspect of relevance is understanding the mechanisms associated with motor and functional amelioration in stroke.

Whereas some studies with the Wii are dedicated to rehabilitating the upper limbs, others focus on the lower limbs. The Wii Fit with a balance board may provide a viable means of improving postural control and balance. In a randomized controlled trial study, the researchers tested therapy programs for 30 individuals with subacute post-stroke [37]. The authors showed improvement in postural control (Step Test and the COP measured on a Wii balance board) for patients submitted to Wii Fit training on a balance board in a standing position. The control group trained with the Wii Sports and Wii Sports Resort in a sitting position showed an improvement in arm function, but it was not significant. In addition to conventional physiotherapy and occupational therapy, both groups trained for three sessions per week, 45 min each, over two to 4 weeks. These results strongly indicate task-specific training effects according to training programs.

Comparing two equivalent physical therapy programs related to lower limb exercises, Barcala and colleagues [38] showed beneficial effects in both groups of physical therapies for individuals post-stroke. Both the physical therapy program combined with activities of Wii Fit and the conventional rehabilitation only led to improvements in body symmetry, balance, and function. The therapy was done in two weekly sessions, 60 min for each session over 5 weeks. Wii Fit balance training lasted an extra 30 min for the combined treatments. The combination of exercises involving muscle strengthening, static and dynamic balance training, training of functional activities (conventional physical therapy), and specific balance exercises with visual feedback that strengthen the sensory-motor integration (Wii Fit exercises) appears to enhance the effect of rehabilitation in individuals post-stroke.

Another randomized controlled trial study with individuals post-stroke demonstrated that the Wii Fit therapy group was more effective than conventional weight-shift training instability in some sensory-challenged positions [39]. However, both groups showed improvement in the TUG and forward reach tests and fear of falling. Physical therapy protocols occurred twice weekly, 30 min each for 12 weeks, and simultaneously with another physical maintenance program. Unlike a previous study, Hung and colleagues [39] ran a follow-up of 3 months. The Wii Fit group did not maintain the training effects regarding stability. In comparison, the weight-shift training (i.e., control group) showed more improvement in weight-bearing symmetry than the Wii Fit group. According to the authors, the gain from Wii Fit training was not enough to be maintained, possibly due to the rapid weight shifting between the legs.

PD affects about 8.5 million people worldwide [40]. PD is a degenerative, chronic, and progressive condition of the central nervous system and causes motor, cognitive, and social impairments. Among the motor symptoms, rigidity, bradykinesia, postural instability, and tremor are the most common. Consequently, individuals with PD are at greater risk of falls, loss of independence, and lower quality of life than people of the same age without PD [41]. Rehabilitation is strongly indicated for people with PD because of exercise principles associated with neuroplasticity, such as the intensity and complexity of activities that promote synaptic plasticity and structural adaptation. Furthermore, exercise stimulates dopamine synthesis in dopaminergic cells, and higher dopamine levels facilitate learning. Consequently, practicing exercise in the early stage of PD can help delay its progression [42].

Individuals with PD may benefit from the intervention based on the Wii gaming system. For example, using Wii Fit games at home for 6 weeks of training for individuals with PD and healthy older adults improved significantly in static and dynamic balance tests, locomotion, and mobility compared to their baseline measures [43]. Another study [44] involving people with PD for 7 weeks showed improved walking, reduced rigidity, and increased functional independence. Overall, the literature review [45, 46] reported that Wii Fit seems effective for people with PD in improving functional and health outcomes related to balance and locomotion. At least 5 weeks of Wii Fit exercises are needed to benefit individuals with PD [46]. These authors suggest better results when patients combine Wii Fit with conventional activities. However, there is a need for consistent and quality methods to standardize the types of games, intensity, and frequency of each kind of individual with PD [45].

Is there an effect of Wii Fit practicing in the long term? That is a relevant question to incorporating video game technology into daily physical exercises or including it as an occasional treatment. A study analyzed the impact of practicing various Wii Fit Plus games compared with conventional intervention over 12 weeks on balance, fatigue, functional capacity, and quality of life of individuals with PD [47]. The results did not indicate changes in functional capacity and quality of life. However, exergaming effectively enhanced balance and reduced fatigue in individuals with PD after 12 weeks of treatment. Still, this benefit was not sustained long-term after 60 days of follow-up. Similar to the results of individuals post-stroke, the rehabilitation of individuals with PD using Wii Fit appears to be effective, either practiced alone or in combination with conventional techniques [48, 49].

Virtual reality dance exercises using Wii gaming have also improved balance and quality of life in people with PD [49]. In this trial, 20 individuals with PD received neurodevelopmental treatment and functional electrical stimulation (FES) five times weekly for 6 weeks. Ten of these patients also engaged in an additional 30-minute dance exercise (K-Pop Dance Festival for the Wii system) per week. Patients were allowed to choose the songs they liked from the package. The results showed that PD patients who performed the dance exercises improved balance (assessed by BBS) and achieved better balance results than those who only received neurodevelopmental treatment and FES. Additionally, the participants who engaged in dancing showed better results in activities of daily living and reduced depressive symptoms after 6 weeks of treatment.

The Wii gaming system appears to provide additional gain, especially on balance disabilities, to individuals post-stroke and with PD [50] and may be part of rehabilitation. The results in the literature suggest that the Wii gaming system may be introduced as physical therapy as soon as possible. The lack of high-quality evidence prevents one from concluding about the effectiveness of the Wii gaming system and other similar systems—such as PlayStation, and Kinect Microsoft—[51, 52]. Wii gaming is still exploratory in clinical settings, and much research is still needed to consolidate some preliminary findings. The protocol incorporating the Wii gaming system requires further research contemplating large-scale samples, randomized control trials, comparable procedures and types of video game systems, complete assessment such as balance, locomotion, health, and activities of daily living, aspects of training related to number of trials, frequency training, intensity, duration period, and long-term follow-up.

Underlying Mechanisms of Motor Learning and Wii Gaming

The Nintendo Wii Fit and Wii Sports are widely spread for health, exercise training, and rehabilitation. Studies using Wii gaming to promote healthy aging and prevent degenerative diseases demonstrated the efficacy of energy expenditure. More recently, Wii gaming has been incorporated into rehabilitating functional and movement recovery of movement impairment patients. The safety and feasibility of Wii gaming for exercise training and rehabilitation (e.g., [51]) are fairly established in research. The Wii gaming system was primarily designed as a consuming product for entertainment purposes for healthy people. The application to healthy aging and rehabilitation should be further examined in terms of adapting the devices for individuals who do not have sufficient hand control or cannot stand on the Wii Fit board because of balance deficits [53].

Wii gaming allows users to interact with a computer-simulated environment in various games and activities. The user produces motor actions in which an avatar on a screen represents him/her in the virtual environment. Playing Wii games requires sensory-motor integration and cognitive effort. The user must capture relevant visual or auditory information from a screen of elements. Moreover, he/she must interpret such information to elaborate a plan and execute the appropriate response. In some of the Wii games, the user does not have the opportunity to correct his/her movement during a play. In these contexts, the user must frequently plan his/her actions before a movement begins and correction is made on the next attempt (e.g., Wii Sports Resorts: archery). In other games, visual or auditory cues (i.e., real-time feedback on performance) may supplement coordination and motor control during play. The user may correct or adjust his/her movement for better performance on ongoing tasks (e.g., Wii Sport: wakeboarding).

Understanding the mechanisms that promote improvements in healthy aging and motor impairments is one of the critical points to consolidating Wii gaming as an exercise program and rehabilitation, respectively. The motor skill performance to play games and exercise in the Wii system demands explicit knowledge to operate Wii devices and the usage of real-time feedback to achieve game or exercise objectives. Feedback plays a significant role in motor skill acquisition and learning [54]. The Wii games provide visual, auditory, and tactile (haptic) feedback [53]. The haptic (e.g., presented in the form of rumbles) and auditory feedback are transmitted through the Wii remote (i.e., the main game controller). At the same time, the visual feedback is shown on the screen [14]. The feedback information reduces the uncertainty of the virtual environment to achieve task goals.

Two main types of feedback are available to learners [54]. Intrinsic feedback refers to the sensory information resulting from moving the body. Intrinsic feedback comes from sources outside of the body (exteroception) and inside the body (proprioception). The former informs about the events in the environment, mainly with vision and hearing. The latter provides information about body movements, such as limb position and the action itself, using the vestibular system, muscle, joint, and cutaneous receptors. Extrinsic feedback is additional information over the content of intrinsic feedback and comes from an outside source (e.g., verbal or written instruction, images of a video played). According to Schmidt and Lee [54], after the completion of a motor action, extrinsic feedback is categorized into the knowledge of results (KR) and knowledge of performance (KP). KR is the feedback about the outcome of the movement relative to the performance's goal, whereas KP is feedback about the movement pattern generated to achieve the goal. According to Deutsch and colleagues [53], KR is the predominant type of feedback in Wii gaming, specifically in the Wii Sports and Wii Fit, compared to the KP.

Feedback provided by the Wii gaming system is abundant and diverse. KR about the partial or total scores or the precise location of a target shooting helps to facilitate performance. Deutsch and colleagues [53] argue that the abundance of KR in Wii gaming may explain the positive outcomes for rehabilitation based on the assumption that KR facilitates learning and skill acquisition. For instance, in the Wii Fit balance exercises, online visual feedback (KR) informs the user about how much and in what direction he/she oscillates while performing balance exercises. Moreover, Wii gaming consistently rewards the user with positive feedback that is not linked to performance but is related to enhancing motivation and engagement [53]. For example, in the Wii games and exercises, there is cheering in the stadium, ribbons, and pleasing music when the user wins a game or succeeds in executing an activity, and stars appear to reward the winners. Feedback, mainly positive or rewarding, may motivate patients to rehabilitation.

A fundamental principle that directly affects motor skill acquisition and learning is practice. Repeated movement or motor action rehearsal may guarantee motor skill acquisition, but it does not ensure the retention of acquisition (i.e., learning) over time [54]. One of the first concerns about rehabilitation and exercise training is organizing practice schedules, such as the frequency per week, the duration of each practice session, and the length of a practice protocol. At first glance, one could argue that providing as much practice as possible would maximize the practice effect. However, there is a limit to the amount of training per day for effective learning, at least for non-patient individuals [54].

An approach in stroke rehabilitation based on intensive massed practice (i.e., Constraint-induced movement therapy—CIMT) restored substantial motor function in individuals post-stroke [55]. This protocol limits the use of the unaffected limb, stimulating the utilization of the affected limb through massed practice (approximately 6 h a day for 2 weeks) in daily activities. Although the CIMT improves upper limb function following stroke compared to alternative or no treatment, it remains controversial in several issues (e.g., [56, 57]). Practice methods not involving physical execution may also improve learning [54]. Intensive massed practice such as

CIMT for stroke rehabilitation may integrate with a technique that does not include physical rehearsals. For example, observing a model executing a task takes the learner to gather all relevant information and think about his/her execution [54]. Similar processing may occur with a mental practice that requires mental effort for imagery processing.

The variable practice of a given task is better for retention and generalizability than constant practice [54]. According to the authors, the variability of a particular task operates on a generalized motor program that defines a movement pattern and its parameters. Neurological patients may benefit from strong, flexible generalized motor programs to recover function and movement over time. A study showed that PD patients could learn and retain performance in various Wii Fit games. Still, they faced difficulties in motor learning when the games required cognitive demands such as divided attention, decision-making, response inhibition, and working memory [58]. Wii gaming system offers a varied and enjoyable exercise training and rehabilitation environment. In such an environment, the chance for individuals to sustain the motivation to practice for an extended period is promising.

The positive effect of the Wii gaming system for individuals post-stroke and with PD is possibly due to brain plasticity [59]. A cortical reorganization and a rewiring of damaged neural circuits occur due to training and practice. You and colleagues [60] showed that cortical reorganization is associated with improvements in lower limb function for individuals post-stroke after VR rehabilitation. Practicing with Wii gaming facilitates motor representation and promotes the reorganization of motor cortical function. A functional magnetic resonance imaging study reported related changes in cortical activity and behavioral improvements in the upper limbs of post-stroke survivors after VR rehabilitation [61]. Similarly, physical therapy with Wii Fit modulated cortical motor excitability of individuals post-stroke and with PD [43], accompanied by improved dynamic balance and balance confidence [62]. Behavioral modifications demonstrated in clinical trials associated with rehabilitation based on Wii gaming need further understanding of the underlying neural circuit changes.

Conclusion

The findings related to using the Wii gaming system suggest that the energy requirements of playing the games correspond to moderate exercise, meeting the recommended guidelines for health and fitness. Wii gaming system is feasible as physical therapy to improve motor control and learning in patients and enhance physiological and functional capacities in healthy aging. Although commercial video games may be complex and challenging for patients, they are still an alternative to adjunctive therapy.

References

1. McIntire JP, Havig PR, Geiselman EE. Stereoscopic 3D displays and human performance: a comprehensive review. Displays. 2014;35(1):18–26.
2. Pouliquen M, Bernard A, Marsot J, Chodorge L. Virtual hands and virtual reality multimodal platform to design safer industrial systems. Comput Ind. 2007;58(1):46–56.
3. Man DWK. Common issues of virtual reality in neuro-rehabilitation. In: Kim J-J, editor. Virtual Real-London. Shanghai: InTech; 2010. p. 419–28.
4. Connelly L, Jia YC, Toro ML, Stoykov ME, Kenyon RV, Kamper DG. A pneumatic glove and immersive virtual reality environment for hand rehabilitative training after stroke. IEEE T Neur Sys Reh. 2010;18(5):551–9.
5. Editorial. Virtual reality is nearly on our doorstep Bangkok, Thailand: The Nation; [cited 2015 20th Apr]. Available from: http://www.nationmultimedia.com/opinion/Virtual-reality-is-nearly-on-our-doorstep-30257950.html.
6. Kye B, Han N, Kim E, Park Y, Jo S. Educational applications of metaverse: possibilities and limitations. J Educ Eval Health Prof. 2021;18:1–13.
7. Holzwarth M, Janiszewski C, Neumann MM. The influence of avatars on online consumer shopping behavior. J Marketing. 2006;70(4):19–36.
8. Nunez J, Krynski L, Otero P. The metaverse in the world of health: the present future. Challenges and opportunities. Arch Argent Pediatr. 2024;122(1):e202202942. https://doi.org/10.5546/aap.2022-02942.eng.
9. Moon HJ, Han S. Perspective: present and future of virtual reality for neurological disorders. Brain Sci. 2022;12(12):6.
10. Allain P, Foloppe DA, Besnard J, Yamaguchi T, Etcharry-Bouyx F, Le Gall D, et al. Detecting everyday action deficits in Alzheimer's disease using a nonimmersive virtual reality kitchen. J Int Neuropsych Soc. 2014;20(5):468–77.
11. Olivieri I, Chiappedi M, Meriggi P, Mazzola M, Grandi A, Angelini L. Rehabilitation of children with hemiparesis: a pilot study on the use of virtual reality. Biomed Res Int. 2013;2013:695935. https://doi.org/10.1155/2013/695935.
12. Sato K, Fukumori S, Matsusaki T, Maruo T, Ishikawa S, Nishie H, et al. Nonimmersive virtual reality mirror visual feedback therapy and its application for the treatment of complex regional pain syndrome: an open-label pilot study. Pain Med. 2010;11(4):622–9.
13. Row H. Codename revolution: The Nintendo Wii platform. New Media Soc. 2015;17(2):312–4.
14. Jones SE, Thiruvathukal GK. Codename revolution: The Nintendo Wii platform. Cambridge, MA: The MIT Press; 2012.
15. Lee JC. Hacking the Nintendo Wii remote. IEEE Pervasive Comput. 2008;7(3):39–45.
16. The TD, Wii N. Technol Rev. 2007;110(4):22–3.
17. Clark RA, Bryant AL, Pua YH, McCrory P, Bennell K, Hunt M. Validity and reliability of the Nintendo Wii balance board for assessment of standing balance. Gait Posture. 2010;31(3):307–10.
18. Sinclair J, Hingston P, Masek M. Considerations for the design of exergames. Graphite 2007: 5th International Conference on Computer Graphics and Interactive Techniques in Australasia and Southern Asia, Proceedings. 2007:289–95.
19. World Health Organization. WHO guidelines on physical activity and sedentary behaviour. Geneva: World Health Organization; 2020.
20. Martinez-Gonzalez MA, Martinez JA, Hu FB, Gibney MJ, Kearney J. Physical inactivity, sedentary lifestyle and obesity in the European Union. Int J Obes Relat Metab Disord. 1999;23(11):1192–201.
21. Sherrington C, Fairhall N, Kwok W, Wallbank G, Tiedemann A, Michaleff ZA, et al. Evidence on physical activity and falls prevention for people aged 65+ years: systematic review to inform the WHO guidelines on physical activity and sedentary behaviour. Int J Behav Nutr Phy. 2020;17(1):144.

22. Graves LEF, Ridgers ND, Williams K, Stratton G, Atkinson G, Cable NT. The physiological cost and enjoyment of Wii fit in adolescents, young adults, and older adults. J Phys Act Health. 2010;7(3):393–401.
23. Guderian B, Borreson LA, Sletten LE, Cable K, Stecker TP, Probst MA, et al. The cardiovascular and metabolic responses to Wii fit video game playing in middle-aged and older adults. J Sport Med Phys Fit. 2010;50(4):436–42.
24. Miyachi M, Yamamoto K, Ohkawara K, Tanaka S. METs in adults while playing active video games: a metabolic chamber study. Med Sci Sport Exer. 2010;42(6):1149–53.
25. Cho GH, Hwangbo G, Shin HS. The effects of virtual reality-based balance training on balance of the elderly. J Phys Ther Sci. 2014;26(4):615–7.
26. Chao YY, Scherer YK, Montgomery CA, Wu Y-W, Lucke KT. Physical and psychosocial effects of Wii fit exergames use in assisted living residents: a pilot study. Clin Nurs Res. 2015;24(6):589–603. https://doi.org/10.1177/1054773814562880.
27. Toulotte C, Toursel C, Olivier N. Wii fit (R) training vs. adapted physical activities: which one is the most appropriate to improve the balance of independent senior subjects? A randomized controlled study. Clin Rehabil. 2012;26(9):827–35.
28. Franco JR, Jacobs K, Inzerillo C, Kluzik J. The effect of the Nintendo Wii fit and exercise in improving balance and quality of life in community dwelling elders. Technol Health Care. 2012;20(2):95–115.
29. Pluchino A, Lee SY, Asfour S, Roos BA, Signorile JF. Pilot study comparing changes in postural control after training using a video game balance board program and 2 standard activity-based balance intervention programs. Arch Phys Med Rehab. 2012;93(7):1138–46.
30. Jung DI, Ko DS, Jeong MA. Kinematic effect of Nintendo Wii(TM) sports program exercise on obstacle gait in elderly women with falling risk. J Phys Ther Sci. 2015;27(5):1397–400.
31. Pacheco TBF, de Medeiros CSP, de Oliveira VHB, Vieira ER, de Cavalcanti FAC. Effectiveness of exergames for improving mobility and balance in older adults: a systematic review and meta-analysis. Syst Rev. 2020;9(1):163.
32. Siriphorn A, Chamonchant D. Wii balance board exercise improves balance and lower limb muscle strength of overweight young adults. J Phys Ther Sci. 2015;27(1):41–6.
33. Chao YY, Scherer YK, Montgomery CA. Effects of using Nintendo Wii exergames in older adults: a review of the literature. J Aging Health. 2015;27(3):379–402.
34. Donnan GA, Fisher M, Macleod M, Davis SM. Stroke. Lancet. 2008;371(9624):1612–23.
35. Langhorne P, Coupar F, Pollock A. Motor recovery after stroke: a systematic review. Lancet Neurol. 2009;8(8):741–54.
36. Laver KE, George S, Thomas S, Deutsch JE, Crotty M. Virtual reality for stroke rehabilitation. Cochrane Database Syst Rev. 2017;11(11):CD008349. https://doi.org/10.1002/14651858.CD008349.pub4.
37. Bower KJ, Clark RA, McGinley JL, Martin CL, Miller KJ. Clinical feasibility of the Nintendo Wii (TM) for balance training post-stroke: a phase II randomized controlled trial in an inpatient setting. Clin Rehabil. 2014;28(9):912–23.
38. Barcala L, Grecco LAC, Colella F, Lucareli PRG, Salgado ASI, Oliveira CS. Visual biofeedback balance training using Wii fit after stroke: a randomized controlled trial. J Phys Ther Sci. 2013;25(8):1027–32.
39. Hung JW, Chou CX, Hsieh YW, Wu WC, Yu MY, Chen PC, et al. Randomized comparison trial of balance training by using exergaming and conventional weight-shift therapy in patients with chronic stroke. Arch Phys Med Rehab. 2014;95(9):1629–37.
40. World Health Organization. Parkinson disease: a public health approach. Technical brief. Geneva: World Health Organization; 2022. Licence: CC BY-NC-SA 3.0 IGO.]. Available from: https://www.who.int/news-room/fact-sheets/detail/parkinson-disease
41. Pelicioni PHS, Menant JC, Latt MD, Lord SR. Falls in Parkinson's disease subtypes: risk factors, locations and circumstances. Int J Environ Res Public Health. 2019;16(12):2216. https://doi.org/10.3390/ijerph16122216.

42. Fox CM, Ramig LO, Ciucci MR, Sapir S, McFarland DH, Farley BG. The science and practice of LSVT/LOUD: neural plasticity-principled approach to treating individuals with Parkinson disease and other neurological disorders. Semin Speech Lang. 2006;27(4):283–99.
43. Esculier JF, Vaudrin J, Beriault P, Gagnon K, Tremblay LE. Home-based balance training programme using Wii fit with balance Board for Parkinson's disease: a pilot study. J Rehabil Med. 2012;44(2):144–50.
44. Gonçalves GB, Leite MA, Orsini M, Pereira JS. Effects of using the Nintendo Wii fit plus platform in the sensorimotor training of gait disorders in Parkinson's disease. Neurol Int. 2014;6(1):5048.
45. Ferraz DD, Trippo K, Dominguez A, Santos A, Oliveira J. Nintendo Wii training on postural balance and mobility rehabilitation of adults with Parkinson's disease: a systematic review. Fisioterapia em Movimento. 2017;30:1–11.
46. Shahhar AZM, Qasheesh M, Shaphe MA. Effectiveness of Nintendo Wii on balance in people with Parkinson's disease: a systematic review. J Lifestyle Med. 2022;12(3):105–12.
47. Ribas CG, Alves da Silva L, Corrêa MR, Teive HG, Valderramas S. Effectiveness of exergaming in improving functional balance, fatigue and quality of life in Parkinson's disease: a pilot randomized controlled trial. Parkinsonism Relat Disord. 2017;38:13–8.
48. Santos P, Machado T, Santos L, Ribeiro N, Melo A. Efficacy of the Nintendo Wii combination with conventional exercises in the rehabilitation of individuals with Parkinson's disease: a randomized clinical trial. NeuroRehabilitation. 2019;45(2):255–63.
49. Lee NY, Lee DK, Song HS. Effect of virtual reality dance exercise on the balance, activities of daily living, and depressive disorder status of Parkinson's disease patients. J Phys Ther Sci. 2015;27(1):145–7.
50. Prosperini L, Tomassini V, Castelli L, Tacchino A, Brichetto G, Cattaneo D, et al. Exergames for balance dysfunction in neurological disability: a meta-analysis with meta-regression. J Neurol. 2021;268(9):3223–37.
51. Thomson K, Pollock A, Bugge C, Brady M. Commercial gaming devices for stroke upper limb rehabilitation: a systematic review. Int J Stroke. 2014;9(4):479–88.
52. Pietrzah E, Cotea C, Pullman S. Using commercial video games for upper limb stroke rehabilitation: is this the way of the future? Top Stroke Rehabil. 2014;21(2):152–62.
53. Deutsch JE, Brettler A, Smith C, Welsh J, John R, Guarrera-Bowlby P, et al. Nintendo Wii sports and Wii fit game analysis, validation, and application to stroke rehabilitation. Top Stroke Rehabil. 2011;18(6):701–19.
54. Schmidt RA, Lee TD. Motor learning and performance. From principles to application. 5th ed. Champaign, IL: Human Kinetics; 2014.
55. Taub E, Miller NE, Novack TA, Cook EW, Fleming WC, Nepomuceno CS, et al. Technique to improve chronic motor deficit after stroke. Arch Phys Med Rehab. 1993;74(4):347–54.
56. Krakauer JW. Motor learning: its relevance to stroke recovery and neurorehabilitation. Curr Opin Neurol. 2006;19(1):84–90.
57. Hakkennes S, Keating JL. Constraint-induced movement therapy following stroke: a systematic review of randomised controlled trials. Aust J Physiother. 2005;51(4):221–31.
58. Mendes FAS, Pompeu JE, Lobo AM, da Silva KG, Oliveira TP, Zomignani AP, et al. Motor learning, retention and transfer after virtual-reality-based training in Parkinson's disease—effect of motor and cognitive demands of games: a longitudinal, controlled clinical study. Physiotherapy. 2012;98(3):217–23.
59. Adamovich SV, August K, Merians A, Tunik E. A virtual reality-based system integrated with fmri to study neural mechanisms of action observation-execution: a proof of concept study. Restor Neurol Neuros. 2009;27(3):209–23.
60. You SH, Jang SH, Kim YH, Hallett M, Ahn SH, Kwon YH, et al. Virtual reality-induced cortical reorganization and associated locomotor recovery in chronic stroke. An experimenter-blind randomized study. Stroke. 2005;36(6):1166–71.

61. Orihuela-Espina F, del Castillo IF, Palafox L, Pasaye E, Sanchez-Villavicencio I, Leder R, et al. Neural reorganization accompanying upper limb motor rehabilitation from stroke with virtual reality-based gesture therapy. Top Stroke Rehabil. 2013;20(3):197–209.
62. Omiyale O, Crowell CR, Madhavan S. Effect of Wii-based balance training on corticomotor excitability post stroke. J Motor Behav. 2015;47(3):190–200.

Towards Context-Aware Free-Living Digital Biomarkers for Gait Assessment

28

Jason Moore, Samuel Stuart, Peter Mcmeekin,
Richard Walker, and Alan Godfrey

Abstract

Inertial measurement units (IMUs) have emerged as popular tools for gait related fall risk analysis due to their low cost, portability, and ability to capture spatial and temporal gait characteristics (e.g., step length and step time, respectively). Free-living analysis using IMUs is an unobtrusive means for wearers to perform daily activities without being confined to a lab setting, enabling habitual data capture. However, the lack of absolute contextual factors in IMU data poses challenges in interpreting gait characteristics accurately. Factors such as terrain, environmental obstacles or even weather conditions can significantly influence gait characteristics and arising fall risk. To address this limitation, wearable cameras have been integrated with IMUs to provide absolute context. Wearable cameras can capture a participant's near complete environment context, enabling researchers to examine video data with corresponding IMU data to determine cause of abnormal gait characteristics such as high step time variability. Although

J. Moore · A. Godfrey (✉)
Department of Computer and Information Sciences, Northumbria University,
Newcastle upon Tyne, UK
e-mail: jason.moore@northumbria.ac.uk; alan.godfrey@northumbria.ac.uk

S. Stuart
Department of Sport, Exercise and Rehabilitation, Northumbria University,
Newcastle upon Tyne, UK

Department of Neurology, Oregon Health and Science University, Portland, Oregon, USA
e-mail: samuel2.stuart@northumbria.ac.uk

P. Mcmeekin
Department of Nursing and Midwifery, Northumbria University, Newcastle upon Tyne, UK
e-mail: peter.mcmeekin@northumbria.ac.uk

R. Walker
Northumbria Healthcare NHS Foundation Trust, North Tyneside, UK
e-mail: richard.walker@northumbria-healthcare.nhs.uk

F. A. Barbieri et al. (eds.), *Locomotion and Posture in Older Adults*,
https://doi.org/10.1007/978-3-031-74123-4_28

wearable cameras offer enhanced contextual information, concerns regarding the time-consuming process of manual review and privacy remain. Machine learning and computer vision techniques show promise in automating the review process and upholding privacy. Incorporating wearable video cameras and advanced algorithms could provide a comprehensive understanding of gait patterns and potential fall risks in free-living analysis.

Introduction

Wearable inertial measurement units (IMUs) are increasingly popular tools for fall risk assessment arising from gait analysis [1]. That is facilitated by their general low cost, portability, and ability to track spatial and temporal gait characteristics such as step length, step time, and cadence in an unobtrusive and efficient manner across a wide timeframe from hours to days [2]. Specifically, IMU-based gait has been used to assess fall risk by measuring asymmetry and variability of spatial and temporal characteristics [2–4]. Typically, fall risk assessment through gait analysis has been performed within the lab. However, key limitations with that approach are (i) the testing environment itself, i.e., a safe lab with little probability of replicating a real world scenario to elicit increased fall risk and (ii) Hawthorne effect, i.e., a participant may walk more optimally when not being observed [3]. To address this issue, free-living analysis using IMUs has become popular, as it allows participants to go about their daily activities, which can provide more informative gait data and better insight to fall risk. However, one challenge of free-living analysis still to be overcome is the lack of contextual information available from the IMU data, making it difficult to determine if observed gait patterns are due to (i) an intrinsic neurological condition(s) or (ii) external environmental factor(s), e.g., tripping hazard. This limitation is due to the inherent "blindness" of IMUs, being that they can provide numerical output of movement but are not capable of providing any insight into the environment in which a participant was navigating at the time. Researchers have aimed to address this limitation using an array of methodologies with the two stand outs being the addition of global positioning system (GPS) devices and the use of wearable cameras to provide additional context to IMU data. While the latter approach has shown promise, there are concerns pertaining to (i) the time-consuming manual review of arising videos and (ii) privacy of the video footage. The following chapter will aim to expand on these issues by providing insight to the current state of research within the field.

IMU-Based Gait Analysis

Prior to the use of IMUs, multiple different technologies such as instrumented walkways [5, 6] or three dimensional (3D) motion capture systems [7, 8] were the defacto for lab-based objective/digital gait assessment. However, those technologies are only applicable within high-resource settings requiring purpose-built labs. The introduction of IMUs has enabled lab-based assessment within a much wider context such as low resource settings. Given the highly portable nature of IMUs, perhaps the key advantage to the integrations of IMUs into gait-based fall risk assessments is their ability to perform habitual data capture from free-living (i.e., everyday) environments.

IMUs typically consist of a combination of accelerometers and gyroscope inertial sensors that can track the orientation and motion of body segments where they are attached [9–11]. Accordingly, inertial sensors have become popular for gait analysis when attached to the lower limbs or waist level [2, 4]. Moreover, IMUs have the ability for wider integration to other peripheral technologies to enable data to be recorded in, e.g., real time in a non-invasive and unobtrusive manner [12]. Current state of the art recommends use of a single IMU worn on the lower back (primarily to ease patient burden) to capture 14 clinically relevant characteristics, aligning to four domains of gait which help aid interpretation and enable possible use in rehabilitation [13, 14].

Free-Living Analysis

Use of IMUs beyond the lab in a free-living context provides a more natural approach to the collection of inertial gait data. That is because the person being assessed is removed from a simulated situation (i.e., scripted lab protocol) while being observed. Accordingly, the person could walk more optimally compared to normal/habitual behaviours in their home and local community. In the context of gait analysis, any altered behaviour could mean unnatural gait characteristics and an inaccurate estimation of fall risk. To date, there is evidence showing that spatial and temporal gait characteristics differ between lab and free-living environment [15], but notable challenges must still be overcome.

IMUs for free-living gait analysis are typically used with high-resolution data capture. That means a very large acquisition of data such as 100 data points/second (i.e., 100 Hertz/Hz) on three planes of movement (sagittal, frontal, and transverse) which defines motion sensing on three axes (mediolateral, anteroposterior, and longitudinal, respectively) [10]. That equates to 300 data points/second. Typically, a person will wear an IMU for 7 days to gather a broad spectrum of behaviours to better inform spatial and temporal characteristics. Accordingly, more than 181 million data points would be collected. This creates a notable challenge to *mine* those data to (i) identify and extract periods of walking before (ii) analysing those extracted periods to quantify spatial and temporal gait characteristics, but approaches exist [16, 17]. Current analytical approaches generally examine statistical outcomes while considering all extracted periods but that is limited as it fails to account for the absolute context during which walks were conducted. For example, during the 7-day data capture period, many extracted gait bouts could have been conducted while walking: (i) with another person and so there may be a deliberate increase or decrease in walking speed; (ii) in very busy environments where the person's gait is forced to be erratic to avoid other pedestrians or obstacles. Accordingly, the field of free-living gait analysis must better understand the extrinsic (environmental) factors which negatively impact gait. Quantifying and understanding extrinsic factors will help better understand intrinsic limitations and arising fall risk [3, 18].

Lack of Contextual Information

Figure 28.1 shows typical IMU accelerometer-based data along the longitudinal axis while worn on the lower back. The data are rich with information pertaining to macro- as well as micro-movements due to the capture frequency (100 Hz). To extract spatial and temporal gait characteristics, several algorithms exist for use with an IMU worn on the lower back [19–21], helping translate raw data (Fig. 28.1a and c) to secondary signals (Fig. 28.1b and d) and arising characteristics such as step time, stance time, and step length as well as subsequent variability and asymmetry outcomes. The process whereby raw IMU data (gathered from the lower back) is translated into useful characteristics is described in detail elsewhere [22] but in short, the raw accelerometer data is filtered twice to derive two signals (Fig. 28.1b and d, red and blue trace) whereby the identification of peaks and troughs (Fig. 28.1b and d, red *x*'s and blue *o*'s) equate to initial contact (IC) and final contact (FC) events. Timed identification of IC's and FC's

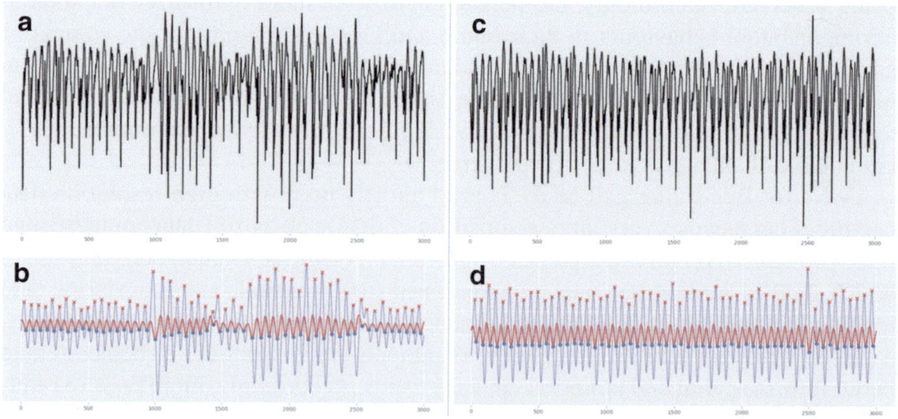

Fig. 28.1 Translating raw IMU data (top) to meaningful points of interest relating to phases of the gait cycle (bottom) from 3000 data points (i.e., 30 s from 100 Hz). Specifically, (**a**) raw accelerometer data acquired from the lower back about the longitudinal axis and (**b**) filtered versions of the acceleration to generate new signals where the peaks and troughs correspond to initial contact and final contact timed events within the gait cycle. (**c**) is a gait period of raw accelerometer data and (**d**) filtered signals but appears more stable (i.e., less erratic). Without understanding the context such as environmental information, complete interpretation of the gait characteristic remains limited. What cause the erratic raw data in (a), was it due to an extrinsic or intrinsic factor?

help estimate step length, step time, stance time, and swing time due to their sequence within one gait cycle [23, 24]. Subsequently, an array of those characteristics captured during a period of walking leads to variability and asymmetry outcomes [25]. All contribute to a thorough understanding of gait and possible fall risk [14].

Accordingly, raw IMU data are extremely useful, but those data alone fail to provide thorough insights as to why any abnormality may arise. Equally, little can be categorically concluded from IC and FC events which may lead to erratic spatial and temporal characteristics. The latter may be deemed to be erratic when compared to ground truth values gathered from the same person in the lab or to normative values in the literature [26]. Examining Fig. 28.1b, why do the amplitudes of the signals/traces fluctuate? For more insight, Fig. 28.2 shows raw accelerometer data and filtered signals from another period of walking but with context. Although algorithms can be applied to both periods of raw data (Fig. 28.1a and c) with gait characteristics quantified, how should both periods be interpreted? Lack of contextual information makes it impossible to determine why the signals fluctuate and why any arising characteristic may seem erratic. Perhaps, IMU data could be complimented with questionnaire and self-reports to try and understand where someone was walking but given the possible number of variables and clarity needed that is not a realistic solution.

Wearable cameras (e.g., GoPro https://gopro.com) have been used to provide insight to free-living gait and compensatory balance reactions [27, 28] but their use remains limited due to size and means of attachment via belts/straps. Moreover, that camera modality could often have the high probability of drawing attention to the wearer meaning lack of adherence during extended wear time. Alternatively, Moore et al. proposed a more contemporary and ergonomic approach by exploring use of video-based tracking glasses [18]. It was suggested that use of that mode of technology could be more user friendly by being a routine donning of a typical accessory worn during daily life. More importantly, video data from the environment could be captured to better inform IMU data while also providing eye-tracking data to examine where the person is looking. That additional means of data capture could help further identify extrinsic and/or intrinsic factors leading to fall risk.

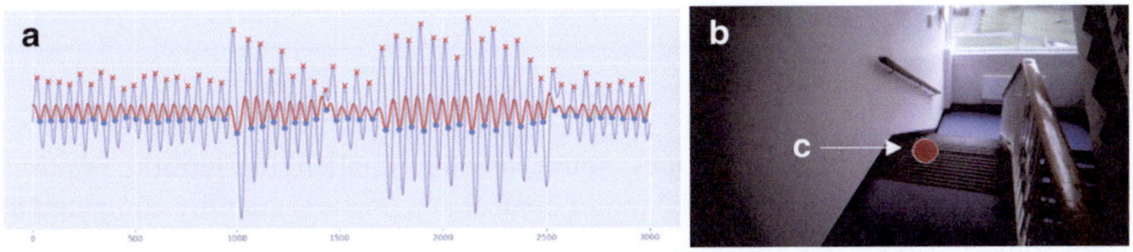

Fig. 28.2 (**a**) context provided for apparent abnormal gait fluctuations, (**b**) explained through stair descent, (**c**) additional eye-tracking data from video glasses provides further details which may help free-living fall risk assessment

Wearable Video-Based Eye-Tracking Glasses

Glasses also offer participants greater "control" as they are much easier to take on and off during periods of recording than having to detach an entire harness. These devices can capture a first-person view of the participant's environment, providing valuable and absolute context to the gait data attained at a specific time point when synchronised to the IMU. Specifically, the exact moment an erratic gait characteristic is captured can be directly matched to the environment at that time. Videos could be reviewed alongside IMU data to determine if observed gait patterns are due to intrinsic or external factors [18]. For example, if high gait variability is quantified during a period of walking, the corresponding video could determine if the person is either walking (i) indoors on a smooth/level terrain or (ii) outdoors on a rocky surface. If the person was indoor on level terrain, then that could allude to some underlying intrinsic factor at that time because their gait variability should be low in that environment and on that terrain. Alternatively, if the person was outdoor and on a challenging terrain, then high gait variability was likely due to an extrinsic factor. Accordingly, absolute clarity on erratic gait characteristics may ultimately help fall prevention strategies [1].

Wearable video glasses could also provide additional information. For instance, the video could provide information on whether the participant is walking on an icy surface or increasing their pace due to precipitation [27]. Equally, whether the participant is walking in a crowded space and having to safely navigate pedestrians or other obstacles that cross their path. This additional context can help researchers better understand why certain gait patterns occur and why certain conditions may increase their fall risk. However, a notable advantage of wearable video capture glasses with embedded eye-tracking capabilities is to provide further context by understanding exactly where a person was looking (their attention) during a period of erratic gait and subsequent elevated fall risk [29]. This mechanism may also help understanding the causes of falls as when performing longer-term free-living analysis, any falls that do occur can have the proceeding footage meticulously analysed for effects such as missed obstacles and the effect it had on the participants gait. This could be especially significant when navigating stairs or pavements and whether the participant was paying attention to the step [30, 31]. Additionally, the technology may be useful to determine what environmental visual cues aid gait and reduce fall risk (e.g., stripes on steps).

Terrain

Walking on uneven surfaces, slopes, stairs, or other challenging terrains imposes additional demands on individuals' motor control and postural stability compared to level walking [32]. Therefore, gait characteristics can vary substantially depending on terrain. Individuals intuitively adjust their gait patterns and adopt specific strategies to navigate different terrains to maintain stability. For instance, they may alter step length, increase step width, or modify gait speed to adapt to uneven or challenging surfaces [27, 33–35]. Considering terrain in free-living gait analysis is critically important to enhance the accuracy and ecological validity of fall risk prediction models. Identifying high-risk terrains or situations could better guide interpretation of gait and targeted interventions, such as gait re-training, balance exercises, or environmental modifications, to mitigate fall risk [36–40].

Previously, GPS devices have been proposed [41] to inform context relating to terrain identification but the approach is flawed due to reliance on third party data pertaining to geographic maps (which could be outdated and not representative of true terrain type) and poor spatial resolution (e.g., 5 m in the UK and 30 m elsewhere). Moreover, the poor resolution will fail to categorically identify new trip hazards such as uneven pavements. Alternatively, machine learning algorithms being applied to the raw IMU signals [42] to the embedding of GPS sensors used in conjunction with satellite imagery [41]. The latter have shown some success in giving accurate estimates of a participant's terrain from ground truth dataset but fails again to provide the required wider and absolute context.

When aiming to provide a well-rounded and high-resolution description of an environment the only suitable methodology is wearable cameras. Previously in this chapter, Fig. 28.1 drew attention to gait assessment without context, two periods, where Fig. 28.1a seems erratic compared to Fig. 28.1b. By augmenting those plots with video data from wearable video-based eye-tracking glasses much more insight is provided, see Fig. 28.2. In this instance, the erratic signals can be explained by the wearer's natural response to an extrinsic factor, i.e., descending stairs. Moreover, the eye-tracking component (Fig. 28.2c) helps provide extra/additional insight. Here, the eye-tracker objectively shows how the person identifies the edge of the upcoming first step, signifying that they have recognised, and are preparing to navigate steps which could help inform free-living fall risk assessment. Weerdesteyn et al previously discussed gait adaptability in relation to manoeuvre planning and described the importance of *looking ahead* to ensure one has sufficient time to plan the type of gait adaptation needed to accommodate environmental demands [43].

Environmental Factors: Hazards and Obstacles

Environmental hazards (e.g., curbs, steps, stairs, uneven surfaces, low/dim lighting) and obstacles (e.g., crowds, animals, furniture) pose challenges for safe gait and therefore increased fall risk. Negotiating both may require individuals to adapt their routine gait pattern [44–46]. An inability to adapt gait to hazards and obstacles may be a manifestation of selectivity and motor control impairments [47]. For example, those with cerebral palsy do not alter their ankle and foot motion [48] while those with Parkinson's disease (PD) present increased gait asymmetry during single obstacle crossing compared to unobstructed walking [49]. Accordingly, it is critical to fully understand environmental factors when quantifying gait to derive absolute certainty from free-living assessment to inform fall risk, particularly in those with gait impairments. Objective clarification of all environmental factors through video data could be used to better interpret IMU gait and what could be better described as reactive adaptions (slips, trips) or proactive adaptions such as navigation and route planning, manoeuvre planning, obstacle crossing, turning, and stair ambulation [43].

Weather Conditions

While terrain and environmental hazards pose the most immediate alterations to a participants gait, other factors such as generalised weather conditions like rain (slippery surfaces) and snow can exacerbate gait instability and elevate fall risk [50]. Individuals may have difficulty maintaining balance and traction on wet or icy surfaces, leading to gait instability [51, 52]. Moreover, extreme temperatures can affect individuals' physical and cognitive functioning [53], potentially compromising gait stability, and increasing fall risk. Cold temperatures may increase gait speed, while hot temperatures can lead to fatigue and decreased gait speed [54]. Considering seasonal variations in gait analysis may be crucial in developing personalised fall prevention strategies tailored to specific weather conditions [55]. Awareness of the challenges posed by different weather conditions enables healthcare professionals to implement targeted interventions and environmental modifications. For example, during periods of inclement weather, individuals may benefit from using assistive devices, wearing appropriate footwear, or modifying their walking routes to avoid slippery surfaces [56]. That could be best informed from IMU gait and video eye-tracking data capture.

Providing Context

The key extrinsic (environmental) factors that could negatively influence free-living gait characteristics are listed. Wearable eye-tracking video glasses could be an appropriate mechanism to provide context to IMU gait, in a nonobtrusive and ergonomic manner. The next question is how can context from video-based glasses be achieved?

Wearable Cameras

Wearable cameras could solve many issues, but some key challenges exist such as privacy and timeliness of analysis [57, 58]. Within free-living video capture, recording a person's view for an extended period can be invasive to privacy, and the use of such devices must be ethically justified. Participants must give their informed consent and be informed about the risks such as gathering of video data during very personal moments or capture of financial information. Timeliness of analysis is more a pragmatic issue pertaining to the manual reviewing of video footage. With current practices a researcher is required to watch and manually label every relevant aspect of the video, such as describing terrain, hazards, and obstacles. The manual process can be extremely time-consuming. In some cases, manual review can take two to three times longer than the actual length of the video. With current practices of manual review and privacy concerns, studies spanning many participants may not be feasible. However, recent advances in hardware and machine learning technologies are beginning to provide solutions to these challenges.

Machine Learning and Computer Vision

Object detection is a crucial task in the field of computer vision that aims to automatically identify and locate objects of interest within images or video frames [59, 60]. This technology has gained significant attention due to its diverse applications, ranging from autonomous vehicles [61] and surveillance systems [62] to medical imaging [63] and gait analysis. One popular family of object detection algorithms is the Region-based convolutional neural networks (R-CNNs) approach [59]. These algorithms work in two steps: First, they propose potential regions in an image that might contain objects. Then, they classify and refine these proposed regions to accurately detect the objects. Although effective, R-CNN methods can be computationally intensive, making real-time applications challenging in certain cases. To address the speed issue, Single Shot Multibox Detector (SSD) [64] and You Only Look Once (YOLO) [60] were introduced. These are known as one-stage detectors because they directly predict object categories and their bounding boxes without requiring the two-step process of region proposals. SSD and YOLO are faster and more efficient, making them suitable for real-time object detection tasks. They have found applications in various areas, including robotics, surveillance, and human movement analysis.

YOLO stands out for its simplicity and speed. It treats object detection as a regression problem and divides the input image into a grid. For each grid cell, YOLO predicts bounding boxes and class probabilities, making it highly efficient. This approach enables YOLO to process images in real-time without sacrificing accuracy significantly. YOLO has undergone several improvements over time, leading to versions like YOLOv4 [65] and YOLOv8 [66], which have enhanced performance and usability. Recent developments within the field of machine learning based computer vision are beginning to show promise in their ability to successfully alleviate many of the issues presented within manual review [67–70]. Contemporary machine learning computer vision algorithms are presenting strong accuracies within tasks like automated detection of obstacles and hazards within a participants view, which when implemented with eye-tracking glasses can automatically detect the overlap between objects and eye location enabling the inference of what a participant is paying attention to. Not only is the automation of this task being accomplished but also the greater and greater efforts into improving the efficiencies of these models [66, 71] mean this automated process can be ran over the course of a video automatically labelling the potential objects / hazards within view in real time [66] drastically reducing the time required to review these videos. This processing time is also dependant on the capabilities of the machine processing the data, meaning more advanced machines could process these videos in as little as a quarter of the length of a given video.

Terrain Detection

Some of the first applications of machine learning and computer vision within free-living gait analysis were the automated contextualisation of surrounding terrain detection. To begin, a model was proposed that utilised wearable cameras aimed directly down at the feet attached at the waist [27]. The proposed model would then iterate over the video frame by frame classifying current terrain type from pavement, gravel, grass, soil, snow, wood, indoor tiles, and high friction materials. Extending from this, a further model was proposed to achieve the same aims but from a first-person perspective using wearable video glasses [72]. This approach, while more challenging, opened the wider context of a participants environment allowing opportunities to investigate areas like eye tracking or external effects on gait such as doorways and stairs [18].

Automated Contextualisation

Moving forward from just the detection of terrain is the automated classification of the wider context a participant navigates within. This is a very challenging task to overcome given the sheer number of variables at play when aiming to classify "everything" within a scene [73, 74]. The first steps into this field have been conducted within free-living based environments across a small cohort of participants utilising wearable eye-tracking glasses. The model showed promising accuracy at detecting the different assortment of objects within the scene (people, obstacles, chair, table, etc.) and more importantly was able to automatically detect what the participant was looking at across the frames and what was in the immediate walking path (Fig. 28.3). While this work showcased the first steps into providing a framework for automating the context of a participant's environment it is preliminary with much more to be done.

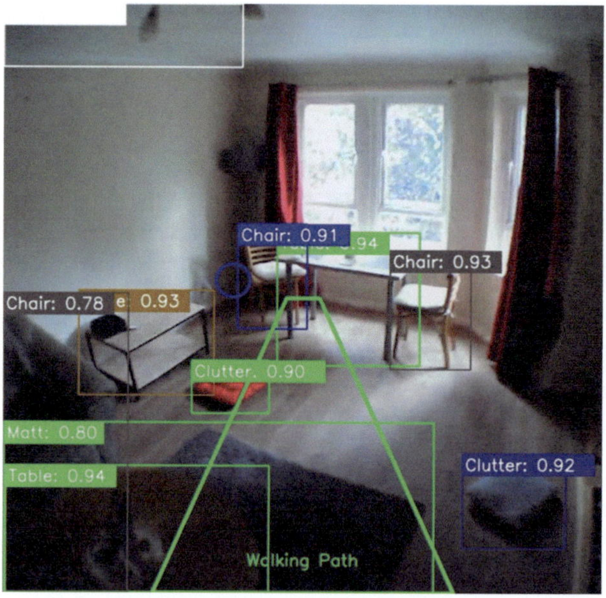

Fig. 28.3 Example output from object detection model showcasing detection of objects and participants attention from blue eye-tracking circle (centre)

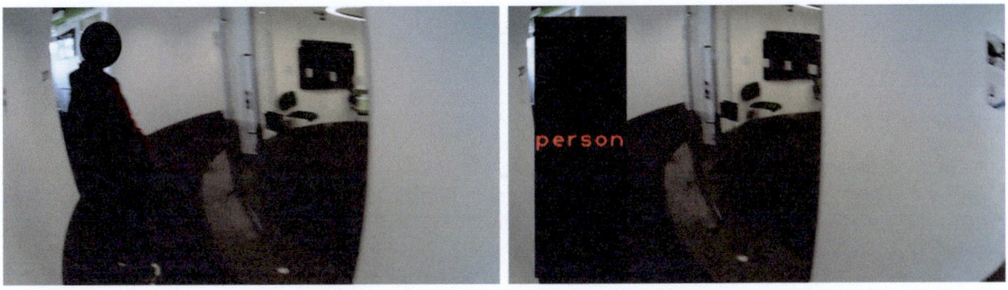

Fig. 28.4 Example output from model used for contextualisation while also applying anonymisation features. Left shows input image to model, right shows output from the model (to preserve privacy the left input image has had face manually removed)

Privacy Protection

Capturing videos within people's own homes creates a huge challenge to overcome, i.e., privacy. While previous studies have relied on manual review of video captured within the home [18, 75], the two main issues of this approach were firstly the cumbersome and time intensive task of manually reviewing all footage and annotating context [75, 76]. Secondly, the serious privacy implications of watching back a participant conduct their normal daily activities. Through use of the AI methodologies discussed here, both issues can be alleviated. As already discussed, due to the increasing efficiencies of object detection algorithms these videos can be processed in real time (≈x3 times faster than manual review) [72] but more importantly the ethical concern of having a human playback the footage is removed as the AI becomes a black-box approach taking in the video and providing output without need for any human intervention. Interestingly, the same algorithms used for detecting the objects within the scene can also be used to provide clinicians with an anonymised version of the video with all sensitive areas blurred out to allow for ethical playback if required, Fig. 28.4.

Synchronisation

Detailed are the potential solutions to context-aware free-living gait analysis using wearable cameras. However, an important aspect to consider is how the two data streams are synchronised. To date, no best practice has been decided upon, however, with typical IMU's (100 Hz) providing millisecond level timestamps and the video files stemming from wearable cameras containing metadata such as the time the video was created at, the process of synchronising data streams remains trivial. Subjectively, beginning IMU capture before video capture is more convenient due to the more granular resolution of the sensors and the ability to place markers within the signal for alignment. For example, having a participant stand completely still before beginning video capture, Fig. 28.5.

This method of alignment not only makes finding the timepoint within an IMU signal that video capture began an easier endeavour but is also more accurate than solely relying on the metadata provided by the video file itself.

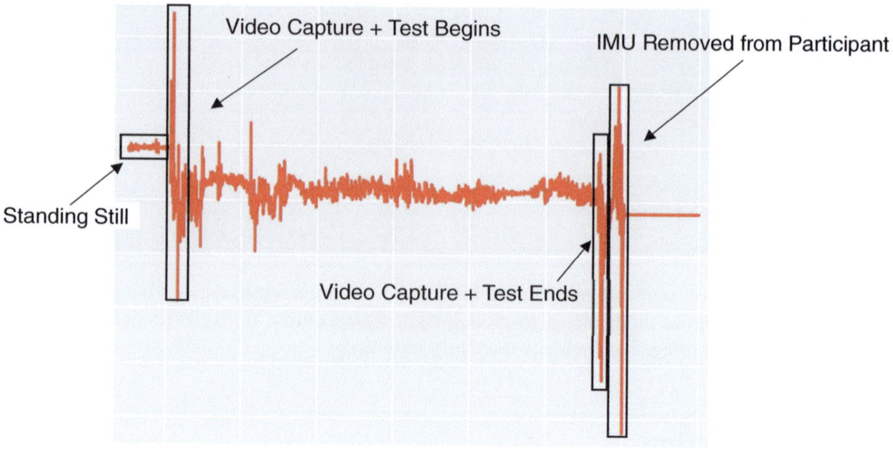

Fig. 28.5 Example output from model used for contextualisation also applying anonymisation features

Step Time	Stance Time	Stride Time	Swing Time	Step Length	Environment	Terrain	Looking At	Within View	Conditions	Temperature
0.55	0.68	1.09	0.38	1.012635	Indoor	Wood	Person	Stairs, Person, Person, Phone	Sunny	20
0.54	0.68	1.11	0.41	1.169108	Indoor	Wood	Person	Stairs, Person, Person, Phone	Sunny	20
0.57	0.76	1.39	0.43	0.979038	Indoor	Wood	Person	Stairs, Person, Person, Phone	Sunny	20
0.82	0.99	1.42	0.63	1.409842	Indoor	Wood	Person	Stairs, Person, Person, Phone	Sunny	20
0.6	0.74	1.21	0.43	1.056472	Indoor	Wood	Person	Stairs, Person, Person, Phone	Sunny	20
0.61	0.77	1.23	0.47	1.129478	Indoor	Wood	Person	Stairs, Person, Person, Phone	Sunny	20

Fig. 28.6 Example output showing resulting CSV file upon video processing completion

Output

With inertial and contextual information synchronised, a pipeline is instantiated and begins to iterate over the provided video. A computer programme is given the video in its standard .mp4 format along with the array of inertial data pertaining to that specific video [72]. After the current video frame has propagated throughout the network, all aspects of necessary context will be stored before moving onto the next video frame. After the entire video has been processed, a finalised CSV file will be available for review, containing all relevant spatio-temporal characteristics along with a high-level overview of the context the participant was navigating within at the specified timepoint (Fig. 28.6).

Alongside, if specified, a new MP4 video will also be available to the clinician containing the original video but with all identified sensitive objects anonymised (Fig. 28.4).

Conclusion

Gait analysis using IMUs has become the de facto method of instrumentation. IMUs provide a valuable tool for assessing gait patterns and fall risk, both within the lab and in free-living analysis. Free-living analysis allows participants to engage in their daily activities, providing a more natural and holistic view of their gait patterns. However, a significant limitation of free-living analysis is the lack of contextual information provided by IMUs. This limitation, referred to as "blindness," hinders the absolute interpretation of gait data and the identification of external factors influencing gait patterns. Several external factors play a crucial role in gait analysis, including terrain, environmental obstacles and hazards, and weather conditions. Terrain variability can significantly influence gait characteristics [18, 75, 76], and individuals adapt their gait patterns to navigate different terrains and maintain stability. Environmental obstacles and hazards, such as curbs or crowded areas, also impact gait stability and safety. Weather conditions, including rain, snow, extreme temperatures, and slippery surfaces, exacerbate fall risk factors and pose challenges to gait stability.

To address the lack of contextual information, researchers have explored various methodologies [77, 78], including the use of GPS sensors and wearable cameras. GPS sensors provide information about the participant's general location and can offer some insights into terrain and outdoor/indoor environments. However, they lack granularity for more specific indicators. Alternatively, wearable cameras, such as head-mounted video capture glasses [18, 75], can provide a first-person view of the participant's environment, offering valuable context to IMU data. Combining IMU data with wearable video footage allows researchers to better understand why certain gait patterns occur and differentiate between intrinsic neurological conditions and external factors. With current advances within machine learning based computer vision algorithms, methodologies are beginning to be developed to provide the absolute context necessary to begin analysing this contextual information in a privacy focused and efficient manner. Considering the contextual information, such as terrain, environmental obstacles, weather conditions, and time of day, is essential in developing personalised fall prevention strategies and optimising gait stability. Understanding how these factors influence gait patterns and fall risk enables healthcare professionals to implement targeted interventions and environmental modifications.

References

1. Godfrey A. Wearables for independent living in older adults: gait and falls. Maturitas. 2017;100:16–26.
2. Del Din S, Godfrey A, Mazzà C, Lord S, Rochester L. Free-living monitoring of Parkinson's disease: lessons from the field. Mov Disord. 2016;31(9):1293–313.
3. Nouredanesh M, Godfrey A, Howcroft J, Lemaire ED, Tung J. Fall risk assessment in the wild: a critical examination of wearable sensor use in free-living conditions. Gait Posture. 2021;85:178–90.
4. Celik Y, Stuart S, Woo WL, Godfrey A. Gait analysis in neurological populations: progression in the use of wearables. Med Eng Phys. 2021;87:9–29.
5. Cutlip RG, Mancinelli C, Huber F, DiPasquale J. Evaluation of an instrumented walkway for measurement of the kinematic parameters of gait. Gait Posture. 2000;12(2):134–8.
6. Van Uden CJ, Besser MP. Test-retest reliability of temporal and spatial gait characteristics measured with an instrumented walkway system (GAITRite®). BMC Musculoskelet Disord. 2004;5(1):1–4.

7. Pfister A, West AM, Bronner S, Noah JA. Comparative abilities of Microsoft Kinect and Vicon 3D motion capture for gait analysis. J Med Eng Technol. 2014;38(5):274–80.
8. Rucco R, Agosti V, Jacini F, Sorrentino P, Varriale P, De Stefano M, et al. Spatio-temporal and kinematic gait analysis in patients with frontotemporal dementia and Alzheimer's disease through 3D motion capture. Gait Posture. 2017;52:312–7.
9. Jarchi D, Pope J, Lee TK, Tamjidi L, Mirzaei A, Sanei S. A review on accelerometry-based gait analysis and emerging clinical applications. IEEE Rev Biomed Eng. 2018;11:177–94.
10. Godfrey A, Conway R, Meagher D, ÓLaighin G. Direct measurement of human movement by accelerometry. Med Eng Phys. 2008;30(10):1364–86.
11. Hutabarat Y, Owaki D, Hayashibe M. Quantitative gait assessment with feature-rich diversity using two IMU sensors. IEEE Trans Med Robot Bionics. 2020;2(4):639–48.
12. Young F, Mason R, Morris RE, Stuart S, Godfrey A. IoT-enabled gait assessment: the next step for habitual monitoring. Sensors. 2023;23(8):4100.
13. Morris R, Hickey A, Del Din S, Godfrey A, Lord S, Rochester L. A model of free-living gait: a factor analysis in Parkinson's disease. Gait Posture. 2017;52:68–71.
14. Morris R, Lord S, Bunce J, Burn D, Rochester L. Gait and cognition: mapping the global and discrete relationships in ageing and neurodegenerative disease. Neurosci Biobehav Rev. 2016;64:326–45.
15. Del Din S, Godfrey A, Galna B, Lord S, Rochester L. Free-living gait characteristics in ageing and Parkinson's disease: impact of environment and ambulatory bout length. J Neuroeng Rehabil. 2016;13(1):1–12.
16. Hickey A, Del Din S, Rochester L, Godfrey A. Detecting free-living steps and walking bouts: validating an algorithm for macro gait analysis. Physiol Meas. 2016;38(1):N1.
17. Weiss A, Brozgol M, Dorfman M, Herman T, Shema S, Giladi N, et al. Does the evaluation of gait quality during daily life provide insight into fall risk? A novel approach using 3-day accelerometer recordings. Neurorehabil Neural Repair. 2013;27(8):742–52.
18. Moore J, Stuart S, McMeekin P, Walker R, Celik Y, Pointon M, et al. Enhancing free-living fall risk assessment: contextualizing mobility based IMU data. Sensors. 2023;23(2):891.
19. Trojaniello D, Ravaschio A, Hausdorff JM, Cereatti A. Comparative assessment of different methods for the estimation of gait temporal parameters using a single inertial sensor: application to elderly, post-stroke, Parkinson's disease and Huntington's disease subjects. Gait Posture. 2015;42(3):310–6.
20. Zijlstra W, Hof AL. Assessment of spatio-temporal gait parameters from trunk accelerations during human walking. Gait Posture. 2003;18(2):1–10.
21. Moe-Nilssen R, Helbostad JL. Estimation of gait cycle characteristics by trunk accelerometry. J Biomech. 2004;37(1):121–6.
22. Godfrey A, Del Din S, Barry G, Mathers JC, Rochester L. Instrumenting gait with an accelerometer: a system and algorithm examination. Med Eng Phys. 2015;37(4):400–7.
23. Harris GF, Wertsch JJ. Procedures for gait analysis. Arch Phys Med Rehabil. 1994;75(2):216–25.
24. Whittle MW. Gait analysis: an introduction. Oxford: Butterworth-Heinemann; 2014.
25. Galna B, Lord S, Rochester L. Is gait variability reliable in older adults and Parkinson's disease? Towards an optimal testing protocol. Gait Posture. 2013;37(4):580–5.
26. Oberg T, Karsznia A, Oberg K. Basic gait parameters: reference data for normal subjects, 10-79 years of age. J Rehabil Res Dev. 1993;30(2):210–23.
27. Nouredanesh M, Godfrey A, Powell D, Tung J. Egocentric vision-based detection of surfaces: towards context-aware free-living digital biomarkers for gait and fall risk assessment. J Neuroeng Rehabil. 2022;19(1):79.
28. Nouredanesh M, Ojeda L, Alexander NB, Godfrey A, Schwenk M, Melek W, et al. Automated detection of older adults' naturally-occurring compensatory balance reactions: translation from laboratory to free-living conditions. IEEE J Trans Eng Health Med. 2022;10:1–13.
29. Stuart S, Parrington L, Martini D, Popa B, Fino PC, King LA. Validation of a velocity-based algorithm to quantify saccades during walking and turning in mild traumatic brain injury and healthy controls. Physiol Meas. 2019;40(4):044006.

30. Wang K, Delbaere K, Brodie MAD, Lovell NH, Kark L, Lord SR, et al. Differences between gait on stairs and flat surfaces in relation to fall risk and future falls. IEEE J Biomed Health Inform. 2017;21(6):1479–86.
31. Francksen N, Ackermans T, Holzer D, Maganaris C, Hollands M, Roys M, et al. Underlying mechanisms of fall risk on stairs with inconsistent going size. Appl Ergon. 2022;101:103678.
32. Lin Y-C, Fok LA, Schache AG, Pandy MG. Muscle coordination of support, progression and balance during stair ambulation. J Biomech. 2015;48(2):340–7.
33. Marigold DS, Patla AE. Age-related changes in gait for multi-surface terrain. Gait Posture. 2008;27(4):689–96.
34. Kowalsky DB, Rebula JR, Ojeda LV, Adamczyk PG, Kuo AD. Human walking in the real world: interactions between terrain type, gait parameters, and energy expenditure. PLoS One. 2021;16(1):e0228682.
35. Celik Y, Stuart S, Woo WL, Sejdic E, Godfrey A. Multi-modal gait: a wearable, algorithm and data fusion approach for clinical and free-living assessment. Information Fusion. 2022;78:57–70.
36. Buchner DM, Cress ME, de Lateur BJ, Esselman PC, Margherita AJ, Price R, et al. The effect of strength and endurance training on gait, balance, fall risk, and health services use in community-living older adults. J Gerontol A Biol Sci Med Sci. 1997;52(4):M218–24.
37. Mirelman A, Maidan I, Herman T, Deutsch JE, Giladi N, Hausdorff JM. Virtual reality for gait training: can it induce motor learning to enhance complex walking and reduce fall risk in patients with Parkinson's disease? J Gerol Ser A Biomed Sci Med Sci. 2011;66(2):234–40.
38. Tofthagen C, Visovsky C, Berry DL. Strength and balance training for adults with peripheral neuropathy and high risk of fall: current evidence and implications for future research. Oncol Nurs Forum. 2012;39(5):E416–24.
39. Ong MF, Soh KL, Saimon R, Wai MW, Mortell M, Soh KG. Fall prevention education to reduce fall risk among community-dwelling older persons: a systematic review. J Nurs Manag. 2021;29(8):2674–88.
40. Tse T. The environment and falls prevention: do environmental modifications make a difference? Aust Occup Ther J. 2005;52(4):271–81.
41. Mazzà C, Alcock L, Aminian K, Becker C, Bertuletti S, Bonci T, et al. Technical validation of real-world monitoring of gait: a multicentric observational study. BMJ Open. 2021;11(12):e050785.
42. Hashmi MZUH, Riaz Q, Hussain M, Shahzad M. What lies beneath one's feet? Terrain classification using inertial data of human walk. Appl Sci. 2019;9(15):3099.
43. Weerdesteyn V, Hollands KL, Hollands MA. Chapter 8—Gait adaptability. In: Day BL, Lord SR, editors. Handbook of clinical neurology, vol. 159. Elsevier; 2018. p. 135–46.
44. Stegemöller EL, Buckley TA, Pitsikoulis C, Barthelemy E, Roemmich R, Hass CJ. Postural instability and gait impairment during obstacle crossing in Parkinson's disease. Arch Phys Med Rehabil. 2012;93(4):703–9.
45. Sparrow W, Shinkfield AJ, Chow S, Begg R. Characteristics of gait in stepping over obstacles. Hum Mov Sci. 1996;15(4):605–22.
46. Chen H-C, Ashton-Miller JA, Alexander NB, Schultz AB. Stepping over obstacles: gait patterns of healthy young and old adults. J Gerontol. 1991;46(6):M196–203.
47. Malone A, Kiernan D, French H, Saunders V, O'Brien T. Do children with cerebral palsy change their gait when walking over uneven ground? Gait Posture. 2015;41(2):716–21.
48. Dussault-Picard C, Mohammadyari SG, Arvisais D, Robert MT, Dixon PC. Gait adaptations of individuals with cerebral palsy on irregular surfaces: a scoping review. Gait Posture. 2022;96:35–46.
49. Barbieri FA, Simieli L, Orcioli-Silva D, Baptista AM, Borkowske Pestana M, Spiandor Beretta V, et al. Obstacle avoidance increases asymmetry of crossing step in individuals with Parkinson's disease and neurologically healthy individuals. J Mot Behav. 2018;50(1):17–25.
50. Ahamed NU, Kobsar D, Benson L, Clermont C, Kohrs R, Osis ST, et al. Using wearable sensors to classify subject-specific running biomechanical gait patterns based on changes in environmental weather conditions. PLoS One. 2018;13(9):e0203839.

51. Gevitz K, Madera R, Newbern C, Lojo J, Johnson CC. Risk of fall-related injury due to adverse weather events, Philadelphia, Pennsylvania, 2006-2011. Public Health Rep. 2017;132(1_suppl):53S–8S.
52. Letts L, Moreland J, Richardson J, Coman L, Edwards M, Ginis KM, et al. The physical environment as a fall risk factor in older adults: systematic review and meta-analysis of cross-sectional and cohort studies. Aust Occup Ther J. 2010;57(1):51–64.
53. Finlay J, Khan A, Gronlund C, Sol K, Jang J, Melendez R, et al. Weather woes? Exploring potential links between precipitation and age-related cognitive decline. Int J Environ Res Public Health. 2020;17(23):9011.
54. Fossum M, Ryeng EO. The walking speed of pedestrians on various pavement surface conditions during winter. Transp Res Part D: Transp Environ. 2021;97:102934.
55. Pillay J, Riva JJ, Tessier LA, Colquhoun H, Lang E, Moore AE, et al. Fall prevention interventions for oldercommunity-dwelling adults: systematic reviews on benefits, harms, and patient values andpreferences. Syst Rev. 2021;10(1):18.
56. Clemson L, Stark S, Pighills AC, Fairhall NJ, Lamb SE, Ali J, et al. Environmental interventions for preventing falls in older people living in the community. Cochrane Database Syst Rev. 2023;3(3):CD013258. https://doi.org/10.1002/14651858.CD013258.pub2.
57. Datta P, Namin AS, Chatterjee M, editors. A Survey of Privacy Concerns in Wearable Devices. 2018 IEEE International Conference on Big Data (Big Data); 2018 10–13 Dec. 2018.
58. Awais M, Palmerini L, Bourke AK, Ihlen EAF, Helbostad JL, Chiari L. Performance evaluation of state of the art Systems for physical activity classification of older subjects using inertial sensors in a real life scenario: a benchmark study. Sensors. 2016;16(12):2105.
59. Ren S, He K, Girshick R, Sun J. Faster R-CNN: towards real-time object detection with region proposal networks. In: Cortes C, Lawrence N, Lee D, Sugiyama M, Garnett R, editors. Advances in Neural Information Processing Systems, vol. 28. San Francisco, CA: Curran Associates, Inc; 2015.
60. Redmon J, Divvala S, Girshick R, Farhadi A, editors. You only look once: Unified, real-time object detection. Proceedings of the IEEE conference on computer vision and pattern recognition; 2016.
61. Feng D, Harakeh A, Waslander SL, Dietmayer K. A review and comparative study on probabilistic object detection in autonomous driving. IEEE Trans Intell Transp Syst. 2021;23(8):9961–80.
62. Raghunandan A, Raghav P, Aradhya HR, editors. Object detection algorithms for video surveillance applications. 2018 International Conference on Communication and Signal Processing (ICCSP); 2018: IEEE.
63. Yang R, Yu Y. Artificial convolutional neural network in object detection and semantic segmentation for medical imaging analysis. Front Oncol. 2021;11:638182.
64. Liu W, Anguelov D, Erhan D, Szegedy C, Reed S, Fu C-Y, et al., editors. Ssd: Single shot multibox detector. Computer Vision–ECCV 2016: 14th European Conference, Amsterdam, The Netherlands, October 11–14, 2016, Proceedings, Part I 14; 2016: Springer.
65. Bochkovskiy A, Wang C-Y, Liao H-YM. Yolov4: Optimal speed and accuracy of object detection. arXiv preprint arXiv:200410934. 2020;
66. Jocher G, Chaurasia A, Qiu J. YOLO by Ultralytics. 2023.
67. Kao PY, Lei Y-J, Chang C-H, Chen C-S, Lee M-S, Hung Y-P, editors. Activity recognition using first-person-view cameras based on sparse optical flows. 2020 25th International Conference on Pattern Recognition (ICPR); 2021: IEEE.
68. Sanal Kumar K, Bhavani R. Human activity recognition in egocentric video using PNN, SVM, kNN and SVM+ kNN classifiers. Clust Comput. 2019;22(Suppl 5):10577–86.
69. Yan Y, Ricci E, Liu G, Sebe N. Egocentric daily activity recognition via multitask clustering. IEEE Trans Image Process. 2015;24(10):2984–95.
70. Itano F, Pires R, de Sousa MAA, Del-Moral-Hernandez E. Human actions recognition in video scenes from multiple camera viewpoints. Cogn Syst Res. 2019;56:223–32.

71. Tan M, Pang R, Le QV, editors. Efficientdet: Scalable and efficient object detection. Proceedings of the IEEE/CVF conference on computer vision and pattern recognition; 2020.
72. Moore J, Stuart S, McMeekin P, Walker R, Tung J, Nouredanesh M, et al. Toward enhanced free-living fall risk assessment: Data mining and deep learning for environment and terrain classification. Intelligence Based Medicine. 2023;8:100103.
73. Xu H-h, Wang X-q, Wang D, Duan B-g, Rui T. Object detection in crowded scenes via joint prediction. Defence Technology. 2021;21:103–15.
74. Deng J, Fan D, Qiu X, Zhou F, editors. Improving crowded object detection via copy-paste. Proceedings of the AAAI conference on artificial intelligence; 2023.
75. Patterson MR, Whelan D, Reginatto B, Caprani N, Walsh L, Smeaton AF, et al., editors. Does external walking environment affect gait patterns? 2014 36th annual international conference of the IEEE engineering in medicine and biology society; 2014, 26–30 Aug. 2014.
76. Celik Y, Stuart S, Woo WL, Godfrey A. Wearable inertial gait algorithms: impact of Wear location and environment in healthy and Parkinson's populations. Sensors. 2021;21(19):6476.
77. Micó-Amigo ME, Bonci T, Paraschiv-Ionescu A, Ullrich M, Kirk C, Soltani A, et al. Assessing real-world gait with digital technology? Validation, insights and recommendations from the mobilise-D consortium. J Neuroeng Rehabil. 2023;20(1):1–26.
78. Claudia M, Lisa A, Kamiar A, Clemens B, Stefano B, Tecla B, et al. Technical validation of real-world monitoring of gait: a multicentric observational study. BMJ Open. 2021;11(12):e050785.

29 Transcranial Direct Current Stimulation Effect on Locomotion and Posture

Edgard Morya, Alexandre H. Okano, Luciane A. Moscaleski, and Alexandre Moreira

Abstract

This chapter explores transcranial direct current stimulation (tDCS) in motor neurorehabilitation for aging and neurological disorders. tDCS uses cathode and anode electrodes on the scalp, delivering low direct current to targeted brain areas. Aging and certain neurological conditions can impact balance control, leading to increased fall risk and reduced mobility. Motor cortex and cerebellum

E. Morya (✉)
Edmond and Lily Safra International Institute of Neuroscience, Santos Dumont Institute, Macaíba, RN, Brazil

Brazilian Institute of Neuroscience and Neurotechnology (BRAINN/CEPID-FAPESP), University of Campinas, Campinas, SP, Brazil

Brazil NAPeN Network (Rede de Núcleos de Assistência e Pesquisa em Neuromodulação), Campinas, SP, Brazil
e-mail: edgard.morya@isd.org.br

A. H. Okano · L. A. Moscaleski
Brazilian Institute of Neuroscience and Neurotechnology (BRAINN/CEPID-FAPESP), University of Campinas, Campinas, SP, Brazil

Brazil NAPeN Network (Rede de Núcleos de Assistência e Pesquisa em Neuromodulação), Campinas, SP, Brazil

Center of Mathematics, Computation, and Cognition, Universidade Federal do ABC, São Bernardo do Campo, SP, Brazil

A. Moreira
Brazilian Institute of Neuroscience and Neurotechnology (BRAINN/CEPID-FAPESP), University of Campinas, Campinas, SP, Brazil

Brazil NAPeN Network (Rede de Núcleos de Assistência e Pesquisa em Neuromodulação), Campinas, SP, Brazil

Department of Sport, School of Physical Education and Sport, University of São Paulo, São Paulo, SP, Brazil

F. A. Barbieri et al. (eds.), *Locomotion and Posture in Older Adults*,
https://doi.org/10.1007/978-3-031-74123-4_29

stimulation may improve motor coordination and stability. Modulation of attention and cognitive processing may enhance cognitive-motor integration. In aging and neurological disorders, tDCS holds promise for gait and balance rehabilitation. Combining safety considerations, individualized approaches, and technological integration are essential to enhance tDCS effect on gait and balance training. Further research is needed to determine optimal stimulation parameters and the long-term effects of tDCS in gait and balance neurorehabilitation.

Introduction

Transcranial direct current stimulation (tDCS) is a non-invasive electrical stimulation method that modulates neuronal activity and alters the excitability of targeted brain regions. This modulation can have downstream effects on the neural circuits involved in gait and balance control. Motor cortex stimulation can influence the activation and synchronization of motor neurons, leading to improved motor coordination during walking [1, 2]. Cerebellum stimulation can enhance the integration of sensory inputs and motor outputs, improving postural stability and balance control [3, 4]. Additionally, modulation of regions involved in attention, spatial perception, or cognitive processing can enhance cognitive-motor integration during gait and balance tasks.

Physiological Basis of tDCS

tDCS is a non-invasive stimulation method that uses a cathode (negative) and an anode (positive) electrode [5] positioned on the scalp according to the 10–20 international system of electroencephalography (EEG) electrode placement [Fig. 29.1].

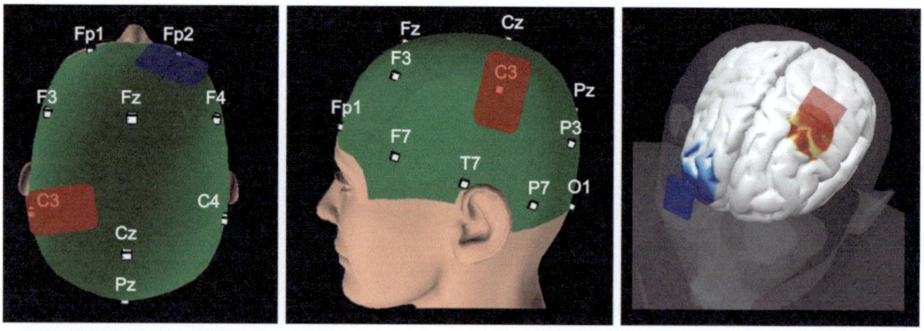

Fig. 29.1 Illustration of top and left view of 10–20 international system of EEG electrode placement with representative tDCS C3 anode and Fp2 cathode electrodes. The letter of the electrode stands for the brain region: Fp (frontal pole), F (frontal), C (central), T (temporal), P (parietal), and O (occipital). The number gives the distance from the midline of the brain (z line), and the hemisphere side (odd—left hemisphere, and even—right hemisphere). Note that the modified 10–10 system replaces the T3/T4 and T5/T6 terms with the T7/T8 and P7/P8, respectively [6]

tDCS devices deliver a low direct current (0.1–4 mA, most studies use 2 mA) through two damp sponge electrode holding bags (e.g., 5 × 7 cm) placed on the scalp for several minutes (e.g., 20 min). A saline solution or, more recently, EEG gel can be used as a conductive substrate to keep a lower impedance (<5 kΩ). Direct current flows from the anode to the cathode [7]. This direction matters since anodal and cathodal stimulation produces different effects on cortical neurons' soma, axon terminals, and dendrites that are also depolarized or hyperpolarized according to the electric field direction [7, 8]. This current flow and electric field direction modulate the spontaneous neuronal activity, facilitating or inhibiting networks related to the task (e.g., gait, balance, or cognitive training). In these cases, tDCS physiological basis is fundamental to support the modulation of brain regions related to gait and balance control. The key physiological processes underlying tDCS are presented in Table 29.1:

Table 29.1 The physiological processes underlying tDCS

Polarization of neuronal targets	tDCS simultaneously polarizes neuronal compartments, depolarizing, and hyperpolarizing. This polarization alters resting membrane potential and affects spontaneous neuronal activity, leading to a more or less likely generation of action potentials [9].
Modulation of neuronal excitability	tDCS influences neuronal excitability by changing the membrane potential of neurons. On the motor cortex, it has been suggested that these excitability changes are polarity dependent, with anodal stimulation increasing excitability and cathodal stimulation decreasing excitability [10, 11].
Synaptic plasticity	tDCS has been associated with the modulation of synaptic plasticity, which refers to the ability of synapses to change their strength in response to activity. Plasticity seems polarity independent as anodal and cathodal stimulation modulate synaptic plasticity. However, tDCS may facilitate long-term potentiation (LTP), a process that strengthens synaptic connections, and may reduce long-term depression (LTD), which weakens synaptic connections [12]. These plasticity changes can persist beyond the stimulation period and contribute to lasting alterations in neural circuits.
Neurotransmitter modulation	tDCS can affect the release and uptake of neurotransmitters in the stimulated brain regions. Anodal stimulation has been shown to increase the release of excitatory neurotransmitters and decrease inhibitory neurotransmitters [13]. These neurotransmitter changes can further modulate neuronal excitability and network activity.
Network effects	The effects of tDCS extend beyond the directly stimulated region, as neuronal networks are anatomically and functionally integrated. Changes in the excitability of a specific brain area can propagate to interconnected regions, leading to widespread effects on the neural networks involved in various cognitive and motor processes. These network effects contribute to the broader impact of tDCS on brain functions [14].

tDCS in Motor Neurorehabilitation for Aging and Neurological Disorders

Aging and neurological disorders can significantly impact balance control, leading to an increased risk of falls, reduced mobility, and diminished quality of life. Indeed, age and age-related illness involve both structural and physiological changes in the body [15]. These changes interact with aging process and impact the functioning of the brain's network [16] and balance control [17]. Targeting the supraspinal elements of balance control through strategic approaches has immense potential for enhancing balance, safety, and independence in older adults [17, 18]. Understanding these effects is therefore crucial for developing effective interventions to mitigate balance impairments and improve the functional outcomes of tDCS, which is a promising strategy to modulate brain network function, which in turn may modulate the supraspinal control of balance in older adults.

Balance Impairments and tDCS

As individuals age, various physiological changes can affect balance control. Age-related declines in balance can result in increased postural sway, compromised postural stability, and decreased ability to recover from perturbations. The underlying mechanisms of balance impairments in aging and neurological disorders are multifaceted and can vary depending on the specific condition. These mechanisms may involve dysfunction in the central nervous system (including areas such as the cerebellum, basal ganglia, and sensorimotor cortex), abnormalities in sensory processing (visual, vestibular, and proprioceptive), alterations in muscle strength and coordination, and deficits in motor planning and execution. Additionally, cognitive factors such as attention, executive function, and visuospatial processing can also influence balance control.

The efficacy of tDCS in addressing balance impairments may depend on individual factors such as the underlying condition, severity of symptoms, and specific deficits. Individualized approaches to tDCS targeting and stimulation parameters are crucial to optimize the outcomes. Identifying the most appropriate brain regions, determining the optimal stimulation intensity and duration, and considering the individual's specific impairments and needs can enhance the effectiveness of tDCS interventions for balance rehabilitation [3, 4, 19–21].

In the aging population, tDCS holds promise as a non-invasive intervention to enhance balance control. Anodal tDCS over the cortical motor area has shown the potential to improve older adults' motor function and postural stability [20]. By modulating neuronal excitability and promoting neuroplasticity, tDCS may enhance motor network activation and sensory input integration, leading to a more robust balance control.

Moreover, considering that non-motor brain areas associated with cognitive function, such as attention, executive function, and visuospatial processing, can influence balance control; other montages (electrodes positioning) rather than modulating cortical motor area might be considered for tDCS application. For instance, Manor et al. [22] conducted a study showcasing how a single session of tDCS aimed at the left dorsolateral prefrontal cortex (DLPFC) led to improved standing and walking performance in healthy older adults. The intervention reduced standing postural sway and increased walking speed, especially when participants were engaged in a simultaneous cognitive task (dual tasking). Several meta-analyses have demonstrated the favorable effects of anodal tDCS applied over the DLPFC using the +F3/-F4 montage. These studies have shown significant improvements in cognitive performance in healthy individuals and in those with neuropsychiatric conditions [23–26]. In addition, the potential use of this bilateral montage (+F3/-F4 montage) over the DLPFC to increase well-being and promote stress attenuation has also been demonstrated in professional athletes [27–29], while changes in brain electrical activity after the application of the high-definition cathodic tDCS were reported in professional female athletes [30]. In conjunction, these behavioral and mechanistic findings suggest that tDCS applied over the DLPFC shows promise for influencing balance control besides applying tDCS over motor brain areas. Nevertheless, future studies with larger and more diverse samples are needed.

Furthermore, despite the demonstrated tDCS potential strategy to modulate balance control in older adults, it is important to highlight some aspects that should be considered. For example, Guo et al. [18] recently conducted a systematic review of the effects of tDCS on balance control in older adults. The authors found that most studies examined in this analysis primarily concentrated on the immediate outcomes of a single session of tDCS, demonstrating that the long-term effects of multi-session tDCS interventions on balance control in older adults still lack clarity. They also reported concerns about the effectiveness of blinding in the assessed studies. Out of the ten studies included in their systematic review, nine utilized a double-blinded design; however, only four reported the effectiveness of blinding. Hence, it is highly recommended that future studies provide detailed reporting of blinding efficacy, as similar sham interventions employed in neuropsychological studies have indicated inadequate blinding effectiveness. Considering this issue, it seems reasonable to suggest that further research is needed to optimize stimulation parameters, identify the most effective target areas, and determine the long-term effects of tDCS in aging individuals.

Several neurological disorders can significantly impact balance control, exacerbating the risk of falls and functional limitations. Conditions such as Parkinson's disease, multiple sclerosis, stroke, peripheral neuropathy, and cerebellar ataxia often manifest with balance impairment as a primary symptom. These disorders can affect various components of balance control, including sensory integration, motor coordination, and postural stability. Understanding the specific effects of each neurological condition is essential for tailoring interventions and developing targeted rehabilitation strategies.

tDCS has been investigated as a potential adjunct therapy for various neurological disorders associated with balance impairment [31], including Parkinson's disease, multiple sclerosis, stroke, and cerebellar ataxia. By targeting specific brain regions involved in motor control and balance processing, tDCS can modulate neural activity and enhance the rehabilitation outcomes in these populations. Studies have shown that tDCS can be combined with conventional rehabilitation or balance training to improve gait, postural stability, and functional outcomes [18, 31–33]. However, the optimal stimulation protocols [32] and previous level of postural control [34] should be considered to achieve long-term effects of tDCS on neurological conditions, and require further investigation.

Gait and tDCS

tDCS can influence gait control by modulating the excitability of specific brain regions involved in motor planning, execution, and coordination. Anodal stimulation over the M1 has been shown to enhance corticospinal excitability and improve motor function. By increasing neuronal excitability in M1, tDCS may facilitate the activation of motor pathways, leading to improved muscle recruitment, coordination, and gait performance. Additionally, tDCS can modulate other areas, such as the supplementary motor area (SMA) and cerebellum, which play vital roles in gait control [1, 3, 20, 35–37].

In the aging population, gait changes are commonly observed, including reduced walking speed, stride length, and balance control. tDCS has shown promise as a potential intervention to enhance gait in older adults. Anodal tDCS over M1 or SMA has been associated with improved gait parameters, such as increased speed, stride length, and symmetry [38]. tDCS may optimize motor control and coordination by enhancing cortical excitability and facilitating neural activation, leading to more efficient and stable gait patterns in older adults.

Neurological disorders such as Parkinson's disease, stroke, multiple sclerosis, and cerebral palsy often present with gait disturbances as prominent considerations. tDCS has been investigated as an adjunctive therapy to conventional rehabilitation interventions for improving gait in these conditions. Studies have shown that tDCS combined with gait training or physical therapy can lead to positive outcomes, including enhanced gait velocity, stride length, and improved gait symmetry [39–41]. By modulating cortical excitability and promoting neuroplasticity, tDCS may facilitate motor recovery, compensate for impaired neural pathways, and optimize gait performance in individuals with neurological disorders.

To maximize the benefits of tDCS for gait improvement, optimal stimulation parameters and target selection are crucial. The specific brain regions targeted, such as M1, SMA, or cerebellum, may vary depending on the underlying condition and associated gait deficits. Stimulation intensity, duration, and electrode montage should be carefully considered to achieve desired effects. Individualized approaches are important for optimizing outcomes.

Technology Integration

While tDCS shows promise for enhancing gait and balance in aging and neurological disorders, combining it with other interventions may further amplify its effects. Future research should investigate the timing, duration, and combination of interventions to maximize gait and balance improvements. Long-term effects, maintenance of gains, and home-based tDCS protocols also warrant further exploration. Combining tDCS with a walkway system to optimize gait and balance may maximize motor training and neuronal modification. Gait and balance features [Fig. 29.2] such as center of pressure (COP) displacement (area, anteroposterior, and mediolateral), stride length, velocity, and acceleration are standard variables that can be analyzed in real time and delivered as visual, tactile or auditory feedback to enhance motor control, improving neuroplasticity, and overall mobility.

The Zeno Walkway system (Protokinetics, USA) is a gait analysis tool that utilizes an electronic walkway with pressure sensors to assess various spatiotemporal parameters during gait. It provides objective measurements of gait parameters, such as step length, cadence, gait speed, and symmetry, allowing for comprehensive gait analysis [Fig. 29.3]. The Zeno Walkway system provides real-time feedback, facilitating gait training, balance exercises, and the evaluation of intervention outcomes. Providing quantitative data and visual feedback enhances the precision and effectiveness of gait and balance rehabilitation programs.

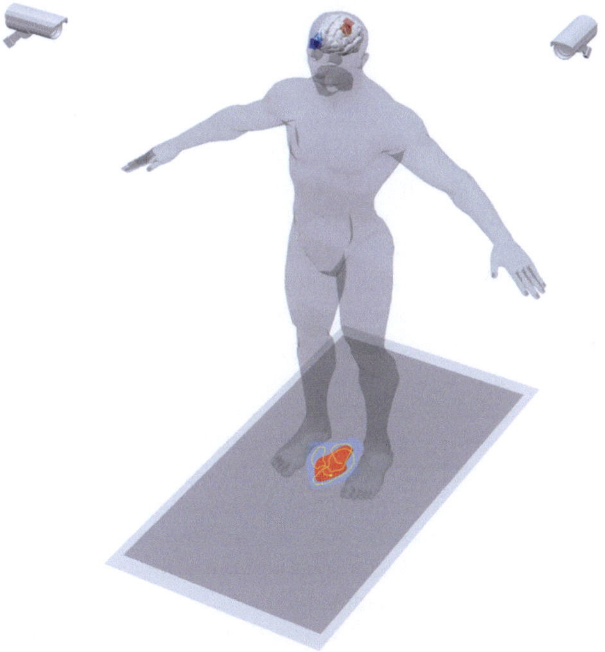

Fig. 29.2 Representation (created with Blender 3.6) of M1 anodal stimulation effect on balance assessment. Several tDCS articles showed evidence of a reduction in anteroposterior and mediolateral center of pressure (COP) displacement (represented by the blue area (sham or before stimulation) and red area (after tDCS stimulation). Illustration of COP trajectory in yellow. Motion capture cameras acquire 3D full-body movements synchronized to balance assessment allowing balance and gait detailed analysis effect of tDCS on aging and neurological disorders (e.g., cerebral palsy, Parkinson, stroke)

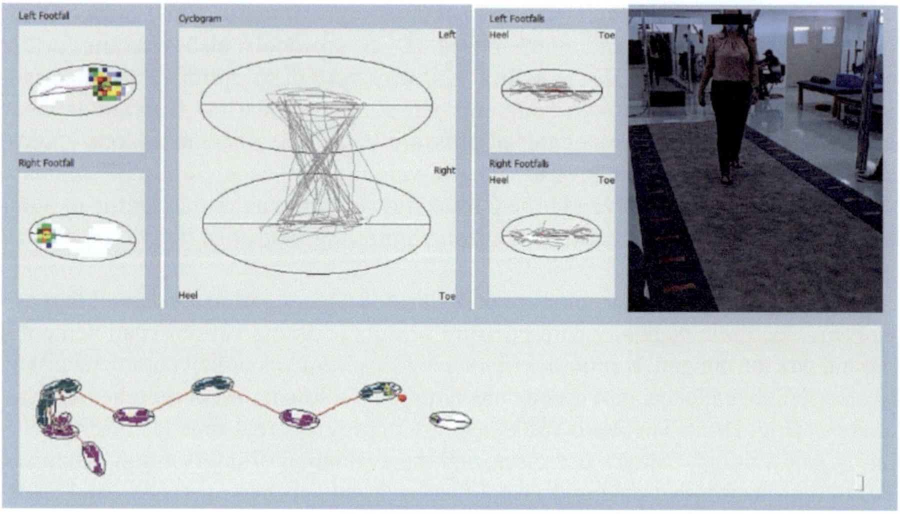

Fig. 29.3 Illustrative print screen of PKMAS Gait Analysis Software with gait data plot of left/right foot. Footfalls show the pressure level (blue to red, lower to higher pressure) in the footprint areas. COP Cyclogram symmetry during left and right stances. Footprints (left-green and right-purple) and COP trajectory in a 6-m gait evaluation (video screenshot). A customized screen can use individual gait variables as real-time visual feedback to the subject to improve gait and balance training

Combining tDCS with gait analysis system can yield synergistic effects in improving gait and balance. Firstly, tDCS can prime the cortical circuits involved in gait and balance control, making the subsequent gait training or balance exercises more effective. Secondly, the Zeno Walkway system provides objective feedback, allowing individuals to adjust their gait patterns and balance strategies in real-time. This immediate feedback facilitates motor learning and promotes the adoption of more stable and efficient movement patterns. Moreover, combining gait training with virtual reality can enhance engagement and motivation during rehabilitation sessions, leading to better adherence and improved treatment outcomes [42].

Individualized approaches are crucial to maximize the benefits of tDCS with combined intervention. This includes tailoring tDCS parameters, such as stimulation intensity, duration, and target selection, based on each movement disorder's specific gait and balance deficits. Similarly, a walkway system can be customized to focus on specific gait parameters that require improvement. A comprehensive assessment of gait and balance and ongoing monitoring can guide the development of a more effective personalized treatment.

The ZeroG System (Aretech, USA) is a dynamic body weight support system that utilizes a harness and an overhead track system during gait training or balance exercises. It provides adjustable levels of body weight support, allowing individuals to practice walking or performing functional activities with reduced gravitational load. The ZeroG System offers a safe and controlled environment for rehabilitation, enabling individuals to focus on improving gait patterns, balance, and overall motor coordination [Fig. 29.4].

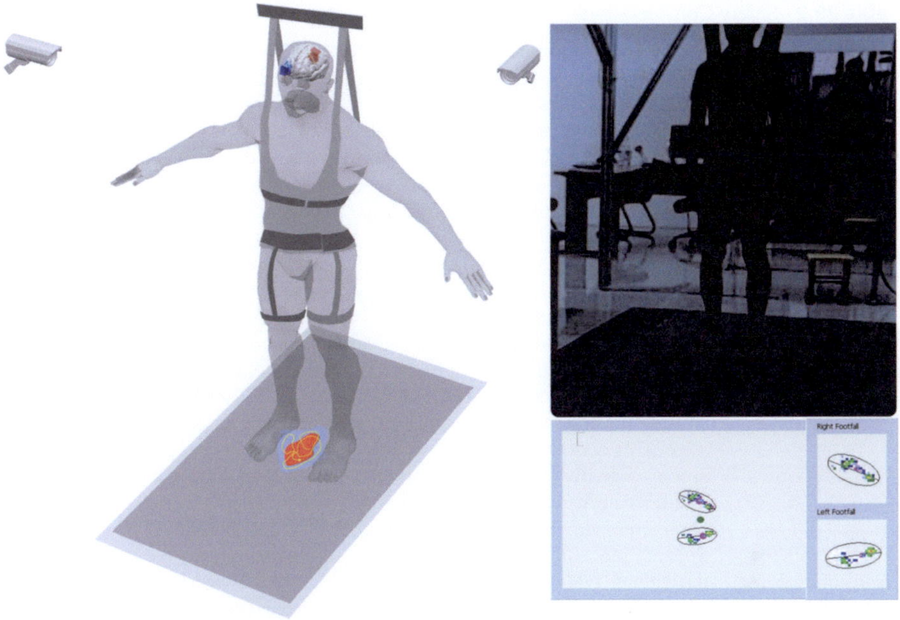

Fig. 29.4 Illustrative body weight support with COP displacement (created with Blender 3.6), and a print screen of a subject wearing a body weight support harness during balance training (extracted from PKMAS Gait Analysis Software). Visual feedback of footprints guides the balance training to keep a green circle between the footprints, and the pressure color level guides the distribution of weight on plantar areas

Providing body weight support or protection from falls reduces the fear of falling, allowing individuals to practice gait and balance tasks with greater confidence and improved postural control. Combining tDCS with a body weight support system can yield synergistic effects. tDCS modulates cortical excitability and enhances the neural substrates underlying motor control and balance. These interventions can improve motor learning, optimize gait parameters, and improve balance control.

tDCS Safety Considerations

tDCS is considered a safe and well-tolerated neuromodulation method with growing interest in enhancing motor and cognitive functioning in older adults [43–44]. Functional decline related to age is a common physiological change that can be worsened by neurological disorders. Although tDCS is not approved by the US Food and Drug Administration (FDA), the FDA has granted Investigational Device Exemption for clinical trials. In Europe there are tDCS devices with CE (European Conformity) marking approval which allows commercialization in countries of Asia and Latin America. Regulatory considerations for the clinical and research use of tDCS have been discussed to regulate its clinical practice by researchers of several

Table 29.2 Safety Considerations

Individual Assessment	Each aging person should undergo a comprehensive assessment to evaluate their suitability for tDCS (e.g., metal implants or devices, skin conditions, epilepsy, and other common medical age conditions).
Stimulation parameters	The selection of appropriate stimulation parameters is crucial for safety and benefits. This includes determining the intensity, duration, and electrode placement.
Electrode placement	Proper electrode placement is essential to ensure safe and effective current flow and avoid current concentration. Precise positioning of the anode and cathode electrodes is important to target the desired brain regions and minimize potential adverse effects (e.g., precaution if seizurogenic focus underlies the anode).
Adverse effects	While tDCS is considered safe, individuals may experience mild and transient adverse effects, such as tingling, itching, mild discomfort, or skin redness at the electrode sites. These effects usually subside shortly after the stimulation session. There is no evidence of an increased risk of serious adverse effects in aging individuals [46]. The response to tDCS can vary among individuals, and it is important to closely monitor each person's tolerance and response to the stimulation. Adjustments to the stimulation parameters may be necessary based on individual needs and tolerability.
Precautions for neurological disorders	Specific precautions should be considered when applying tDCS to individuals with neurological disorders (e.g., in individuals with epilepsy may increase the risk of seizure, but there is also evidence that anodal stimulation does not increase epileptiform discharges at the stimulation site [49]). Close monitoring and individualized adjustments may be necessary to ensure safety.
Cognitive impairment	Age individuals with significant cognitive impairments may have difficulty providing informed consent, monitoring their safety during tDCS application, and following motor or cognitive demands. Caregiver involvement and appropriate supervision are needed.
Coraindications	Although there are no absolute contraindications for tDCS, some considerations in aging and neurological disorders should be considered. These include active scalp lesions (common age-related skin issues), intracranial abnormalities/surgeries, implanted devices near the stimulation site (e.g., tDCS and DBS presence [50], and a history of seizures or epilepsy [49]).

countries, such as Australia, Brazil, Canada, France, Germany, India, Iran, Italy, Portugal, South Korea, Taiwan, and US [45–48]. Thus, for individuals with aging and/or neurological disorders, certain safety considerations are presented in Table 29.2.

Conclusion

tDCS studies have demonstrated functional improvements in gait and balance. Technological integration can potentiate tDCS effects on healthy and disabled subjects. Therefore, further studies with tDCS and real-time gait and posture will contribute to novel rehabilitation clinical practice.

References

1. Grecco LAC, Oliveira CS, Duarte NA, Lima VL, Zanon N, Fregni F. Cerebellar transcranial direct current stimulation in children with ataxic cerebral palsy: a sham-controlled, crossover, pilot study. Dev Neurorehabil. 2017;20:142–8.
2. Lang N, Siebner HR, Ward NS, Lee L, Nitsche MA, Paulus W, Rothwell JC, Lemon RN, Frackowiak RS. How does transcranial DC stimulation of the primary motor cortex alter regional neuronal activity in the human brain? Eur J Neurosci. 2005;22:495–504.
3. Ehsani F, Samaei A, Zoghi M, Hedayati R, Jaberzadeh S. The effects of cerebellar transcranial direct current stimulation on static and dynamic postural stability in older individuals: a randomized double-blind sham-controlled study. Eur J Neurosci. 2017;46:2875–84.
4. Yosephi MH, Ehsani F, Zoghi M, Jaberzadeh S. Multi-session anodal tDCS enhances the effects of postural training on balance and postural stability in older adults with high fall risk: primary motor cortex versus cerebellar stimulation. Brain Stimul. 2018;11:1239–50.
5. Priori A. Brain polarization in humans: a reappraisal of an old tool for prolonged non-invasive modulation of brain excitability. Clin Neurophysiol. 2003;114:589–95.
6. Acharya JN, Hani AJ, Cheek J, Thirumala P, Tsuchida TN. American clinical neurophysiology society guideline 2: guidelines for standard electrode position nomenclature. Neurodiagn J. 2016;56:245–52.
7. Morya E, Monte-Silva K, Bikson M, et al. Beyond the target area: an integrative view of tDCS-induced motor cortex modulation in patients and athletes. J Neuroeng Rehabil. 2019;16:141.
8. Stagg CJ, Antal A, Nitsche MA. Physiology of transcranial direct current stimulation. J ECT. 2018;34:144–52.
9. Bikson M, Inoue M, Akiyama H, Deans JK, Fox JE, Miyakawa H, Jefferys JGR. Effects of uniform extracellular DC electric fields on excitability in rat hippocampal slices in vitro. J Physiol. 2004;557:175–90.
10. Nitsche MA, Paulus W. Sustained excitability elevations induced by transcranial DC motor cortex stimulation in humans. Neurology. 2001;57:1899–901.
11. Nitsche MA, Seeber A, Frommann K, et al. Modulating parameters of excitability during and after transcranial direct current stimulation of the human motor cortex. J Physiol. 2005;568:291–303.
12. Kronberg G, Bridi M, Abel T, Bikson M, Parra LC. Direct current stimulation modulates LTP and LTD: activity dependence and dendritic effects. Brain Stimul. 2017;10:51–8.
13. Alvarez-Alvarado S, Boutzoukas EM, Kraft JN, et al. Impact of transcranial direct current stimulation and cognitive training on frontal lobe neurotransmitter concentrations. Front Aging Neurosci. 2021;13:761348.
14. Polanía R, Nitsche MA, Paulus W. Modulating functional connectivity patterns and topological functional organization of the human brain with transcranial direct current stimulation. Hum Brain Mapp. 2011;32:1236–49.
15. Chu J-S, Liu T-H, Wang K-L, Han C-L, Liu Y-P, Michitomo S, Zhang J-G, Fang T, Meng F-G. The metabolic activity of caudate and prefrontal cortex negatively correlates with the severity of idiopathic Parkinson's disease. Aging Dis. 2019;10:847–53.
16. Fjell AM, Walhovd KB, Fennema-Notestine C, McEvoy LK, Hagler DJ, Holland D, Brewer JB, Dale AM. One-year brain atrophy evident in healthy aging. J Neurosci. 2009;29:15223–31.
17. Beheshti I, Mishra S, Sone D, Khanna P, Matsuda H. T1-weighted MRI-driven brain age estimation in Alzheimer's disease and Parkinson's disease. Aging Dis. 2020;11:618–28.
18. Guo Z, Bao D, Manor B, Zhou J. The effects of transcranial direct current stimulation (tDCS) on balance control in older adults: a systematic review and meta-analysis. Front Aging Neurosci. 2020;12:275.
19. Kaminski E, Steele CJ, Hoff M, Gundlach C, Rjosk V, Sehm B, Villringer A, Ragert P. Transcranial direct current stimulation (tDCS) over primary motor cortex leg area promotes dynamic balance task performance. Clin Neurophysiol. 2016;127:2455–62.

20. Baharlouei H, Sadeghi-demneh E, Mehravar M, Manzari P, Shaterzadeh Yazdi MJ, Joghataei MT, Jaberzadeh S. Comparison of transcranial direct current stimulation of the primary motor cortex and cerebellum on static balance in older adults. Iran Red Crescent Med J. 2020;22(3):e96259. https://doi.org/10.5812/ircmj.96259.
21. Saeys W, Vereeck L, Lafosse C, Truijen S, Wuyts FL, Van De Heyning P. Transcranial direct current stimulation in the recovery of postural control after stroke: a pilot study. Disabil Rehabil. 2015;37:1857–63.
22. Manor B, Zhou J, Jor'dan A, Zhang J, Fang J, Pascual-Leone A. Reduction of dual-task costs by noninvasive modulation of prefrontal activity in healthy elders. J Cogn Neurosci. 2016;28:275–81.
23. Brunoni AR, Vanderhasselt M-A. Working memory improvement with non-invasive brain stimulation of the dorsolateral prefrontal cortex: a systematic review and meta-analysis. Brain Cogn. 2014;86:1–9.
24. Dedoncker J, Brunoni AR, Baeken C, Vanderhasselt M-A. The effect of the interval-between-sessions on prefrontal transcranial direct current stimulation (tDCS) on cognitive outcomes: a systematic review and meta-analysis. J Neural Transm. 2016;123:1159–72.
25. Dedoncker J, Brunoni AR, Baeken C, Vanderhasselt M-A. A systematic review and meta-analysis of the effects of transcranial direct current stimulation (tDCS) over the dorsolateral prefrontal cortex in healthy and neuropsychiatric samples: influence of stimulation parameters. Brain Stimul. 2016;9:501–17.
26. Hill AT, Fitzgerald PB, Hoy KE. Effects of anodal transcranial direct current stimulation on working memory: a systematic review and meta-analysis of findings from healthy and neuropsychiatric populations. Brain Stimul. 2016;9:197–208.
27. Moreira A, DGDS M, Moscaleski L, et al. Effect of tDCS on Well-being and autonomic function in professional male players after official soccer matches. Physiol Behav. 2021;233:113351.
28. Moreira A, DGDS M, Bikson M, Unal G, Bradley PS, Moscaleski L, Costa T, GCSG K, Chao LW, Baptista AF, Morya E, Okano AH. Effect of transcranial direct current stimulation on professional female soccer players' recovery following official matches. Percept Mot Skills. 2021;128(4):1504–29.
29. Moreira A, Moscaleski L, DGDS M, Bikson M, Unal G, Bradley PS, Cevada T, FTGD S, Baptista AF, Morya E, Okano AH. Transcranial direct current stimulation during a prolonged cognitive task: the effect on cognitive and shooting performances in professional female basketball players. Ergonomics. 2023;66:492–505.
30. Moscaleski LA, Fonseca A, Brito R, Morya E, Morgans R, Moreira A, Okano AH. Does high-definition transcranial direct current stimulation change brain electrical activity in professional female basketball players during free-throw shooting? Front Neuroergon. 2022;3:932542. https://doi.org/10.3389/fnrgo.2022.932542.
31. Beretta VS, Santos PCR, Orcioli-Silva D, Zampier VC, Vitório R, Gobbi LTB. Transcranial direct current stimulation for balance rehabilitation in neurological disorders: a systematic review and meta-analysis. Ageing Res Rev. 2022;81:101736. https://doi.org/10.1016/j.arr.2022.101736.
32. Beretta VS, Vitório R, Nóbrega-Sousa P, Conceição NR, Orcioli-Silva D, Pereira MP, Gobbi LTB. Effect of different intensities of transcranial direct current stimulation on postural response to external perturbation in patients with Parkinson's disease. Neurorehabil Neural Repair. 2020;34(11):1009–19. https://doi.org/10.1177/1545968320962513.
33. de Oliveira PCA, de Araújo TAB, DGDS M, Rodrigues AC, Bikson M, Andrade SM, Okano AH, Simplicio H, Pegado R, Morya E. Transcranial direct current stimulation on Parkinson's disease: systematic review and meta-analysis. Front Neurol. 2021;12:794784.
34. Beretta VS, Orcioli-Silva D, Conceição NR, Nóbrega-Sousa P, Pereira MP, Gobbi LTB, Vitório R. tDCS application for postural control in Parkinson's disease: effects are associated with baseline characteristics. Parkinsonism Relat Disord. 2021;93:62–5. https://doi.org/10.1016/j.parkreldis.2021.11.012.
35. Hou J, Nitsche MA, Yi L, Kong Z, Qi F. Effects of transcranial direct current stimulation over the primary motor cortex in improving postural stability in healthy young adults. Biology (Basel). 2022;11(9):1370. https://doi.org/10.3390/biology11091370.

36. de Duarte NAC, LAC G, Galli M, Fregni F, Oliveira CS. Effect of transcranial direct-current stimulation combined with treadmill training on balance and functional performance in children with cerebral palsy: a double-blind randomized controlled trial. PLoS One. 2014;9(8):e105777. https://doi.org/10.1371/journal.pone.0105777.
37. Kaski D, Dominguez RO, Allum JH, Islam AF, Bronstein AM. Combining physical training with transcranial direct current stimulation to improve gait in Parkinson's disease: a pilot randomized controlled study. Clin Rehabil. 2014;28:1115–24.
38. Grecco LAC, Duarte NAC, Zanon N, Galli M, Fregni F, Oliveira CS. Effect of a single session of transcranial direct-current stimulation on balance and spatiotemporal gait variables in children with cerebral palsy: a randomized sham-controlled study. Braz J Phys Ther. 2014;18:419–27.
39. Beretta VS, Conceição NR, Nóbrega-Sousa P, Orcioli-Silva D, Dantas LKBF, Gobbi LTB, Vitório R. Transcranial direct current stimulation combined with physical or cognitive training in people with Parkinson's disease: a systematic review. J Neuroeng Rehabil. 2020;17(1):74. https://doi.org/10.1186/s12984-020-00701-6.
40. Mishra RK, Thrasher AT. Transcranial direct current stimulation of dorsolateral prefrontal cortex improves dual-task gait performance in patients with Parkinson's disease: a double blind, sham-controlled study. Gait Posture. 2021;84:11–6. https://doi.org/10.1016/j.gaitpost.2020.11.012.
41. Conceição NR, Gobbi LTB, Nóbrega-Sousa P, Orcioli-Silva D, Beretta VS, Lirani-Silva E, Okano AH, Vitório R. Aerobic exercise combined with transcranial direct current stimulation over the prefrontal cortex in Parkinson disease: effects on cortical activity, gait, and cognition. Neurorehabil Neural Repair. 2021;35(8):717–28. https://doi.org/10.1177/15459683211019344.
42. Silva PMM, Silva LWM, Vieira ER, Cavalvanti FAC, Morya E. Go across immersive technology: a preliminary study of the design and development of a system for gait training using virtual reality. Games Health J. 2023;12(6):472–9. https://doi.org/10.1089/g4h.2023.0101.
43. Hsu W-Y, Ku Y, Zanto TP, Gazzaley A. Effects of noninvasive brain stimulation on cognitive function in healthy aging and Alzheimer's disease: a systematic review and meta-analysis. Neurobiol Aging. 2015;36:2348–59.
44. Elder GJ, Taylor J-P. Transcranial magnetic stimulation and transcranial direct current stimulation: treatments for cognitive and neuropsychiatric symptoms in the neurodegenerative dementias? Alzheimers Res Ther. 2014;6:74.
45. Fregni F, Nitsche MA, Loo CK, Brunoni AR, Marangolo P, Leite J, Carvalho S, Bolognini N, Caumo W, Paik NJ, Simis M, Ueda K, Ekhitari H, Luu P, Tucker DM, Tyler WJ, Brunelin J, Datta A, Juan CH, Venkatasubramanian G, Boggio PS, Bikson M. Regulatory considerations for the clinical and research use of transcranial direct current stimulation (tDCS): review and recommendations from an expert panel. Clin Res Regul Aff. 2015;32(1):22–35. https://doi.org/10.3109/10601333.2015.980944. PMID: 25983531; PMCID: PMC4431691
46. Bikson M, Grossman P, Thomas C, et al. Safety of transcranial direct current stimulation: evidence based update 2016. Brain Stimul. 2016;9:641–61.
47. Buchanan DM, Bogdanowicz T, Khanna N, Lockman-Dufour G, Robaey P, D'Angiulli A. Systematic review on the safety and tolerability of transcranial direct current stimulation in children and adolescents. Brain Sci. 2021;11(2):212. https://doi.org/10.3390/brainsci11020212.
48. Buchanan DM, Amare S, Gaumond G, D'Angiulli A, Robaey P. Safety and tolerability of tDCS across different ages, sexes, diagnoses, and amperages: a randomized double-blind controlled study. J Clin Med. 2023;12(13):4346. https://doi.org/10.3390/jcm12134346.
49. Fregni F, Thome-Souza S, Nitsche MA, Freedman SD, Valente KD, Pascual-Leone A. A controlled clinical trial of cathodal DC polarization in patients with refractory epilepsy. Epilepsia. 2006;47:335–42.
50. Iannone A, Allam N, Brasil-Neto JP. Safety of transcranial direct current stimulation in a patient with deep brain stimulation electrodes. Arq Neuropsiquiatr. 2019;77:174–8.

Using mHealth Technology to Monitor People with Parkinson's Disease

30

Camila Torriani-Pasin, Vitoria Leite Domingues, Tatiana Beline de Freitas, and Shashwati Geed

Abstract

Parkinson's disease (PD) is a complex disorder that presents both motor and nonmotor symptoms, impacting their physical performance, functional independence, and overall quality of life. The integration of mobile health (mHealth) technologies has emerged as a crucial asset in the ongoing monitoring and management of individuals with PD. Among the various mHealth tools, accelerometers have proven indispensable for their ability to precisely measure activity levels and gait patterns. Smartphone applications play a pivotal role in remote monitoring, offering a means to adjust therapeutic interventions and providing valuable data for rehabilitation planning beyond clinical settings. Despite challenges in accurately measuring step count at lower speeds, recent reviews underscore the promise of specific wearables and smartphone applications in reliably monitoring gait and mobility in PD. Moreover, these technological applications extend their utility to tracking motor symptoms, with tremor emerging as the most frequently monitored aspect. People with PD express satisfaction with

C. Torriani-Pasin (✉)
Department of Physical Therapy and Movement Sciences, The University of Texas at El Paso, El Paso, TX, USA

School of Physical Education and Sport, University of Sao Paulo, São Paulo, São Paulo, Brazil
e-mail: ctorrianip@utep.edu

V. L. Domingues · T. B. de Freitas
School of Physical Education and Sport, University of Sao Paulo, São Paulo, São Paulo, Brazil

S. Geed
Department of Physical Therapy and Movement Sciences, The University of Texas at El Paso, El Paso, TX, USA

Department of Rehabilitation Medicine, MedStar National Rehabilitation Hospital and Georgetown University, Washington, DC, USA

F. A. Barbieri et al. (eds.), *Locomotion and Posture in Older Adults*,
https://doi.org/10.1007/978-3-031-74123-4_30

discreet and small mHealth devices, appreciating their accessibility and cost-effectiveness. In summary, the widespread use of mHealth devices, encompassing accelerometers and smartphone applications, represents a transformative approach to PD management. This not only enhances rehabilitation strategies but also empowers patients to monitor themselves. Looking ahead, it is imperative for future research to prioritize user-friendliness and explore integrated technologies, potentially revolutionizing the landscape of PD care. This chapter explores mHealth applications for monitoring various aspects of PD, emphasizing its role in enhancing clinical decision-making and improving the overall management of individuals with PD.

Introduction

Parkinson's disease (PD) is a multisystem disease caused by the loss of dopaminergic cells in the substantia nigra pars compacta of the basal ganglia [1–3], disorders in the cholinergic systems [4], in addition to the presence of Lewis corpuscles in the cytoplasm of the remaining neural cells in the substantia nigra pars compacta [1, 5, 6]. Age is the most significant risk factor for developing PD, and men are more susceptible than women with a prevalence ratio of approximately 3:2 [7].

The disease is characterized by motor symptoms (tremor at rest, bradykinesia, rigidity, and postural instability) and nonmotor symptoms (cognitive, emotional, and psychiatric alterations) [3]. The characteristic symptoms of PD can lead to impaired physical performance [2], loss or decrease in functional independence, increased social isolation, restriction in social participation, and low level of physical activity [8]. As the disease progresses, individuals experience a deterioration of bodily function and daily activities and a decline in mobility. This can lead to increased dependence, inactivity, and social isolation, resulting in a reduced quality of life [9].

Individuals with PD exhibit additional functional impairments, i.e., changes in gait pattern [3] showing variability [10] intensified with the progression of the disease [11]. The gait pattern of most people with PD is characterized by a reduced stride length [11], reduced automaticity, increased double-support time, and cadence [12], and asymmetrical reduction in arm swing and a stooped posture [11]. As the disease progresses, an increasing reduction in stride length becomes evident, leading to a drastically reduced walking speed [11].

One way of monitoring the changes that occurred over the course of the PD progression is using mobile health (mHealth). According to the World Health Organization [13], mHealth refers to the utilization of mobile devices like mobile phones, patient monitoring devices, personal digital assistants, and other wireless gadgets to support medical and public health practices. mHealth devices offer professionals and researchers more reliable and objective evaluations of PD outcomes, thereby enhancing shared clinical decision-making.

mHealth devices are considered one of the most valuable and highly recommended methods for monitoring active behavior, especially when utilizing wearable sensors for movement [14]. Among the movement sensors, pedometers and accelerometers have demonstrated themselves as the most precise and comprehensive devices for measuring daily life activity [15, 16]. Pedometers are devices capable of counting the number of steps taken in a horizontal movement, and some more technologically advanced models are capable of estimating time in activity and steps counting [16]. Conversely, accelerometers are devices able to record the body's accelerations during movement (including number of steps), sedentary behavior, and energy expenditure. They capture frequency, duration, and intensity of movements in 1, 2, or 3 planes (vertical, anteroposterior, and mediolateral), being called uni-, bi-, or triaxial, respectively [15]. Besides, as smartphones have accelerometers, they can capture similar information. However, validity and reliability studies are necessary to investigate its usefulness in each clinical population.

Novel smartphone applications can provide one-time or continuous data to monitor people with PD in person or remotely. This may support precise therapeutic adjustments and management decisions. While the smartphone's sensors can effectively monitor motor symptoms, monitoring nonmotor symptoms typically requires manual entry, which can be susceptible to confounding factors, such as fatigue and mood [17].

People with PD generally express high satisfaction with mHealth devices, particularly when the devices have a discrete and simple design [18, 19]. The widespread accessibility of such devices underscores the potential of using smartphones as effective health monitoring tools. This is attributed to the ease of collecting and sharing real-time data, offering a fast, accessible, and cost-effective service, which can save both money and travel [20]. These devices have proven to be useful in monitoring daily physical activity and sedentary behavior [15, 18, 21], assessment of gait and mobility [11], and monitoring the disease symptoms to help PD diagnosis and treatment [19, 22, 23].

In this chapter, we address the use of mHealth technologies to monitor physical activity, sedentary behavior, gait, mobility, and monitor motor/nonmotor symptoms in PD individuals.

Monitoring Physical Activity and Sedentary Behavior

People with PD have low physical activity level, even when compared to older individuals with no chronic illnesses [24, 25] due to physical limitations, fatigue, and apathy related to the disease [26]. When comparing the patterns of physical activity levels between people with PD and healthy older individuals, it is observed that people with PD not only engage in fewer activities but also exhibit a decrease in daily energy expenditure, reduced physical conditioning, and an increased instances of sedentary behavior [27, 28]. The literature points out that people with PD spent less than 7% of their waking hours in moderate-to-vigorous physical activity [24, 29–32], and more than 70% of their day in sedentary behavior [24, 29, 32–34], reaching up to 98% of the day [30]. In other words, they spent a significant part of their day on sedentary behavior and did not achieve the weekly recommendations of moderate-to-vigorous physical activity [21].

Although low adherence to physical activity is a problem for all people in different age groups and physical conditions, those with disabilities tend to be at greater risk of developing health-related problems because of physical inactivity [27]. Additionally, it is well established in the literature that a more active lifestyle provides several benefits. The benefits are related to the prevention and treatment of other chronic diseases, management of PD symptoms, and slow the progression of the PD [35–38]. Moreover, leading an inactive lifestyle can exacerbate disease symptoms, creating a vicious cycle, in which increasingly severe symptoms can slow or prevent movement, thereby further worsening the symptoms [26, 39]. Using the mHealth devices allows the monitoring of the physical activity level and sedentary behavior of people with PD through their daily steps count, activity/inactive time, or energy expenditure [15, 21, 40]. This information becomes valuable during the rehabilitation process to outline specific objectives and the most appropriate intervention program. In addition, it helps the health professional to outline a strategy to be carried out outside the therapeutic environment.

Monitoring Gait and Mobility

The mHealth devices have proven to be viable for monitoring gait parameters in the home and laboratory environment [41–44]. However, a comparison between laboratory measurements and free-living assessments revealed that people with PD exhibited reduced stride, increased pace, greater variability, and asymmetry in the laboratory setting [45]. Consequently, assessments conducted in real-world environments are becoming increasingly crucial, enhancing the ecological validity of the data.

Although mHealth devices can measure the step count, mHealth devices are reported to be inaccurate for individuals who walk at low speed [15, 16, 18]. There is much interest in monitoring and measurement of gait and mobility outcomes in PD, given the disabling limitations imposed by gait and mobility impairments in this population [3]. A recent systematic review has revealed that smartphone applications serve as promising mHealth tools for assessing both gait and balance, demonstrating robust validity and reliability in both home and laboratory settings [46]. Additionally, another systematic review identified 22 mHealth wearable devices employed in PD for measuring various parameters such as gait, fall incidents, and symptoms [47]. In the realm of gait and falls, the authors recommended only five of these devices based on their established validity and reliability: Mobility Lab System (APDM), Physilog, StepWatch 3, McRoberts DynaPort, and Axivity AX3. To facilitate the monitoring of gait and mobility aspects, these mHealth devices are utilized to measure parameters including gait variability [42, 45, 48], gait asymmetry [45, 48–50], cadence [28, 41, 42], step length [42, 45, 51], and gait or step velocity [41, 42, 48, 51].

Monitoring Motor and Nonmotor Symptoms

PD is considered a complex and heterogeneous disease; therefore, it is mandatory to constantly monitor the symptoms of the disease, analyze the fluctuations of symptoms, and identify the worsening of symptoms and progression of the disease [52]. There have been numerous studies focusing on the measurement of both motor and nonmotor symptoms of people with PD, although quantifying certain symptoms using technology is a highly challenging task [22].

A systematic review on the utilization of smartphone applications in PD revealed that tremor is the most frequently monitored symptom, followed by bradykinesia, postural instability, and gait [19]. This finding is consistent with other investigations employing mHealth devices, with the purpose of providing awareness for daily posture detection [38, 39] and tremor [53, 54] as key areas of monitoring. Furthermore, Lee and colleagues' [19] systematic review also identified studies monitoring additional PD-related characteristics (i.e., rigidity, speech difficulty, dyskinesia, neuropsychiatric symptoms, sleep disorders, and constipation). These symptoms can be monitored through various methods, including self-reporting, finger tapping, or movement analysis using accelerometers and gyroscopes [19, 22, 23]. By employing mHealth for symptom tracking, clinicians can regularly monitor patients' symptoms over time and potentially complement conventional face-to-face interactions. Additionally, mHealth (particularly smartphone applications) is reported to assist in disease management by improving medication adherence [55, 56] and promoting a more active lifestyle [57–59]. Consequently, mHealth devices enable patients to engage with healthcare professionals not only through ongoing symptom monitoring in their daily lives but also by facilitating remote communication.

There is evidence supporting effectiveness when directly monitoring the disease's motor symptoms, tremor [19, 22], and postural instability [22, 60], whereas bradykinesia [19, 22] can only be monitored indirectly. However, measuring rigidity remains a significant challenge due to its reliance on passive movement-based assessment [22].

A systematic review conducted by Rovini et al. [22] indicates that mHealth devices can indeed be effective in monitoring resting tremor. However, achieving a more detailed investigation of this symptom often requires the use of triaxial inertial sensors. Tremor data were also collected through activities such as ball games or rapid alternating movements of the hand holding a smartphone [19]. The accelerometer-based approach can help to measure postural instability, especially for the retropulsion test in MDS-UPDRS [60], offering a more accessible alternative to force plates. This approach is particularly useful for the early stages of the disease assessment and evaluating changes during ON and OFF states of medication [22]. Bradykinesia can be measured indirectly through timed-up-and-go and walking assessments with the use of accelerometers, gyroscopes, or smartphone-equipped triaxial accelerometers to measure spatiotemporal gait changes, i.e., step length and speed [22]. Alternatively, finger tapping within a 9-hole peg game is also utilized [19].

To address the importance of measuring motor symptoms, Antoni et al. [61] validated the PDMonitor® system developed by PD Neurotechnology®. This class IIa CE-marked medical device is designed for continuous home monitoring of PD patients. Placed on wrists, torso, and ankles, PDMonitor® employs accelerometers, gyroscopes, and magnetometers to comprehensively measure motor symptoms in people with PD.

The measurement of motor symptoms through technology-based assessment has pros and cons. Advantages include quantifiable data, continuous monitoring, and versatile technology platforms. Disadvantages encompass potential high costs, increased risks from medical devices, limited applicability for daily clinical use, and a lack of large prospective clinical trials for accurate diagnosis. Standardization of setups and criteria remains absent [62].

The assessment of nonmotor symptoms was performed by a limited number of studies, and its effectiveness remains modest [19]. According to Lee et al. [19], all data on nonmotor symptom were obtained via self-reporting questionnaires, except for sleep and cognitive symptoms, which were investigated objectively using wearable devices and task performance, respectively. Sleep data, including duration and wakefulness, was automatically collected through wearable devices, such as accelerometers and smartwatches. Sleep quality is effectively measured by nighttime accelerometers by screening for abnormal axial and limb movements, which may account for REM behavior disorder and/or nocturnal hypokinesia [63]. Cognition data were collected using task performance, involving cognitive interference tests, memory assessments, and cognitive games [19]. Individuals with PD may experience autonomic dysfunction, with some presenting orthostatic hypotension. This condition is effectively evaluated using 24-hour ambulatory blood pressure monitoring [63].

Wearable Sensors Commonly Used in People with PD

Accelerometers are one of the most common mHealth devices used to monitor PD symptoms, physical activity levels, and gait in PD. The ActiGraph GT3X (ActiGraph, Pensacola) and activPAL 3™ (PAL Technologies Ltd., Glasgow, UK) are two accelerometers with wide use and acceptance by studies with PD individuals. Figure 30.1 shows a summary of the main information, including the devices and research findings.

The ActiGraph GT3X is a triaxial accelerometer that is able to record acceleration in three planes (vertical, anteroposterior, and mediolateral). The outcome of the acceleration of this device is expressed in counts (number of accelerations per unit of time) or in vector magnitude. The counts are an arbitrary unit used to compose the amount of physical activity, number of steps, and energy expenditure. The vector magnitude is used to distinguish the body posture by attributing a number from 0 to 3—0 is not wearing it; 1 is standing; 2 is lying; and 3 is sitting [64].

The body placement of the ActiGraph GT3X can be on the wrist [65, 66] when measuring upper extremity (UE) function like tremors or physical activity level, but

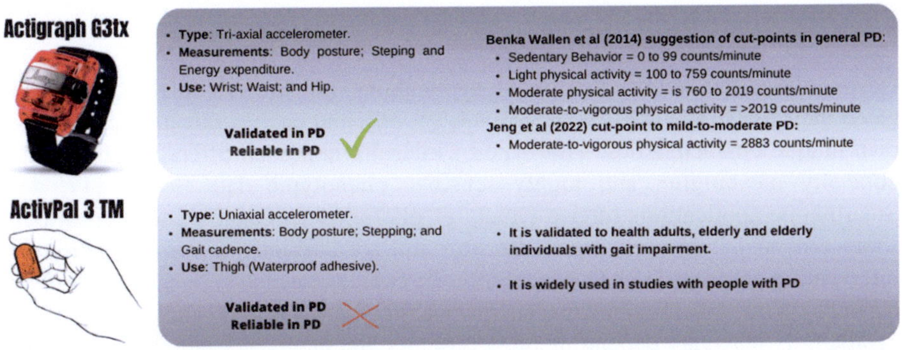

Fig. 30.1 Overview of the two most often mHealth devices selected in research with Parkinson's disease monitoring. (PD: Parkinson's disease)

it is notably situated predominantly at the waist or hip level for full body/torso movements like gait [29, 67–71]. The monitoring length usually is 7 days long [69, 71–74], but it depends on the study objective. The most recent study, which examines cut-points for moderate-to-vigorous physical activity in PD using ActiGraph GT3X, reports a value of 2883 (871) counts per minute [66]. The sample was composed of 26 individuals with mild-to-moderate PD (Hoehn and Yahr stages 2-3), and they used the accelerometer on the more affected wrist. Based on prior studies, Wallén et al. [69] suggest the cutoff of physical activity levels in people with PD. The cutoff for sedentary behavior is 0–99 counts per minute; for light physical activity, it is 100–759 counts per minute; for moderate physical activity, it is 760–2019 counts per minute; and for moderate-to-vigorous physical activity, it is more than 2019 counts per minute.

The activPAL 3™ is a thigh-worn uniaxial device that monitors the postural body positions. It is a small and slim monitor that needs to be fixed on the anterior tight. Through proprietary algorithms, the accelerometer-derived information can properly determine sitting, lying, and upright positions, transitions between these postures, stepping, and cadence—which the energy expenditure can be inferred [75].

The body placement of the activPAL 3™ is always on the anterior thigh because the measurement is specific to this positioning. Most of the studies that use this device in PD individuals monitor them for 7 days [28, 31, 33, 34, 73]. The activPAL is a small device that is normally attached to the thigh using waterproof adhesive tape. Because of this, some studies do not ask to remove the device during the monitoring period [28, 33, 76]; however, other studies provide extra tape and ask to remove it when the individual engages in water activities (i.e., bathing and swimming) [34, 77]. The activPAL 3™ has undergone validation in both healthy adults [78] and the older individuals [79]. Furthermore, this device has been validated for use in older individuals with gait impairment [80]; however, its sensitivity is limited when gait speed falls below 0.47 meters per second. Despite the lack of specific validation studies or established cutoff points for the PD population, this device is extensively utilized in PD individuals [28, 31, 33, 34, 73, 76, 79, 81, 82].

Smartphone Applications

Despite the utilization of smartphone applications, numerous studies have investigated their use in PD [17, 19, 22, 23, 44, 55, 56], and each application exhibits its own unique characteristics. This type of mHealth approach offers reliable, valid, clinically meaningful, and highly sensitive phenotypic data in PD [17, 44]. Smartphone applications offer a variety of platforms that enable meaningful both short-term and long-term data collection and are currently under evaluation for intervention purposes [17]. Consequently, the choice of which application to employ depends on the specific objective (i.e., what is being measured), the country of use (availability may vary depending on the country and language), and the smartphone available for use. To the best of our knowledge, our research did not identify any standout smartphone application, providing these distinct features.

Smartphone applications are also targeted to monitor disease progression, manage medication, modulate remote movement, and provide treatment, typically implemented over a period ranging from 3 to 6 months [17]. Smartwatches, however, can measure tremors, detect motor fluctuations, track dyskinesias [83], as well as monitor steps count [12, 84]. They are utilized for healthcare interventions lasting from 90 days to 12 months [83], offering valuable insights into long-term trends and patient outcomes.

Conclusion

In conclusion, the extensive utilization of mHealth devices, encompassing accelerometers and smartphone applications, has significantly impacted the field of PD management. While not all devices have attained validity and reliability standards, some of them have met these criteria, showcasing their potential. These devices have emerged as great tools for rehabilitation professionals, facilitating a closer connection between the clinician and the individual. This enhanced proximity empowers the rehabilitation professional to tailor an effective rehabilitation strategy according to the updated needs of each patient. Moreover, these devices empower individuals by enabling them to actively engage in activities while efficiently managing their symptoms. Furthermore, the integration of mHealth devices augments the rehabilitation professional's comprehension of the individual's daily life experiences, allowing for a more comprehensive and holistic approach to treatment.

While the validation of mHealth devices for PD is significant, the scope of future research extends well beyond this topic. As technological progress rapidly evolves, upholding the user-friendliness and accessibility of mHealth devices remains necessary. Given the abundance of smartphone applications for people with PD, the strategic enhancement and consolidation of existing applications, potentially through the integration of diverse technologies, emerge as a promising avenue for exploration. The integration of mHealth devices with telemedicine platforms has the potential to reshape the landscape of PD care.

References

1. Balestrino R, Schapira AHV. Parkinson disease. Eur J Neurol. 2020;27:27–42.
2. Hamani C, Lozano AM. Physiology and pathophysiology of Parkinson's disease. Ann N Y Acad Sci [Internet]. 2003;991:15–21. Available from: www.pdflib.com
3. Rodriguez-Oroz MC, Jahanshahi M, Krack P, Litvan I, Macias R, Bezard E, et al. Initial clinical manifestations of Parkinson's disease: features and pathophysiological mechanisms. Lancet Neurol. 2009;8(12):1128–39.
4. Duchesne C, Lungu O, Nadeau A, Robillard ME, Boré A, Bobeuf F, et al. Enhancing both motor and cognitive functioning in Parkinson's disease: aerobic exercise as a rehabilitative intervention. Brain Cogn. 2015 Oct;1(99):68–77.
5. Braak H, del Tredici K, Rüb U, de Vos RAI, Jansen Steur ENH, Braak E. Staging of brain pathology related to sporadic Parkinson's disease. Neurobiol Aging. 2003;24(2):197–211. https://doi.org/10.1016/s0197-4580(02)00065-9.
6. Pereira MP, Batistela RA, Simieli L. Fisiopatologia, sinais e sintomas da Doença de Parkinson. In: Gobbi LTB, Barbieri FA, Vitório R, editors. Doença de Parkinson e exercício físico. 1st ed. Curitiba: Editora CRV; 2014. p. 1–21.
7. Tolosa E, Garrido A, Scholz SW, Poewe W. Challenges in the diagnosis of Parkinson's disease. Lancet Neurol. 2021;20:385–97.
8. Keus S, Muneke M, Graziano M, Paltamas J, Pelosin E, Domingos J. European physiotherapy guideline for Parkinson disease, vol. 1. 1st ed. Nijmegen: ParkinsonNet; 2014. p. 1–29.
9. Nag N, Jelinek GA. A narrative review of lifestyle factors associated with Parkinson's disease risk and progression. Neurodegener Dis. 2019;19(2):51–9. https://doi.org/10.1159/000502292.
10. Mak MKY, Pang MYC, Mok V. Gait difficulty, postural instability, and muscle weakness are associated with fear of falling in people with Parkinson's disease. Parkinson's Dis. 2012;2012:901721. https://doi.org/10.1155/2012/901721.
11. Debû B, De Oliveira GC, Lino JC, Moro E. Managing gait, balance, and posture in Parkinson's disease. Curr Neurol Neurosci Rep. 2018;18(5):23. https://doi.org/10.1007/s11910-018-0828-4.
12. Bianchini E, Caliò B, Alborghetti M, Rinaldi D, Hansen C, Vuillerme N, et al. Step-counting accuracy of a commercial smartwatch in mild-to-moderate PD patients and effect of spatiotemporal gait parameters, laterality of symptoms, pharmacological state, and clinical variables. Sensors (Basel). 2023;23(1):214. https://doi.org/10.3390/s23010214.
13. WHO Global Observatory for eHealth. MHealth: new horizons for health through mobile technologies. [Internet]. World Health Organization; 2011. [cited 2023 Jul 19]. Available from: https://apps.who.int/iris/handle/10665/44607
14. Skender S, Ose J, Chang-Claude J, Paskow M, Brühmann B, Siegel EM, et al. Accelerometry and physical activity questionnaires—a systematic review. BMC Public Health [Internet]. 2016;16(1):1–10. https://doi.org/10.1186/s12889-016-3172-0.
15. Strath SJ, Kaminsky LA, Ainsworth BE, Ekelund U, Freedson PS, Gary RA, et al. Guide to the assessment of physical activity: clinical and research applications: a scientific statement from the American Heart association. Circulation. 2013;128(20):2259–79.
16. Sylvia LG, Bernstein EE, Hubbard JL, Keating L, Anderson EJ. Practical guide to measuring physical activity. J Acad Nutr Diet. 2014;114(2):199–208.
17. Tripathi S, Malhotra A, Qazi M, Chou J, Wang F, Barkan S, et al. Clinical review of smartphone applications in Parkinson's disease. Neurologist. 2022;27(4):183–93. https://doi.org/10.1097/NRL.0000000000000413.
18. Block VAJ, Pitsch E, Tahir P, Cree BAC, Allen DD, Gelfand JM. Remote physical activity monitoring in neurological disease: a systematic review. PLoS One. 2016;11(4):e0154335.
19. Lee JH, Yeom I, Chung ML, Kim Y, Yoo S, Kim E. Use of Mobile apps for self-care in people with Parkinson disease: systematic review. JMIR Mhealth Uhealth. 2022;10(1):e33944. https://doi.org/10.2196/33944.

20. Alam MZ, Hoque MR, Hu W, Barua Z. Factors influencing the adoption of mHealth services in a developing country: a patient-centric study. Int J Inf Manag. 2020 Feb;1(50):128–43.
21. Bouça-Machado R, Rosário A, Caldeira D, Castro Caldas A, Guerreiro D, Venturelli M, et al. Physical activity, exercise, and physiotherapy in Parkinson's disease: defining the concepts. Mov Disord Clin Pract. 2020;7(1):7–15.
22. Rovini E, Maremmani C, Cavallo F. How wearable sensors can support Parkinson's disease diagnosis and treatment: a systematic review. Front Neurosci. 2017;11:555. https://doi.org/10.3389/fnins.2017.00555.
23. Morgan C, Rolinski M, McNaney R, Jones B, Rochester L, Maetzler W, et al. Systematic review looking at the use of technology to measure free-living symptom and activity outcomes in Parkinson's disease in the home or a home-like environment. J Parkinsons Dis. 2020;10:429–54.
24. Pradhan S, Kelly VE. Quantifying physical activity in early Parkinson disease using a commercial activity monitor. Parkinsonism Relat Disord [Internet]. 2019;66(July):171–5. https://doi.org/10.1016/j.parkreldis.2019.08.001.
25. Prusynski RA, Kelly VE, Fogelberg DJ, Pradhan S. The association between sleep deficits and sedentary behavior in people with mild Parkinson disease. Disabil Rehabil. 2022;44(19):5585–91.
26. Nimwegen M, Speelman AD, Hofman-van Rossum EJM, Overeem S, Deeg DJH, Borm GF, et al. Physical inactivity in Parkinson's disease. J Neurol [Internet]. 2011;258(12):2214–21. https://doi.org/10.1007/s00415-011-6097-7.
27. Ellis T, Motl RW. Physical activity behavior change in persons with neurologic disorders: overview and examples from Parkinson disease and multiple sclerosis. J Neurol Phys Ther. 2013;37(2):85–90.
28. Klenk J, Srulijes K, Schatton C, Schwickert L, Maetzler W, Becker C, et al. Ambulatory activity components deteriorate differently across neurodegenerative diseases: a cross-sectional sensor-based study. Neurodegener Dis. 2016;16(5–6):317–23.
29. Benka Wallén M, Franzén E, Nero H, Hagströmer M. Levels and patterns of physical activity and sedentary behavior in elderly people with mild to moderate Parkinson disease. Phys Ther [Internet]. 2015;95(8):1135–41. Available from: https://academic.oup.com/ptj/article/95/8/1135/2686470
30. Dontje M, de Greef M, Speelman A, van Nimwegen M, Krijnen W, Stolk R, et al. Determinants of daily physical activity in inactive Parkinson's disease patients. J Sci Med Sport. 2013;15:S79.
31. Lord S, Godfrey A, Galna B, Mhiripiri D, Burn D, Rochester L. Ambulatory activity in incident Parkinson's: more than meets the eye? J Neurol. 2013;260(12):2964–72.
32. Cerff B, Maetzler W, Sulzer P, Kampmeyer M, Prinzen J, Hobert MA, et al. Home-based physical behavior in late stage Parkinson disease dementia: differences between cognitive subtypes. Neurodegener Dis. 2017;17(4–5):135–44.
33. Chastin SFM, Baker K, Jones D, Burn D, Granat MH, Rochester L. The pattern of habitual sedentary behavior is different in advanced Parkinson's disease. Mov Disord. 2010;25(13):2114–20.
34. Hiorth YH, Larsen JP, Lode K, Tysnes OB, Godfrey A, Lord S, et al. Impact of falls on physical activity in people with Parkinson's disease. J Parkinsons Dis. 2016;6(1):175–82.
35. Fox CM, Raming LO, Ciucci MR, Sapir S, McFarland DH, Farley BG. The science and practice of LSVT/LOUD: neural plasticity—principled approach to treating individuals with Parkinson disease and other neurological disorders. Semin Speech Lang. 2006;27(4):283–99.
36. Okun MS. Management of Parkinson Disease in 2017: personalized approaches for patient-specific needs. JAMA. 2017;318(9):791–2. https://doi.org/10.1001/jama.2017.7914.
37. Sutoo D, Akiyama K. Regulation of brain function by exercise. Neurobiol Dis. 2003;13(1):1–14.
38. Warburton DER, Nicol CW, Bredin SSD. Health benefits of physical activity: the evidence. CMAJ: Canadian Med Assoc J. 2006;174(6):801–9.
39. Speelman AD, Van De Warrenburg BP, Van Nimwegen M, Petzinger GM, Munneke M, Bloem BR. How might physical activity benefit patients with Parkinson disease? Nat Rev Neurol [Internet]. 2011;7(9):528–34. https://doi.org/10.1038/nrneurol.2011.107.

40. Tudor-Locke C, Craig CL, Aoyagi Y, Bell RC, Croteau KA, De Bourdeaudhuij I, et al. How many steps/day are enough? For older adults and special populations. Int J Behav Nutr Phys Activity [Internet]. 2011;8(1):80. Available from:http://www.ijbnpa.org/content/8/1/80
41. Zago M, Sforza C, Pacifici I, Cimolin V, Camerota F, Celletti C, et al. Gait evaluation using inertial measurement units in subjects with Parkinson's disease. J Electromyogr Kinesiol. 2018;42:44–8.
42. Schlachetzki JCM, Barth J, Marxreiter F, Gossler J, Kohl Z, Reinfelder S, et al. Wearable sensors objectively measure gait parameters in Parkinson's disease. PLoS One. 2017;12(10):e0183989. https://doi.org/10.1371/journal.pone.0183989.
43. Kluge F, Gaßner H, Hannink J, Pasluosta C, Klucken J, Eskofier BM. Towards mobile gait analysis: concurrent validity and test-retest reliability of an inertial measurement system for the assessment of spatio-temporal gait parameters. Sensors (Switzerland). 2017;17(7):1522. https://doi.org/10.3390/s17071522.
44. Lipsmeier F, Taylor KI, Kilchenmann T, Wolf D, Scotland A, Schjodt-Eriksen J, et al. Evaluation of smartphone-based testing to generate exploratory outcome measures in a phase 1 Parkinson's disease clinical trial. Movement disorders [internet]. Mov Disord. 2018;33(8):1287–97. https://doi.org/10.1002/mds.27376.
45. Del Din S, Godfrey A, Galna B, Lord S, Rochester L. Free-living gait characteristics in ageing and Parkinson's disease: impact of environment and ambulatory bout length. J Neuroeng Rehabil. 2016;13(1):46.
46. Abou L, Peters J, Wong E, Akers R, Dossou MS, Sosnoff JJ, et al. Gait and balance assessments using smartphone applications in Parkinson's disease: a systematic review. J Med Syst. 2021;45(9):87. https://doi.org/10.1007/s10916-021-01760-5.
47. Godinho C, Domingos J, Cunha G, Santos AT, Fernandes RM, Abreu D, et al. A systematic review of the characteristics and validity of monitoring technologies to assess Parkinson's disease. J Neuroeng Rehabil. 2016;13:24. https://doi.org/10.1186/s12984-016-0136-7.
48. Bettecken K, Bernhard F, Sartor J, Hobert MA, Hofmann M, Gladow T, et al. No relevant association of kinematic gait parameters with health-related quality of life in Parkinson's disease. PLoS One. 2017;12(5):e0176816. https://doi.org/10.1371/journal.pone.0176816.
49. Perumal SV, Sankar R. Gait and tremor assessment for patients with Parkinson's disease using wearable sensors. ICT Express. 2016;2(4):168–74.
50. Santanna A, Salarian A, Wickstrom N. A new measure of movement symmetry in early Parkinson's disease patients using symbolic processing of inertial sensor data. IEEE Trans Biomed Eng. 2011;58(7):2127–35.
51. Ghassemi NH, Hannink J, Roth N, Gaßner H, Marxreiter F, Klucken J, et al. Turning analysis during standardized test using on-shoe wearable sensors in Parkinson's disease. Sensors (Switzerland). 2019;19(14):3103.
52. Godoi BB, Amorim GD, Quiroga DG, Holanda VM, Júlio T, Tournier MB. Parkinson's disease and wearable devices, new perspectives for a public health issue: an integrative literature review. Rev Assoc Med Bras. 2019;65(11):1413–20.
53. Kostikis N, Hristu-Varsakelis D, Arnaoutoglou M, Kotsavasiloglou C. A smartphone-based tool for assessing parkinsonian hand tremor. IEEE J Biomed Health Inform. 2015;19(6):1835–42.
54. Daneault JF, Carignan B, Codère CÉ, Sadikot AF, Duval C. Using a smart phone as a standalone platform for detection and monitoring of pathological tremors. Front Hum Neurosci. 2012;6:357.
55. Elm JJ, Daeschler M, Bataille L, Schneider R, Amara A, Espay AJ, et al. Feasibility and utility of a clinician dashboard from wearable and mobile application Parkinson's disease data. NPJ Digit Med. 2019;2(1):95. https://doi.org/10.1038/s41746-019-0169-y.
56. Lakshminarayana R, Wang D, Burn D, Ray Chaudhuri K, Galtrey C, Valle Guzman N, et al. Erratum: author correction: using a smartphone-based self-management platform to support medication adherence and clinical consultation in Parkinson's disease. NPJ Parkinson's Disease. 2017;3:32. https://doi.org/10.1038/s41531-017-0034-0.
57. Ellis TD, Cavanaugh JT, Deangelis T, Hendron K, Thomas CA, Saint-Hilaire M, et al. Comparative effectiveness of mHealth-supported exercise compared with exercise

alone for people with Parkinson disease: randomized controlled pilot study. Phys Ther. 2018;99(2):203–2016.
58. Landers MR, Ellis TD. A mobile app specifically designed to facilitate exercise in Parkinson disease: single-cohort pilot study on feasibility, safety, and signal of efficacy. JMIR Mhealth Uhealth. 2020;8(10):e18985. https://doi.org/10.2196/18985.
59. Horin AP, McNeely ME, Harrison EC, Myers PS, Sutter EN, Rawson KS, et al. Usability of a daily mHealth application designed to address mobility, speech and dexterity in Parkinson's disease. Neurodegener Dis Manag. 2019;9(2):97–105.
60. Goetz CG, Tilley BC, Shaftman SR, Stebbins GT, Fahn S, Martinez-Martin P, et al. Movement Disorder Society-sponsored revision of the unified Parkinson's disease rating scale (MDS-UPDRS): scale presentation and clinimetric testing results. Mov Disord. 2008;23(15):2129–70.
61. Antonini A, Reichmann H, Gentile G, Garon M, Tedesco C, Frank A, et al. Toward objective monitoring of Parkinson's disease motor symptoms using a wearable device: wearability and performance evaluation of PDMonitor®. Front Neurol. 2023;14:1080752. https://doi.org/10.3389/fneur.2023.1080752.
62. Bhidayasiri R, Martinez-Martin P. Clinical assessments in Parkinson's disease: scales and monitoring. Int Rev Neurobiol. 2017;132:129–82. https://doi.org/10.1016/bs.irn.2017.01.001.
63. Klingelhoefer L, Jitkritsadakul O, Bhidayasiri R. Objective measurement and monitoring of nonmotor symptoms in Parkinson's disease. Int Rev Neurobiol. 2017;133:347–87. https://doi.org/10.1016/bs.irn.2017.04.004.
64. John D, Freedson P. ActiGraph and actical physical activity monitors: a peek under the hood. Med Sci Sports Exerc. 2012;44(1 SUPPL. 1):S86–9. https://doi.org/10.1249/MSS.0b013e3182399f5e.
65. Porta M, Pilloni G, Pili R, Casula C, Murgia M, Cossu G, et al. Association between objectively measured physical activity and gait patterns in people with Parkinson's disease: results from a 3-month monitoring. Parkinsons Dis. 2018;2018:7806574. https://doi.org/10.1155/2018/7806574.
66. Jeng B, Cederberg KLJ, Lai B, Sasaki JE, Bamman MM, Motl RW. Wrist-based accelerometer cut-points for quantifying moderate-to-vigorous intensity physical activity in Parkinson's disease. Gait Posture. 2022;91:235–9.
67. Christiansen C, Moore C, Schenkman M, Kluger B, Kohrt W, Delitto A, et al. Factors associated with ambulatory activity in De novo Parkinson disease. J Neurol Phys Ther [Internet]. 2017;41(2):93–100. Available from: http://insights.ovid.com/crossref?an=01253086-201704000-00002
68. Mantri S, Wood S, Duda JE, Morley JF. Comparing self-reported and objective monitoring of physical activity in Parkinson disease. Parkinsonism Relat Disord [Internet]. 2019;67(September):56–9. https://doi.org/10.1016/j.parkreldis.2019.09.004.
69. Wallén MB, Nero H, Franzén E, Hagströmer M. Comparison of two accelerometer filter settings in individuals with Parkinson's disease. Physiol Meas [Internet]. 2014;35:2287–96. Available from: http://stacks.iop.org/0967-3334/35/i=11/a=2287?key=crossref.e46f9488013f745074a41f00e45fdff5
70. Nero H, Wallén MB, Franzén E, Ståhle A, Hagströmer M. Accelerometer cut points for physical activity assessment of older adults with Parkinson's disease. PLoS One. 2015;10(9):1–11.
71. Nero H, Benka Wallén M, Franzén E, Conradsson D, Ståhle A, Hagströmer M. Objectively assessed physical activity and its association with balance, physical function and dyskinesia in Parkinson's disease. J Parkinsons Dis. 2016;6(4):833–40. https://doi.org/10.3233/JPD-160826.
72. Donahue EK, Venkadesh S, Bui V, Tuazon AC, Wang RK, Haase D, et al. Physical activity intensity is associated with cognition and functional connectivity in Parkinson's disease. Parkinsonism Relat Disord. 2022 Nov;1(104):7–14.
73. Ellingson LD, Zaman A, Stegemöller EL. Sedentary behavior and quality of life in individuals with Parkinson's disease. Neurorehabil Neural Repair. 2019;33(8):595–601.
74. Mantri S, Wood S, Duda JE, Morley JF. Understanding physical activity in veterans with Parkinson disease : a mixed-methods approach. Parkinsonism Relat Disord. 2019;61:156–60.

75. Edwardson CL, Winkler EAH, Bodicoat DH, Yates T, Davies MJ, Dunstan DW, et al. Considerations when using the activPAL monitor in field-based research with adult populations. J Sport Health Sci. 2017;6:162–78.
76. Lamont RM, Daniel HL, Payne CL, Brauer SG. Accuracy of wearable physical activity trackers in people with Parkinson's disease. Gait Posture [Internet]. 2018;63:104–8. https://doi.org/10.1016/j.gaitpost.2018.04.034.
77. Godfrey A, Morris R, Hickey A, Del Din S. Beyond the front end: investigating a thigh worn accelerometer device for step count and bout detection in Parkinson's disease. Med Eng Phys. 2016;38(12):1524–9.
78. Lyden K, Kozey Keadle SL, Staudenmayer JW, Freedson PS. Validity of two wearable monitors to estimate breaks from sedentary time. Med Sci Sports Exerc. 2012;44(11):2243–52.
79. Godfrey A, Culhane KM, Lyons GM. Comparison of the performance of the activPAL™ professional physical activity logger to a discrete accelerometer-based activity monitor. Med Eng Phys. 2007;29(8):930–4.
80. Taraldsen K, Askim T, Sletvold O, Einarsen EK, Bjåstad KG, Indredavik B, et al. Evaluation of a body-worn sensor system to measure physical activity in older people with impaired function. Phys Ther. 2011;91(2):277–85.
81. Cavanaught JT, Ellis TD, Earhart GM, Ford MP, Foreman KB, Dibble LE. Capturing ambulatory activity decline in Parkinson disease. J Neurol Phys Ther. 2012;36(2):51–7.
82. Lamont RM, Morris ME, Woollacott MH, Brauer SG. Ambulatory activity in people with early Parkinson's disease. Brain Impairment. 2016;17(1):87–98.
83. Adams JL, Kangarloo T, Tracey B, O'Donnell P, Volfson D, Latzman RD, et al. Using a smartwatch and smartphone to assess early Parkinson's disease in the WATCH-PD study. NPJ Parkinsons Dis. 2023;9(1):64. https://doi.org/10.1038/s41531-023-00497-x.
84. de Lima ALS, Evers LJW, Hahn T, de Vries NM, Daeschler M, Boroojerdi B, et al. Impact of motor fluctuations on real-life gait in Parkinson's patients. Gait Posture [Internet]. 2018;62:388–94. https://doi.org/10.1016/j.gaitpost.2018.03.045.

31 Remote Balance and Gait Assessment Via Telehealth: Are We Ready for This?

Paulo Henrique Silva Pelicioni, Renato Barbosa dos Santos, Carolina Tsen, and Larissa Pires de Andrade

Abstract

The use of telehealth has grown in the last two decades; however, its "boom" happened during the COVID-19 pandemic. With that, clinicians and researchers shifted their assessments and treatment sessions to telehealth. However, most of these assessments have not been previously investigated to determine whether they were feasible, reliable, and valid to be used via telehealth, especially gait and balance assessments, once they are challenging to administer and perform in older adults and people with neurological disorders. In this chapter, we discussed the use of balance and gait assessments via telehealth and how clinicians and researchers have adapted these assessments to be undertaken remotely. In this in-depth-discussed chapter, we argue whether these assessments are safe to be used remotely, and we, as researchers and clinicians, are ready for this.

Background

Telehealth is defined as the "delivery of healthcare services where patients and providers are separated by a distance" [1]. The World Health Organization (WHO) also defines that "telehealth uses information and communication technologies for the exchange of information for the diagnosis and treatment of diseases and injuries,

P. H. S. Pelicioni (✉)
School of Health Sciences, University of New South Wales, Sydney, NSW, Australia
e-mail: paulo.silvapelicioni@unsw.edu.au

R. B. dos Santos
Rehabilitation Sciences Institute, University of Toronto, Toronto, ON, Canada
e-mail: renatob.santos@utoronto.ca

C. Tsen · L. P. de Andrade
Physiotherapy Department, Federal University of São Carlos, São Paulo, Brazil
e-mail: carolina.tsen@estudante.ufscar.br; larissa.andrade@ufscar.br

F. A. Barbieri et al. (eds.), *Locomotion and Posture in Older Adults*,
https://doi.org/10.1007/978-3-031-74123-4_31

research and evaluation and the continuing education of health professionals" [1]. Telehealth first emerged in Europe during the middle ages, when a doctor isolated himself during the plague due to the risk of contamination and communicated with a community worker to provide instructions and guidance for treatment and has been increasingly popular, even more during the COVID-19 pandemic [2].

Due to the COVID-19 pandemic and its fast spread, the WHO recommended lockdowns to prevent the spread of COVID-19 [3]. These measures, however, prevented the population from accessing health services, exerting negative impacts on functional capacity, mental health, and quality of life [3–8], particularly for older adults [9] and people with neurological disorders [10]. To mitigate the impacts of the COVID-19 pandemic, health professionals sought to apply "Actions at a distance" in clinical practice, using telehealth to provide health services to the general population, especially to the most vulnerable ones [9–11].

Telehealth brings many advantages, such as increasing access to health services, improving treatment delivery, promoting adherence to treatments, promoting self-care, providing remote transmission of care, and providing information quickly accessible through technology. These advantages are significant for the rural population or people in remote areas with little access to health services [12–17]. This method can be performed synchronously when there is real-time communication (live) between health professionals and clients/patients/consumers, such as video and audio calls. Also, it can be carried out asynchronously, which occurs offline by receiving guidance and information provided by professionals [12, 18]. Additionally, telehealth can be delivered using websites, apps, sensors, and accessories technology, among others [19].

The use of telehealth is observed in studies focusing on screenings or assessments with different methods and even using remote sensors [20–22] in reliability analyses comparing virtual and face-to-face assessments and interventions, analysis of the effects, and effectiveness of the use of telehealth in the prevention of falls, improvements in activities of daily living, physical functioning, participation, and adherence to rehabilitation [21, 23, 24], especially in assessments of balance and gait of these individuals.

In recent years, telehealth has been widely used for delivering interventions synchronously or asynchronously, monitoring patients, undertaking cognitive, quality of life and physical assessments, and investigating interventions' effects on balance and gait [15, 25, 26]. Some populations involved in studies using telehealth comprised older adults and people with neurological disorders, such as stroke survivors, Parkinson's disease (PD), dementias, and other age-related pathologies [21, 22, 26, 27]. In this chapter, we focus our discussion on the use of telehealth to assess balance and gait when an interaction happens between clients/patients/ consumers and therapists/clinicians/health professionals, rather than using sensors or apps which could also be used in clinical practice.

Telehealth in Aging

In the aging process, functional decline occurs, and greater chances of loss of independence may increase with the accumulation of comorbidities. The COVID-19 pandemic has disproportionately impacted the health of older adults worldwide. The increased use of telehealth for this population during the pandemic, and new information about this modality was explored [28]. Although telehealth can be seen as important and promising for the implementation of interventions, it should be noted that its use can be complex, especially in older adults, as some factors may hinder the expansion of services. Patient safety, lack of data reliability, lack of face-to-face physical examination by health professionals, lack of access to technology, legal restrictions, and ambiguous health insurance coverage policies [29] comprise a list of concerns regarding the use of telehealth in older adults. In addition, health professionals need to take into account, when considering telehealth sessions, the lack of technological literacy in older adults and the need for adjustments for possible cognitive decline or natural auditory and/or visual deficits during the course of aging [30].

Wildenbos et al. [31] carried out a scoping review to summarize the main physical and functional barriers to the use of telehealth in older adults. The authors identified four main categories of aging barriers: cognition, motivation, physical ability, and perception. The effective and satisfactory use of telehealth by older adults is hampered by cognitive and motivational barriers. Physical ability and perceptual barriers further increase the risk of user errors and failure to perceive important interaction tasks. Furthermore, complexities of medical conditions, such as visual impairment related to diabetes or impaired motor skills, can cause errors in user interaction [31].

Concerns regarding the rapid increase in the use of telehealth during COVID-19 include the quality of the assessments undertaken, which could not be reliable nor valid to assess what these measures were supposed to measure, especially balance and gait, which are related to fall risk. So, inaccurate information to patients could affect the progression and efficacy of their treatments. To evaluate the effectiveness of physical performance, mainly balance and gait, which could be delivered via telehealth, it is important to consider whether these assessments are reliable and valid. In a previous study, Pelicioni et al. investigated whether balance and gait measurements used in clinical practice are reliable and valid when remotely used via telehealth in 15 older adults [32]. The authors evaluated various tests that are usually undertaken in face-to-face clinical practice, such as the Timed Up and Go (TUG), simple and with dual cognitive and motor tasks; Berg Balance Scale (BBS), Functional Gait Assessment and Dynamic Gait Index. The tests were administered on two different dates, using different modalities: (i) face-to-face (ii) and remote assessment via videoconference. The results showed that all tests presented good reliability when comparing face-to-face and real-time telehealth (ICC = 0.79–0.87) and also when comparing face-to-face and telehealth after being recorded and re-watched (ICC = 0.78–0.88). For the recorded telehealth assessments, the authors observed good to excellent interrater reliability (ICC = 0.80–1.00) for all tests examined. Finally, they observed that these tests were correlated with a measurement of fall risk, the physiological profile assessment. These correlations were significant for real time (r = −0.68–0.64) and recorded (r = −0.69–0.71) telehealth assessments, indicating that even when gold standard assessments of balance and gait are used remotely, they are valid to measure fall risk. These results showed good reliability between face-to-face and remote measurements, together with moderate validity of these measures to assess fall risk. Thus, health professionals could use these measures to evaluate the balance and gait of older adults remotely.

Overall, studies show that the use of telehealth in older adults is promising, but more research is needed, including research focusing on usability, participation, and the investigation of reliability in other tests highly used in clinical practice [e.g., Short Physical Performance Battery (SPPB)] [33]. There is now growing optimism about the global use of telehealth services in various specialties, not different for geriatric care. Optimizing telehealth services that can be accessed by older adults requires greater government investment and active engagement through broader participation by older adults, their families and caregivers, healthcare professionals, technology experts, and health managers.

Telehealth in Neurological Disorders and Age-Related Pathologies

The scientific literature on telehealth in neurological disorders and age-related pathologies suggests that it holds promise as a convenient and effective approach for assessing outcomes and managing and treating these conditions. The drastic changes imposed by the COVID-19 pandemic, which greatly impacted the delivery of health services, propelled the uptake of telehealth for assessment, service delivery (including prevention, rehabilitation, supervision, support, and education) and evaluation.

Several studies have explored the use of telehealth interventions in various neurological disorders, such as stroke [34, 35], PD [36, 37], multiple sclerosis [38], and dementia [39]. These studies have used various telecommunication technologies, such as the internet, videoconferencing, telephone, and virtual reality and found positive outcomes in terms of improved functional outcomes, including balance and gait. Balance and gait assessments are crucial components of rehabilitation for patients with neurological conditions. Traditionally, these assessments have been performed in person by healthcare professionals using specialized equipment and standardized measures. The use of validated assessment tools to evaluate balance and gait is a recommended best practice in rehabilitation to evaluate the magnitude of the deficit, inform treatment selection, patient education and goal setting, and monitor response to treatment [40]. Several measures of balance and gait have demonstrated evidence of reliability, validity, and sensitivity to change when administered in person by clinicians. In the next sections, we provide an overview of the literature on remote assessment of balance and gait via telehealth in stroke survivors, people with PD, people with dementia, and people affected by other aging-related pathologies.

Stroke

The current literature suggests that telehealth in stroke rehabilitation can be feasible and effective compared with in-person appointments [34]. Recently published systematic reviews indicate that telehealth produces similar effects on outcomes such as balance, motor function, and performance of activities of daily living, as well as high patient satisfaction when compared to conventional in-person rehabilitation [34, 35]. Furthermore, some programs offered via telehealth have shown the advantage of potentially being less costly than in-person therapy.

A recent review of ten stroke clinical practice guidelines worldwide identified recommendations for the use of over 25 unique standardized tools for assessing balance and mobility (including gait) [41]. For people with stroke, guidelines most commonly recommend using the BBS to evaluate standing balance, 6-Minute Walk Test (6MWT) to evaluate functional walking capacity, the TUG as a measure of functional mobility, and the 10-Meter Walk Test (10mWT) for assessing gait speed. These tests can be incorporated in a telehealth setting if adequate equipment and space are available.

While some assessment tools that evaluate balance and gait may not be feasible or safe to use in a virtual assessment due to a lack of safeguarding from a therapist and inadequate space and equipment, others may be suitable. Selected tests for telehealth use should have low equipment/technology requirements, brief administration time, easy-to-understand instructions, and performance tasks that could be viewed using a webcam or a camera from cell phones or tablets. The Canadian Stroke Best Practice Recommendations: Virtual Stroke Rehabilitation Interim Consensus Statement 2022 recommends that assessment tools selected for use via telehealth should have evidence of validity for the method of virtual administration and be administered by trained personnel using a structured process [42].

To date, only a limited number of studies have examined the validity and reliability of balance and gait assessment when administered remotely using telehealth in stroke survivors [43, 44]. Of these tests, one study compared the performance of 20 community-dwelling stroke survivors on the BBS administered in person and using telehealth [43]. In this study, a pair of trained physical and occupational therapists administered the BBS, and a trained therapy assistant was present at the participant's home. The findings showed that agreement of total scores (range of total score: 20–56 points) was excellent between the telehealth and in-person assessment methods ($\kappa = 0.97$; 95% CI: 0.96, 0.99). Interrater reliability estimates were excellent for all BBS items except two, which the estimates were good for turning to look behind (item 10), (ICC = 0.84, 95% CI: 0.61, 0.94), and tandem stance (item 13) (ICC = 0.81, 95% CI: 0.52, 0.93). In addition, responses regarding patients' perceived hearing and understanding of instructions as well as perceived safety, were comparable between both modes of assessments. However, the generalizability of study findings is limited since participants were provided with a laptop with a motorized camera that evaluators could remotely control, and a therapy assistant was present in the home to assist with the assessments.

In another study examining 21 community-dwelling stroke survivors (> 1-year post-stroke), the authors estimated the reliability, validity, and feasibility of using five measures to assess stroke survivors via videoconferencing (i.e., Zoom®). Assessments were the 5-times Sit-to-Stand (5STS), widely used to evaluate lower extremity strength for older adults and as a predictor of falls and dependence in activities of daily living [45]; the Functional Reach Test (FRT) [46], a task included in the BBS to evaluate the maximum distance an individual can reach forward while standing in a fixed position; the tandem stance (TS), a measure of standing balance also a task among the BBS items; the TUG; and the 30-second sit-to-stand (30STS) which measures subjects' lower extremity muscle strength and balance capacity. In this study, a trained physiotherapist conducted three sessions. The first session included orienting the participant to the Zoom® platform and preparing the evaluation environment (i.e., identifying the 3-m route for conducting TUG in the participant's home, ensuring the safety of the environment, and optimizing the camera view). In the second session, the physiotherapist conducted virtual balance and mobility assessments over videoconferencing. In the third session, a week later, all the virtual assessments were administered again by the same physiotherapist. The intra-rater reliability was excellent for the TUG (ICC = 0.97; 95% CI 0.90, 0.99) and the 30STS (ICC = 0.90, 95% CI 0.78, 0.96). Good intra-rater reliability was found for the 5STS (ICC = 0.77, 95% CI 0.51, 0.90). The lowest reliability of the clinical measures was observed for the FRT (ICC = 0.54, 95% CI 0.12, 0.79) and TS tests (ICC = 0.50, 95% CI 0.09, 0.77).

Regarding the feasibility of administering balance and gait assessments via telehealth, participants faced technical challenges and internet connection difficulties. However, they generally felt safe while performing the tasks. The orientation session proved helpful in familiarizing them with the setup and videoconferencing platform, and the physiotherapist's explicit instruction and demonstration provided clarity during the assessments. The physiotherapist emphasized certain important factors for conducting the assessment effectively. Firstly, for conducting an initial session to familiarize the participant with the platform and determine the evaluation setup in their home environment. Secondly, using a safety check-in list to ensure the clinician's comfort in remotely challenging participants' balance. Thirdly, to ensure that the participants watched the physiotherapist's task demonstration before attempting it themselves. Lastly, avoiding talking to participants while they focused on performing the timed task, therefore minimizing interruptions or diverting their attention to the videoconferencing device. Concerning the safety of each measure, the physiotherapist expressed particular concern regarding the safety of the FRT, as it raised the most concern for potential loss of balance during the assessment since participants perform this test excursing over their limits of stability.

Overall, telehealth has shown to be a feasible and effective option for stroke rehabilitation, including balance and gait assessments. While some assessments may not be suitable for virtual administration due to a lack of supervision and limited space/equipment, others can be adapted. Limited studies have explored the validity and reliability of remote balance and gait assessments, but preliminary findings indicate promising results. Despite technical challenges and internet difficulties, participants generally felt safe and benefited from the orientation session and explicit instructions provided by the physiotherapist. Important considerations for effective telehealth assessments include initial orientation, safety checks, task demonstrations, and minimizing distractions.

Parkinson's Disease

Even before the COVID-19 pandemic, clinicians considered that telehealth was a good quality modality to examine people with PD [47] since both physicians and patients were highly satisfied with telehealth services for people with PD. Despite patients' satisfaction, there is not much evidence regarding the use of telehealth to assess the balance and gait of people with PD. The only study undertaken to examine the reliability of gait and balance assessment in people with PD was undertaken over ten years ago, using a cohort of only 12 participants (Hoehn and Yahr stages from 1 to 4) [48]. In this study, Russel et al. [49] undertook assessments in person and remotely, although the assessors were still in the same building. The authors examined balance and gait assessments' interrater (baseline versus telehealth) and intra-rater (for telehealth only) reliability: time stance test, TUG, step test, number of steps taken to turn 360 degrees, BBS, lateral and forward FRT. The authors obtained excellent intra-rater (ICC > 0.98) and interrater (ICC >0.96) for all assessments. When the authors examined the reliability of each BBS item, all items showed excellent reliability (Kappa scores ranging from 0.77 to 1.00) except for the item "standing on one leg." Due to the small sample size and the fact that these participants did not perform these tests remotely at home and always with a presence of a therapist, these results might not be generalizable.

Ashfari et al. [50] examined 5STS and 360-degree rapid turn tests remotely in 15 people with mild to moderate PD (Hoehn and Yahr 2 and 3). These participants undertook four telehealth visits (at their home environment) every 2 weeks after the initial assessment in person. The authors did not examine the reliability of these tests remotely; however, they found out that 22% of the 5STS assessments determined individuals at fall risk (score > 16 s or the use of a support to perform the test) and 55% of the assessments were sensitive to capture freezing of gait in these participants during the 360-degree rapid turn test. The authors did not find any limitations to undertaking these tests at home, and participants did not exhibit any near falls or fall during the assessments.

The main PD clinical assessment for measuring patients' motor impairments, the Movement Disorders Society—Unified Parkinson's Disease Rating Scale (MDS-UPDRS) [51], was initially not encouraged to be used remotely via telehealth since clinicians cannot assess patients' rigidity and neither their postural reflexes because these assessment items require a clinician/ patient in-person interaction [52]. On the other hand, Luo et al. [53] found out that the MDS-UPDRS part III (for motor impairments assessment) total score still correlates with the sum of part III's score without rigidity and postural reflexes assessment items. However, if the progression of rigidity and balance recovery is important for examining certain patients, clinicians must examine them in person to overcome this limitation. Given that there is no way to remotely assess the entire MDS-UPDRS part III due to the limitation of not assessing rigidity and postural reflexes, as mentioned above, researchers created an abbreviated version of the MDS-UPDRS to be undertaken remotely [54]. This abbreviated version of the MDS-UPDRS comprises eight items from parts I (non-motor experiences of daily living), II (motor experiences of daily living) and III, including assessments of walking and balance (item 12, part II) and arising from a chair (item 9 from part III). The MDS-UPDRS abbreviated version highly correlated with the full version of the assessment ($r = 0.919/p < 0.0001$), indicating this tool is promising for remote assessment.

The assessment of balance and gait remotely via telehealth in people with PD is promising; however, there are no reliable and valid tools to assess people with PD remotely. The only study undertaken so far to examine the reliability of gait and balance assessments [49], unfortunately, is underpowered and did not examine people in their home environment. Yet, the results are promising since the tools used in these assessments are highly used in clinical practice and are highly reliable and valid for assessing fall risk in older adults without PD [32]. Moreover, the possibility to undertake MDS-UPDRS remotely, either entire or abbreviated, adds some robust information to examine the clinical aspects of PD fully and consequently gives a thorough clinical examination to be used as outcomes for interventions focusing on balance and gait rehabilitation.

Dementia

In people with dementia, non-pharmacological interventions, such as physical and cognitive exercises, have been used in-person to improve mental health [55, 56] and functional capacity in these populations [57, 58]. These types of interventions seem to be feasible alternatives to deliver via telehealth for people with dementia compared to in-person care [5, 11, 59, 60].

In a pilot study comparing the effect of telehealth and face-to-face rehabilitation on the cognitive performance of people with dementia, Jelcic et al. [61] observed that telehealth had positive effects on cognition. It seems then that telehealth, if used in intensive care is well accepted by this population. In a recent systematic review [60], authors examined the impact of telehealth on health outcomes in people with dementia living in rural areas. The authors observed that telehealth is a potentially promising solution to overcome barriers imposed by the COVID-19 pandemic to access conventional healthcare. Moreover, older adults, their families, and healthcare professionals were satisfied with telehealth. In the study conducted by Menengi et al. [62], the use of telehealth in people with Alzheimer's disease could provide significant changes in cognition and mobility, resulting in greater independence. Finally, due to the positive effects of telehealth use on people with dementia, Tsen et al. are examining the impacts of physical activity delivered through telehealth on the functional capacity, mental health and quality of life of people with dementia [39].

Unfortunately, no study thus far has investigated the reliability and validity of balance and gait assessments administered via telehealth in people with dementia. Therefore, interventions using telehealth in this population have used assessments that are reliable and valid in older populations without dementia, such as the assessments previously investigated by Pelicioni et al. [32]. Thus, when assessing people with dementia, we must be careful in assuming the safety of tools used to assess populations without dementia. Measures of safety should be adopted (e.g., having caregivers support throughout the entire assessment) and assessments that are of easy instruction (e.g., TUG) could present a viable option to assess the balance and gait of these individuals via telehealth. More studies should be undertaken to address this important clinical gap.

Aged-Related Pathologies

In addition to the neurological disorders discussed above, it is worth mentioning other clinical conditions that affect older adults. In the systematic review by Walsh et al. [63], the authors investigated the psychometric properties of measures based on the performance of the physical function in individuals with chronic health conditions, including balance and gait assessments such as TUG and the 6MWT. The authors did not observe strong evidence to affirm the reliability of the tests; however, the authors state that the quality of the included studies was low, associated with the low sample number and absence of optimized analyzes [63]. Although these studies have contributed to the advancement of knowledge about psychometric results in remote assessments, most studies carried out remote assessments in healthy older adults [32], people with PD [49], cancer patients [64] or people who had heart failure [65]. Examining the use of telehealth in other populations, such as people with knee osteoarthritis or people with mild cognitive impairment, should be investigated in order to guarantee safe and reliable assessments for a broad spectrum of older adults suffering from many diverse conditions, including musculoskeletal, neurological, and cardiac diseases/disorders.

Challenges, Solutions, and Future Directions

While the WHO has suggested the adoption of telehealth as a means for achieving the equitable provision of health-related services, older adults and people with neurological disorders experience difficulties and barriers accessing and using virtually-delivered remote services. Below we highlight some of the challenges and potential solutions for administering gait and balance assessment remotely via telehealth [1].

1. Technical limitations: older adults and people with neurological disorders may have limited experience or familiarity with technology, making it challenging for them to navigate the telehealth platform or use the required devices for balance and gait assessments. Technical difficulties such as poor internet connectivity,

audio or video lag, problems with equipment handling (e.g., poor dexterity to click small cell phone buttons), or equipment setup issues can also hinder the assessment process.

2. Environmental constraints: Assessing gait and balance remotely may be limited by the physical environment of these patients' home environment. Limited space, obstacles, or uneven surfaces for performing specific tasks can impact the accuracy and reliability of the assessments.
3. Lack of physical presence: Assessing gait and balance remotely eliminates the ability of a healthcare professional to provide hands-on assistance or support during the assessment. This can make it challenging to ensure proper positioning, technique, or safety measures during the evaluation. This can be more harmful in tests requiring transitions, fast responses and tasks that could elicit some unwanted responses (e.g., a 360-degree fast turn could trigger an episode of freezing of gait in people with PD).
4. Lack of standardized protocols: The absence of standardized protocols for conducting gait and balance assessments through telehealth can make it challenging to ensure consistency and reliability across different healthcare providers or settings. This can impact the comparability of results and hinder the ability to track progress or make accurate treatment decisions.
5. Safety concerns: Safety is a crucial aspect of gait and balance assessments, especially in populations who may be at a higher risk of falls (e.g., an older adult frequent faller, a person with moderate PD, etc.). Ensuring adequate supervision, monitoring, and safeguards during remote assessments can be challenging, potentially compromising patients' safety.
6. Social-economic barriers: the use of devices, such as tablets and Smartphones, has increased, even in populations of low-social economic status. However, assuming that all people will equally have access to technology is not equitable. Thus, we must be careful in considering the use of telehealth assessments and treatments in people from low social, economic status, including those living in rural and remote areas, since in some remote places, Internet signal can be poor, therefore not benefiting these individuals.

Addressing these challenges requires careful consideration and adaptations in telehealth protocols and practices. The selection of tests that have low equipment/technology requirements, brief administration time, easy-to-understand instructions, and performance tasks that could be viewed using a webcam is highly recommended. To overcome these challenges, clinicians might consider providing technical support, such as an orientation session (either in-person or remote) or having someone familiar with the technology to support the patient during the assessments that could also help in positioning the camera to provide an optimal view for the evaluator. In addition, modifying assessment procedures to suit the virtual environment and developing standardized protocols for administration could be considered, as long as it does not change the characteristics of the tests, consequently reducing their reliability. The implementation of safety measures to mitigate risks, such as clearing the space and having emergency contacts in hand, is crucial. Finally, ongoing research and the adaptation or development of reliable and validated assessment tools specific to be used via telehealth to assess gait and balance in older adults and people with neurological disorders can help overcome these challenges and improve the feasibility and reliability of remote assessments.

References

1. World Health Organisation. WHO-ITU global standard for accessibility of telehealth services 2022. Available on https://www.who.int/publications/i/item/9789240050464.
2. Seid AA, Aychiluhm SB, Mohammed AA. Effectiveness and feasibility of telerehabilitation in patients with COVID-19: a systematic review and meta-analysis. BMJ Open. 2022;12:e063961.
3. World Health Organization. Critical preparedness, readiness and response actions for COVID-19: interim guidance. Available from https://www.Who.Int/Publications-Detail/Critical-Preparedness-Readiness-And-Response-Actions-For-Covid-19.
4. Azevedo LVS, Calandri IL, Slachevsky A, Graviotto HG, Santos-Vieira MC, Andrade CBD, et al. Impact of social isolation on people with dementia and their family caregivers. J Alzheimers Dis. 2021;81:607–17.
5. Di Lorito C, Masud T, Gladman J, Godfrey M, Dunlop M, Harwood RH. Deconditioning in people living with dementia during the COVID-19 pandemic: qualitative study from the promoting activity, Independence and stability in early dementia (PrAISED) process evaluation. BMC Geriatr. 2021;21:529.
6. Kumar A, Salinas J. The long-term public health impact of social distancing on brain health: topical review. Int J Environ Res Public Health. 2021;18:7307.
7. Rokstad AMM, Røsvik J, Fossberg M, Eriksen S. The COVID-19 pandemic as experienced by the spouses of home-dwelling people with dementia–a qualitative study. BMC Geriatr. 2021;21:583.
8. Verity R, Okell LC, Dorigatti I, Winskill P, Whittaker C, Imai N, et al. Estimates of the severity of coronavirus disease 2019: a model-based analysis. Lancet Infect Dis. 2020;20:669–77.
9. Pelicioni PHS, Lord SR. COVID-19 will severely impact older people's lives, and in many more ways than you think! Braz J Phys Ther. 2020;24:293–4.
10. Pelicioni PHS, Schulz-Moore JS, Hale L, Canning CG, Lord SR. Lockdown during COVID-19 pandemic and the increase of frailty in people with neurological conditions. Front Neurol. 2020;11:604299.
11. Nicol GE, Piccirillo JF, Mulsant BH, Lenze EJ. Action at a distance: geriatric research during a pandemic. J Am Geriatr Soc. 2020;68:922–5.
12. Cary MP Jr, Spencer M, Carroll A, Hand DH, Amis K, Karan E, et al. Benefits and challenges of delivering tele-rehabilitation services to rural veterans. Home Health Now. 2016;34:440–6.
13. Xu L, Li F, Zhou C, Li J, Hong C, Tong Q. The effect of mobile applications for improving adherence in cardiac rehabilitation: a systematic review and meta-analysis. BMC Cardiovasc Disord. 2019;19:166.
14. Smith AC, Thomas E, Snoswell CL, Haydon H, Mehrotra A, Clemensen J, et al. Telehealth for global emergencies: implications for coronavirus disease 2019 (COVID-19). J Telemed Telecare. 2020;26:309–13.
15. McDonnell JM, Ahern DP, Ross TD, Gibbons D, Synnott KA, Butler JS. The efficacy of remote virtual care in comparison to traditional clinical visits for elective orthopaedic patients: a meta-analysis of prospective randomised controlled trials. Surgeon. 2022;20:177–86.
16. Zischke C, Simas V, Hing W, Milne N, Spittle A, Pope R. The utility of physiotherapy assessments delivered by telehealth: a systematic review. J Glob Health. 2021;11:04072.
17. Xie L, Zhang S, Xin M, Zhu M, Lu W, Mo PKH. Electronic health literacy and health-related outcomes among older adults: a systematic review. Prev Med. 2022;157:106997.

18. Jaswal S, Lo J, Sithamparanathan G, Nowrouzi-Kia B. The era of technology in healthcare: an evaluation of telerehabilitation on patient outcomes—a systematic review and meta-analysis protocol. Syst Rev. 2023;12:76.
19. Tossaint-Schoenmakers R, Versluis A, Chavannes N, Talboom-Kamp E, Kasteleyn M. The challenge of integrating eHealth into health care: systematic literature review of the Donabedian model of structure, process, and outcome. J Med Internet Res. 2021;23:e27180.
20. Gaspar AGM, Lapão LV. eHealth for addressing balance disorders in the elderly: systematic review. J Med Internet Res. 2021;23:e22215.
21. Kraaijkamp JJ, van Dam van Isselt EF, Persoon A, Verslui A, Chavannes NH, Achterberg WP. eHealth in geriatric rehabilitation: systematic review of effectiveness, feasibility, and usability. J Med Internet Res. 2021;23:e24015.
22. Saito T, Izawa KP. Effectiveness and feasibility of home-based telerehabilitation for community-dwelling elderly people in southeast Asian countries and regions: a systematic review. Aging Clin Exp Res. 2021;33:2657–69.
23. Yerrakalva D, Yerrakalva D, Hajna S, Griffin S. Effects of mobile health app interventions on sedentary time, physical activity, and fitness in older adults: systematic review and meta-analysis. J Med Internet Res. 2019;21:e14343.
24. Lu AD, Veet CA, Aljundi O, Whitaker E, Smith WB, Smith JE. A systematic review of physical examination components adapted for telemedicine. Telemed J E Health. 2022;28:1764–85.
25. Wang K, Varma DS, Prosperi M. A systematic review of the effectiveness of mobile apps for monitoring and management of mental health symptoms or disorders. J Psychiatr Res. 2018;107:73–8.
26. Abou L, Peters J, Wong E, Akers R, Dossou MS, Sosnoff JJ, et al. Gait and balance assessments using smartphone applications in Parkinson's disease: a systematic review. J Med Syst. 2021;45:87.
27. Sarfo FS, Ulasavets U, Opare-Sem OK, Ovbiagele B. Tele-rehabilitation after stroke: an updated systematic review of the literature. J Stroke Cerebrovasc Dis. 2018;27:2306–18.
28. Doraiswamy S, Jithesh A, Mamtani R, Abraham A, Cheema S. Telehealth use in geriatrics care during the COVID-19 pandemic — a scoping review and evidence synthesis. Int J Environ Res Public Health. 2021;18:1755.
29. Lustig TA. The role of telehealth in an evolving health care environment: workshop summary. Washington, DC: National Academies Press; 2012.
30. Foster MV, Sethares KA. Facilitators and barriers to the adoption of telehealth in older adults: an integrative review. Comput Inform Nurs. 2014;32:523–33.
31. Wildenbos GA, Peute L, Jaspers M. Aging barriers influencing mobile health usability for older adults: a literature based framework (MOLD-US). Int J Med Inform. 2018;114:66–75.
32. Pelicioni PHS, Waters DL, Still A, Hale L. A pilot investigation of reliability and validity of balance and gait assessments using telehealth with healthy older adults. Exp Gerontol. 2022;162:111747.
33. Guralnik JM, Seeman TE, Tinetti ME, et al. Validation and use of performance measures of functioning in a non-disabled older population: MacArthur studies of successful aging. Aging. 1994;6:410–9.
34. Laver KE, Schoene D, Crotty M, George S, Lannin NA, Sherrington C. Telerehabilitation services for stroke. Cochrane Database Syst Rev. 2013;2013:CD010255.
35. Tchero H, Teguo MT, Lannuzel A, Rusch E. Telerehabilitation for stroke survivors: systematic review and meta-analysis. J Med Internet Res. 2018;20:e10867.
36. Flynn A, Preston E, Dennis S, Canning CG, Allen NE. Home-based exercise monitored with telehealth is feasible and acceptable compared to Centre-based exercise in Parkinson's disease: a randomized pilot study. Clin Rehabil. 2021;35:728–39.
37. Bianchini E, Onelli C, Morabito C, Alborghetti M, Rinaldi D, Anibaldi P, et al. Feasibility, safety, and effectiveness of telerehabilitation in mild-to-moderate Parkinson's disease. Front Neurol. 2022;13:909197.
38. Khan F, Amatya B, Kesselring J, Galea M. Telerehabilitation for persons with multiple sclerosis. Cochrane Database Syst Rev. 2015;2015:CD010508.

39. Tsen C, Andreatto CADA, Aily JB, Pelicioni PHS, Neto DB, Mattiello SM, et al. Effects of telehealth on functional capacity, mental health and quality of life among older people with dementia: LAPESI telehealth protocol for a randomized controlled trial. Physiother Res Int. 2023;28:e1981.
40. Moore JL, Potter K, Blankshain K, Kaplan SL, O'Dwyer LC, Sullivan JE. A core set of outcome measures for adults with neurologic conditions undergoing rehabilitation: a clinical practice guideline. J Neurol Phys Ther. 2018;42:174–220.
41. Dos Santos RB, Fiedler A, Badwal A, Legasto-Mulvale JM, Sibley KM, Olaleye OA, et al. Standardized tools for assessing balance and mobility in stroke clinical practice guidelines worldwide: a scoping review. Front Rehabil Sci. 2023;4:1084085.
42. Salbach NM, Mountain A, Lindsay MP, Blacquiere D, McGuff R, Foley N, et al. Canadian stroke best practice recommendations: virtual stroke rehabilitation interim consensus statement 2022. Am J Phys Med Rehabil. 2022;101:1076–82.
43. Gillespie D, MacLellan C, Ferguson-Pell M, Taeger A, Manns PJ. Balancing access with technology: comparing in-person and telerehabilitation berg balance scale scores among stroke survivors. Physiother Can. 2021;73:276–85.
44. Peng T-H, Harris A, Tang A, Sakakibara B, Eng JJ, Pollock CL. Clinical measures of balance and walking ability in people with stroke for assessment via videoconferencing. Physiother Can. 2023;2023:e20220039. https://doi.org/10.3138/ptc-2022-0039.
45. Bohannon RW. Reference values for the five-repetition sit-to-stand test: a descriptive meta-analysis of data from elders. Percept Mot Skills. 2006;103:215–22.
46. Duncan PW, Weiner DK, Chandler J, Studenski S. Functional reach: a new clinical measure of balance. J Gerontol. 1990;45:M192–7.
47. Hanson RE, Truesdell M, Stebbins GT, Weathers AL, Goetz CG. Telemedicine vs office visits in a movement disorders clinic: comparative satisfaction of physicians and patients. Mov Disord Clin Pract. 2019;6:65–9.
48. Hoehn MM, Yahr MD. Parkinsonism: onset, progression, and mortality. Neurology. 1967;17:427.
49. Russell TG, Hoffmann TC, Nelson M, Thompson L, Vincent A. Internet-based physical assessment of people with Parkinson disease is accurate and reliable: a pilot study. J Rehabil Res Dev. 2013;50:643–50.
50. Ashfari M, Hernandez AV, Nonnekes J, Bloem BR, Goetz CG. Are virtual objective assessments of fall-risk feasible and safe for people with Parkinson's disease? Mov Disord Clin Pract. 2022;9:799–804.
51. Goetz CG, Tilley BC, Shaftman SR, Stebbins GT, Fahn S, Martinez-Martin P, et al. Movement disorder society-sponsored revision of the unified Parkinson's disease rating scale (MDS-UPDRS): scale presentation and clinimetric testing results. Mov Disord. 2008;23:2129–70.
52. Goetz CG, Stebbins GT, Luo S. Movement disorder society–unified Parkinson's disease rating scale use in the COVID-19 era. Mov Disord. 2020;35:911.
53. Luo S, Goetz CG, Choi D, Aggarwal S, Mestre TA, Stebbins GT. Resolving missing data from the movement disorder society unified Parkinson's disease rating scale: implications for telemedicine. Mov Disord. 2022;37:1749–55.
54. Morinan G, Hauser RA, Scharg A, Tang J, O'Keefe J. Abbreviated MDS-UPDRS for remote monitoring in PD identified using exhaustive computational search. Parkinsons Dis. 2022;2022:2920255.
55. Du Z, Li Y, Li J, Zhou C, Li F, Yang X. Physical activity can improve cognition in patients with Alzheimer's disease: a systematic review and meta-analysis of randomized controlled trials. Clin Interv Aging. 2018;13:1593.
56. Hernandez SSS, Vital TM, Gobbi S, Costa JLR, Stella F. Atividade física e sintomas neuropsiquiátricos em pacientes com demência de Alzheimer. Motriz: Rev Educ Fis. 2011;17:533–43.
57. Canonici AP, Andrade LPD, Gobbi S, Santos-Galduroz RF, Gobbi LTB, Stella F. Functional dependence and caregiver burden in Alzheimer's disease: a controlled trial on the benefits of motor intervention. Psychogeriatrics. 2012;12:186–92.

58. Santos JGD, Andrade LPD, Pereira JR, Stein AM, Pedroso RV, Costa JLR. Análise de protocolos com intervenção motora domiciliar para pacientes com doença de Alzheimer: uma revisão sistemática. Rev Bras Geriatr Gerontol. 2013;16:615–31.
59. Dinesen B, Nonnecke B, Lindeman D, Toft E, Kidholm K, Jethwani K, et al. Personalized telehealth in the future: a global research agenda. J Med Internet Res. 2016;18:e53.
60. Sekhon H, Sekhon K, Launay C, Afililo M, Innocente N, Vahia I, et al. Telemedicine and the rural dementia population: a systematic review. Maturitas. 2021;143:105–14.
61. Jelcic N, Agostini M, Meneghello F, Bussè C, Parise S, Galano A, et al. Feasibility and efficacy of cognitive telerehabilitation in early Alzheimer's disease: a pilot study. Clin Interv Aging. 2014;9:1605–11.
62. Kübra Nur Menengi Ç, Yeldan İ, Çınar N, Şahiner T. Effectiveness of motor-cognitive dual-task exercise via telerehabilitation in Alzheimer's disease: an online pilot randomized controlled study. Clin Neurol Neurosurg. 2022;223:107501.
63. Walsh CB, Cahalan R, Hinman RS, O'Sullivan K. Psychometric properties of performance-based measures of physical function administered via telehealth among people with chronic conditions: a systematic review. PLoS One. 2022;17:e0274349.
64. Bowman A, Denehy L, Benjemaa A, Crowe J, Bruns E, Hall T, et al. Feasibility and safety of the 30-second sit-to-stand test delivered via telehealth: an observational study. PM R. 2023;15:31–40.
65. Hwang R, Mandrusiak A, Morris NR, Peters R, Korczyk D, Russell T. Assessing functional exercise capacity using telehealth: is it valid and reliable in patients with chronic heart failure? J Telemed Telecare. 2017;23:225–32.

Artificial Intelligence to Locomotion in Movement Disorders

32

Marcela de Oliveira
and Marta Isabel Azevedo Sol Neves Ferreira

Abstract

Parkinson's disease is a chronic and progressive neurodegenerative disease characterized by a reduction in the number of dopaminergic neurons in the par's compacta area of the substantia nigra. In this disease, non-motor symptoms manifest initially, and as the disease advances, motor symptoms emerge. However, motor symptoms are a hallmark of the disease. Unfortunately, Parkinson's disease has no cure and early diagnosis remains a significant challenge. In fact, it is only possible to make a diagnosis when motor symptoms appear, at a stage equivalent to a loss of around 60–70% of dopaminergic neurons. This diagnosis is essentially based on clinical observation and qualitative gait assessment, which may contribute to the existence of inconsistent diagnoses. In this sense, artificial intelligence (AI) offers potential solutions to overcome these limitations, allowing objective and accurate analysis of patients' movements. More specifically, machine learning, a subset of AI, has gained recognition for its effectiveness in analyzing locomotion in populations affected by movement disorders. Thus, this chapter aims to explore the application of machine learning concepts in the study of movement disorders, with a particular focus on Parkinson's disease.

M. de Oliveira (✉)
Bauru College of Technology (FATEC) and School of Sciences, São Paulo, Brazil

Faculdades Integradas de Bauru (FIB), Bauru, Brazil
e-mail: marcela.oliveira@unesp.br

M. I. A. S. N. Ferreira
Faculty of Engineering of the University of Porto, Porto, Portugal

F. A. Barbieri et al. (eds.), *Locomotion and Posture in Older Adults*,
https://doi.org/10.1007/978-3-031-74123-4_32

Introduction

Artificial Intelligence (AI) is becoming increasingly integral to the field of medicine and our understanding of neurological disorders, particularly those related to movement. The use of AI in the realm of locomotion and movement disorders holds the potential to revolutionize the diagnosis and treatment of these conditions, ultimately leading to an improvement in the quality of life for patients.

Movement disorders, such as Parkinson's disease (PD), dystonia, and ataxia, are characterized by alterations in coordination and motor control, significantly affecting patients' ability to walk and perform daily tasks. Traditionally, the evaluation of these disorders relies primarily on clinical observation of movements and the experience of the specialist physician. However, this approach may lead to certain limitations, such as delayed diagnoses and inter- and intra-observer variations. Therefore, AI offers a promising solution to address these limitations and complement clinical diagnoses, enabling an objective and accurate analysis of patients' movements.

One of the most promising approaches is the use of machine learning systems, which are capable of processing vast amounts of data and identifying subtle patterns that might be challenging for the human eye to discern. In general, these systems can be trained with data from both patients with and without movement disorders, using technologies such as wearable sensors, video cameras, or force platforms. Consequently, through the analysis of gait, posture, and other movement aspects, AI can identify distinctive features that differentiate patients with movement disorders from neurologically healthy individuals.

Beyond diagnosis, AI can also play a crucial role in the continuous monitoring of patients over time. With real-time data collection, it is possible to detect subtle changes in locomotion that may indicate disease progression or response to treatment. This facilitates a more personalized approach and enables timely therapeutic adjustments, maximizing patient benefits. Another promising application of AI in locomotion in movement disorders is robot-assisted rehabilitation. Robotic systems can be designed to assist patients during gait training, providing adaptive support and real-time feedback based on information collected by the AI system. This approach can enhance the effectiveness of rehabilitation and expedite functional recovery. Therefore, in this chapter, we will explore in greater detail the characteristics of AI and its application in studying movement disorders.

Overview of Artificial Intelligence

AI is a comprehensive concept that involves the use of a computer to model intelligent behaviors with minimal human intervention [1]. Although AI is a broad field, its recent growth has been significantly driven by new advances and improvements in the machine learning (ML) [1, 2]. ML is a subset of AI and represents powerful mathematical algorithms that enable systems to explore and identify patterns in data, classifying and predicting outcomes based on learning experiences [1, 2].

Recently, ML has received considerable attention due to its ability to accurately predict a wide variety of complex phenomena [3].

In general, there are three types of ML methods: (i) supervised, involving classification and prediction algorithms based on previously presented examples; (ii) unsupervised, with the ability to recognize patterns in data without predefined labels; and (iii) reinforcement learning, based on sequences of rewards and punishments to formulate a strategy for operating in a specific problem space. Additionally, some authors consider the existence of a fourth category consisting of a combination of supervised and unsupervised learning techniques (semi-supervised learning) [4]. Thus, ML comprises a set of computational techniques designed to approximate real-world mathematical functions based on historical data (Fig. 32.1).

Mathematically, when presented with a collection of input (X) and output (Y) data, humans typically possess the ability to discern a relationship between X and Y in the form of a function Y(X). However, when the input involves multiple variables ranging from X_0 to X_n and the output from Y_0 to Y_n, the complexities can quickly overwhelm humans capabilities. Nevertheless, computer algorithms can step in and take the place of humans by "analyzing" the input and output data and "predicting" an approximate function that relates them [5]. The ML model created by these algorithms is an approximate representation of the relationship between input and output. As the amount of input and output data increases, the ML model becomes more precise and accurate. This methodology is commonly referred to as mapping or supervised learning. Thus, in supervised learning, the training set consists of input and desired output pairs (labels). Moreover, this type of ML model only applies to

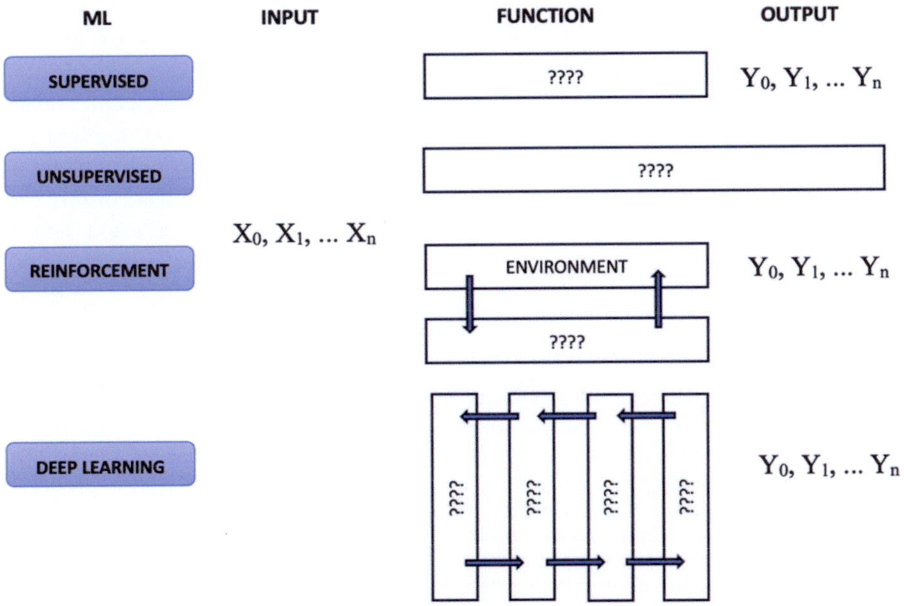

Fig. 32.1 Types of ML methods. (Modified from An et al. [5])

data with associated labels, implying that there is human interaction to label the data [6].

On the other hand, in unsupervised learning, the output (Y) is not provided; instead, the computer algorithms must autonomously determine the output, which could manifest as patterns, clusters, or relationships within the input data (X_0, X_1, … X_n). Consequently, this approach is particularly effective for revealing hidden patterns or relationships within the data. Thus, in this category, the objective is to group sets of input points that are closest to each other and assign a label to each point. Finally, another ML approach is reinforcement learning, where both input (X_0, X_1, … X_n) and output (Y_0, Y_1, … Y_n) are known. In this method, the algorithms aim to discover the functions linking X and Y, similar to supervised ML. However, the learning process involves dynamic interactions with another testing algorithm known as the environment. The environment provides rewards or punishments for the agent's trial-and-error learning, encouraging the ML model to improve its predictions by maximizing the rewards received [5]. Moreover, another comparable approach is deep learning, where trained learning algorithms possess multiple concealed layers and are consistently employed on fresh datasets instead of adaptively modifying the agent's actions based on continuous feedback.

Each machine learning approach has a wide range of algorithms to choose from, and the specific techniques associated with each method are detailed in Table 32.1.

The implementation of an ML model must include the following steps: the choice of the dataset, selection of features, choice of learning algorithm, and an evaluation module [8], as shown in Fig. 32.2. The dataset serves as the input for an ML model, which will be divided into a training set and a test set. After choosing and acquiring the dataset, the data undergoes a feature extraction process. The feature selection process is used to build a small subset of highly predictive features and avoid overfitting the training data [8].

There are two types of feature selection methods, also known as feature space dimensionality reduction methods: the Filter method and the Wrapper method [9]. The Filter method (Fig. 32.3) performs a feature selection process independent of the learning algorithm. In this case, only the attributes that rank high according to a certain selection criterion are chosen. It employs a relevance criterion and is

Table 32.1 Specific techniques in each ML method

Machine learning methods	Main specific techniques
Unsupervised	k-means, generative adversarial networks, expectation-maximization algorithm, Hebbian Learning, self-organizing map, adaptive resonance theory
Supervised	Decision trees, logistic regression, decision forests, support vector machines, kernel machines, Bayesian classifiers
Reinforcement	Monte Carlo, Q-learning, Soft Actor-Critic, proximal policy optimization, Trust Region Policy Optimization, Deep Q-Network, deep deterministic policy gradient

Modified from Yu and Jiang [7]

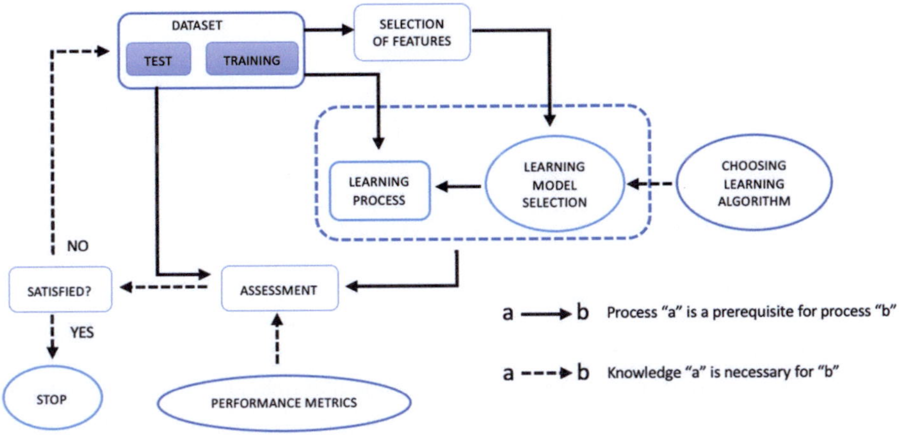

Fig. 32.2 ML model example. (Modified from Mason et al. [8])

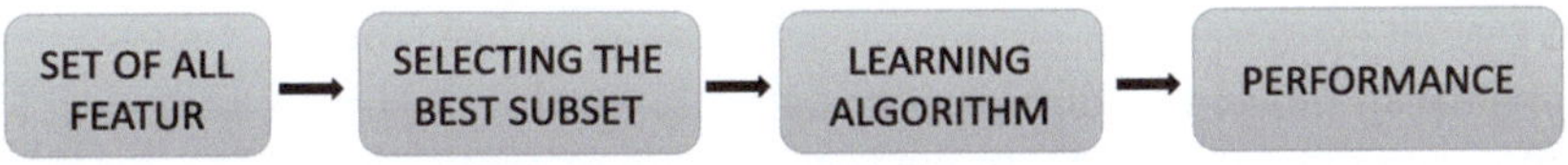

Fig. 32.3 Filter method example. (Modified from Kaushik [10])

typically used a pre-processing step. This method is known for its speed but tends to select large subsets of features [11, 12].

On the other hand, the Wrapper method (Fig. 32.4) uses an approach that iteratively selects, through a feedback loop, the attributes that improve the performance of the learning algorithm used to train the model. Unlike the Filter method, each set is evaluated in the specific context of the learning algorithm. It has the advantage of accuracy but with slow execution, and each classification problem requires a new selection of a subset [11, 12]. Both methods are independent of the type of ML technique [13].

In addition to the aforementioned methods, there is also the embedded method that combines the advantages of the Filter method with the Wrapper method [14]. In this method, feature selection is an integral part of the classification model, based on the score calculated by the model. The classification model is built using a training set and by evaluating the accuracy obtained in the prediction on the test set. The classification model that was built provides the performance value for each characteristic. Features with the lowest scores are removed, and the highest scores remain. However, unlike the Filter method, the performance measure of the features is calculated by the ranking model. Because the model is built only once to determine the score, it has a lower computational cost compared to the Wrapper method, which requires building multiple models due to the iterative process [15]. Therefore, feature selection allows the removal of independent variables that may be strongly correlated with each other and ensures the maintenance of independent variables that may be strongly correlated with the predicted or dependent variable [12].

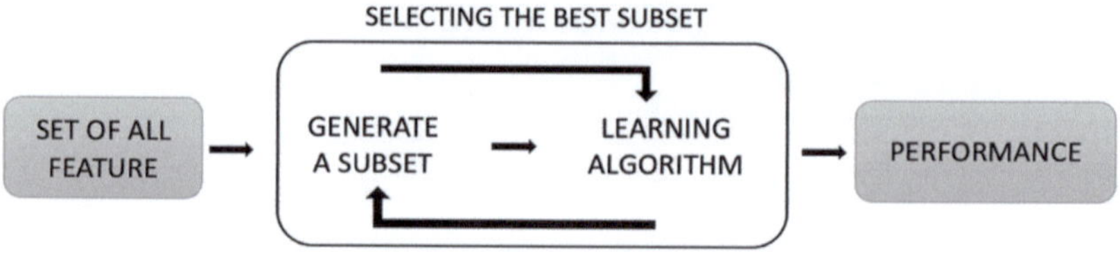

Fig. 32.4 Wrapper method example. (Modified from Kaushik [10])

After the characteristics have been selected, these will be used in the training of the learning algorithm, adjusting various specific parameters values. For each parameter value, the algorithm will select a different hypothesis from a set of hypotheses. The chosen hypothesis will be the one that manages to achieve the best performance on the test set. This performance can be evaluated using a cost function associated with a given task. This function measures the difference between the label predicted by the model and the true label. Finally, using this hypothesis, it will be possible to predict the labels of the samples in the test set [16].

Some of these specific techniques of learning algorithms have been used in the context of movement disorders, specifically for the purpose of analyzing locomotion, including gait in PD. In the specific case of application in PD, for the first step of these computational ML techniques, data belonging to PD patients and healthy individuals are initially acquired, followed by pre-processing. Subsequently, the most relevant characteristics are selected. These characteristics will provide the requisite information that allows us to distinguish parkinsonian gait from non-parkinsonian gait. Finally, the computer system performs an utomated classification to ascertain whether an individual belongs to the cohort of patients with PD or the healthy control group. The final performance of this classification is evaluated in accordance with established evaluation metrics. In the scientific literature, there is a remarkable number of ML models that are capable of identifying PD and predicting the level of severity at an early stage. Thus, in the next section, a brief review of ML applied in movement disorders will be presente.

Applying Machine Learning to Locomotion Analysis in Movement Disorders

Due to recent technological advancements, the identification of abnormal health conditions has become of paramount importance. In the case of movement disorders, the primary assessment focuses on the patient's motor symptoms. Specifically for PD, a clinical diagnosis is based on a series of tests (e.g., magnetic resonance imaging, electroencephalogram, among others), which assess the individual's motor symptoms associated with a level of severity, based on a scale (UPDRS—Unified Parkinson's Disease Rating Scale or HY—Hoehn and Yahr Scale) [17]. Therefore, a higher score on these scales is indicative of a greater degree of disability associated with the disease. However, the symptoms are analyzed based on the individual judgment of the assessor, especially neurologists, and may be susceptible to intra and inter-observer variations. Additionally, the score for this scale is calculated during health center visits, which introduces a potential source of error. Therefore, there is a need to assess patient motor performance in a more automated manner for consistent and efficient symptom checking and following-up [18]. In order to diagnose and analyze PD in a more objective manner, studies have utilized quantitative methods, such as the analysis of gait parameters. These methods are developed by applying machine learning techniques, which are responsible for identifying the gait patterns of people in different stages of PD and distinguishing them from those without neurological disease [18]. Thus, in this present session, the application of diverse computer diagnostic technologies to analysis of gait patterns in patients with PD is investigated and evaluated.

In general, symptoms associated with PD can be classified into two main categories: motor and non-motor. Considering the symptoms that diagnose PD, and the type and origin of data, it is possible to use computer-assisted diagnostic technologies for classifying, predicting, and monitoring patients. In this context, the analysis of data from both wearable and non-wearable systems has emerged as a prevalent category of computational techniques in PD. The analysis of data from wearable and non-wearable systems encompasses a range of motor symptoms, including gait changes [18]. Non-wearable systems are stationary and require the implementation of sensors that acquire gait data while the subject walks. On the other hand, wearable systems permit the acquisition and analysis of gait data outside the laboratory, during daily routine activities. Additionally, a hybrid system that incorporates both methods has been developed [19]. Thus, various computer technologies have been applied to assist clinicians in measuring motor symptoms with greater precision than is possible through subjective clinical assessment [18]. Below, each category system will be addressed specifically.

Non-wearable Systems

Unlike traditional wearable devices, non-wearable systems employ sophisticated technologies such as computer vision, artificial intelligence, and ambient sensors to monitor and assess Parkinson's symptoms. Buongiorno and colleagues [20] developed a low-cost system to analyze spatiotemporal and angular parameters, using the Microsoft Kinect v2 sensor, with the objective of identifying and classifying PD severity. The study involved 16 patients with PD, whose assessment of PD severity was carried out according to the Movement Disorders Society (MDS)-UPDRS scale, and 14 neurologically healthy individuals. Twenty-five reflector markers were strategically positioned facilitate the accurate localization and recording of body position. One of the analyzed tasks was walking. While the participant was walking, a camera (Kinect sensor) positioned 3.5 m away from the starting point of the gait, captured their movement. Using the Microsoft SDK, the 3D positions of the 25 markers were automatically constructed, and 16 features were extracted (temporal, spatial, and angular parameters). Two sets of data were trained for feature classification. The first set consisted of six features, and the second set of nine features. The features were selected from the Weka software using the *CfsSubsetEval* classifier and the *BestFirst* search method. To evaluate the trained model, cross-validation (CV) five-*fold* was used. The artificial neural network (ANN) algorithm demonstrated superior performance, with an accuracy (ACC) of 89.4% (for 9 features) and 95% (for 6 features).

On the other hand, Wahid et al. [21] conducted a study with the primary objective of normalizing spatiotemporal characteristics through the application of dimensionless standard equations and multiple linear regression. The aim was to identify differences between patients with PD and the control group. Subsequently, the study tested the efficacy of employing ML tools for the classification of Parkinsonian gait. the normalization took into account the patient's characteristics, including age, height, body mass, gender, and preferred walking speed. For the study, 23 patients with PD and 26 healthy subjects (control group) with equivalent ages were selected. Fifteen reflector markers were used, following the modified Helen Hayes model. Each individual performed ten trials of 8 m of walking at a self-selected speed. Then, a system comprising eight motion analysis video cameras (Vicon, Oxford Metrics, Ltd., Oxford) was used, with data acquisition occurring simultaneously with two force platforms to obtain the ground reaction force. The results obtained using data normalized by multiple linear regression were found to be superior to those obtained by the other method. The accuracy obtained in the random forest (RF) algorithm was 92.6% compared to 80.4% in the support vector machine (SVM), 86.2% in the Kernel fisher discriminant (KFD), 84.4% in the K-nearest neighbors (KNN), and 82.0% in the Naive Bayes (NB). The internal parameters of the classifiers were optimized using the Grid Search method and the ten-*fold* cross-validation.

Rehman et al. [22] conducted a study to determine the spatial gait characteristics that should be considered for clinical PD classification. The purpose of this study was to develop an ML model that could distinguish between neurologically healthy individuals and patients with PD, as well as identify the best combination of characteristics for early-phase PD classification. In this study, 303 individuals, including 119 patients with PD and 184 neurologically healthy individuals, participated. The motor symptoms of DP were evaluated according to the MDS-UPDRS-III and HY scales, while cognition was assessed using the Mini-Mental State Examination (MMSE) questionnaire. Each participant was instructed to walk at a self-selected speed for 2 min continuously in a 25-m oval circuit that included an instrumented rug (Gaitrite®). A total of 16 characteristics were extracted from Microsoft Access. For the classification, 12 algorithms were tested with the assistance of CV ten-fold. In the end, three models from disparatet domains (RF, logistic regression—LR, and SVM with kernel radial basis function—RBF) were chosen, and the five most relevant characteristics were identified: step velocity, step length, step length variability, step width, and step width variability. The DP classification in the initial phase obtained an ACC that ranged from 73% to 97%, a recall between 63% and 100%, and a specificity (SPEC) of between 79% and 94%.

Urcuqui and colleagues [23] developed an ML model to classify gait in individuals diagnosed with PD. Spatial-temporal parameters were extracted from RGBD (red, green, blue, and depth data) chambers (MS Kinect) for motion capture, and the walking was performed in a corridor equipped with Kinect. Sixty volunteers participated in the study, comprising 24 women and 36 men aged between 44 and 88 years old, grouped by gender and age. The PD group consisted of 18 men and 12 women. Each participant repeated the walking task three times, and the data were collected from three points located on each ankle. The algorithms chosen for qualification were LR, NB, RF, and decision trees (DT). The RF algorithm obtained a better ACC (82%), with a low false positive rate (12%), and a low true positive rate (23%). Past length and age were the best variables to train the DT model, with a 94% ACC.

More recently, a study carried out by Ferreira and collaborators [24] used ML algorithms to (i) distinguish people with PD vs. matched-healthy individuals; and (ii) to discriminate PD stages, based on selected spatial-temporal parameters, including variability and asymmetry. Gait data acquired from 63 people with PD with different severity levels of PD motor symptoms and 63 matched control subjects, during self-selected walking speed, were studied in the experiments. As a result, the researchers achieved an ACC of 84.6% in diagnosing PD, with precision of 92.3% and a recall of 80.0%, using the NB algorithm. Furthermore, the researchers found four significant gait characteristics that are useful for diagnosing PD: step length, speed and width, and step width variability. Regarding the identification of

Table 32.2 Summary of studies found in the scientific literature related to gait analysis using non-wearable systems

Reference	Analysis technique	Gait parameters	Algorithm	Attributes No.	*ACC* (%)	*Recall* (%)	*SPEC* (%)
Buongiorno et al. [20]	Marker-based motion capture	Spatiotemporal and angular	SVM	9	78.5	81.7	74.8
				6	88.7	78.9	96.3
			ANN	9	89.4	87.0	91.8
				6	95.0	90.0	99.0
Wahid et al. [21]	Marker-based motion capture and power platform	Spatiotemporal	RF	9	92.6	96	90
			SVM		80.4	73	100
			KFD		86.2	86	91
			NB		82.0	85	81
			KNN		84.4	69	100
Rehman et al. [22]	Instrumented rug (GAITRite®)	Spatiotemporal	RF	16	94.28	100	89
			LR	5	97.14	100	94
			SVM-	16	82.85	71	89
			RBF	5	84.99	76	94
				16	81.92	71	89
				5	85.71	79	94
Urcuqui et al. [23]	Capture of motion without marked	Spatiotemporal and cinematic	RF	17	82	88.2	76.5
			DT	2	94	76.5	35.3
Ferreira et al. [24]	Vicon Motion Systems®	Spatiotemporal and cinematic	RF	12	69.2	53.3	88.9
			NB	4	84.6	80.0	92.3
			LR	6	76.9	66.7	90.9
			SVM	4	80.8	73.3	91.7

the PD stage, RF demonstrated superior performance compared to the other ML algorithms under consideration, reaching an area under the ROC curve of 78.6%. Finally, the authors found two relevant gait characteristics in identifying the PD stage: step width variability and double step support time variability.

Table 32.2 presents a summary of the studies that used non-wearable systems, including a description of the technique used in the analysis, the gait parameters extracted, and the results of the classification obtained, according to the algorithm and the number of attributes.

Wearable Systems

ML techniques have also been utilized in the development of wearable systems for the detection and evaluation of PD motor and gait symptoms. Aich and colleagues [25] developed and validated an algorithm based on data acquired by an accelerometer during the act of walking. This study includes an examination of signal characteristics and spatiotemporal parameters. Through these characteristics, they intended to classify the medication state (i.e., under—ON—or without—OFF—medication state) in 20 patients with PD. To estimate the severity of the disease, the UPDRS-III and HY scales were used. The data were extracted under two conditions: ON state, 1–1.5 hours after taking the dopaminergic medication, and OFF state—at least 12 hours after the administration of dopaminergic medication. For each task, a triaxial accelerometer was placed on each knee of the participant. From the accelerometer, two types of characteristics were acquired: statistical characteristics (mean, standard deviation, median, minimum, maximum, energy, interquartile interval, signal magnitude, skewness, and kurtosis) and gait parameters (step and stride length, duration, and speed). To validate the model, it was employed using the CV LOSO (Leave-One-Subject-Out) approach. The ML algorithms covered were RF, SVM, KNN, and NB. The RF classifier obtained the most optimal performance, achieving an ACC of 96.72%, a 97.35% recall, and an average precision of 96.92% in the detection of the two states.

Mittra and Rustagi [27] published a study in which gait was analyzed to distinguish patients with PD from neurologically healthy individuals. To carry out this research, 93 patients with PD and 73 neurologically healthy individuals participated in the study. The gait characteristics were extracted from eight sensors placed on each plantar surface of the participant's feet, thereby calculating the vertical component of ground reaction force. Each participant was instructed to walk for 2 minutes. In order to reduce data volume, statistical functions were applied, followed by the data normalization to the range of −1 to 1. The KNN algorithm obtained the best ACC (93.08%) compared to the DT, RF, SVM (with linear kernel, RBF, and polynomial), and logistic regression. Precision (PREC), recall, and F1-Score obtained by KNN were 89.58%, 84.31%, and 86.86%, respectively.

In another study, the authors [28] used the same database that [27] for the purpose of automatically diagnosing PD and determining the level of the disease. This database contains information on patients who are in the early or intermediate stages of the disease. A total of ten patients were classified at level 3 on the HY scale, 28 at level 2.5, and 55 at level 2. From the 16 sensors placed on the feet, spatiotemporal parameters were extracted. To find the best set of characteristics, a correlation-based characteristics selection technique (through the Pearson coefficient) was applied. At the outset of the study, a statistical analysis of the sensor data was performed to differentiate the control group from PD patients. Then, to evaluate the efficiency of the classifiers, ten-fold CV was used. Furthermore, the Shapiro-Wilk test was applied with a significance level of 5% to ascertain the normal distribution of gait attributes. In this study, the authors found that cadence, stride length, duration, and speed were the parameters with the greatest difference between the two groups. The tested classifiers were DT, SVM, EC (Ensemble Classifier), and Bayes Classifier (BC). The DT classifier was built to divide the severity of PD into four levels, based on the HY scale: healthy (expected value <1), light (expected value ≥ 1 and < 2.25), medium (expected value ≥ 2.25 and < 2.75), and high (predicted value ≥ 2.75). In addition, the DT classifier distinguishes between the light level and the middle based on the sensor value (light: value ≥ 122.418, and medium: value <122.418). Regarding the results, both the DT and SVM classifiers obtained the best ACC with 99.4%, as well as the best recall with 99.6% and SPEC with 99.8%.

Table 32.3 presents a summary of the main points found in the previously exploited studies for gait analysis using wearable systems.

Table 32.3 Summary of studies found in the scientific literature related to gait analysis using wearable systems

Reference	Sensor type	Gait parameters	Algorithm	ACC (%)	*Recall* (%)	SPEC (%)	Validation (%)
Aich et al. [26, 25]	Triaxial accelerometers	Spatiotemporal	RF	96	97	–	VC LOSO
			SVM	93	92	–	
			KNN	86	84	–	
			NB	88	86	–	
Mittra & Rustagi [27]	Power	Cinematic	KNN	93.08	84.31	–	–
			DT	87.78	92.00	–	
			RF	90.39	90.91	–	
			SVM-linear	89.95	87.86	–	
			SVM-RBF	90.39	90.38	–	
			SVM-Poly*	88.64	94.44	–	
			LR	90.06	87.76	–	
Balaji et al. [28]	Power	Spatiotemporal	DT	99.4	99.6	99.8	VC ten-*fold*
			SVM	97.6	95.2	99.2	
			EC	95.1	91.5	98.2	
			BC	69.7	46.0	89.2	

Poly*—polynomial

Combination of Wearable and Non-wearable Systems

There are also studies that combine wearable systems with non-wearable systems. In a related study, Aich and collaborators [26] proposed a system that receives data acquired by wearable accelerometers to estimate the gait characteristics, in conjunction with a 3D Movement Analysis Capture System (Vicon®, Oxford, UK). The study was validated by the Tinetti mobility test. This system includes an ML algorithm to distinguish 48 patients with PD from a group of neurologically healthy individuals (22 men and 18 women). To ascertain the severity of the disease, UPDRS and HY scales were used. The accelerometers were placed on both knees of the participants, at a distance of 34 cm from the ground. Each participant walked 6 meters, and five gait characteristics were acquired: step and stride time, step and stride length, and gait speed. For the classification, five algorithms were tested, using five-fold in cross-validation. The DT algorithm achieved better ACC with 88.46%. Recall and SPEC were 92.86% and 90.91%, respectively.

Comparison of Machine Learning Methods

In the scientific literature, there is a remarkable number of ML models that are capable of identifying PD and predicting the level of severity at an early stage. Given the multiplicity of motor and non-motor symptoms associated with PD, various ML methods have been adapted to accommodate different types of data. In the context of gait alterations, some researchers have chosen to employ wearable systems in their studies, while others have opted for non-wearable systems or a combination of both. For instance, Balaji and colleagues [28] utilized wearable force sensors and achieved the highest accuracy, recall, and specificity values of 99.4%, 99.6%, and 99.8%, respectively, when applying the DT classifier. It is noteworthy that other studies conducted with wearable systems also demonstrated high accuracy values. In the study by Mittra and Rustagi [27], the KNN algorithm yielded the best accuracy of 93.08%, while in Aich's et al. [26, 25] investigation, the RF algorithm exhibited the best performance.

In the realm of the learning algorithms employing non-wearable systems, the RF classifier demonstrated the performance with an accuracy of 97.14%. The ten-fold cross-validation technique was frequently mentioned in the literature as the preferred method for model validation. Additionally, spatiotemporal parameters such as step length, stride length, stride duration, and step duration were commonly featured in the literature. Furthermore, step width variability was also considered as one of the most clinically relevant gait parameters in identifying early stage PD by Rehman et al. [22]. The asymmetry of the step speed and the asymmetry of the duration of simple step support were chosen by the LR and RF algorithms, holding less relevant positions. These findings align with the conclusions drawn by Rehman et al. [22], as asymmetry similarly occupies a less significant role in their study. On the other hand, anthropometric and clinical parameters remain limited in the literature.

However, it is important acknowledge that the ML methods discussed in this chapter have some limitations. Many studies utilized relatively small datasets, which may potentially compromise the reliability of the developed systems. Furthermore, increasing the number of samples offers the advantage of implementing deep learning techniques. Another limitation in some studies relates to the use of unbalanced datasets, especially regarding gender distribution.

On a positive note, further research should explore the development of ML methods capable of predicting PD by considering both motor and non-motor symptoms. Regarding studies analyzing gait parameters based on wearable systems, it is essential to conduct testing in a home environment, given that the majority of acquired data was obtained in a clinical context. For non-wearable systems, there is a need to develop more low-cost solutions for gait analysis.

Final Remarks

Due to its capacity for automated pattern extraction and classification, ML is a valuable tool for diagnosis PD and assessing the level of severity. In recent years, several computer-assisted technologies have been developed for the diagnosis and treatment of PD, including gait analysis using both wearable and non-wearable systems. The models developed for this analysis demonstrated superior performance when trained by supervised learning algorithms, focusing solely on spatiotemporal parameters. A PD classification system involves the following phases: data acquisition, data pre-processing, feature extraction and/or selection, classification, and results. While the interest among researchers in this area has grown in recent years and promising results have been achieved, there are still aspects that need further improvement. Despite the exciting prospects, it is crucial to recognize that AI in the field of locomotion in movement disorders is still in the developmental stage. Furthermore, multidisciplinary collaboration between AI experts, clinicians, engineers, and computer scientists is essential to propel progress in this field.

In conclusion, the application of artificial intelligence to locomotion in movement disorders has the potential to transform medical practice by providing more accurate, effective, and individualized approaches to the diagnosis and treatment of these conditions. Thus, AI can serve as a complementary tool for diagnosing and monitoring disease progression, thereby benefiting clinicians. Moreover, with the continuous advancement of technology and interdisciplinary collaboration across different areas, it is plausible to envisage a future in which AI becomes an indispensable ally in the care of patients with movement disorders.

References

1. Hamet P, Tremblay J. Artificial intelligence in medicine. Metabolism. 2017;69:S36–40. https://doi.org/10.1016/j.metabol.2017.01.011.
2. Belić M, Bobić V, Badža M, Šolaja N, Đurić-Jovičić M, Kostić VS. Artificial intelligence for assisting diagnostics and assessment of Parkinson's disease—a review. Clin Neurol Neurosurg. 2019;184:105442. https://doi.org/10.1016/j.clineuro.2019.105442.
3. Murdoch WJ, Singh C, Kumbier K, Abbasi-Asl R, Yu B. Definitions, methods, and applications in interpretable machine learning. Proc Natl Acad Sci. 2019;116(44):22071–80. https://doi.org/10.1073/pnas.1900654116.
4. Saravanan R, Sujatha P. A state of art techniques on machine learning algorithms: a perspective of supervised learning approaches in data classification. In 2018 Second International Conference on Intelligent Computing and Control Systems (ICICCS), p. 945–949; 2018. https://doi.org/10.1109/ICCONS.2018.8663155.
5. An J, Chua CK, Mironov V. Application of machine learning in 3D bioprinting: focus on development of big data and digital twin. Int J Bioprint. 2021;7(1):342. https://doi.org/10.18063/ijb.v7i1.342.
6. Cielen D, Meysman ADB, Ali M. Introducing data science. 1st ed. New York: Manning Publications; 2016.
7. Yu C, Jiang J. A perspective on using machine learning in 3D bioprinting. Int J Bioprint. 2020;6(1):253. https://doi.org/10.18063/ijb.v6i1.253.
8. Mason EJ, Traoré I, Woungang I. Machine learning techniques for gait biometric recognition: using the ground reaction force. 1st ed. Cham: Springer; 2016.
9. Maglogiannis IG. Emerging artificial intelligence applications in computer engineering: real word AI systems with applications in EHealth, HCI, information retrieval and pervasive technologies. IOS Press; 2007. https://books.google.com.br/books?id=vLiTXDHr_sYC
10. Kaushik S. Introduction to Feature Selection methods with an example (or how to select the right variables?). 2016. https://www.analyticsvidhya.com/blog/2016/12/introduction-to-feature-selection-methods-with-an-example-or-how-to-select-the-right-variables/.
11. Dumortier A, Beckjord E, Shiffman S, Sejdić E. Classifying smoking urges via machine learning. Comput Methods Prog Biomed. 2016;137:203–13. https://doi.org/10.1016/j.cmpb.2016.09.016.
12. Kotu V, Deshpande B. Predictive analytics and data mining: concepts and practice with RapidMiner. Elsevier Science; 2014. https://books.google.com.br/books?id=dRHoAwAAQBAJ
13. Suto J, Oniga S, Sitar PP. Comparison of wrapper and filter feature selection algorithms on human activity recognition. In 2016 6th International Conference on Computers Communications and Control (ICCCC), p. 124–129; 2016. https://doi.org/10.1109/ICCCC.2016.7496749.
14. Wang S, Zhang Y, Zhan T, Phillips P, Zhang Y-D, Liu G, Lu S, Wu X. Pathological brain detection by artificial intelligence in magnetic resonance imaging scanning (invited review). Prog Electromagn Res. 2016;156:105–33. https://doi.org/10.2528/PIER16070801.
15. Suppers A, van Gool A, Wessels H. Integrated chemometrics and statistics to drive successful proteomics biomarker discovery. Proteomes. 2018;6(2):20. https://doi.org/10.3390/proteomes6020020.
16. Mohri M, Rostamizadeh A, Talwalkar A. Foundations of machine learning. 2nd ed. MIT Press; 2018. https://books.google.com.br/books?id=V2B9DwAAQBAJ
17. Kour N, Sunanda, Arora S. Computer-vision based diagnosis of Parkinson's disease via gait: a survey. IEEE Access. 2019;7:156620–45. https://doi.org/10.1109/ACCESS.2019.2949744.
18. Goyal J, Khandnor P, Aseri TC. Classification, prediction, and monitoring of Parkinson's disease using computer assisted technologies: a comparative analysis. Eng Appl Artif Intell. 2020;96:103955. https://doi.org/10.1016/j.engappai.2020.103955.
19. Khandpur RS. Compendium of biomedical instrumentation, 3 volume set. Wiley; 2020. https://books.google.com.br/books?id=xBC9DwAAQBAJ

20. Buongiorno D, Bortone I, Cascarano GD, Trotta GF, Brunetti A, Bevilacqua V. A low-cost vision system based on the analysis of motor features for recognition and severity rating of Parkinson's disease. BMC Med Inform Decis Mak. 2019;19(S9):243. https://doi.org/10.1186/s12911-019-0987-5.
21. Wahid F, Begg RK, Hass CJ, Halgamuge S, Ackland DC. Classification of Parkinson's disease gait using spatial-temporal gait features. IEEE J Biomed Health Inform. 2015;19(6):1794–802. https://doi.org/10.1109/JBHI.2015.2450232.
22. Rehman RZU, Del Din S, Guan Y, Yarnall AJ, Shi JQ, Rochester L. Selecting clinically relevant gait characteristics for classification of early Parkinson's disease: a comprehensive machine learning approach. Sci Rep. 2019;9(1):17269. https://doi.org/10.1038/s41598-019-53656-7.
23. Urcuqui C, Castaño Y, Delgado J, Navarro A, Diaz J, Muñoz B, Orozco JL. Exploring machine learning to analyze Parkinson's disease patients. In 2018 14th international conference on semantics, knowledge and grids (SKG), p. 160–166; 2018. https://api.semanticscholar.org/CorpusID:145049803
24. Ferreira MIAS, Barbieri FA, Moreno VC, Penedo T, Tavares JMRS. Machine learning models for Parkinson's disease detection and stage classification based on spatial-temporal gait parameters. Gait Posture. 2022;98:49–55. https://doi.org/10.1016/j.gaitpost.2022.08.014.
25. Aich S, Youn J, Chakraborty S, Pradhan PM, Park J, Park S, Park J. A supervised machine learning approach to detect the on/off state in Parkinson's disease using wearable based gait signals. Diagnostics. 2020b;10(6):421. https://doi.org/10.3390/diagnostics10060421.
26. Aich S, Pradhan PM, Chakraborty S, Kim H-C, Kim H-T, Lee H-G, Kim IH, Joo M, Jong Seong S, Park J. Design of a machine learning-assisted wearable accelerometer-based automated system for studying the effect of dopaminergic medicine on gait characteristics of Parkinson's patients. J Healthcare Eng. 2020a;2020:1–11. https://doi.org/10.1155/2020/1823268.
27. Mittra Y, Rustagi V. Classification of subjects with Parkinson's disease using gait data analysis. In 2018 International Conference on Automation and Computational Engineering (ICACE), p. 84–89; 2018. https://api.semanticscholar.org/CorpusID:115199179.
28. Balaji E, Brindha D, Balakrishnan R. Supervised machine learning based gait classification system for early detection and stage classification of Parkinson's disease. Appl Soft Comput. 2020;94:106494. https://doi.org/10.1016/j.asoc.2020.106494.

Using mHealth Technology to Monitor Arm-Use Behavior, Gait, and Physical Activity in Stroke Survivors

33

Camila Torriani-Pasin, Gisele Carla dos Santos Palma, Leonardo Vinícius Thomé Teixeira da Silva, and Shashwati Geed

Abstract

This chapter advocates for the deployment of monitoring devices to assess the movement behaviors and physical activity of individuals recovering from stroke. The proposed approached encompasses the utilization of these devices in diverse settings, as laboratory and natural environments, and different stages of the recovery trajectory after stroke. This multifaceted monitoring strategy aims to provide a comprehensive understanding of the dynamic and evolving nature of movement patterns throughout the recovery journey, offering insights for personalized and effective rehabilitation interventions. Mobile health (mHealth) refers to the use of technologies (i.e., mobile phones, personal digital assistants,

C. Torriani-Pasin (✉)
Department of Physical Therapy and Movement Sciences, The University of Texas at El Paso, El Paso, TX, USA

School of Physical Education and Sport, University of Sao Paulo, São Paulo, São Paulo, Brazil
e-mail: ctorrianip@utep.edu

G. C. dos Santos Palma
School of Physical Education and Sport, University of Sao Paulo, São Paulo, São Paulo, Brazil

L. V. T. T. da Silva
Department of Physical Therapy and Movement Sciences, The University of Texas at El Paso, El Paso, TX, USA

S. Geed
Department of Physical Therapy and Movement Sciences, The University of Texas at El Paso, El Paso, TX, USA

Department of Rehabilitation Medicine, MedStar National Rehabilitation Hospital and Georgetown University, Washington, DC, USA

F. A. Barbieri et al. (eds.), *Locomotion and Posture in Older Adults*,
https://doi.org/10.1007/978-3-031-74123-4_33

wearable sensors) to provide health care services and information. Digital technologies like mHealth have the potential to revolutionize the interactions among populations and national health services. MHealth technologies (i.e., smartphones, mobile programs, and smartwatches) are available to monitor and encourage health-promoting behaviors that may reduce disability in stroke survivors and provide useful information about functional behaviors, physical activity levels, and metrics of intensity, and have the potential to increase awareness about human–environment interactions and encourage health-promoting behavior. The use of mHealth technology emerges as a good possibility to define each intensity category. As a result, a variety of devices can be used to monitor the use of more affected limb in daily-life activity, to monitor the different levels of physical activity, energy expenditure, sedentary behavior, and parameters of gait.

Introduction

The World Health Organization (WHO) defines eHealth as an approach to health that utilizes information and communication technologies [1, 2]. Under the umbrella of eHealth, *mobile health* (mHealth) refers to the use of technologies (i.e., mobile phones, personal digital assistants, wearable sensors) to provide health care services and information. mHealth services may include, but are not limited to, health monitoring [3], recording or reporting of disease, encouraging health-promoting behaviors to reduce disability in stroke survivors [4], and transmission of information related to healthy behaviors [5].

mHealth interventions can help patients manage chronic conditions by: (a) keeping track of their health, (b) creating social and support networks for patients, (c) telling the care network or provider team about their health, (d) providing feedback, (e) making education and intervention needs more specific, and (f) improving interprofessional communication [6]. In addition, using mHealth apps that focus on users and getting health care providers to use apps as part of a plan to manage health can make health better [7].

Digital technologies like mHealth have the potential to revolutionize the interactions among populations and national health services. Therefore, they are becoming an important resource for health services delivery and public health. Mobile wireless technologies are particularly relevant because of their ease, extensive reach, and widespread acceptance. Digital health, and specifically mHealth, has been shown to improve the quality and coverage of medical care, improve access to health information, services, and skills, and promote positive changes in health behaviors related to the prevention and onset of acute and chronic diseases [8, 9].

The implementation of mHealth stands out as a crucial strategy in the realm of healthcare. Its primary objective is to enhance access to high-quality services, addressing a fundamental aspect of healthcare provision. Moreover, mHealth is strategically positioned to contribute to the reduction of premature mortality associated with noncommunicable diseases and their comorbidities. This health-focused approach aligns with the broader goal of improving overall health outcomes.

Additionally, mHealth plays a vital role in elevating the safety and quality of care provided, ensuring that healthcare services meet optimal standards. Furthermore, the implementation of mHealth extends beyond clinical settings, aiming to improve engagement not only at a patient level but also involving families and communities. By fostering active participation and promoting healthy behaviors, mHealth becomes a comprehensive solution to advancing healthcare delivery and community well-being [1, 9].

The scientific production in this theme has been growing exponentially. A general search on PubMed including keywords *stroke, health technology, telehealth, and mobile health* combined) reveals that, on average, just over 2000 articles/year until 2018 have been published. After 2020, the number of publications was over 12,000, and it continues to grow yearly.

Ecological Momentary Assessment (EMA) and Ecological Momentary Intervention (EMI) Approaches

Access to quality health services is only possible through effective and timely sharing of health data. According to the WHO, the combination of specialized devices and sensors with the capability of mobile technologies defines a more comprehensive manner of diagnosing, monitoring, managing, and researching diseases [9]. Specialized devices include wearable sensors, monitors, smartphone applications and devices, including accelerometers, gyroscope, and inclinometers. These specialized devices can unobtrusively record large quantities of data in the background while the individuals continue to perform their day-to-day lives [10]. Therefore, mHealth devices and the technology to process longitudinal data can accurately capture motor function recovery after stroke. Recent publications point at mHealth technology as reliable and psychometrically valid to measure motor performance in individuals' natural environments [11–16].

While conventional clinical function tests, like the Upper-Extremity Fugl-Meyer [17] and the Action Research Arm Test [18], capture motor function and impairment in the clinic, rehabilitationists are interested in how much of that improvement translates to the individuals' own environments. Understanding day-to-day (and moment-to-moment) assessment of and improvement in function is crucial to better understand post-stroke recovery. Ecological momentary assessment (EMA) refers to a diverse range of methods to repeatedly collect real-time data about subjects' experiences and behaviors in their natural environment [19] (e.g., physical symptoms, behaviors, contexts, beliefs, attitudes, or perceptions) [20]. EMA combines the assessment of events of interest by random time sampling, with the use of technologies. EMA varies from written diaries and telephones to electronic diaries and physiological sensors. EMA approach, thereby, abdicates recall bias and is well suited to address behavior changes over time and across contexts [19]. Beyond recall bias minimization and ecological validity maximization, EMA aims to allow the study of micro-processes that influence behavior in real-world contexts [20], ensuring a more comprehensive perspective of motor recovery.

Ecological momentary intervention (EMI) refers to a framework for interventions for individuals during their everyday lives—in real time and in natural settings [21]. EMI ranges from unstructured clinical recommendations to more formalized and structured interventions and can be implemented on its own or as a supplement to existing interventions or ongoing treatments [20]. One of the primary areas in which EMI has been used is in the promotion of healthy behaviors.

Initial studies have suggested that tailoring EMIs based on EMAs may lead to higher engagement and intervention effectiveness [4, 21, 22]. The use of mobile technologies to collect EMAs and deliver EMIs is growing [22]. Previous systematic reviews and scoping reviews have focused on sedentary behavior, physical activity, diet, specific health conditions, and EMA media for data collection, such as smartphones, mobile technologies, and accelerometers, among others. The use of EMAs and EMIs to monitor and manage stroke health-related [12] is the focus of this book chapter.

EMA and EMI in Stroke Rehabilitation

Individuals may not incorporate the impaired upper extremity (UE) in everyday use even when the UE is nearly fully recovered [12]. Shifting the use of activities to the unimpaired UE occurs as early as the first-week post-stroke [23]; thus, although the impaired UE can perform tested tasks in the laboratory setting (capacity), spontaneous use of the impaired UE in the individuals' own environments is limited (performance). Capacity refers to what individuals can do, while performance refers to how individuals do (e.g., their daily-life activities) [12, 20].

To address the lack of performance related to the arm/hand behavior of stroke survivors, contextually relevant assessment methods (e.g., EMA) and treatment interventions delivered under challenging but natural circumstances (e.g., EMI) are essential. These approaches provide valuable information about how to personalize recovery-promoting interventions and transfer the skills acquired in therapy to the natural environment [12, 20].

Despite the evident significance of contextually relevant EMAs and EMIs in addressing arm/hand behavior issues among stroke survivors, both approaches are yet to be fully embraced in the stroke recovery and rehabilitation field [20]. Nevertheless, there is a promising perspective supported by theoretical frameworks for the combined and synergistic use of EMA and EMI to promote person-centered, recovery-based, durable changes in functional movement behaviors of stroke survivors [12, 20, 24].

A variety of factors (i.e., self-efficacy, mood, and social environment) impact the translation of arm/hand capacity into performance and need to be better understood to guarantee a comprehensive and effective management of stroke rehabilitation. In this regard, Chen et al. [12] investigated the feasibility of a novel combination of accelerometry and EMA to assess paretic arm/hand behavior and related psycho-contextual information in individuals with stroke in their natural environment. The authors established measurement validity of using an accelerometer for ~80% of the waking hours and ~85% of responses to the EMA prompts, a combined method for accurate assessment of function. The combined methodology has been shown to be a feasible tool, with good measurement validity, expressed by the absence of response bias and immediate effect of EMA measurement reactivity, both to chronic stroke survivors, for at least a 5-day period of observation.

The EMAs and EMIs have the potential to be one solution to promote rehabilitation outside clinical settings. However, literature has provided consistent information about EMA. Hence, EMI still need significant efforts from the research groups in the future. In this chapter, we claim that by using EMA research studies, we may understand how stroke survivors perform tasks and purposeful movements at home and in the community (i.e., use the paretic arm in their activities) which will help clinicians to guide personalized clinical interventions.

Applications of mHealth Technologies to Monitoring of Activities, Movement Patterns, and Physical Activity in Stroke Survivors

Stroke impairments reduce the mobility and ability to participate in physical activity. Muscle weakness [25], impaired peripheral blood flow [26], balance impairments, reduced gait velocity [27], fatigue [26], and decreased energy efficiency [28] may affect activity level. Physical deconditioning after stroke increases the risk of cardiovascular disease and is associated with higher mortality and morbidity rates [26]. Unfortunately, stroke survivors perform less than half of the PA levels of age-matched normative values, and an estimated 58% do not meet guidelines recommendation [28–33].

A potential contributing factor to the diminished levels of physical activity observed in stroke survivors is the presence of physical impairments [34]. MHealth technologies, such as smartphones, mobile programs, and smartwatches, are available to monitor and encourage health-promoting behaviors. Emerging evidence suggests that mHealth technologies provide useful information about functional behaviors, physical activity levels, and metrics of intensity [5]. MHealth also has the potential to increase awareness about human-environment interactions and encourage health-promoting behaviors.

Stroke survivors present lower levels of physical activity than community-matched healthy older adults and those with other chronic diseases [35]. Additionally, individuals after a stroke are highly sedentary [36] and more sedentary than healthy sex- and age-matched controls (10.9 versus 8.2 h/waking day, respectively [37]. This occurrence is prevalent among both stroke patients currently hospitalized and those who have been discharged to their homes [38]. In general, wearable devices can measure walking activity, sedentary behavior, and the use of the UE in daily activities. Wearable sensors can be used as a tool to incentivize stroke survivors to engage in physical activity and reduce sedentary behavior [39].

The body of literature using mHealth systems is more consistent and robust in monitoring the stroke survivor's activity [1, 5]. Recent body literature has consistently shown that although stroke survivors are less active than non-neurological impaired health controls, most stroke survivors report undertaking physical activity based on the daily recommendations from WHO [30]. This information is surprisingly positive and includes the stroke survivors who were physically inactive before stroke [29–32]. Hence, the use of these devices can be useful to encourage a healthy lifestyle and monitor the rehabilitation process of stroke survivors.

However, the literature has little evidence of the use of these devices as effective intervention strategies in a structured rehabilitation program context [40]. Most of the studies use these devices to quantify the body movement (i.e., body position (lying, sitting, standing), UE paretic use (activities of daily living) or parameters of gait (i.e., spatial-temporal parameters of gait; step count/ number of walking steps, going up and down stairs).

There is an increased number of studies aiming to encourage the decrease of sedentary behavior in stroke survivors (e.g., Refs [37, 41, 42]). However, this research field is surrounded by heterogeneity of results. Surprisingly, the most recent systematic review found that, despite extensive research efforts, no intervention strategy—whether involving mHealth technologies or not—successfully reduced sedentary behavior. Additionally, it was found a high and unclear risk of bias throughout the systematic review. This shows the importance of this topic to public health and the gap still needing to be filled in between clinical intervention to reduce sedentary behavior and data produced by the recent research. Therefore, this field still lacks evidence of the use of mHealth to reduce sedentary behavior, cardiovascular risk, and risk of recurrent stroke, among other secondary complications [43].

Below, we will address the use of mHealth based on the EMA-use, which will include the purpose of monitoring the use of UE, gait, physical activity level, and sedentary behavior in stroke survivors.

Purpose of Monitoring

Monitor UE and Its Use in Daily-Life Activities

The functional limitation of the UE is among the most prevalent disabilities following a stroke. Importantly, measurement of motor capacity through clinical assessment in the clinic may not index UE use in activities (and instrumental) activities of daily living.

The monitoring of movement behavior is a useful tool for informing clinician's professionals about the paretic limb use and its engagement in daily-life activities. Chen et al. [11] used the accelerometer to monitor arms use during daily activities. They monitored 82 chronic stroke survivors during 3 days before starting the rehabilitation program. The findings demonstrated that the most affected arm activity (measured by the accelerometer) before treatment was significantly correlated with the arm function and participation in daily activities as measured by the Motor Activity Log [44, 45], Stroke Impact Scale [46], and Nottingham Extended Activities of Daily Living [47] after treatment in patients with chronic stroke. This finding suggests that the paretic arm activity measured by the arm accelerometer before treatment, predicts arm function and participation in daily activities [13, 23, 48–50]. However, there is more nuance to what is measured with conventional accelerometry and its relationship to motor function recovery. Conventional accelerometry measures "counts" of arm movements/unit of time (number of accelerations recorded by the sensor over a unit of time). When accelerometry counts and clinical function tests were factor analyzed to determine if they measured a single construct, Barth et al. reported that conventional accelerometry measures a distinct construct, "quantity of movement," separate from a "quality of movement" construct measured by clinical function scales [23]. Thus, generic movement of the limb does not simply translate to purposeful activities or instrumental activities of daily living. A revised machine learning approach based on training accelerometry data on activities and instrumental activities of daily living [51] predicts motor function, impairment, and dexterity [13].

Given the differences between motor function capacity versus performance, the ceiling and floor effects found in conventional clinical scales, mHealth technology such as accelerometers have the potential to measure motor function recovery post-stroke more accurately and sensitively. While recent publications report psychometrically valid and reliable algorithms to interpret intensive accelerometry data, these need to be validated in the context of phase II, and III stroke rehabilitation trials to establish their true utility. Additionally, we need to establish the minimal clinically important difference (MCID: the minimum unit change perceived to result in significant improvement by the patient) values in acute, subacute, and chronic stroke for specific accelerometry algorithms, to extend their use in stroke rehabilitation trials.

Parameters of Gait

Walking is an important activity to improve the quality of life and social participation of stroke survivors [52]. Approximately, 30% of patients do not regain their ability to walk independently during the chronic phase following the stroke, and nearly 65% of them perceive their social participation as limited [53]. The most common parameters used to measure gait in a social environment are speed and distance.

Duclos et al. [54] objectively assessed and compared the accuracy of an activity monitor in counting steps among stroke survivors. They recruited 20 chronic stroke survivors, who performed a 6MWT, ramps, and stairs in the lab and a circuit inside the shopping mall (in a realistic environment). They concluded there was a higher presence of inconsistency during data collected in the realistic environment. Therefore, counting steps might be inaccurately counted during natural environment activities (i.e., stairs among slower walkers and long periods of walking among faster walkers).

The monitoring of walking activity after stroke is limited; however, some studies related important findings. Individuals in the lowest ambulation level (such as household ambulators or basal activity) got the lowest values for steps per day, bouts per day, steps per bout, or both [55, 56]. Additionally, for stroke survivors walking below 0.4 m/s there is no valid and accurate wearable sensor able to step count [57]. There is currently limited evidence of effective interventions that increase free-living walking after stroke, even when stroke survivors engage in activities [58]. Thus, targeting increased walking bouts of any length may serve as an alternative strategy for increasing stepping after stroke.

Sedentary Behavior and Physical Activity

Sedentary behavior is defined as any waking behavior in a sitting, reclining, or lying posture that is characterized by low energy expenditure (less than or equal to 1.5 metabolic equivalents (METs) [59]. Recently, the importance of sedentary behavior for health has emerged. High levels of sedentary behavior are associated with an increased risk of premature death, cardiovascular disease, metabolic disorders, and cancer [60]. Stroke survivors present higher prevalence of sedentary behavior compared to age-matched controls [37] Sedentary behavior is known to be detrimental to health, increasing the risk of heart attacks and strokes, and increasing the chance of death [38].

There is an increased number of studies aiming to reduce sedentary behavior in stroke survivors [37, 40, 61]. found very low certainty in reducing sedentary behavior after intervention programs in stroke survivors. They attributed the heterogeneity in measuring sedentary behavior with valid and accurate self-reported outcomes measures as one of the reasons for the low certainty. We assume, in the next years, we may see more studies investigating sedentary behavior after stroke, since the physical activity levels were quite well established for this population.

Physical activity participation is a modifiable lifestyle factor that can reduce recurrent stroke risk [29, 30]. A systematic review of 26 studies (983 participants) demonstrated that community-dwelling stroke survivors' step counts were less than 50% of their age-matched controls and sedentary time occupied 63% to 87% of reported monitoring periods [62]. Stroke survivors spend less time daily in light physical activity and moderate to vigorous physical activity (MVPA) in comparison with age-matched healthy control participants [37]; individuals affected by stroke allocate 4.9 (standard deviation (SD) 5.8) minutes per day, whereas control participants dedicate 38 (SD 31.0) minutes per day in MVPA. Reducing sedentary time following a stroke may lower the risk of experiencing a heart attack and recurrent stroke events. If sedentary time is decreased, it inherently implies an increase in PA, such as standing or walking. However, this statement comes from common sense and not from research, since [40] were not able to identify the effectiveness of any intervention able to reduce sedentary behavior after stroke. Ideally, interventions to reduce sedentary behavior has the potential to not only mitigate health risks but also enhance the health status and mobility of individuals recovering from a stroke [38].

Future studies, therefore, need to focus on the effects of intervention programs able to encourage breaking up long uninterrupted bouts of sedentary behavior to induce substantial health benefit after stroke [36].

Exercise Prescription, Intensity, and Sensors Placement

Exercise prescription needs a clear measurement of intensity, frequency, and duration. The use of mHealth technology emerges as a good possibility to define each intensity category. Connell et al. [63] used three measures of intensity (a) time, (b) repetitions, and (c) wrist accelerometers to describe the intensity of exercise carried out during a session using the Graded Repetitive Arm Supplementary Program (GRASP).

The GRASP exercises were categorized as passive, active, non-purposeful, resisted, and purposeful exercises. Purposeful exercises refer to systematically designed and executed activities undertaken with explicit objective, such as task-oriented (i.e., dropping and catching a ball) and reflective of activity of daily (i.e., taking the lid of a jam jar) tasks. They recruited 13 stroke survivors and monitored the GRASP with Actical® accelerometer that was placed on both wrists. The authors concluded that stroke survivors were not actively engaged in exercises for approximately one-third of the exercise session. They concluded time, therefore, may not be the most accurate measure of intensity in stroke rehabilitation.

Compagnat et al. [64] aimed to explore the validity of the Actigraph and the influence of the placement of the sensor when estimating the active energy expenditure in four common daily activities (transfers, manual tasks, overground walking, and walking up and down stairs) in stroke survivors. The results showed substantial differences between the active energy expenditure, as estimated by the Actigraph, and the values provided by Metamax for a sequence of common ADL. The best estimation was obtained when the Actigraph was placed on the wrist of the non-affected side.

Lee et al. [65] used the accelerometer to measure physical activity and estimate energy expenditure during 3 days of monitoring in 24 subacute stroke survivors. Authors concluded that of activities at light to moderate intensities, ankle accelerometers correlated with behavior mappings stronger than wrist accelerometers, and the physical activity related energy expenditure discrepancy between paretic and non-paretic sides was major in lower limbs.

Most of the studies that are on this topic recruited more chronic stroke survivors, which makes sense because the impairments caused by the chronic stroke are permanent and these individuals remain for a long period of time in care at the health service. Thus, most of the literature used in this chapter was based on chronic, while more studies in acute and subacute stroke survivors are needed.

A recent scoping review [4] investigated intensity (in terms of energy expenditure, physical activity, and time in body position) as an important aspect of physical activity that can have significant health benefits. By measuring intensity, researchers can better understand the level of physical activity and sedentary behavior of stroke survivors, which can help in informing the development of personalized intervention programs and potentially accelerate recovery [4, 62, 66, 67].

Models and Sensor Placement of mHealth Devices

A variety of devices can be used to monitor the use of more affected limb in daily-life activity, to monitor the different levels of physical activity, energy expenditure, sedentary behavior, and parameters of gait. These devices can be commercial or non-commercial. Smartphone applications, pedometers, accelerometers are the most common examples. A recent scoping review related a variety of models and types of sensors to monitor movement wearable sensors (Actical, Crossbow iMote2, Actigraph, Actiwatch, AW7, and Micro-mini motion logger); smartphone applications (Google Fit, Health, STEPZ, PACER, X sensor Pro); pedometers (Actigraph GT3X, FITBit One, Garmin VivoFit, OMRON) [4, 32]. The choice of type of wearable and the sensors body placement can be decided based on the purpose of use. Due to the notable varied accuracy (ranging from poor to good) sensor placement can be described as a barrier to mHealth device selection [4] Sensors for measuring UE movement can be used on the paretic or non-paretic wrist or arm; locomotion can be monitored using sensors placed on the ankle on paretic or non-paretic side, hip, or wrist [4, 68]. To monitor UE movement, a wrist body placement is desirable, either on the more or less affected arm, depending on the purpose [4]. In stroke, the amount of use of the paretic arm is expressed as the "use ratio" the amount of movement by the paretic arm/non-paretic arm to control for learned non-use of the paretic side; therefore, it is essential to place accelerometers on both wrists [4, 69]. For locomotion, monitoring the number of steps and intensity levels of physical activity can be achieved by placing sensors on the ankle, hip, or wrist on the less affected side [4, 70].

Costa et al. [71] conducted a validity study analyzing Google Fit, Health, STEPZ, Pacer, and Fitbit Ultra to estimate the number of steps in chronic stroke survivors. They compared whether the number of steps measured using mHealth devices was affected by body sensor placement (more and less affected leg) on the individual. They recruited 55 individuals, and the number of steps was measured by mHealth devices, as smartphone applications (Google Fit, Health, STEPZ, and Pacer) during a Two-Minute Walk Test with habitual speed. The authors conclude that mHealth devices (Pacer– iPhone, Fitbit Ultra, Google Fit, and Pacer–Android) provided a valid and reliable measure of step count in chronic stroke survivors. Additionally, the placement of the smartphone (more and less affected hip) did not influence the accuracy of the step count.

Pedometer is an easy-to-use mHealth technology and Compagnat et al. [64] investigated its accuracy in monitoring steps and distance walked using this device. They recruited 35 stroke survivors' participants. The pedometer, that was placed in the same location as ActiGraph (hip on the less affected side) provided a better estimate of the walked distance than the ActiGraph.

Ecological Validity and Measurement Properties in mHealth

Ecological Validity of a functional assessment tool refers to the capability of the instrument of measuring skills and behaviors in a relevant and significant manner to a person's real life and environment [72]. Thus, results obtained by the instrument must reflect the person's functional status in activities (and instrumental activities) of daily living in the real-world context, rather than only in controlled environments such as laboratories and rehabilitation centers [20].

To ensure ecological validity in functional assessment tools, they must be designed considering the individuals living environment and the significance of daily tasks and activities [73]. Trained professionals should administer these tools, identifying specific features and needs unique to each assessed individual [74]. When these tools exhibit high ecological validity, they provide valuable insights into how health conditions impact patients' functionality in real-life situations, spanning home, work, and community settings. In their design, it is imperative to consider the diverse functional demands individuals face in real-life activities, ranging from basic tasks like dressing and eating to more complex activities such as shopping and participating in social interactions [72, 75].

Ecological validity is also related to the generalization of the acquired skills during rehabilitation [76]. That is, if the assessment tool precisely assesses the functional performance in real-world environments, it will help to reassure that the abilities or skills obtained through the treatment will be performed outside of the controlled environment of a rehabilitation center [12, 20, 24]. It is crucial that the professionals are well-trained in the proper use of the assessment, so the accuracy of the collected data is increased [77]. Functional evaluation requires careful observation and an in-depth understanding of the patient's capacity and performance, precisely meaning their real functionality [24].

The ecological validity of a functional assessment tool is a critical feature of informed decision-making in health care and rehabilitation [72]. The capability of precisely assessing how a person performs his/her ADL promotes a solid foundation for planning interventions and searching for better results related to patients' functional improvements [78].

Measurement Properties of mHealth Technology

The key measurement properties for evaluating mHealth functional assessment tools, as described by COSMIN, are reliability, validity, responsiveness, and accuracy [79].

Reliability assesses the consistency and stability of the tool's measurements over time across different administrations [80]. It involves examining both test–retest reliability (consistency of results when the assessment is repeated at different time points) and inter-rater reliability (consistency of results when different raters administer the tool to the same subject) [80, 81]. High reliability ensures that the mHealth tool produces consistent and dependable results, regardless of when or by whom it is administered [82].

Validity is the extent to which mHealth functional assessment tool measures what it intends to measure. It can be analyzed from three components: content validity, construct validity, and criterion validity [80, 81, 83]. Content validity ensures that the tool comprehensively and accurately covers the relevant aspects of the functional abilities of the target population [80, 84, 85]. Construct validity examines how well the tool aligns with theoretical constructs or known relationships with other related measures [80, 81, 86]. Criterion validity assesses how well the mHealth tool compares to a gold standard or established assessment of functional abilities [80, 81, 87]. Strong validity ensures that the tool provides meaningful and accurate information about the patients' functional status [80].

Responsiveness is the ability of the mHealth tool to detect meaningful changes in functional abilities over time [88]. It is especially important for tracking changes in patients' functional status during rehabilitation or health interventions [89]. A responsive tool should be capable of detecting improvements or deteriorations in the patients' functional abilities promptly and equally throughout the range of impairment, allowing healthcare providers to adapt strategic treatments accordingly [89, 90].

Accuracy refers to how closely the measurements obtained from these mHealth assessment tools align with the true or actual values of the targeted health parameters or outcomes [91]. It is a critical aspect to ensure the reliability and validity of the information collected through these mHealth applications [92]. Some factors are known to influence the accuracy of mHealth assessment tools, which are: sensor technology, calibration and validation, data quality and signal processing, algorithm accuracy, user compliance and engagement, contextual factors, clinical validation, and data transmission and storage [93]. Maintaining high accuracy in mHealth assessment tools is critical to enable reliable health monitoring, improve patient care, and support evidence-based decision-making in healthcare settings [94].

The measurement properties of mHealth functional assessment tools in stroke survivors play a crucial role in their successful integration into stroke rehabilitation and healthcare practices [95]. A recent scoping review [4] provided an initial foundation for this emerging field and provided a set of recommendations to clinicians and researchers about how best to choose mHealth technologies according to the objective to be achieved. They conducted a comprehensive review of the measurement properties of the mHealth assessments for stroke survivors and identified facilitators and barriers inherent to these assessments in research and clinical practice settings [4].

When evaluating stroke survivors, studies are analyzing functional skills in terms of locomotion (i.e., lower limbs), movement intensity (in terms of energy expenditure, levels of physical activity, and/or time in body positions) and object-interaction activities (i.e., UEs) [4]. The validity of applications used to measure locomotion, when compared to a criterion-standard measure ranged from poor to good and depended on smartphone operating system [4, 96, 97]. Test-retest reliability ranged between poor and good, also varying according to the smartphone operating system

[96]. Intra- and inter-rater reliability of one specific application (Xsensor Pro) is good [4, 98]. Validity and reliability of the commercially identified technologies to assess locomotion ranged from poor to excellent, while their accuracy ranged from poor to good, depending on sensor positioning and walking speed [4, 43, 54, 64, 99]. Responsiveness was not reported for either commercially or non-commercial available devices [4]. Validity and reliability values can be detailed described in [4].

The validity of the application used to assess the movement intensity showed no association between expenditure estimated by the application (Google Fit) and the gold-standard measure [4, 100]. Reliability, accuracy nor responsiveness were not reported [4]. When considering the commercial devices used to assess movement intensity, validity and reliability ranged from poor to good [63–65, 101–108] and no data was available about their responsiveness [4].

The validity of object-interaction UE behavior measured with non-commercial wearable sensors was assessed in eight studies, and it was reported to range from poor to excellent [4]. No data has been provided on the validity of commercial wearable sensors for assessing object-interaction activities. There is high inter-rater reliability for Actigraph [109] and good accuracy of Crossbow iMote2 [4, 110].

An overall view of the above-mentioned scoping review allows us to state that the most investigated measurement properties, for both commercial and non-commercial devices, are validity and accuracy [4]. Validity is also listed as the most important property necessary for clinical or research purposes [4]. The choice of sensor placement site can interfere with accuracy [4]. It is shown that the devices placed in less affected limb have better accuracy [4]. The lack of data related to responsiveness represents an obvious gap in the literature related to clinical practice, as clinicians often use assessment tools to monitor changes over time in response to an intervention [4].

Recently [32], recommended the following devices:

For use in research to monitor physical activity in stroke survivors:

1. For physical activity **intensity** (e.g., energy expenditure), the Actigraph, Actical, and Activ8;
2. For physical activity **duration** (e.g., time spent in postures, sedentary behavior), the ***ActivPAL*** device is recommended.
3. For physical activity **frequency** (e.g., step count), the ***Step Activity Monitor*** is recommended.

For use in clinical practice to monitor physical activity in stroke survivors:

1. For measuring physical activity **frequency, intensity, and duration**, the ***Fitbit*** (worn on the ankle for research) is recommended.

Figure 33.1 shows a synthesis of model devices, purpose, and measurement properties available to use in research and clinical practice with stroke survivors.

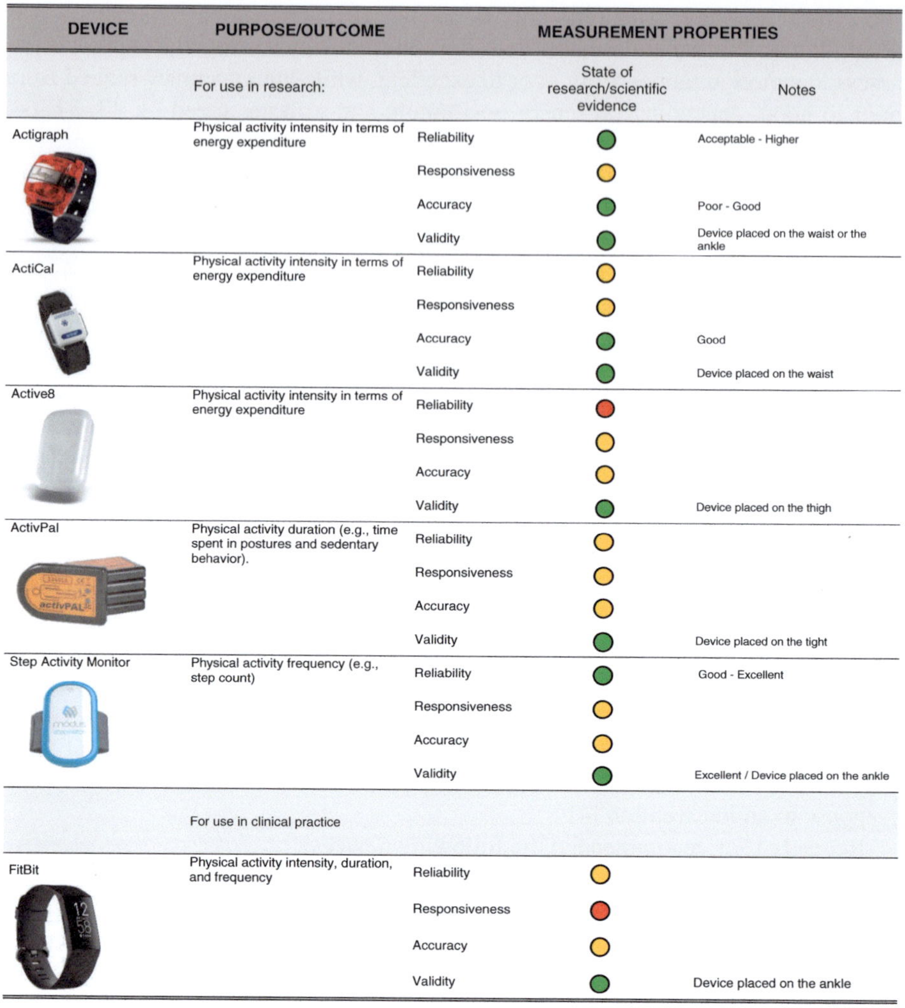

DEVICE	PURPOSE/OUTCOME	MEASUREMENT PROPERTIES	State of research/scientific evidence	Notes
	For use in research:			
Actigraph	Physical activity intensity in terms of energy expenditure	Reliability	🟢	Acceptable - Higher
		Responsiveness	🟡	
		Accuracy	🟢	Poor - Good
		Validity	🟢	Device placed on the waist or the ankle
ActiCal	Physical activity intensity in terms of energy expenditure	Reliability	🟡	
		Responsiveness	🟡	
		Accuracy	🟢	Good
		Validity	🟢	Device placed on the waist
Active8	Physical activity intensity in terms of energy expenditure	Reliability	🔴	
		Responsiveness	🟡	
		Accuracy	🟡	
		Validity	🟢	Device placed on the thigh
ActivPal	Physical activity duration (e.g., time spent in postures and sedentary behavior).	Reliability	🟡	
		Responsiveness	🟡	
		Accuracy	🟡	
		Validity	🟢	Device placed on the tight
Step Activity Monitor	Physical activity frequency (e.g., step count)	Reliability	🟢	Good - Excellent
		Responsiveness	🟡	
		Accuracy	🟡	
		Validity	🟢	Excellent / Device placed on the ankle
	For use in clinical practice			
FitBit	Physical activity intensity, duration, and frequency	Reliability	🟡	
		Responsiveness	🔴	
		Accuracy	🟡	
		Validity	🟢	Device placed on the ankle

Fig. 33.1 Overview of mHealth Devices: Purpose, Outcomes, and Measurement Properties

Functional Outcomes in mHealth for Stroke Survivors

Common functional outcomes currently used in mHealth studies for stroke survivors are focused on investigating features related to activities of daily living, mobility/locomotion and walking, mobility/object-interaction UE and balance and coordination [111]. The most investigated functional outcomes in research using mHealth is mobility, particularly gait in stroke survivors. Monitoring gait by using mHealth applications and wearable devices is being used to evaluate step count, gait speed, step length and stride length, balance and stability, gait symmetry, endurance and walking distance, sit-to-stand transfers, dual-task walking, and gait kinematic analysis [4, 112].

However, functional outcomes related to activity of daily living aim to identify the independence level of the patient in activities (i.e., dressing, grooming and personal hygiene, feeding, bathing/showering, toileting, functional mobility, transferring, and ambulation) [78]. Those functional outcomes are typically assessed using a combination of observation, self-report, and standardized assessment tools [113]. By assessing the level of independence of a patient, healthcare providers can identify areas of weakness, design targeted intervention plans, and track individuals' progress over time [114].

Functional outcomes related to gait are frequently measured using motion sensors, accelerometer, and other wearable devices that can provide real-time data on gait parameters [115, 116]. These outcomes are essential to healthcare professionals and stroke survivors when considering the rehabilitation tracking progress, and the tailoring of objectives to optimize locomotion recovery [115–118].

In mHealth, functional outcomes related to mobility and object-interaction of UE are crucial to characterize the individual's ability to perform daily activities, explore independence, and participate in community activities [12, 119]. These outcomes focus on assessing motor control, coordination, and dexterity of the UE and may allow us to comprehend meaningful interactions with objects in the environment [12, 119, 120]. All of them can be clustered into the amount of use of the UE during the activities of daily living [4, 12, 121].

The functional outcomes explored by a systematic review investigating the use of mHealth included randomized controlled trials and non-randomized controlled trials [122]. They monitored several outcome measurements, namely: balance, mobility, upper extremity recovery, walking and lower extremity function [112, 123]. The assessment tools used to assess the functional outcomes related to balance were the Mini-BESTest, Berg Balance Scale and postural control measures [112, 124–127]. The overall findings regarding the balance outcomes were mixed and not consistently significant [112]. Mobility was investigated by the Timed Up and Go test, the Barthel Index, modified Barthel Index, and Stroke Impact Scale-mobility [112, 126–128]. For the evaluation of the upper extremity recovery, various assessments used, including manual muscle testing of the UE or wrist and fingers, Fugl-Meyer Assessment of the Upper Extremity, Brunnstrom stage for the arm and hand, Manual Functional Test, and Purdue Pegboard Test [112, 125, 129]. The improvements were achieved by the patients through gaming and finger tapping applications [112, 129]. The measurements used to evaluate the walking outcome were 10-Meter Walking Test for walking speed, 6-Minute Walking Test for walking endurance and TUG for mobility and risk of falling [112, 124–128]. Lower extremity function was assessed by the Fugl-Meyer Assessment of the lower extremity and the Motricity Index of the lower extremity leg [112, 127].

Functional outcomes related to self-efficacy for stroke survivors are critical in stroke rehabilitation [130, 131]. Self-efficacy refers to an individual's belief in their ability to successfully perform specific tasks or behaviors, even when facing challenges [132]. It plays a significant role in the recovery process as it influences the patients' motivation, engagement in therapy, and overall well-being [133]. Stroke survivors with higher self-efficacy are more likely to actively participate in rehabilitation sessions and adhere to their therapy programs, demonstrating perseverance and effort in their recovery [131]. Higher self-efficacy is also associated with a greater likelihood of setting and achieving realistic rehabilitation goals, and better functional recovery, including improved mobility, balance, and coordination [134].

Functional outcomes related to self-efficacy can be assessed through validated self-report measures, interviews or questionnaires that evaluate the subjects' beliefs in their abilities to perform specific tasks [135]. Interventions related to self-efficacy may include goal setting, positive reinforcement, motivational strategies, and cognitive-behavioral techniques [136, 137]. By addressing self-efficacy as a functional outcome, healthcare professional can tailor rehabilitation programs to foster a sense of confidence and empowerment in stroke survivors, ultimately promoting greater engagement, improved functional outcomes, and a significant participation in their communities [138]. Acknowledging the fundamental role of self-efficacy in shaping users' adoption behavior toward mHealth, as highlighted by Zhang et al. [139], Alam et al. [140] identified a positive association between self-efficacy and mHealth adoption intentions. These findings underscore the influential link between users' confidence in their capability and their willingness to adopt mHealth technologies.

Limitations Related to mHealth

The deployment of sensors for monitoring physical activity, while promising, is accompanied by several limitations. Accessibility remains a notable concern, as certain populations may face challenges in obtaining or utilizing these devices due to financial constraints or limited technological literacy [141]. Familiarization issues arise as users may struggles to adapt to the intricacies of sensors-based systems, affecting the accurate representation of their PA levels and/or sedentary behavior [142]. Technical challenges, encompassing sensor accuracy, calibration, and reliability, can impact the precision of data collected [143].

Additionally, the proficiency of professionals tasked with managing the extensive datasets generated by these devices is crucial. Inadequate training in data interpretation and utilization may hinder the effective extraction of meaningful insights, limiting the overall utility of sensor-based monitoring in the field of physical activity level and sedentary behavior assessment [144]. Addressing these limitations is imperative to enhance the practicality and effectiveness of sensor technologies in the quantifying and analyzing physical activity levels and sedentary behavior data.

Gaps in the Literature

Smartphone advancements have transformed health care, offering fresh strategies to boost health and wellness. New smartphone applications are becoming more commonly available and can help people with stroke with self-management needs [145]. Although studies on mHealth are growing, and it is a new perspective in the area, there is still much to be researched. This is especially true with respect to their validity, reliability, and responsiveness across the spectrum of impairment severity and time since stroke. Additionally, the time frame to monitor human behavior varies tremendously. Few studies have a longitudinal analysis, or a follow-up time, either when doing EMA or EMI [145]. Finally, other limitation is related to the accessibility to the sensors due to cost as well as familiarization and training required by the professionals to educate patients while wearing the devices.

Conclusion

This chapter recommends the use of devices on monitoring the movement behavior and physical activity of stroke survivors in the laboratory setting, natural environment, and throughout different phases of recovery. Many devices were recommended to monitor stroke survivors' movement behaviors and physical activity, using commercially, and non-commercially available technologies, provided by smartphones, accelerometers, and inclinometers. However, the technology is evolving rapidly, and there is an envision of a near future change in those recommendations. We can anticipate an increase in research investigating property measurements of smartphone applications to monitor human behavior after stroke due to its easy-to-use and accessibility in low- and middle-income countries.

Measurement properties of the sensors are important for clinical, home/community, and research use. Validity and accuracy were the most investigated properties, both for commercial and non-commercial devices. From a practical standpoint, it makes sense that validity should be established before determining accuracy or responsiveness. Sensor placements interfere with accuracy of commercially available devices. For these, non-paretic limb placement has better accuracy. Responsiveness was rarely reported, revealing an obvious knowledge gap. Responsiveness is important in practice, to monitor changes over time or in response to an intervention.

Finally, the criteria to decide about the use of mHealth devices will depend on the human behavior purpose of measurement, user-knowledge, resources, and setting (clinical, research in laboratory or natural environment). Recommendations were provided by the literature, as well as based on the authors experience. Research still needs to evolve and assess the real impact of monitoring human behavior on sedentary behavior and secondary health conditions caused by stroke (e.g., recurrent stroke).

References

1. Moss RJ, Süle A, Kohl S. eHealth and mHealth. Eur J Hosp Pharm. 2019;26(1):57–8. https://doi.org/10.1136/EJHPHARM-2018-001819.

2. World Health Organization. WHO EMRO | eHealth | Health topics. 2023. https://www.emro.who.int/health-topics/ehealth/.
3. Eng JJ, Pastva AM. Advances in remote monitoring for stroke recovery. Stroke. 2022;53(8):2658–61. https://doi.org/10.1161/STROKEAHA.122.038885.
4. Torriani-Pasin C, Demers M, Polese JC, Bishop L, Wade E, Hempel S, Winstein C. mHealth technologies used to capture walking and arm use behavior in adult stroke survivors: a scoping review beyond measurement properties. Disabil Rehabil. 2022;44(20):6094–106. https://doi.org/10.1080/09638288.2021.1953623/SUPPL_FILE/IDRE_A_1953623_SM8264.DOCX.
5. Early J, Gonzalez C, Gordon-Dseagu V, Robles-Calderon L. Use of mobile health (mHealth) technologies and interventions among community health workers globally: a scoping review. Health Promot Pract. 2019;20(6):805–17. https://doi.org/10.1177/1524839919855391.
6. Matthew-Maich N, Harris L, Ploeg J, Markle-Reid M, Valaitis R, Ibrahim S, Gafni A, Isaacs S. Designing, implementing, and evaluating mobile health technologies for managing chronic conditions in older adults: a scoping review. JMIR Mhealth Uhealth. 2016;4(2):e29. https://doi.org/10.2196/MHEALTH.5127.
7. Jeffrey B, Bagala M, Creighton A, Leavey T, Nicholls S, Wood C, Longman J, Barker J, Pit S. Mobile phone applications and their use in the self-management of type 2 diabetes mellitus: a qualitative study among app users and non-app users. Diabetol Metab Syndr. 2019;11(1):1–17. https://doi.org/10.1186/S13098-019-0480-4/TABLES/6.
8. Vo V, Auroy L, Sarradon-Eck A. Patients' perceptions of mHealth apps: meta-ethnographic review of qualitative studies. JMIR Mhealth Uhealth. 2019;7(7):e13817. https://doi.org/10.2196/13817.
9. Executive Board, 142. mHealth: use of appropriate digital technologies for public health: report by the Director-General. World Health Organization; 2017. https://apps.who.int/iris/handle/10665/274134.
10. Fan C, Gao F. Enhanced human activity recognition using wearable sensors via a hybrid feature selection method. Sensors (Basel). 2021;21(19):6434. https://doi.org/10.3390/s21196434. PMID: 34640754; PMCID: PMC8512389.
11. Chen HL, Lin KC, Hsieh YW, Wu CY, Liing RJ, Chen CL. A study of predictive validity, responsiveness, and minimal clinically important difference of arm accelerometer in real-world activity of patients with chronic stroke. Clin Rehabil. 2018;32(1):75–83. https://doi.org/10.1177/0269215517712042.
12. Chen Y-A, Demers M, Lewthwaite R, Schweighofer N, Monterosso JR, Fisher BE, Winstein C. A novel combination of accelerometry and ecological momentary assessment for post-stroke paretic arm/hand use: feasibility and validity. J Clin Med. 2021;10(6):1328. https://doi.org/10.3390/jcm10061328.
13. Geed S, Grainger ML, Mitchell A, Anderson CC, Schmaulfuss HL, Culp SA, McCormick ER, McGarry MR, Delgado MN, Noccioli AD, Shelepov J, Dromerick AW, Lum PS. Concurrent validity of machine learning-classified functional upper extremity use from accelerometry in chronic stroke. Front Physiol. 2023;14:1116878. https://doi.org/10.3389/FPHYS.2023.1116878.
14. Kim GJ, Parnandi A, Eva S, Schambra H. The use of wearable sensors to assess and treat the upper extremity after stroke: a scoping review. Disabil Rehabil. 2022;44(20):6119–38. https://doi.org/10.1080/09638288.2021.1957027.
15. Parnandi A, Kaku A, Venkatesan A, Pandit N, Wirtanen A, Rajamohan H, Venkataramanan K, Nilsen D, Fernandez-Granda C, Schambra H. PrimSeq: a deep learning-based pipeline to quantitate rehabilitation training. PLOS Digital Health. 2022;1(6):e0000044. https://doi.org/10.1371/JOURNAL.PDIG.0000044.
16. Sequeira SB, Grainger ML, Mitchell AM, Anderson CC, Geed S, Lum P, Giladi AM. Machine learning improves functional upper extremity use capture in distal radius fracture patients. Plast Reconstr Surg Glob Open. 2022;10(8):E4472. https://doi.org/10.1097/GOX.0000000000004472.

17. Fugl-Meyer AR, Jääskö L, Leyman I, Olsson S, Steglind S. The post-stroke hemiplegic patient. 1. A method for evaluation of physical performance. Scand J Rehabil Med. 1975;7(1):13–31. http://www.ncbi.nlm.nih.gov/pubmed/1135616
18. Lyle RC. A performance test for assessment of UE function in physical rehabilitation treatment and research. Int J Rehabil Res Internationale Zeitschrift Fur Rehabilitationsforschung/ Revue Internationale de Recherches de Readaptation. 1981;4(4):483–92. https://doi.org/10.1097/00004356-198112000-00001.
19. Shiffman S, Stone AA, Hufford MR. Ecological momentary assessment. Annu Rev Clin Psychol. 2008;4:1–32. https://doi.org/10.1146/ANNUREV.CLINPSY.3.022806.091415.
20. Demers M, Winstein CJ. A perspective on the use of ecological momentary assessment and intervention to promote stroke recovery and rehabilitation. Top Stroke Rehabil. 2021;28(8):594–605. https://doi.org/10.1080/10749357.2020.1856557.
21. Heron KE, Smyth JM. Ecological momentary interventions: incorporating mobile technology into psychosocial and health behavior treatments. Br J Health Psychol. 2010;15(Pt 1):1. https://doi.org/10.1348/135910709X466063.
22. Dao KP, de Cocker K, Tong HL, Kocaballi AB, Chow C, Laranjo L. Smartphone-delivered ecological momentary interventions based on ecological momentary assessments to promote health behaviors: systematic review and adapted checklist for reporting ecological momentary assessment and intervention studies. JMIR Mhealth Uhealth. 2021;9(11):e22890. https://doi.org/10.2196/22890.
23. Barth J, Geed S, Mitchell A, Lum PS, Edwards DF, Dromerick AW. Characterizing upper extremity motor behavior in the first week after stroke. PLoS One. 2020;15(8):e0221668. https://doi.org/10.1371/JOURNAL.PONE.0221668.
24. Chen YA, Lewthwaite R, Schweighofer N, Monterosso JR, Fisher BE, Winstein C. Essential role of social context and self-efficacy in daily paretic arm/hand use after stroke: an ecological momentary assessment study with accelerometry. Arch Phys Med Rehabil. 2023;104(3):390–402. https://doi.org/10.1016/J.APMR.2022.09.003.
25. Wist S, Clivaz J, Sattelmayer M. Muscle strengthening for hemiparesis after stroke: a meta-analysis. Ann Phys Rehabil Med. 2016;59(2):114–24. https://doi.org/10.1016/J.REHAB.2016.02.001.
26. Tsao CW, Aday AW, Almarzooq ZI, Anderson CAM, Arora P, Avery CL, Baker-Smith CM, Beaton AZ, Boehme AK, Buxton AE, Commodore-Mensah Y, Elkind MSV, Evenson KR, Eze-Nliam C, Fugar S, Generoso G, Heard DG, Hiremath S, Ho JE, et al. Heart disease and stroke Statistics-2023 update: a report from the American Heart Association. Circulation. 2023;147(8):E93–E621. https://doi.org/10.1161/CIR.0000000000001123.
27. Yu HX, Wang ZX, Liu CB, Dai P, Lan Y, Xu GQ. Effect of cognitive function on balance and posture control after stroke. Neural Plast. 2021;2021:6636999. https://doi.org/10.1155/2021/6636999.
28. Fonte G, Schreiber C, Areno G, Masson X, Chantraine F, Schütz G, Dierick F. Metabolic energy expenditure and accelerometer-determined physical activity levels in post-stroke hemiparetic patients. J Stroke Cerebrovasc Dis. 2022;31(5):106397. https://doi.org/10.1016/J.JSTROKECEREBROVASDIS.2022.106397.
29. Fini NA, Bernhardt J, Churilov L, Clark R, Holland AE. Adherence to physical activity and cardiovascular recommendations during the 2 years after stroke rehabilitation discharge. Ann Phys Rehabil Med. 2021;64(2):101455. https://doi.org/10.1016/j.rehab.2020.03.018.
30. Fini NA, Bernhardt J, Holland AE. Types of physical activity performed pre and post stroke. Braz J Phys Ther. 2022;26(3):100412. https://doi.org/10.1016/J.BJPT.2022.100412.
31. Fini NA, Bernhardt J, Said CM, Billinger SA. How to address physical activity participation after stroke in research and clinical practice. Stroke. 2021;52(6):e274. https://doi.org/10.1161/STROKEAHA.121.034557.
32. Fini NA, Simpson D, Moore SA, Mahendran N, Eng JJ, Borschmann K, Moulaee Conradsson D, Chastin S, Churilov L, English C. How should we measure physical activity after stroke? An international consensus. Int J Stroke. 2023;18(9):1132–42. https://doi.org/10.1177/17474930231184108.

33. Prior PL, Suskin N. Exercise for stroke prevention. Stroke Vasc Neurol. 2018;3(2):59–68. https://doi.org/10.1136/svn-2018-000155. PMID: 30191075; PMCID: PMC6122300.
34. Saunders DH, Sanderson M, Hayes S, Kilrane M, Greig CA, Brazzelli M, Mead GE. Physical fitness training for stroke patients. Cochrane Database Syst Rev. 2016;3(3):CD003316. https://doi.org/10.1002/14651858.CD003316.pub6. Update in: Cochrane Database Syst Rev. 2020;3:CD003316. PMID: 27010219; PMCID: PMC6464717.
35. Ashe MC, Miller WC, Eng JJ, Noreau L. Older adults, chronic disease and leisure-time physical activity. Gerontology. 2009;55(1):64–72. https://doi.org/10.1159/000141518.
36. Hall J, Morton S, Fitzsimons CF, Hall JF, Corepal R, English C, Forster A, Lawton R, Patel A, Mead G, Clarke DJ. Factors influencing sedentary behaviours after stroke: findings from qualitative observations and interviews with stroke survivors and their caregivers. BMC Public Health. 2020;20(1):1–15. https://doi.org/10.1186/S12889-020-09113-6/TABLES/3.
37. English C, Healy GN, Coates A, Lewis L, Olds T, Bernhardt J. Sitting and activity time in people with stroke. Phys Ther. 2016;96(2):193–201. https://doi.org/10.2522/PTJ.20140522.
38. Saunders DH, Sanderson M, Hayes S, Johnso L, Kramer S, Carter DD, Jarvis H, Brazzelli M, Mead GE. Physical fitness training for stroke patients. Cochrane Database Syst Rev. 2020;2020(3):1–3. https://doi.org/10.1002/14651858.CD003316.pub7.
39. Sullivan J, Espe L, Kelly A, Veilbig L, Kwasny M. Feasibility and outcomes of a community-based, pedometer-monitored walking program in chronic stroke: a pilot study. Top Stroke Rehabil. 2014;21(2):101–10. https://doi.org/10.1310/TSR2102-101.
40. Saunders DH, Mead GE, Fitzsimons C, Kelly P, van Wijck F, Verschuren O, Backx K, English C. Interventions for reducing sedentary behaviour in people with stroke. Cochrane Database Syst Rev. 2021;6(6):CD012996. https://doi.org/10.1002/14651858.CD012996.PUB2.
41. Juengst SB, Terhorst L, Nabasny A, Wallace T, Weaver JA, Osborne CL, Burns SP, Wright B, Wen PS, Kew CL, Morris J. Use of mHealth technology for patient-reported outcomes in community-dwelling adults with acquired brain injuries: a scoping review. Int J Environ Res Public Health. 2021;18(4):2173. https://doi.org/10.3390/IJERPH18042173.
42. Neff AJ, Lee Y, Metts CL, Wong AWK. Ecological momentary assessment of social interactions: associations with depression, anxiety, pain, and fatigue in individuals with mild stroke. Arch Phys Med Rehabil. 2021;102(3):395–405. https://doi.org/10.1016/J.APMR.2020.08.007.
43. Klassen TD, Simpson LA, Lim SB, Louie DR, Parappilly B, Sakakibara BM, Zbogar D, Eng JJ. "Stepping up" activity poststroke: ankle-positioned accelerometer can accurately record steps during slow walking. Phys Ther. 2016;96(3):355. https://doi.org/10.2522/PTJ.20140611.
44. Uswatte G, Taub E, Morris D, Light K, Thompson PA. The Motor Activity Log-28: assessing daily use of the hemiparetic arm after stroke. Neurology. 2006;67(7):1189–94. https://doi.org/10.1212/01.WNL.0000238164.90657.C2.
45. Uswatte G, Taub E, Morris D, Vignolo M, McCulloch K. Reliability and validity of the upper-extremity Motor Activity Log-14 for measuring real-world arm use. Stroke. 2005;36(11):2493–6. https://doi.org/10.1161/01.STR.0000185928.90848.2E.
46. Duncan PW, Wallace D, Lai SM, Johnson D, Embretson S, Laster LJ. The stroke impact scale version 2.0. Evaluation of reliability, validity, and sensitivity to change. Stroke. 1999;30(10):2131–40. https://doi.org/10.1161/01.STR.30.10.2131.
47. Nouri FM, Lincoln NB. An extended activities of daily living scale for stroke patients. Clin Rehabil. 1987;1(4):301–5. https://doi.org/10.1177/026921558700100409.
48. Gebruers N, Truijen S, Engelborghs S, De Deyn PP. Predictive value of upper-limb accelerometry in acute stroke with hemiparesis. J Rehabil Res Dev. 2013;50(8):1099–106. https://doi.org/10.1682/JRRD.2012.09.0166.
49. Gebruers N, Truijen S, Engelborghs S, De Deyn PP. Prediction of UE recovery, general disability, and rehabilitation status by activity measurements assessed by accelerometers or the Fugl-Meyer score in acute stroke. Am J Phys Med Rehabil. 2014;93(3):245–52. https://doi.org/10.1097/PHM.0000000000000045.
50. Gebruers N, Vanroy C, Truijen S, Engelborghs S, De Deyn PP. Monitoring of physical activity after stroke: a systematic review of accelerometry-based measures. Arch Phys Med Rehabil. 2010;91(2):288–97. https://doi.org/10.1016/J.APMR.2009.10.025.

51. Lum PS, Shu L, Bochniewicz EM, Tran T, Chang LC, Barth J, Dromerick AW. Improving accelerometry-based measurement of functional use of the upper extremity after stroke: machine learning versus counts threshold method. Neurorehabil Neural Repair. 2020;34(12):1078–87. https://doi.org/10.1177/1545968320962483.
52. Lee J, Stone AJ. Combined aerobic and resistance training for cardiorespiratory fitness, muscle strength, and walking capacity after stroke: a systematic review and meta-analysis. J Stroke Cerebrovas Dis. 2020;29(1):104498. https://doi.org/10.1016/J.JSTROKECEREBROVASDIS.2019.104498.
53. Mayo NE, Wood-Dauphinee S, Côté R, Durcan L, Carlton J. Activity, participation, and quality of life 6 months poststroke. Arch Phys Med Rehabil. 2002;83(8):1035–42. https://doi.org/10.1053/APMR.2002.33984.
54. Duclos NC, Aguiar LT, Aissaoui R, Faria CDCM, Nadeau S, Duclos C. Activity monitor placed at the nonparetic ankle is accurate in measuring step counts during community walking in Poststroke individuals: a validation study. PM & R. 2019;11(9):963–71. https://doi.org/10.1002/PMRJ.12080.
55. Handlery R, Fulk G, Pellegrini C, Stewart JC, Monroe C, Fritz S. Stepping after stroke: walking characteristics in people with chronic stroke differ on the basis of walking speed, walking endurance, and daily steps. Phys Ther. 2020;100(5):807–17. https://doi.org/10.1093/PTJ/PZAA020.
56. Schaffer SD, Holzapfel SD, Fulk G, Bosch PR. Step count accuracy and reliability of two activity tracking devices in people after stroke. Physiother Theory Pract. 2017;33(10):788–96. https://doi.org/10.1080/09593985.2017.1354412.
57. Compagnat M, Batcho CS, David R, Vuillerme N, Salle JY, Daviet JC, Mandigout S. Validity of the walked distance estimated by wearable devices in stroke individuals. Sensors (Basel). 2019;19(11):2497. https://doi.org/10.3390/s19112497. PMID: 31159246; PMCID: PMC6604102.
58. Fulk GD, He Y, Boyne P, Dunning K. Predicting home and community walking activity poststroke. Stroke. 2017;48(2):406–11. https://doi.org/10.1161/STROKEAHA.116.015309.
59. Tremblay MS, Aubert S, Barnes JD, Saunders TJ, Carson V, Latimer-Cheung AE, Chastin SFM, Altenburg TM, Chinapaw MJM, Aminian S, Arundell L, Hinkley T, Hnatiuk J, Atkin AJ, Belanger K, Chaput JP, Gunnell K, Larouche R, Manyanga T, et al. Sedentary Behavior Research Network (SBRN)—Terminology Consensus Project process and outcome. Int J Behav Nutr Phys Act. 2017;14(1):1–17. https://doi.org/10.1186/S12966-017-0525-8/FIGURES/3.
60. Biswas D, Cranny A, Gupta N, Maharatna K, Achner J, Klemke J, Jöbges M, Ortmann S. Recognizing UE movements with wrist worn inertial sensors using k-means clustering classification. Hum Mov Sci. 2015;40:59–76. https://doi.org/10.1016/J.HUMOV.2014.11.013.
61. Ezeugwu VE, Garga N, Manns PJ. Reducing sedentary behaviour after stroke: perspectives of ambulatory individuals with stroke. Disabil Rehabil. 2017;39(25):2551–8. https://doi.org/10.1080/09638288.2016.1239764.
62. English C, Manns PJ, Tucak C, Bernhardt J. Physical activity and sedentary behaviors in people with stroke living in the community: a systematic review. Phys Ther. 2014;94(2):185–96. https://doi.org/10.2522/PTJ.20130175.
63. Connell LA, McMahon NE, Simpson LA, Watkins CL, Eng JJ. Investigating measures of intensity during a structured UE exercise program in stroke rehabilitation: an exploratory study. Arch Phys Med Rehabil. 2014;95(12):2410–9. https://doi.org/10.1016/J.APMR.2014.05.025.
64. Compagnat M, Mandigout S, Chaparro D, Daviet JC, Salle JY. Validity of the Actigraph GT3x and influence of the sensor positioning for the assessment of active energy expenditure during four activities of daily living in stroke subjects. Clin Rehabil. 2018;32(12):1696–704. https://doi.org/10.1177/0269215518788116.
65. Lee JY, Kwon SY, Kim WS, Hahn SJ, Park J, Paik NJ. Feasibility, reliability, and validity of using accelerometers to measure physical activities of patients with stroke during inpatient rehabilitation. PLoS One. 2018;13(12):e0209607. https://doi.org/10.1371/JOURNAL.PONE.0209607.

66. Fini NA, Holland AE, Keating J, Simek J, Bernhardt J. How physically active are people following stroke? Systematic review and quantitative synthesis. Phys Ther. 2017;97(7):707–17. https://doi.org/10.1093/ptj/pzx038.
67. Thilarajah S, Mentiplay BF, Bower KJ, Tan D, Yong Hao P, Williams G, Koh G, Clark RA. Factors associated with post-stroke physical activity: a systematic review and meta-analysis. Arch Phys Med Rehabil. 2018;99(9):1876–89. https://doi.org/10.1016/j.apmr.2017.09.117.
68. Pohl J, Ryser A, Veerbeek JM, Verheyden G, Vogt JE, Luft AR, Easthope CA. Accuracy of gait and posture classification using movement sensors in individuals with mobility impairment after stroke. Front Physiol. 2022;13:933987. https://doi.org/10.3389/fphys.2022.933987. PMID: 36225292; PMCID: PMC9549863.
69. Otaki R, Oouchida Y, Aizu N, Sudo T, Sasahara H, Saito Y, Takemura S, Izumi SI. Relationship between body-specific attention to a paretic limb and real-world arm use in stroke patients: a longitudinal study. Front Syst Neurosci. 2022;15:806257. https://doi.org/10.3389/fnsys.2021.806257. PMID: 35273480; PMCID: PMC8902799.
70. Marshall MR, Montoye AHK, Conway MR, Schlaff RA, Pfeiffer KA, Pivarnik JM. Location, location, location: accelerometer placement affects steps-based physical activity outcomes during pregnancy and postpartum. Am J Lifestyle Med. 2021;17(1):123–30. https://doi.org/10.1177/15598276211030472. PMID: 36636394; PMCID: PMC9830244.
71. Costa PHV, de Jesus TPD, Winstein C, Torriani-Pasin C, Polese JC. An investigation into the validity and reliability of mHealth devices for counting steps in chronic stroke survivors. Clin Rehabil. 2020;34(3):394–403. https://doi.org/10.1177/0269215519895796.
72. Spooner DM, Pachana NA. Ecological validity in neuropsychological assessment: a case for greater consideration in research with neurologically intact populations. Arch Clin Neuropsychol. 2006;21(4):327–37. https://doi.org/10.1016/J.ACN.2006.04.004.
73. Naumann S, Byrne ML, de la Fuente A, Harrewijn A, Nugiel T, Rosen M, van Atteveldt N, Matusz PJ. Assessing the degree of ecological validity of your study: introducing the Multidimensional Assessment of Research in Context (MARC) tool. Mind Brain Educ. 2022;16(3):228–38. https://doi.org/10.1111/MBE.12318.
74. American Psychological Association, APA task force on psychological assessment and evaluation guidelines. APA guidelines for psychological assessment and evaluation. 2020. Retrieved from https://www.apa.org/about/policy/guidelines-psychological-assessment-evaluation.pdf
75. Pashmdarfard M, Azad A. Assessment tools to evaluate Activities of Daily Living (ADL) and Instrumental Activities of Daily Living (IADL) in older adults: a systematic review. Med J Islam Repub Iran. 2020;34(1):33. https://doi.org/10.34171/MJIRI.34.33.
76. Zimmermann N, De Oliveira Cardoso C, Kochhann R, Jacobsen G, Fonseca RP. Contributions of the ecological approach to the neuropsychology of executive functions. Temas Em Psicologia. 2014;22(3):639–54. https://doi.org/10.9788/TP2014.3-09.
77. Andrade HL. A critical review of research on student self-assessment. Frontiers in Education. 2019;4:468374. https://doi.org/10.3389/FEDUC.2019.00087/BIBTEX.
78. Edemekong PF, Bomgaars DL, Sukumaran S, Schoo C. Activities of daily living. In: Encyclopedia of the neurological sciences; 2022. p. 47–8. https://doi.org/10.1016/B978-0-12-385157-4.00464-4.
79. Prinsen CAC, Mokkink LB, Bouter LM, Alonso J, Patrick DL, de Vet HCW, Terwee CB. COSMIN guideline for systematic reviews of patient-reported outcome measures. Qual Life Res. 2018;27(5):1147–57. https://doi.org/10.1007/S11136-018-1798-3.
80. Mohajan H. Two criteria for good measurements in research: validity and reliability. Annals Spiru Haret Univ. 2017;17(3):58–82.
81. Chiang ICA, Jhangiani RS, Price PC. Research methods of psychology—2nd Canadian edition. Victoria: BCcampus; 2015.
82. Chassin MR, Loeb JM. High-reliability health care: getting there from here. Milbank Q. 2013;91(3):459. https://doi.org/10.1111/1468-0009.12023.

83. Echevarría-Guanilo ME, Gonçalves N, Romanoski PJ. Propriedades psicométricas de instrumentos de medidas: bases conceituais emétodos de avaliação—Parte I. Texto Contexto Enferm. 2017;26(4):1–11.
84. Taherdoost H. Validity and reliability of the research instrument; how to test the validation of a questionnaire/survey in a research. Int J Acad Res Manag (IJARM). 2016;5(3):28–36. https://hal.science/hal-02546799
85. Taherdoost H. Validity and reliability of the research instrument; how to test the validation of a questionnaire/survey in a research. SSRN Electron J. 2016;5(3):28–36. Available at SSRN: https://ssrn.com/abstract=3205040 or https://doi.org/10.2139/ssrn.3205040.
86. Strauss ME, Smith GT. Construct validity: advances in theory and methodology. Annu Rev Clin Psychol. 2009;5:1–25. https://doi.org/10.1146/annurev.clinpsy.032408.153639. PMID: 19086835; PMCID: PMC2739261.
87. Jung A, Balzer J, Braun T, Luedtke K. Identification of tools used to assess the external validity of randomized controlled trials in reviews: a systematic review of measurement properties. BMC Med Res Methodol. 2022;22(1):100. https://doi.org/10.1186/s12874-022-01561-5.
88. Braun T, Thiel C, Schulz RJ, et al. Responsiveness and interpretability of commonly used outcome assessments of mobility capacity in older hospital patients with cognitive spectrum disorders. Health Qual Life Outcomes. 2021;19:68. https://doi.org/10.1186/s12955-021-01690-3.
89. National Committee on Vital and Health Statistics. Classifying and reporting functional status: Subcommittee on Populations. U.S. Department of Health and Human Services. 2001. Available from: https://www.ncvhs.hhs.gov/wpcontent/uploads/2017/08/010617rp.pdf.
90. Bohr A, Memarzadeh K. The rise of artificial intelligence in healthcare applications. Artificial Intelligence in Healthcare. 2020:25–60. https://doi.org/10.1016/B978-0-12-818438-7.00002-2. Epub 2020 Jun 26. PMCID: PMC7325854.
91. Antipova D, Eadie L, Macaden A, et al. Diagnostic accuracy of clinical tools for assessment of acute stroke: a systematic review. BMC Emerg Med. 2019;19:49. https://doi.org/10.1186/s12873-019-0262-1.
92. Nouri R, R Niakan Kalhori S, Ghazisaeedi M, Marchand G, Yasini M. Criteria for assessing thequality of mHealth apps: a systematic review. J Am Med Inform Assoc. 2018;25(8):1089–98. https://doi.org/10.1093/jamia/ocy050. PMID: 29788283; PMCID: PMC7646896.
93. Ellis LA, Meulenbroeks I, Churruca K, Pomare C, Hatem S, Harrison R, Zurynski Y, Braithwaite J. The application of E-mental health in response to COVID-19: scoping review and bibliometric analysis. JMIR Ment Health. 2021;8:e32948. https://doi.org/10.2196/32948.
94. Zamzam AH, Abdul Wahab AK, Azizan MM, Satapathy SC, Lai KW, Hasikin K. A systematic review of medical equipment reliability assessment in improving the quality of healthcare services. Front Public Health. 2021;9:753951. https://doi.org/10.3389/fpubh.2021.753951. PMID: 34646808; PMCID: PMC8503610.
95. Slatyer S, Toye C, Burton E, Jacinto AF, Hill KD. Measurement properties of self-report instruments to assess health literacy in older adults: a systematic review. Disabil Rehabil. 2022;44(11):2241–57. https://doi.org/10.1080/09638288.2020.1836044. Epub 2020 Nov 9. PMID: 33164591.
96. Costa S, Ogilvie D, Dalton A, Westgate K, Brage S, Panter J. Quantifying the physical activity energy expenditure of commuters using a combination of global positioning system and combined heart rate and movement sensors. Prev Med. 2015;81:339–44.
97. Polese M, Chiariotti F, Bonetto E, Rigotto F, Zanella A, Zorzi M. A survey on recent advances in transport layer protocols. IEEE Commun Surv Tutor. 2019;21(4):3584–608.
98. Merchán-Baeza JA, González-Sánchez M, Cuesta-Vargas AI. Using smartphones to collect quantitative data on lower limb functionality in people who have suffered a stroke. J Stroke Cerebrovasc Dis. 2018;27(12):3555–62.
99. Campos C, DePaul VG, Knorr S, et al. Validity of the ActiGraph activity monitor for individuals who walk slowly post-stroke. Top Stroke Rehabil. 2018;25(4):295–304.
100. Faria GS, Polese JC, Ribeiro-Samora GA, Scianni AA, Faria CDCM, Teixeira-Salmela LF. Validity of the accelerometer and smartphone application in estimating energy

expenditure in individuals with chronic stroke. Braz J Phys Ther. 2019;23(3):236–43. https://doi.org/10.1016/j.bjpt.2018.08.003. Epub 2018 Aug 20. PMID: 30143357; PMCID: PMC6531636.

101. Falk Neto JH, Kennedy MD. The multimodal nature of high-intensity functional training: potential applications to improve sport performance. Sports (Basel). 2019;7(2):33. https://doi.org/10.3390/sports7020033. PMID: 30699906; PMCID: PMC6409553.
102. Fanchamps MHJ, Horemans HLD, Ribbers GM, Stam HJ, Bussmann JBJ. The accuracy of the detection of body postures and movements using a physical activity monitor in people after a stroke. Sensors (Basel). 2018;18(7):2167. https://doi.org/10.3390/s18072167. PMID: 29976900; PMCID: PMC6069255.
103. Haeuber E, Shaughnessy M, Forrester LW, Coleman KL, Macko RF. Accelerometer monitoring of home- and community-based ambulatory activity after stroke. Arch Phys Med Rehabil. 2004;85(12):1997–2001. https://doi.org/10.1016/j.apmr.2003.11.035. PMID: 15605339.
104. Jayaraman C, Mummidisetty CK, Mannix-Slobig A, McGee KL, Jayaraman A. Variables influencing wearable sensor outcome estimates in individuals with stroke and incomplete spinal cord injury: a pilot investigation validating two research grade sensors. J Neuroeng Rehabil. 2018;15:19. https://doi.org/10.1186/s12984-018-0358-y.
105. Mandigout S, Lacroix J, Ferry B, Vuillerme N, Compagnat M, Daviet J-C. Can energy expenditure be accurately assessed using accelerometry-based wearable motion detectors for physical activity monitoring in post-stroke patients in the subacute phase? Eur J Prev Cardiol. 2020;24(18):2009–16.
106. Serra MC, Balraj E, DiSanzo BL, Ivey FM, Hafer-Macko CE, Treuth MS, Ryan AS. Validating accelerometry as a measure of physical activity and energy expenditure in chronic stroke. Top Stroke Rehabil. 2017;24(1):18–23. https://doi.org/10.1080/10749357.2016.1183866. Epub 2016 Jun 20. PMID: 27322733; PMCID: PMC5125839.
107. Shimizu N, Hashidate H, Ota T, Saito A. The known-groups validity of intensity-based physical activity measurement using an accelerometer in people with subacute stroke. J Phys Ther Sci. 2018;30(4):507–13. https://doi.org/10.1589/jpts.30.507. Epub 2018 Apr 13. PMID: 29706696; PMCID: PMC5908992.
108. Vanroy C, Vissers D, Cras P, Beyne S, Feys H, Vanlandewijck Y, Truijen S. Physical activity monitoring in stroke: SenseWear Pro2 activity accelerometer versus Yamax Digi-Walker SW-200 pedometer. Disabil Rehabil. 2014;36(20):1695–703. https://doi.org/10.3109/09638288.2013.859307. Epub 2013 Nov 27. PMID: 24279597.
109. Sokal B, Uswatte G, Barman J, Brewer M, Byrom E, Latten J, et al. Network of movement and proximity sensors for monitoring upper-extremity motor activity after stroke: proof of principle. Arch Phys Med Rehabil. 2014;95(3):499–505.
110. Gubbi J, Rao AS, Fang K, et al. Motor recovery monitoring using acceleration measurements in post acute stroke patients. Biomed Eng Online. 2013;12:33. https://doi.org/10.1186/1475-925X-12-33.
111. McGlinchey MP, James J, McKevitt C, Douiri A, Sackley C. The effect of rehabilitation interventions on physical function and immobility-related complications in severe stroke: a systematic review. BMJ Open. 2020;10(2):e033642. https://doi.org/10.1136/bmjopen-2019-033642. PMID: 32029489; PMCID: PMC7045156.
112. Rintala A, Kossi O, Bonnechère B, Evers L, Printemps E, Feys P. Mobile health applications for improving physical function, physical activity, and quality of life in stroke survivors: a systematic review. Disabil Rehabil. 2022;45(24):4001–15. https://doi.org/10.1080/09638288.2022.2140844. PMID: 36325613.
113. Kasper JD, Chan KS, Freedman VA. Measuring physical capacity: an assessment of a composite measure using self-report and performance-based items. J Aging Health. 2017;29(2):289–309. https://doi.org/10.1177/0898264316635566.
114. World Health Organization. Monitoring the building blocks of health systems: a handbook of indicators and their measurement strategies. Geneva: WHO; 2010. http://apps.who.int/iris/bitstream/handle/10665/258734/9789241564052-eng.pdf

115. Peters DM, O'Brien ES, Kamrud KE, et al. Utilization of wearable technology to assess gait and mobility post-stroke: a systematic review. J NeuroEngineering Rehabil. 2021;18:67. https://doi.org/10.1186/s12984-021-00863-x.
116. Tao W, Liu T, Zheng R, Feng H. Gait analysis using wearable sensors. Sensors (Basel). 2012;12(2):2255–83. https://doi.org/10.3390/s120202255. Epub 2012 Feb 16. PMID: 22438763; PMCID: PMC3304165.
117. Hatem SM, Saussez G, Della Faille M, Prist V, Zhang X, Dispa D, Bleyenheuft Y. Rehabilitation of motor function after stroke: a multiple systematic review focused on techniques to stimulate upper extremity recovery. Front Hum Neurosci. 2016;10:442. https://doi.org/10.3389/fnhum.2016.00442. PMID: 27679565; PMCID: PMC5020059.
118. Lin SH, Dionne TP. Interventions to improve movement and functional outcomes in adult stroke rehabilitation: review and evidence summary. J Particip Med. 2018;10(1):e3. https://doi.org/10.2196/jopm.8929. PMID: 33052128; PMCID: PMC7434068.
119. Pollock A, Baer G, Campbell P, Choo PL, Forster A, Morris J, Pomeroy VM, Langhorne P. Physical rehabilitation approaches for the recovery of function and mobility following stroke. Cochrane Database Syst Rev. 2014;2014(4):CD001920. https://doi.org/10.1002/14651858.CD001920.pub3. PMID: 24756870; PMCID: PMC6465059.
120. Muratori LM, Lamberg EM, Quinn L, Duff SV. Applying principles of motor learning and control to upper extremity rehabilitation. J Hand Ther. 2013;26(2):94–102; quiz 103. https://doi.org/10.1016/j.jht.2012.12.007. PMID: 23598082; PMCID: PMC3773509.
121. Karagiannis C, Savva C, Mamais I, Adamide T, Georgiou A, Xanthos T. Upper limb exercise training and activities of daily living in patients with COPD: a systematic review of randomized controlled trials. J Bras Pneumol. 2020;46(6):e20190370. https://doi.org/10.36416/1806-3756/e20190370.
122. Rowland SP, Fitzgerald JE, Holme T, Powell J, McGregor A. What is the clinical value of mHealth for patients? NPJ Digit Med. 2020;3:4. https://doi.org/10.1038/s41746-019-0206-x. PMID: 31970289; PMCID: PMC6957674.
123. Bonanno M, De Luca R, Torregrossa W, Tonin P, Calabrò RS. Moving toward appropriate motor assessment tools in people affected by severe acquired brain injury: a scoping review with clinical advices. Healthcare. 2022;10:1115. https://doi.org/10.3390/healthcare10061111.
124. Burgos PI, Lara O, Lavado A, Rojas-Sepúlveda I, Delgado C, Bravo E, Kamisato C, Torres J, Castañeda V, Cerda M. Exergames and telerehabilitation on smartphones to improve balance in stroke patients. Brain Sci. 2020;10(11):773. https://doi.org/10.3390/brainsci10110773. PMID: 33114245; PMCID: PMC7690853.
125. Choi YH, Paik NJ. Mobile game-based virtual reality program for upper extremity stroke rehabilitation. J Vis Exp. 2018;133:56241. https://doi.org/10.3791/56241. PMID: 29578520; PMCID: PMC5931529.
126. Grau-Pellicer M, Lalanza JF, Jovell-Fernández E, Capdevila L. Impact of mHealth technology on adherence to healthy PA after stroke: a randomized study. Top Stroke Rehabil. 2020;27(5):354–68. https://doi.org/10.1080/10749357.2019.1691816. Epub 2019 Dec 2. PMID: 31790639.
127. Vloothuis JDM, Mulder M, Nijland RHM, Goedhart QS, Konijnenbelt M, Mulder H, Hertogh CMPM, van Tulder M, van Wegen EEH, Kwakkel G. Caregiver-mediated exercises with e-health support for early supported discharge after STROKE (CARE4STROKE): a randomized controlled trial. PLoS One. 2019;14(4):e0214241. https://doi.org/10.1371/journal.pone.0214241. PMID: 30958833; PMCID: PMC6453481.
128. Paul L, Wyke S, Brewster S, Sattar N, Gill JM, Alexander G, Rafferty D, McFadyen AK, Ramsay A, Dybus A. Increasing physical activity in stroke survivors using STARFISH, an interactive mobile phone application: a pilot study. Top Stroke Rehabil. 2016;23(3):170–7. https://doi.org/10.1080/10749357.2015.1122266. Epub 2016 Jan 8. PMID: 27077973.
129. Jang SH, Jang WH. The effect of a finger training application using a tablet PC in chronic hemiparetic stroke patients. Somatosens Mot Res. 2016;33(2):124–9. https://doi.org/10.1080/08990220.2016.1197117. Epub 2016 Jun 29. PMID: 27357969.

130. Pui Kei C, Mohd Nordin NA, Abdul Aziz AF. The effectiveness of home-based therapy on functional outcome, self-efficacy and anxiety among discharged stroke survivors. Medicine (Baltimore). 2020;99(47):e23296. https://doi.org/10.1097/MD.0000000000023296. PMID: 33217861; PMCID: PMC7676535.
131. Szczepańska-Gieracha J, Mazurek J. The role of self-efficacy in the recovery process of stroke survivors. Psychol Res Behav Manag. 2020;13:897–906. https://doi.org/10.2147/PRBM.S273009. PMID: 33177896; PMCID: PMC7649225.
132. Bandura A. Self-efficacy: toward a unifying theory of behavioral change. Psychol Rev. 1977;84(2):191–215. http://psycnet.apa.org/journals/rev/84/2/191/
133. Medalia A, Saperstein A. The role of motivation for treatment success. Schizophr Bull. 2011;37 Suppl 2(Suppl 2):S122–8. https://doi.org/10.1093/schbul/sbr063. PMID: 21860041; PMCID: PMC3160119.
134. Gangwani R, Cain A, Collins A, Cassidy JM. Leveraging factors of self-efficacy and motivation to optimize stroke recovery. Front Neurol. 2022;13:823202. https://doi.org/10.3389/fneur.2022.823202.
135. Bandura A. The primacy of self-regulation in health promotion. Appl Psychol. 2005;54:245–54. https://doi.org/10.1111/j.1464-0597.2005.00208.x.
136. Naar-King S, Outlaw AY, Sarr M, Parsons JT, Belzer M, Macdonell K, et al. Motivational Enhancement System for Adherence (MESA): a randomized pilot trial of a brief computer-delivered prevention intervention for youth initiating antiretroviral treatment. J Pediatr Psychol. 2013;38(6):638–48.
137. Warner L, French D. Self-efficacy interventions. In: Hagger M, Cameron L, Hamilton K, Hankonen N, Lintunen T, editors. The handbook of behavior change (Cambridge handbooks in phsycology). Cambridge: Cambridge University Press; 2020. p. 461–78. https://doi.org/10.1017/9781108677318.032.
138. Fugazzaro S, Denti M, Accogli MA, Costi S, Pagliacci D, Calugi S, Cavalli E, Taricco M, Bardelli R. On behalf of look after yourself project. self-management in stroke survivors: development and implementation of the Look after Yourself (LAY) intervention. Int J Environ Res Public Health. 2021;18(11):5925. https://doi.org/10.3390/ijerph18115925. PMID: 34072998; PMCID: PMC8198104.
139. Zhang X, Han X, Dang Y, Meng F, Guo X, Lin J. User acceptance of mobile health services from users' perspectives: the role of self-efficacy and response-efficacy in technology acceptance. Inform Health Soc Care. 2017;42(2):194–206. https://doi.org/10.1080/17538157.2016.1200053. Epub 2016 Aug 26. PMID: 27564428.
140. Alam MZ, Hu W, Abdul KM, Rakibul HM, Alam MMD. Understanding the determinants of mHealth apps adoption in Bangladesh: a SEM-neural network approach. Technol Soc. 2020;61:101255.
141. Kaihlanen AM, Virtanen L, Buchert U, Safarov N, Valkonen P, Hietapakka L, Hörhammer I, Kujala S, Kouvonen A, Heponiemi T. Towards digital health equity—a qualitative study of the challenges experienced by vulnerable groups in using digital health services in the COVID-19 era. BMC Health Serv Res. 2022;22(1):188. https://doi.org/10.1186/s12913-022-07584-4. PMID: 35151302; PMCID: PMC8840681.
142. Tariq U, Ahmed I, Bashir AK, Shaukat K. A critical cybersecurity analysis and future research directions for the internet of things: a comprehensive review. Sensors. 2023;23:4117. https://doi.org/10.3390/s23084117.
143. Teh HY, Kempa-Liehr AW, Wang KIK. Sensor data quality: a systematic review. J Big Data. 2020;7:11. https://doi.org/10.1186/s40537-020-0285-1.
144. Diaz C, Caillaud C, Yacef K. Mining sensor data to assess changes in physical activity behaviors in health interventions: systematic review. JMIR Med Inform. 2023;11:e41153. https://doi.org/10.2196/41153. PMID: 36877559; PMCID: PMC10028506.
145. Burns SP, Terblanche M, MacKinen A, DeLaPena C, Fielder JDP. Smartphone and mHealth use after stroke: results from a pilot survey. OTJR (Thorofare N J). 2022;42(2):127–36. https://doi.org/10.1177/15394492211068851.

Mental Practice for Gait Improvement 34

Maria Elisa Pimentel Piemonte
and Karina Yumi Tashima Honda

Abstract

Mental practice (MP) aims to improve motor performance through mental movement training, and its potential is being demonstrated in several areas. This chapter aims to provide a general understanding of MP and the main evidence on gait improvement in neurological disorders. The literature considers that MP activates cognitive and motor components, promoting motor learning through an internal control model. It has been considered as a promising tool in gait rehabilitation in stroke survivors, people with Parkinson's disease and multiple sclerosis. The findings so far are positive, suggesting further investigations, since there are still gaps in knowledge due to methodological heterogeneity and diversity in the characteristics of the samples currently.

Introduction

"Practice makes perfection." This has been the golden rule for improving motor performance in healthy people or people living with motor dysfunction who need rehabilitation. But would it be possible to improve motor performance without physical practice? Would it be possible to improve the motor performance by mental rehearsal only?

Several evidences from different fields as sports, music, and rehabilitation, suggest that it is possible. However, despite the growing evidence, the clinical

M. E. P. Piemonte (✉)
Department of Physiotherapy, Speech Therapy and Occupational Therapy, Faculty of Medical Science, University of São Paulo, São Paulo, SP, Brazil
e-mail: elisapp@usp.br

K. Y. T. Honda
Department of Experimental Psychology—Neurosciences and Behavior, Institute of Psychology, University of São Paulo, São Paulo, SP, Brazil

F. A. Barbieri et al. (eds.), *Locomotion and Posture in Older Adults*,
https://doi.org/10.1007/978-3-031-74123-4_34

utilization of mental practice for repair remains very limited. Why? Considering its safe and low cost, why have not the physiotherapists, occupational and speech therapists used this kind of intervention largely?

This chapter aims to offer a general understanding of mechanisms behind the mental practice and show the main evidence of its results in improving the gait performance in people with neurological dysfunction.

We hope this chapter can increase the enthusiasm of the professionals to study and experience this kind of training in their intervention program.

Mental Practice

Motor imagery is the mental performance of an action without its actual physical execution; it is an active process during which the representation of an action is reproduced internally. *Mental practice (MP) or motor imagery practice* is the repetition or mental rehearsal of movement, from the perspective of the first or third person in the absence of any real movement, with the intention of improving performance in a motor task [1]. The MP can be of the visual type, in which the motor act is imagined as if it were watching the scene, or the kinesthetic type, where the individual is stimulated to "feel the movement" in a first-person perspective. The kinesthetic modality has shown a better correlation with the form and time of real movements by the greater activation of neural motor areas [2, 3].

Its effects on performance and motor skills, combined with *physical practice (PP),* have been demonstrated in several areas: sports, music, orthopedic rehabilitation, and neurological rehabilitation [4–6]. Among the advantages of MP as a rehabilitation method are the absence of risk of physical injuries, independence of the level of motor capacity, high availability and accessibility, low financial cost, and no need for equipment [4]. The MP offers an opportunity to increase the number of repetitions safely and autonomously, wherever, and whenever the individual wants, without physical fatigue, also enabling the performance of more demanding or complex motor tasks when PP is impossible or very difficult [7].

In addition to targeting motor aspects, MP can target non-motor aspects of performance, i.e., sensory and cognitive, including improved attention to movement, reduced anxiety, and increased self-confidence [8].

However, despite these advantages, MP is a complex and multidimensional mental process that is not easily integrated into clinical practice [1], and the individual capacity of motor imagination can generate differences in the learning effect [9].

Fundamentals of Mental Practice as an Intervention to Improve Gait

The beneficial effects of MP on physical performance have been suggested due to the close temporal association between motor rehearsal and physical performance [10]. It is suggested that MP induces an efficient process of motor learning and not just a transient change in motor performance [11]. In addition, it is proposed that the motor skills trained by MP become more flexible and adaptable than PP, transferable to similar tasks or untrained segments, being less susceptible to negative interference from other tasks [12].

The mechanisms activated by MP, although not yet fully understood, involve cognitive and motor components. Cognitive components include facilitating skill-related cognitive elements, such as identifying and sequentially activating the subcomponents of a task and increasing attentional focus on movement, which facilitate learning more efficient movement strategies. The broader involvement of non-motor areas in MP has justified its inclusion as a cognitive-motor rehabilitation strategy [13–15].

Motor components during MP involve the activation of brain areas common to PP, such as the premotor area, supplementary motor area, cingular cortex, parietal cortex, basal nuclei, and cerebellum [2]. Corticospinal excitability increases with the complexity of the task in both motor imagination and motor execution [16].

Although they predominantly activate the same brain areas, some studies have shown important differences, suggesting that the processes involved in MP and PP may be distinct. In PP, there is greater activation of ventral premotor cortex, middle temporal gyrus, SMA, cerebellum, and somatosensory cortex. In MP, there is an additional activation of the visual association cortex, posterior cingulate cortex, precuneus, frontal-parietal cortex, inferior frontal cortex, and midbrain [12]. These differences may be associated with the distinct construction of the internal representation of MP and PP [9].

While the representation of PP is based on the feedback of the sensory results of the movements performed, resulting in an internal model of bottom-up, or effector-dependent, control, the internal representation developed by the MP is based on the motor and sensory estimation of the planned movement, generating a prospective internal model, or top-down control [10]. That is, in MP, the neural system internally simulates motor output commands and predicts or estimates their sensory consequence based on previous experiences [17].

MP goes beyond remembering or responding to information, as it is able to activate and reorganize the cerebral cortex, influencing the learning of motor skills by reinforcing existing neural connections and making them more efficient with training [18].

Figure 34.1 represents the motor learning model based on anticipatory internal models promoted by MP proposed by Rodrigues and Piemonte [19]. When we intend to perform a movement, signals from motor cortical areas activate motor commands to plan and execute the desired movement by recruiting subcortical and peripheral motor systems. In parallel, a motor efference copy is processed internally, simulating the same movements through implicit mental process. When the motor action does not occur, this motor efference copy activates an inverse control model that allows the estimation of somatosensory and perceptual consequences of the imaged movement based on previous similar motor experiences. The somatosensory and perceptual prediction of imaged movement will allow error correction by forward control. This correction of the estimated errors will improve the motor

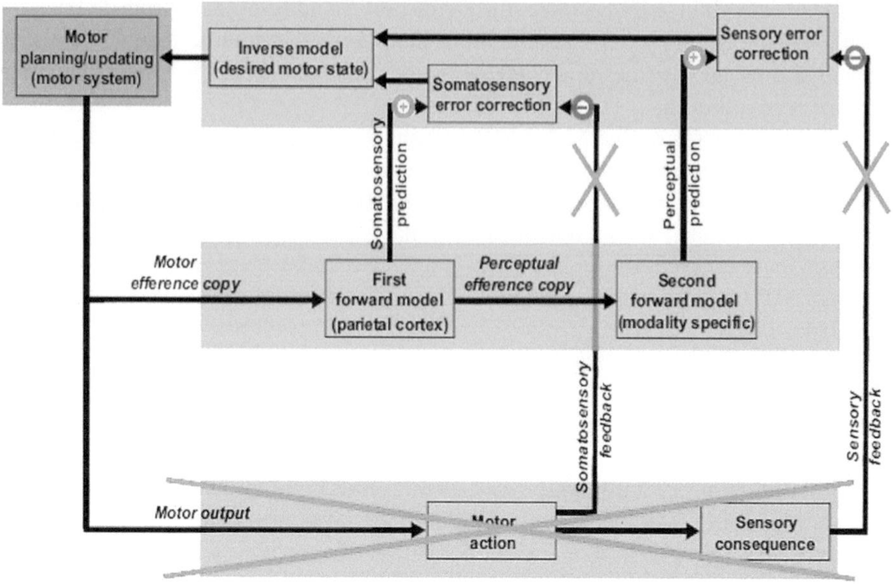

Fig. 34.1 Representation of the motor learning model based on anticipatory internal models promoted by the MP [19]

plan for the next movement. If this process is repeated several times, it will promote proper motor learning.

Although most of studies have investigated the MP for upper limbs rehabilitation, there is a growing interest in verifying the effects of MP in treating gait disorders [1]. The studies are based on neurophysiological and brain imaging findings demonstrating similarities between real and imagined locomotor activities. For example, the change in heart and respiratory rate of healthy individuals when they imagine themselves walking on the treadmill at different speeds [20, 21]; the temporal coupling between the duration of a real and imagined walk at different distances [22, 23] and also when obstacles and alternations are added in the course (e.g., hills and narrow roads) the time of the real and imagined task are also decreased [24]. In addition, during the imagination of complex bodily activities (e.g., swimming, dancing), cortical brain activation overlaps with real activities [25–27].

Functional gait is a complex process that involves the interaction of volitional, emotional, and automatic control. The integration between the motor cortex, basal nuclei, and cerebellum contribute to a constant recalibration of gait, ensuring adaptation to different environments and tasks, requiring volition, cognition, attention, and prediction. Meanwhile, information processing between the basal ganglia, cerebellum, and brainstem allows the automatic regulation of muscle tone and rhythmic limb movements, even in the absence of conscious control [28–30].

Considering the forward control activated by MP, this kind of intervention may be particularly advantageous to improve the top-down gait control to minimize the lack in automatic gait control associated to aging process [31] and neurogenerative disease such as PD [32, 33].

In this context, MP has been studied by several researchers who believe that this may be a new proposed approach in gait training for its potential to accelerate motor skills gains [1, 8, 34–36].

Mental Practice for Gait Improvement in Parkinson's Disease

PD is a neurodegenerative disease with the early death of dopaminergic neurons of the substantia nigra pars compacta in the basal nuclei, leading to a decrease in the processing of information essential for motor control [37].

Although with heterogeneous presentations, individuals with PD are often affected by bradykinesia, muscle rigidity, tremor, postural instability, freezing of gait, and sensory and autonomic changes [38, 39]. The gait is characterized by the reduced amplitude of arm swing and dissociation of trunk movements, decrease in step length, increase in step length variability, and decrease in speed [40]. This gait and balance disorder limit mobility and results in falls, generating disabilities and worsening quality of life [41, 42].

Authors have suggested that MP is a promising and emerging tool in PD rehabilitation [2, 43, 44]. The studies that showed that people with PD maintain the ability to create mental images of gait vividly and accurately correlated with the actual performance of walking support the viability and potentiality of MP to improve the gait changes characteristic of the disease [45, 46]. Neurophysiological changes associated with episodes of gait freezing are also present during imaginative gait [47, 48], and the vividness of the motor imagination is similar between the on and off state of dopaminergic medication [49].

On the effects of MP on gait: (1) Tamir, Dickstein, and Huberman (2007) [50]—concluded that MP integrated with PP can reduce bradykinesia and increase gait speed in those with PD (improvement in the performance of "timed up and go test", $p = 0.0005$); (2) Braun et al. (2011) [51]—find no difference between the experimental group and relaxation intervention; (3) El-Wishy and Fayez (2013) [52]—demonstrate that MP associated with physiotherapy promoted an increase in step length ($p = 0.0025$) and improved gait speed ($p = 0.0001$); (4) Santiago et al. (2015) [53]—report not having found improvement in gait after a single session of MP compared to PP exclusively; (5) Pikel et al. (2015) [54]—demonstrate that a MP associated to PP improved gait stability in people living in mild to moderate PD stages (improvement in the BESTest, $p = 0.01$, ES = 0.80); (6) Abraham et al. (2018) [55]—find improvement in in the UPDRS-III ($p = 0.05$), the TUG-manual ($p = 0.05$), time and number of steps to turn 360° ($p = 0.01$) and the reactive postural control ($p = 0.02$); (7) Bezerra et al. (2022) [56]—conclude that the combination of AOT with MP did not obtain superior results than PP in FOG; (8) Kashif et al. (2022) [57]—combine virtual reality, MP and PP obtaining improvements in motor function and balance (tremor at rest and rigidity at 16th week, $p = 0.001$; posture at 6th week, $p = 0.004$; gait at the 6th week, $p = 0.034$).

The lack of congruence in the results obtained is due to the diversity in the samples' characteristics, the method, and the experimental protocols established. There is still limited literature on MP in PD, and more studies are needed to specify the training dosage and the short- and long-term efficacy of the different MP approaches in subgroups of people with PD [8].

Mental Practice to Improve Stroke Gait

Stroke is an acute event caused by a blockage or bleeding that impedes blood flow in the brain, resulting in motor and non-motor symptoms, representing one of the leading causes of mortality and disability [58].

After a stroke, many survivors have chronic, usually complex and heterogeneous sequelae, including hemiparesis, spasticity, pain, parkinsonism, loss of dexterity, and impaired gait and balance, which can lead to greater dependence [59, 60], and a high risk of falls [61, 62]. For an effective return to activities of daily living and community, one of the most critical goals in post-stroke treatment is gait rehabilitation [63].

The systematic review of Silva et al. (2020) [64], when investigating the effects of MP on gait, includes 21 randomized controlled trials that used MP alone or associated with *action observation therapy (AOT)* or PP. It presents that MP can favor gait speed in the short term. However, it is impossible to conclude long-term effects because of the study's heterogeneity and low quality of evidence. It finds that only one study evaluated walking resistance, observing a significant difference comparing the experimental group to the control group in the 6-minute walk test [65].

A meta-analysis of randomized clinical trial between 2015 and 2020 [66] analyzing the effects of MP on post-stroke rehabilitation reveals a wide range of protocols combined with a wide diversity of interventions. There was no consensus on the duration of the intervention and frequency of sessions, where the studies presented training times between 30 and 180 minutes and an intervention period between the first and 12th month after stroke. This extreme disparity undermines conclusions or comparisons; however, their data show an improvement in gait speed (SMD = 0.42 [95% CI,–0.34–1.17], $p = 0.09$, $I^2 = 65\%$) and the Fugl-Meyer Assessment (FMA) (SMD = 2.32 [95% CI,–1.19–5.83], $p < 0.00001$, $I^2 = 91\%$).

These findings corroborate a more recent randomized clinical trial meta-analysis [67], which includes only protocols that combine MP and PP, concluding that this training has more benefits than PP alone, bringing a positive impact on the lower extremity assessment of AMF and the Barthel index in the acute phase of stroke (1–7 days), walking ability, stride length and cadence in the subacute phase (7 days–6 months), and walking speed in the chronic stage (more than 6 months). However, there was no data available on long-term follow-up, and only 43% of the included studies were rated as having good methodological quality.

A still remaining question is about the capacity of motor imagination in stroke survivors; some studies do not find any impairment [68, 69], while others note an impaired general capacity after stroke [70], or only of specific aspects [71, 72].

However, this divergence can be explained by the difference in the populations investigated, the individual characteristics, and the established methodologies [73].

Although there is still conflicting evidence about the usefulness and effectiveness of MP in the rehabilitation of stroke survivors, the recommendations are in favor of the intervention [74].

Mental Practice for Gait Improvement in Multiple Sclerosis

Multiple sclerosis (*MS*) is a neurodegenerative autoimmune disease that affects the central nervous system through the degradation of the myelin sheath, resulting in cognitive and motor deficits in young adults [75]. People with MS (pwMS) often have problems with memory, attention, information processing speed, visuospatial ability, and mental flexibility [76]. Motor symptoms include muscle weakness, spasticity, incoordination, fatigue, gait, and balance disturbance, leading to functional limitations and increased risk of falls [77, 78].

The MP in MS has recently been studied; however, since pwMS presents cognitive and motor dysfunctions, one of the considerations about the applicability of MP is whether these individuals would be able to generate accurate and vivid motor images. In this sense, Heremans et al. (2012) [79] demonstrate that the vivacity of the motor image in pwMS did not differ from the controls, but having been evaluated by a self-assessment questionnaire makes a caveat about the possibility of overestimation of the answers, and that pwMS present lower accuracy of the images and in the temporal organization, being correlated with cognitive impairments regardless of motor function. Wajda et al. (2021) [80] conclude that pwMS have lower motor imagination capacity and lower ability to update estimated time in the mental gait chronometry after performing the actual task. There are limitations to the applicability of MP in those with the presence of cognitive impairments [81].

A recent systematic review that included only studies investigating MP alone [82] finds five studies showing positive effects: significant improvement in gait speed, walking distance, fatigue, and quality of life, also points to benefits in dynamic balance and perception of gait ability. Notably, the intervention protocols were heterogeneous, with significant variations in the MP time and number of sessions.

In addition, MP associated with auditory and rhythmic cues seems to affect gait and balance in pwMS positively [83, 84].

Although the results are positive, the literature lacks more studies to analyze the effects of the intervention in pwMS.

Final Considerations

There is growing evidence showing the positive effects of MP for gait rehabilitation of people with neurological diseases, highlighting its potential as a safe and inexpensive cognitive-motor intervention to promote the motor learning and neuroplasticity, not only when physical execution is not possible, but to improve the rehabilitation results.

However, further studies are needed to determine the best recommendations related to the duration and frequency of sessions, the total time of intervention, the ideal time to start interventions after injuries and established diagnoses, and the long-term effects of MP.

The studies present diversity in the intervention modalities, associating with other interventions such as AOT and virtual reality, suggesting versatility and practicality in the application of MP in rehabilitation protocols. Some studies suggest that the association of AOT may bring additional benefits to rehabilitation with MP [2, 5], and the integration of peripheral sensory stimulation seems to promote improvement in the consolidation of acquisitions [85, 86].

A relevant issue for neurorehabilitation is whether the ability of imagination is a determinant for the improvement of motor performance by MP. Subjective assessment through questionnaires may not be a reliable predictor [79, 87], although some authors find that the more the subjects are good performers of motor imagination, the more the practice of MP is effective in modifying performance [9]. It is also worth mentioning that age and gender interfere with the individual's imaginative capacity [88].

The findings so far are promising, considering that MP has positive effects on gait rehabilitation as a tool associated with PP, however, the literature is not unanimous and there are still gaps in knowledge, thus requiring the continuity of investigations in the area.

References

1. Malouin F, Richards CL. Mental practice for relearning locomotor skills. Phys Ther. 2010;90(2):240–51.
2. Abbruzzese G, Avanzino L, Marchese R, Pelosin E. Action observation and motor imagery: innovative cognitive tools in the rehabilitation of Parkinson's disease. Parkinson's Disease. 2015;2015:1–9.
3. Guillot A, Collet C, Nguyen VA, Malouin F, Richards C, Doyon J. Brain activity during visual versus kinesthetic imagery: an fMRI study. Hum Brain Mapp. 2009;30(7):2157–72.
4. Braun S, Kleynen M, van Heel T, Kruithof N, Wade D, Beurskens A. The effects of mental practice in neurological rehabilitation; a systematic review and meta-analysis. Front Hum Neurosci. 2013;7:390. https://doi.org/10.3389/fnhum.2013.00390.
5. Herranz-Gómez A, Gaudiosi C, Angulo-Díaz-Parreño S, Suso-Martí L, La Touche R, Cuenca-Martínez F. Effectiveness of motor imagery and action observation on functional variables: an umbrella and mapping review with meta-meta-analysis. Neurosci Biobehav Rev. 2020;118:828–45.
6. Schuster C, Hilfiker R, Amft O, Scheidhauer A, Andrews B, Butler J, et al. Best practice for motor imagery: a systematic literature review on motor imagery training elements in five different disciplines. BMC Med. 2011;9(1):75. https://doi.org/10.1186/1741-7015-9-75.
7. Malouin F, Jackson PL, Richards CL. Towards the integration of mental practice in rehabilitation programs. A critical review. Front Hum Neurosci. 2013;7:576. https://doi.org/10.3389/fnhum.2013.00576.

8. Abraham A, Duncan RP, Earhart GM. The role of mental imagery in Parkinson's disease rehabilitation. Brain Sci. 2021;11(2):185.
9. Avanzino L, Lagravinese G, Abbruzzese G, Pelosin E. Relationships between gait and emotion in Parkinson's disease: a narrative review. Gait Posture. 2018;65:57–64.
10. Avanzino L, Giannini A, Tacchino A, Pelosin E, Ruggeri P, Bove M. Motor imagery influences the execution of repetitive finger opposition movements. Neurosci Lett. 2009;466(1):11–5.
11. Gentili R, Han CE, Schweighofer N, Papaxanthis C. Motor learning without doing: trial-by-trial improvement in motor performance during mental training. J Neurophysiol. 2010;104(2):774–83.
12. Asa SKP, Melo MCS, Piemonte MEP. Effects of mental and physical practice on a finger opposition task among children. Res Q Exerc Sport. 2014;85(3):308–15.
13. Hanakawa T, Immisch I, Toma K, Dimyan MA, Van Gelderen P, Hallett M. Functional properties of brain areas associated with motor execution and imagery. J Neurophysiol. 2003;89(2):989–1002.
14. Kim YK, Park E, Lee A, Im CH, Kim YH. Changes in network connectivity during motor imagery and execution. PLoS One. 2018;13(1):e0190715.
15. Mulder T. Motor imagery and action observation: cognitive tools for rehabilitation. J Neural Transm. 2007;114(10):1265–78.
16. Mizuguchi N, Kanosue K. Changes in brain activity during action observation and motor imagery: their relationship with motor learning. Prog Brain Res. 2017;234:189–204.
17. Tian X, Poeppel D. Mental imagery of speech: linking motor and perceptual systems through internal simulation and estimation. Front Hum Neurosci. 2012;6:314. https://doi.org/10.3389/fnhum.2012.00314.
18. Hong IK, Choi JB, Lee JH. Cortical changes after mental imagery training combined with electromyography-triggered electrical stimulation in patients with chronic stroke. Stroke. 2012;43(9):2506–9.
19. Rodrigues AS, Piemonte MEP. Efeitos de um treinamento de prática mental associada à prática física sobre o desempenho da marcha em pessoas com Doença de Parkinson [Dissertation (Master)]. University of São Paulo; 2018. p. 98.
20. Fusi S, Cutuli D, Valente MR, Bergonzi P, Porro CA, Di Prampero PE. Cardioventilatory responses during real or imagined walking at low speed. Arch Ital Biol. 2005;143(3–4):223–8.
21. Pellicano A, Mingoia G, Ritter CA, Buccino G, Binkofski F. Respiratory function modulated during execution, observation, and imagination of walking via SII. Sci Rep. 2021;11(1):23752. https://doi.org/10.1038/s41598-021-03147-5.
22. Bakker M, Floris SJA, Toni I, Bloem BR. Motor imagery of gait: a quantitative approach. Exp Brain Res. 2007;179(3):497–504.
23. Courtine G, Papaxanthis C, Gentili R, Pozzo T. Gait-dependent motor memory facilitation in covert movement execution. Cogn Brain Res. 2004;22(1):67–75.
24. Bakker M, De Lange FP, Helmich RC, Scheeringa R, Bloem BR, Toni I. Cerebral correlates of motor imagery of normal and precision gait. NeuroImage. 2008;41(3):998–1010.
25. Malouin F, Richards CL, Jackson PL, Dumas F, Doyon J. Brain activations during motor imagery of locomotor-related tasks: a PET study. Hum Brain Mapp. 2003;19(1):47–62.
26. Szameitat AJ, Shen S, Sterr A. Motor imagery of complex everyday movements. An fMRI study. NeuroImage. 2007;34(2):702–13.
27. Wagner J, Stephan T, Kalla R, Brückmann H, Strupp M, Brandt T, et al. Mind the bend: cerebral activations associated with mental imagery of walking along a curved path. Exp Brain Res. 2008;191(2):247–55.
28. Al-Yahya E, Dawes H, Smith L, Dennis A, Howells K, Cockburn J. Cognitive motor interference while walking: a systematic review and meta-analysis. Neurosci Biobehav Rev. 2011;35(3):715–28.
29. Beyaert C, Vasa R, Frykberg GE. Gait post-stroke: pathophysiology and rehabilitation strategies. Neurophysiologie Clinique/Clin Neurophysiol. 2015;45(4–5):335–55.
30. Takakusaki K. Neurophysiology of gait: from the spinal cord to the frontal lobe. Mov Disord. 2013;28(11):1483–91.

31. Wu T, Hallett M. The influence of normal human ageing on automatic movements. J Physiol. 2005;562(2):605–15.
32. Pikel MR. Efeitos de um treinamento de prática mental associada à prática física sobre o desempenho da marcha em pessoas com Doença de Parkinson [Dissertation (Master)]. University of São Paulo; 2017. p. 83.
33. Pimentel Piemonte ME, Okamoto E. Improvement in gait performance after training based on declarative memory cues in patients with Parkinsons disease: a randomized clinical trial. J Novel Physiother. 2015;5(6):277. https://doi.org/10.4172/2165-7025.1000277.
34. Dickstein R, Deutsch JE. Motor imagery in physical therapist practice. Phys Ther. 2007;87(7):942–53.
35. Jackson PL, Lafleur MF, Malouin F, Richards C, Doyon J. Potential role of mental practice using motor imagery in neurologic rehabilitation. Arch Phys Med Rehabil. 2001;82(8):1133–41.
36. Oostra K, Oomen A, Vanderstraeten G, Vingerhoets G. Influence of motor imagery training on gait rehabilitation in sub-acute stroke: a randomized controlled trial. J Rehabil Med. 2015;47(3):204–9.
37. Balestrino R, Schapira AHV. Parkinson disease. Eur J Neurol. 2019;27(1):27–42.
38. Grabli D, Karachi C, Welter ML, Lau B, Hirsch EC, Vidailhet M, et al. Normal and pathological gait: what we learn from Parkinson's disease: figure 1. J Neurol Neurosurg Psychiatry. 2012;83(10):979–85.
39. Jankovic J, Tarakad A. Diagnosis and management of Parkinson's disease. Semin Neurol. 2017;37(02):118–26.
40. Brognara L, Palumbo P, Grimm B, Palmerini L. Assessing gait in Parkinson's disease using wearable motion sensors: a systematic review. Diseases. 2019;7(1):18.
41. Andreadou E, Anagnostouli M, Vasdekis V, Kararizou E, Rentzos M, Kontaxis T, et al. The impact of comorbidity and other clinical and sociodemographic factors on health-related quality of life in Greek patients with Parkinson's disease. Aging Ment Health. 2011;15(7):913–21.
42. Creaby MW, Cole MH. Gait characteristics and falls in Parkinson's disease: a systematic review and meta-analysis. Parkinsonism Relat Disord. 2018;57:1–8.
43. Caligiore D, Mustile M, Spalletta G, Baldassarre G. Action observation and motor imagery for rehabilitation in Parkinson's disease: a systematic review and an integrative hypothesis. Neurosci Biobehav Rev. 2017;72:210–22.
44. Lahuerta-Martín S, Llamas-Ramos R, Llamas-Ramos I. Effectiveness of therapies based on mirror neuron system to treat gait in patients with Parkinson's disease—a systematic review. J Clin Med. 2022;11(14):4236.
45. Heremans E, Feys P, Nieuwboer A, Vercruysse S, Vandenberghe W, Sharma N, et al. Motor imagery ability in patients with early- and mid-stage Parkinson disease. Neurorehabil Neural Repair. 2011;25(2):168–77.
46. Pickett KA, Peterson DS, Earhart GM. Motor imagery of gait tasks in individuals with Parkinson disease. J Parkinsons Dis. 2012;2(1):19–22.
47. Cohen RG, Nutt JG, Horak FB. Recovery from multiple APAs delays gait initiation in Parkinson's disease. Front Hum Neurosci. 2017;11:60. https://doi.org/10.3389/fnhum.2017.00060.
48. Snijders AH, Leunissen I, Bakker M, Overeem S, Helmich RC, Bloem BR, et al. Gait-related cerebral alterations in patients with Parkinson's disease with freezing of gait. Brain. 2010;134(1):59–72.
49. Peterson DS, Smulders K, Mancini M, Nutt JG, Horak FB, Fling BW. Relating response inhibition, brain connectivity, and freezing of gait in people with Parkinson's disease. J Int Neuropsychol Soc. 2020;27(7):733–43.
50. Tamir R, Dickstein R, Huberman M. Integration of motor imagery and physical practice in group treatment applied to subjects with Parkinson's disease. Neurorehabil Neural Repair. 2007;21(1):68–75.
51. Braun S, Beurskens A, Kleynen M, Schols J, Wade D. Rehabilitation with mental practice has similar effects on mobility as rehabilitation with relaxation in people with Parkinson's disease: a multicentre randomised trial. J Physiother. 2011;57(1):27–34.

52. El-Wishy AA, Fayez ES. Effect of locomotor imagery training added to physical therapy program on gait performance in Parkinson patients: a randomized controlled study. Egypt J Neurol Psychiat Neurosurg. 2013;50(1):31–7.
53. Santiago LM, de Oliveira DA, de Macêdo Ferreira LG, de Brito Pinto HY, Spaniol AP, de Lucena Trigueiro LC, Ribeiro TS, de Sousa AV, Piemonte ME, Lindquist AR. Immediate effects of adding mental practice to physical practice on the gait of individuals with Parkinson's disease: randomized clinical trial. NeuroRehabilitation. 2015;37(2):263–71.
54. Pikel MR, Costa ALD, Nogueira LM, Okamoto E, Piemonte MEP. Mental practice may improve the gait stability in patients with Parkinson's disease: a single-blind, randomised clinical trial. Physiotherapy. 2015;101:e1208–9.
55. Abraham A, Hart A, Andrade I, Hackney ME. Dynamic neuro-cognitive imagery improves mental imagery ability, disease severity, and motor and cognitive functions in people with Parkinson's disease. Neural Plast. 2018;2018:6168507. https://doi.org/10.1155/2018/6168507.
56. Bezerra PT, Santiago LM, Silva IA, Souza AA, Pegado CL, Damascena CM, et al. Action observation and motor imagery have no effect on balance and freezing of gait in Parkinson's disease: a randomized controlled trial. Eur J Phys Rehabil Med. 2022;58(5):715–22.
57. Kashif M, Ahmad A, Bandpei MAM, Gilani SA, Hanif A, Iram H. Combined effects of virtual reality techniques and motor imagery on balance, motor function and activities of daily living in patients with Parkinson's disease: a randomized controlled trial. BMC Geriatr. 2022;22(1):381. https://doi.org/10.1186/s12877-022-03035-1.
58. Wafa HA, Wolfe CDA, Emmett E, Roth GA, Johnson CO, Wang Y. Burden of stroke in Europe. Stroke. 2020;51(8):2418–27.
59. Gladstone DJ, Lindsay MP, Douketis J, Smith EE, Dowlatshahi D, Wein T, et al. Canadian stroke best practice recommendations: secondary prevention of stroke update 2020. Can J Neurol Sci. 2022;49(3):315–37.
60. Suri R, Rodriguez-Porcel F, Donohue K, Jesse E, Lovera L, Dwivedi AK, et al. Post-stroke movement disorders: the clinical, neuroanatomic, and demographic portrait of 284 published cases. J Stroke Cerebrovasc Dis. 2018;27(9):2388–97.
61. Abdollahi M, Whitton N, Zand R, Dombovy M, Parnianpour M, Khalaf K, et al. A systematic review of fall risk factors in stroke survivors: towards improved assessment platforms and protocols. Front Bioeng Biotechnol. 2022;10:910698. https://doi.org/10.3389/fbioe.2022.910698.
62. Weerdesteyn V, De Niet M, Van Duijnhoven H, Geurts A. Falls in individuals with stroke. J Rehabil Res Dev. 2008;45(8):1195–214.
63. Selves C, Stoquart G, Lejeune T. Gait rehabilitation after stroke: review of the evidence of predictors, clinical outcomes and timing for interventions. Acta Neurol Belg. 2020;120(4):783–90. https://doi.org/10.1007/s13760-020-01320-7.
64. Silva S, Borges LR, Santiago L, Lucena L, Lindquist AR, Ribeiro T. Motor imagery for gait rehabilitation after stroke. Cochrane Database Syst Rev. 2020;9(9):CD013019. https://doi.org/10.1002/14651858.CD013019.pub2.
65. Verma R, Narayan Arya K, Garg RK, Singh T. Task-oriented circuit class training program with motor imagery for gait rehabilitation in poststroke patients: a randomized controlled trial. Top Stroke Rehabil. 2011;18(suppl 1):620–32.
66. Monteiro KB, Cardoso MDS, Cabral VRDC, Santos AOBD, Silva PSD, Castro JBP, Vale RGS. Effects of motor imagery as a complementary resource on the rehabilitation of stroke patients: a meta-analysis of randomized trials. J Stroke Cerebrovasc Dis. 2021;30(8):105876.
67. Zhao LJ, Jiang LH, Zhang L, Li Y, Sun P, Liu Y, et al. Effects of motor imagery training for lower limb dysfunction in patients with stroke: a systematic review and meta-analysis of randomized controlled trials. Am J Phys Med Rehabil. 2023;102(5):409–18. https://doi.org/10.1097/PHM.0000000000002107.
68. Johnson SH. Imagining the impossible. Neuroreport. 2000;11(4):729–32.
69. Johnson SH, Sprehn G, Saykin AJ. Intact motor imagery in chronic upper limb hemiplegics: evidence for activity-independent action representations. J Cogn Neurosci. 2002;14(6):841–52.
70. Malouin F, Richards CL, Desrosiers J, Doyon J. Bilateral slowing of mentally simulated actions after stroke. Neuroreport. 2004;15(8):1349–53.

71. Liepert J, Büsching I, Sehle A, Schoenfeld MA. Mental chronometry and mental rotation abilities in stroke patients with different degrees of sensory deficit. Restor Neurol Neurosci. 2016;34(6):907–14.
72. Vries S, Tepper M, Feenstra W, Oosterveld H, Boonstra AM, Otten B. Motor imagery ability in stroke patients: the relationship between implicit and explicit motor imagery measures. Front Hum Neurosci. 2013;7:790. https://doi.org/10.3389/fnhum.2013.00790.
73. Braun N, Kranczioch C, Liepert J, Dettmers C, Zich C, Büsching I, et al. Motor imagery impairment in postacute stroke patients. Neural Plast. 2017;2017:1–13.
74. Minelli C, Luvizutto GJ, Cacho RO, Neves LO, Magalhães SCSA, Pedatella MTA, Mendonça LIZ, Ortiz KZ, Lange MC, Ribeiro PW, Souza LAPS, Milani C, Cruz DMCD, Costa RDMD, Conforto AB, Carvalho FMM, Ci+arlini BS, Frota NAF, Almeida KJ, Schochat E, Oliveira TP, Miranda C, Piemonte MEP, Lopes LCG, Lopes CG, Tosin MHS, Oliveira BC, Oliveira BGRB, Castro SS, Andrade JBC, Silva GS, Pontes-Neto OM, Carvalho JJF, Martins SCO, Bazan R. Brazilian practice guidelines for stroke rehabilitation: part II. Arq Neuropsiquiatr. 2022;80(07):741–58.
75. Ghasemi N, Razavi S, Nikzad E. Multiple sclerosis: pathogenesis, symptoms, diagnoses and cell-based therapy. Cell J. 2017;19(1):1–10.
76. Benedict RHB, Holtzer R, Motl RW, Foley FW, Kaur S, Hojnacki D, et al. Upper and lower extremity motor function and cognitive impairment in multiple sclerosis. J Int Neuropsychol Soc. 2011;17(4):643–53.
77. Abou L, Peters J, Fritz N, Sosnoff JJ, Kratz AL. Motor cognitive dual-task testing to predict future falls in multiple sclerosis: a systematic review. Neurorehabil Neural Repair. 2022;36(12):757–69.
78. Cameron MH, Nilsagard Y. Balance, gait, and falls in multiple sclerosis. Handb Clin Neurol. 2018;159:237–50.
79. Heremans E, Nieuwboer A, Feys P, Vercruysse S, Vandenberghe W, Sharma N, et al. External cueing improves motor imagery quality in patients with Parkinson disease. Neurorehabil Neural Repair. 2011;26(1):27–35.
80. Wajda DA, Zanotto T, Sosnoff JJ. Motor imagery of walking in people living with and without multiple sclerosis: a cross-sectional comparison of mental chronometry. Brain Sci. 2021;11(9):1131.
81. Tabrizi YM, Mazhari S, Nazari MA, Zangiabadi N, Sheibani V, Azarang S. Compromised motor imagery ability in individuals with multiple sclerosis and mild physical disability: an ERP study. Clin Neurol Neurosurg. 2013;115(9):1738–44.
82. Gil-Bermejo-Bernardez-Zerpa A, Moral-Munoz JA, Lucena-Anton D, Luque-Moreno C. Effectiveness of motor imagery on motor recovery in patients with multiple sclerosis: systematic review. Int J Environ Res Public Health. 2021;18(2):498.
83. Seebacher B, Kuisma R, Glynn A, Berger T. The effect of rhythmic-cued motor imagery on walking, fatigue and quality of life in people with multiple sclerosis: a randomized controlled trial. Mult Scler J. 2016;23(2):286–96.
84. Seebacher B, Kuisma R, Glynn A, Berger T. Effects and mechanisms of differently cued and non-cued motor imagery in people with multiple sclerosis: a randomised controlled trial. Mult Scler. 2019;25(12):1593–604.
85. Bonassi G, Biggio M, Bisio A, Ruggeri P, Bove M, Avanzino L. Provision of somatosensory inputs during motor imagery enhances learning-induced plasticity in human motor cortex. Sci Rep. 2017;7(1):9300.
86. Bonassi G, Lagravinese G, Bisio A, Ruggeri P, Pelosin E, Bove M, et al. Consolidation and retention of motor skill after motor imagery training. Neuropsychologia. 2020;143:107472.
87. Ruffino C, Papaxanthis C, Lebon F. The influence of imagery capacity in motor performance improvement. Exp Brain Res. 2017;235(10):3049–57.
88. Subirats L, Allali G, Briansoulet M, Salle JY, Perrochon A. Age and gender differences in motor imagery. J Neurol Sci. 2018 Aug;391:114–7.

Index

F. A. Barbieri et al. (eds.), *Locomotion and Posture in Older Adults*, https://doi.org/10.1007/978-3-031-74123-4

MIX
Papier aus verantwortungsvollen Quellen
Paper from responsible sources
FSC® C105338

If you have any concerns about our products,
you can contact us on
ProductSafety@springernature.com

In case Publisher is established outside the EU,
the EU authorized representative is:
Springer Nature Customer Service Center GmbH
Europaplatz 3, 69115 Heidelberg, Germany

Printed by Libri Plureos GmbH
in Hamburg, Germany